TEXTBOOK OF ANATOMY

UPPER LIMB AND THORAX

TEXTBOOK OF ANATOMY
UPPER LIMB AND THORAX
Volume I

Fourth Edition

Vishram Singh, MBBS, MS(LKO), PhD(hc), MICPS, FASI, FIMSA

Adjunct Professor, Department of Anatomy, KMC, Manipal Academy of Higher Education (MAHE), Mangalore, Karnataka, India

Editor-in-chief, *Journal of the Anatomical Society of India*

Chairman Expert Group, Research-in-Anatomy
Indian Council of Medical Research (ICMR), New Delhi

Member, Federative International Committee
on Scientific Publications (FICSP) of IFAA, Geneva

Member, COPE Council (England and Wales)

Former Professor and Head, Department of Anatomy
Santosh Medical College
Member, Academic Council and Core Committee, PhD Course
Santosh Deemed to be University, Ghaziabad, NCR, Delhi

Project Editor, BI Churchill Livingstone, New Delhi

Examiner in National and International Universities; Member, Editorial Board
Indian Journal of Otology; Journal of Anatomy and Cell Biology; and *National Journal of Clinical Anatomy*
Ex-Vice President, Anatomical Society of India
Medicolegal Advisor, ICPS, India
Consulting Editor, ABI, North Carolina, USA
Associate Editor, Acta Medica International
Member British Association of Clinical Anatomists (BACA)

Formerly at: King George's Medical College, Lucknow
GSVM Medical College, Kanpur
Al-Arab Medical University, Benghazi (Libya)
All India Institute of Medical Sciences, New Delhi

ELSEVIER

ELSEVIER

RELX India Pvt. Ltd.

Registered Office: 818, 8th Floor, Indraprakash Building, 21, Barakhamba Road, New Delhi 110 001
Corporate Office: 14th Floor, Building No. 10B, DLF Cyber City, Phase II, Gurgaon-122 002, Haryana, India

Textbook of Anatomy: Upper Limb and Thorax, Volume I, Fourth Edition, Vishram Singh

ISBN: 978-81-312-6481-2
eISBN: 978-81-312-6482-9

First Printed in India 2023, Reprinted 2023

Head–Content Strategy, Education: Arvind Koul
Content Project Manager: Goldy Bhatnagar
Sr Production Executive: Dhan Singh Rana
Sr Graphic Designer: Milind Majgaonkar

Typeset by

Printed in India by Sanat Printers

Dedicated to

My Parents
Late Smt Ganga Devi Singh and **Late Shri HR Singh,**
an ever-guiding force in my life

My Elder Sister
Late Smt Susheela Singh
for her help and cooperation during my student life

My Elder Brother
Shri Kaptan Singh
for his sacrifice for me

My Wife
Late Smt Manorama Rani Singh
for her unending support and cooperation of my pursuits

My Students
Past, and Present

Preface to the Fourth Edition

It is a matter of great pride to present before you all the fourth edition of *Textbook of Anatomy: Upper Limb and Thorax, Volume I* to view. This book is widely used not only in India but abroad also by the undergraduate and postgraduate students of anatomy. The popularity of this book reflects the appeal of its concept-building approach and easy to understand language with clearly drawn figures. This approach has been retained in this edition as well. Based on a large number of suggestions, criticisms and comments received from the students and fellow academicians, the following major changes have been done.

The competency codes are integrated within the text in accordance with the competency-based curriculum of anatomy as per the revised guidelines of National Medical Commission (NMC).

In this edition new features such as addition of competencies along with codes in learning objectives, new facts to remember, new line diagrams, half-tone diagrams, ultrasonographs, CT scans, MRIs, tables, and flowcharts have been included.

Most of the diagrams are completely revised and redrawn by the Author himself for easy understanding and reproducibility in the exam.

The chapters on Bones of the Upper Limb; Pectoral Region; Axilla; Cutaneous Innervation, Motor Innervation, Venous Drainage and Lymphatic Drainage; Arm; Forearm; Hand; Wrist Joint, Joints of the Hand, and Movements of the Hand; Major Nerves of the Upper Limb; Bones and Joints of the Thorax; Lungs; Pericardium and Heart; Thoracic Duct, Azygos and Hemiazygos Veins, and Thoracic Sympathetic Trunks have been significantly revised.

The clinical correlations providing anatomical basis of common clinical conditions have been presented in boxes, to provide clinical orientation to students, which will help them immensely during their clinical years.

Anatomical, embryological, histological and radiological basis of case studies are discussed at the end of each chapter to help students during their early clinical exposure.

In addition, complimentary access to online chapter-wise image bank along with complete e-book is also provided.

I sincerely hope that with changes made in this edition will make this book more interesting and useful than the previous one. I would highly appreciate to receive fair comments, both good and bad, from students and teachers.

"Anatomy Provides Basis of Clinical Practice."

Vishram Singh

Preface to the First Edition

This textbook on upper limb and thorax has been carefully planned for the 1st year MBBS students. It follows the revised anatomy curriculum of the Medical Council of India. Following the current trends of clinically oriented study of anatomy, I have adopted a parallel approach—that for imparting basic anatomical knowledge to students and simultaneously providing them its applied aspects.

To help students score high in examinations, the text is written in simple language. It is arranged in easily understandable small sections. While anatomical details of little clinical relevance, phylogenetic discussions and comparative analogies have been omitted; all clinically important topics are described in detail. Brief accounts of histological features and developmental aspects have been given only where they aid in understanding of gross form and function of organs and appearance of common congenital anomalies. The tables and flowcharts summarise important and complex information into digestible knowledge capsules. Multiple-choice questions have been given chapterwise at the end of the book to test the level of understanding and memory recall of the students. The numerous simple four-colour illustrations further assist in fast comprehension and retention of complicated information. All the illustrations are drawn by the author himself to ensure accuracy.

Throughout the preparation of this book, one thing I have kept in mind is that anatomical knowledge is required by clinicians and surgeons for physical examination, diagnostic tests and surgical procedures. Therefore, topographical anatomy relevant to diagnostic and surgical procedures is clinically correlated throughout the text. Further, clinical case study is provided at the end of each chapter for problem-based learning (PBL) so that the students could use their anatomical knowledge in clinical situations. Moreover, the information is arranged regionally because while assessing lesions and performing surgical procedures, the clinicians encounter region-based anatomical features. Due to propensity of fractures, dislocations and peripheral nerve lesions in the upper limb, there is in-depth discussion on joints and peripheral nerves.

As a teacher, I have tried my best to make the book easy to understand and interesting to read. For further improvement of this book, I would greatly welcome comments and suggestions from the readers.

Vishram Singh

Acknowledgements

At the outset, I would like to express my gratitude to Prof (Dr) A. Halim, my teacher and former Prof. and Head of the Department of Anatomy, King George's Medical University, Lucknow, for creating my interest in anatomy. I learned not only the art of good teaching but also the art of drawing good, simple and technically accurate line diagrams from him. May God bless him with long life.

I sincerely thank my colleagues in the Department, especially Prof Rajanigandha Vadgaonkar (HOD), Prof Mangala M Pai, Prof Latha V Prabhu, Dr B V Murlimanju and others for their cooperation and appreciation of my work.

I highly appreciate the help provided in proof reading the whole text, by Dr C S Ramesh Babu, Former Professor and HOD of Anatomy, Lala Lajpat Rai Memorial Medical College, Meerut, UP.

I gratefully acknowledge the feedback and support of all my fellow colleagues in Anatomy throughout India, particularly:

- Profs Punita Manik (HOD), Anita Rani, Jyoti Chopra, Archana Rani, Rakesh Kumar Dewan, R K Verma and others King George Medical University, Lucknow, UP.
- Prof A Shariff (HOD), AIIMS, New Delhi.
- Prof Vandana Sharma (HOD), Gandhi Medical College, Bhopal, MP.
- Profs S K Jain (HOD) Nidhi Sharma and others, Teerthanker Mahaveer Medical College, Moradabad, UP.
- Prof Ruchira Sethi (HOD), Uma Nath Singh Medical College, Jaunpur, UP.
- Profs Yogesh Yadav (HOD) and Pratishtha Potdar, NIIMS, Greater Noida, UP.
- Prof L Peter Ericson (HOD) and Dr D Krishna Chaitanya Reddy, Assistant Professor, KAMSRC, Hyderabad.
- Prof Bipin Khade (HOD) Chirayu Medical College, Bhopal, MP.
- Prof T S Roy (HOD) and Dr Preeti Shrivastava (Associate Professor), NDMC Medical College and Hindu Rao Hospital, Delhi.
- Prof N C Goel, Vice Principal and Dr Shweta Singh, Acting HOD, Hind Institute of Medical Sciences, Barabanki, Lucknow, UP.
- Prof (Emeritus) P K Sharma, Era Medical College, Lucknow, UP.
- Prof Poonam Kharb (HOD), ITS Dental College, Ghaziabad, UP.
- Prof T C Singel, Dr M K Shah Medical College, Gandhinagar, Ahmedabad, Gujarat.
- Profs Vandana Mehta (HOD) and Hitendra Lohiya, Vardhman Mahavir Medical College, New Delhi.
- Prof Sneh Agrawal (HOD), Lady Harding Medical College, New Delhi.
- Prof Shashi Raheja (HOD), Dr Baba Sahib Ambedkar Medical College, Rohini, New Delhi.
- Prof Vanita Gupta (HOD), GS Medical College, Hapur, UP.
- Profs S L Jethani (Medical Superintendent) and Deepa Singh (HOD) and Akshya Dubey, Himalayan Institute of Medical Sciences, Jolly Grant, Dehradun, Uttarakhand.
- Prof W M S Johnson (Dean) and Dr Jaya Kumari, Sree Balaji Medical College, Chennai.
- Prof Suniti Pandey (HOD), GSVM Medical College, Kanpur, UP.
- Prof G M Mahesh, Basaveshwara Medical College, Chitradurga, Karnataka.
- Prof Deepti Shastri (Dean), VMKVMC & Hospital, Salem, Tamil Nadu.
- Profs L C Prasanna (HOD), Sneha Guruprasad Kalthur and Dr Prakash Babu, KMC, Manipal, MAHE, Karnataka.
- Dr S D Joshi, Director Professor of Anatomy, Sri Aurobindo Medical College.

I would also like to express my deep sense of regards to renowned anatomists of India, especially to Prof A C Das, my teacher (Anatomist, Surgeon and Radiologist), Prof Inderbir Singh, Prof Mahdi Hasan, Prof Indra Bhargava, Prof Shamer Singh, Prof A K Datta and Dr B D Chaurasia, who had inspired me a lot during my student life and teaching carrier.

Lastly, I thank my daughter Dr Rashi Singh, son Dr Gaurav Singh and daughter-in-law Ms Anupama Singh for helping me in the preparation of this manuscript. I gratefully acknowledge the help and cooperation received from the staff of RELX India Pvt Ltd, especially Arvind Koul (Sr Content Strategist), Shabina Nasim (Head of Content Project Management) and Goldy Bhatnagar (Content Project Manager), in completing the project on time.

Reviewers

I would like to give special thanks to those who have reviewed the digital copies of this book, before publication.

- Dr C S Ramesh Babu, Former Professor and HOD of Anatomy, LLRM Medical College, Meerut, UP.
- Dr T S Roy, Former Professor and HOD of Anatomy, AIIMS, New Delhi.
- Dr Garima Sehgal, Professor of Anatomy, King George's Medical College, Lucknow, UP.
- Dr Ajai Nene, Professor and HOD of Anatomy, ESIC Medical College, Faridabad, Haryana.
- Dr Vipin Khade, Professor and HOD of Anatomy, Chirayu Medical College, Bhopal, MP.
- Dr Preeti Shrivastava, Associate Professor, NDMC Medical College, Delhi.

Contents

Competency Map: Upper Limb and Thorax

Competency code	Competency	Core (Y/N)	Chapter Nos.	Page Nos.
UPPER LIMB				
Topic: Features of Individual Bones (Upper Limb)				
AN 8.1	Identify the given bone, its side, important features and keep it in anatomical position.	Y	2	9–33
AN 8.2	Identify and describe joints formed by the given bone.	Y	2	9–33
AN 8.3	Enumerate peculiarities of clavicle.	Y	2	10
AN 8.4	Demonstrate important muscle attachment on the given bone.	Y	2	9–33
AN 8.5	Identify and name various bones in articulated hand, Specify the parts of metacarpals and phalanges and enumerate the peculiarities of pisiform.	Y	2	29–32
AN 8.6	Describe scaphoid fracture and explain the anatomical basis of avascular necrosis.	N	2	29
Topic: Pectoral Region				
AN 9.1	Describe attachment, nerve supply and action of pectoralis major and pectoralis minor.	Y	3	34–37
AN 9.2	Describe the location, extent, deep relations, structure, age changes, blood supply, lymphatic drainage, microanatomy and applied anatomy of breast.	Y	3	39–47
AN 9.3	Describe development of breast.	N	3	45
Topic: Axilla, Shoulder and Scapular Region				
AN 10.1	Identify and describe boundaries and contents of axilla.	Y	4	48–49
AN 10.2	Identify, describe and demonstrate the origin, extent, course, parts, relations and branches of axillary artery and tributaries of vein.	Y	4	49–53
AN 10.3	Describe, identify and demonstrate formation, branches, relations, area of supply of branches, course and relations of terminal branches of brachial plexus.	Y	4	54–58
AN 10.4	Describe the anatomical groups of axillary lymph nodes and specify their areas of drainage.	Y	4	53

(Continued)

Competency code	Competency	Core (Y/N)	Chapter Nos.	Page Nos.
AN 10.5	Explain variations in formation of brachial plexus.	Y	4	54
AN 10.6	Explain the anatomical basis of clinical features of Erb's palsy and Klumpke's paralysis.	N	4	56
AN 10.7	Explain anatomical basis of enlarged axillary lymph nodes.	N	4	54
AN 10.8	Describe, identify and demonstrate the position, attachment, nerve supply and actions of trapezius and latissimus dorsi.	Y	5	62–63
AN 10.9	Describe the arterial anastomosis around the scapula and mention the boundaries of triangle of auscultation.	N	4, 5	51–52, 64–65
AN 10.10	Describe and identify the deltoid and rotator cuff muscles.	Y	5	65–68
AN 10.11	Describe and demonstrate attachment of serratus anterior with its action.	Y	3	37–38
AN 10.12	Describe and demonstrate shoulder joint for– type, articular surfaces, capsule, synovial membrane, ligaments, relations, movements, muscles involved, blood supply, nerve supply and applied anatomy.	Y	6	73–82
AN 10.13	Explain anatomical basis of Injury to axillary nerve during intramuscular injections.	N	5	66
Topic: Arm and Cubital Fossa				
AN 11.1	Describe and demonstrate muscle groups of upper arm with emphasis on biceps and triceps brachii.	Y	8	92–95, 103–104
AN 11.2	Identify and describe origin, course, relations, branches (or tributaries), termination of important nerves and vessels in arm.	Y	8	95–101
AN 11.3	Describe the anatomical basis of Venepuncture of cubital veins.	Y	8	102–103
AN 11.4	Describe the anatomical basis of Saturday night paralysis.	Y	13	174–175
AN 11.5	Identify and describe boundaries and contents of cubital fossa.	Y	8	100–102
AN 11.6	Describe the anastomosis around the elbow joint.	N	8	98
Topic: Forearm and Hand				
AN 12.1	Describe and demonstrate important muscle groups of ventral with attachments, nerve supply and actions forearm.	Y	9	108–114
AN 12.2	Identify and describe origin, course, relations, branches (or tributaries), termination of important nerves and vessels of forearm.	Y	9	114–118

Competency code	Competency	Core (Y/N)	Chapter Nos.	Page Nos.
AN 12.3	Identify and describe fl exor retinaculum with its attachments.	Y	11	140–141
AN 12.4	Explain anatomical basis of carpal tunnel syndrome.	Y	11	178
AN 12.5	Identify and describe small muscles of hand.	Y	11	145–149
AN 12.6	Describe and demonstrate movements of thumb and muscles involved.	Y	12	167–169
AN 12.7	Identify and describe course and branches of important blood vessels and nerves in hand.	Y	11	149–153
AN 12.8	Describe anatomical basis of claw hand.	Y	13	180
AN 12.9	Identify and describe fibrous flexor sheaths, ulnar bursa, radial bursa and digital synovial sheaths.	Y	11	142–144
AN 12.10	Explain infection of fascial spaces of palm.	N	11	154
AN 12.11	Identify, describe and demonstrate important muscle groups of dorsal forearm with attachments, nerve supply and actions.	Y	9	118–122
AN 12.12	Identify and describe origin, course, relations, branches (or tributaries), termination of important nerves and vessels of back of forearm.	Y	9	122–124
AN 12.13	Describe the anatomical basis of wrist drop.	Y	13	174
AN 12.14	Identify and describe compartments deep to extensor retinaculum.	Y	9	122–124
AN 12.15	Identify and describe extensor expansion formation	Y	11	156
Topic: General Features, Joints, Radiographs and Surface Marking				
AN 13.1	Describe and explain fascia of upper limb and compartments, veins of upper limb and its lymphatic drainage.	Y	7	83–90
AN 13.2	Describe dermatomes of upper limb.	N	7	85–86
AN 13.3	Identify and describe the type, articular surfaces, capsule, synovial membrane, ligaments, relations, movements, blood and nerve supply of elbow joint, proximal and distal radio-ulnar joints, wrist joint and first carpometacarpal joint.	Y	10, 12	128–137, 160
AN 13.4	Describe sternoclavicular joint, acromioclavicular joint, carpometacarpal joints and metacarpophalangeal joint.	N	6, 12	80–81, 164–165
AN 13.5	Identify the bones and joints of upper limb seen in anteroposterior and lateral view radiographs of shoulder region, arm, elbow, forearm and hand.	Y	2, 6, 10, 12	29–32, 128, 160
AN 13.6	Identify and demonstrate important bony landmarks of upper limb: jugular notch, sternal angle, acromial angle, spine of the scapula, vertebral level of the medial end, inferior angle of the scapula.	Y	3, 5	34, 59–60

(Continued)

Competency code	Competency	Core (Y/N)	Chapter Nos.	Page Nos.
AN 13.7	Identify and demonstrate surface projection of: cephalic and basilic vein, palpation of brachial artery, radial artery, testing of muscles: trapezius, pectoralis major, serratus anterior, latissimus dorsi, deltoid, biceps brachii, brachioradialis.	Y	3, 7, 8, 9, 14	35, 36, 38, 62, 91, 184–186
AN 13.8	Describe development of upper limb.	N	Refer *Textbook of Clinical Embryology* by Vishram Singh, 134–136	
THORAX				
AN 21.1	Identify and describe the salient features of sternum, typical rib, Ist rib and typical thoracic vertebra.	Y	16	203–206, 207–209
AN 21.2	Identify and describe the features of 2nd, 11th and 12th ribs, 1st, 11th and 12th thoracic vertebrae.	N	16	209–210, 213–214
AN 21.3	Describe and demonstrate the boundaries of thoracic inlet, cavity and outlet.	Y	15	193–200
AN 21.4	Describe and demonstrate extent, attachments, direction of fibres, nerve supply and actions of intercostal muscles.	Y	17	219–222
AN 21.5	Describe and demonstrate origin, course, relations and branches of a typical intercostal nerve.	Y	17	222–223
AN 21.6	Mention origin, course and branches/ tributaries of: 1) anterior and posterior intercostal vessels, 2) internal thoracic vessels.	Y	17	224–227
AN 21.7	Mention the origin, course, relations and branches of: 1) atypical intercostal nerve, 2) superior intercostal artery, subcostal artery.	N	17	223–224
AN 21.8	Describe and demonstrate type, articular surfaces and movements of manubriosternal, costovertebral, costotransverse and xiphisternal joints.	Y	16	215–216
AN 21.9	Describe and demonstrate mechanics and types of respiration.	Y	17	228–230
AN 21.10	Describe costochondral and interchondral joints.	N	16	216
AN 21.11	Mention boundaries and contents of the superior, anterior, middle and posterior mediastinum.	Y	20	255–256
AN 22.1	Describe and demonstrate subdivisions, sinuses in pericardium, blood supply and nerve supply of pericardium.	Y	21	262–265
AN 22.2	Describe and demonstrate external and internal features of each chamber of heart.	Y	21	265–276
AN 22.3	Describe and demonstrate origin, course and branches of coronary arteries.	Y	21	278–280

Competency code	Competency	Core (Y/N)	Chapter Nos.	Page Nos.
AN 22.4	Describe anatomical basis of ischaemic heart disease.	Y	21	280–281
AN 22.5	Describe and demonstrate the formation, course, tributaries and termination of coronary sinus.	Y	21	281–283
AN 22.6	Describe the fibrous skeleton of heart.	Y	21	277
AN 22.7	Mention the parts, position and arterial supply of the conducting system of heart.	Y	21	277–278
Topic: Mediastinum				
AN 23.1	Describe and demonstrate the external appearance, relations, blood supply, nerve supply, lymphatic drainage and applied anatomy of oesophagus.	Y	23	298–303
AN 23.2	Describe and demonstrate the extent, relations tributaries of thoracic duct and enumerate its applied anatomy.	Y	24	305–307
AN 23.3	Describe and demonstrate origin, course, relations, tributaries and termination of superior venacava, azygos, hemiazygos and accessory hemiazygos veins.	Y	22, 24	287–289, 308–309
AN 23.4	Mention the extent, branches and relations of arch of aorta and descending thoracic aorta.	Y	22	289–295
AN 23.5	Identify and Mention the location and extent of thoracic sympathetic chain.	Y	24	309–310
AN 23.6	Describe the splanchnic nerves.	N	24	309–310
AN 23.7	Mention the extent, relations and applied anatomy of lymphatic duct.	Y	24	305–307
Topic: Lungs and Trachea				
AN 24.1	Mention the blood supply, lymphatic drainage and nerve supply of pleura, extent of pleura and describe the pleural recesses and their applied anatomy.	Y	18	233–238
AN 24.2	Identify side, external features and relations of structures which form root of lung and bronchial tree and their clinical correlate.	Y	19	244–251
AN 24.3	Describe a bronchopulmonary segment.	Y	19	251–253
AN 24.4	Identify phrenic nerve and describe its formation and distribution.	Y	Refer *Textbook of Anatomy: Head, Neck and Brain,* Vol 3, 3e by Vishram Singh, 170, 334, 336	
AN 24.5	Mention the blood supply, lymphatic drainage and nerve supply of lungs.	Y	19	249–251
AN 24.6	Describe the extent, length, relations, blood supply, lymphatic drainage and nerve supply of trachea.	N	23	296–298

(Continued)

Competency code	Competency	Core (Y/N)	Chapter Nos.	Page Nos.
Topic: Thorax				
AN 25.1	Identify, draw and label a slide of trachea and lung.	Y	23	297
AN 25.2	Describe development of pleura, lung and heart.	Y	Refer *Textbook of Clinical Embryology,* 3e by Vishram Singh, 216–224, 236–251	
AN 25.3	Describe fetal circulation and changes occurring at birth.	Y	Refer *Textbook of General Embryology,* 3e by Vishram Singh, 269–270	
AN 25.4	Describe embryological basis of: 1) atrial septal defect, 2) ventricular septal defect, 3) Fallot's tetralogy and 4) tracheo-oesophageal fistula.	Y	Refer *Textbook of Clinical Embryology*, 3e by Vishram Singh, 243, 247, 218, 219	
AN 25.5	Describe developmental basis of congenital anomalies, transposition of great vessels, dextrocardia, patent ductus arteriosus and coarctation of aorta.	Y	Refer *Textbook of Clinical Embryology* 3rd edit. by Vishram Singh, 258	
AN 25.6	Mention development of aortic arch arteries, SVC, IVC and coronary sinus.	N	Refer *Textbook of Clinical Embryology,* 3e by Vishram Singh, 253–259, 264–269	
AN 25.7	Identify structures seen on a plain x-ray chest (PA view).	Y	21	268–269
AN 25.8	Identify and describe in brief a barium swallow.	N	23	303
AN 25.9	Demonstrate surface marking of lines of pleural reflection, lung borders and fissures, trachea, heart borders, apex beat and surface projection of valves of heart.	Y	25, 19, 21	239, 262, 312–314

SECTION I
UPPER LIMB

CHAPTER 1

Introduction to the Upper Limb

SPECIFIC LEARNING OBJECTIVES

After studying this chapter, the student should be able to:

- Define the upper limb and tell its main functions.
- Enumerate evolutionary changes in the human upper limb to make it suitable for prehensile activities.
- Compare the homologous parts of the upper and lower limbs.
- Discuss the differences between the upper and lower limbs.
- Trace the route of transmission of force from hand to the axial skeleton.

The upper limb (or upper extremity) is an appendage of the body, responsible for prehensile/manual activities. It extends on either side from shoulder region proximally to the hand distally. It is freely movable, especially its distal segment—the hand, which is adapted for grasping and manipulating objects.

A brief description of the comparative anatomy of the limbs would facilitate the understanding of their structure and function.

All the terrestrial vertebrates possess four limbs—a pair of forelimbs and a pair of hindlimbs. In quadrupeds such as dogs and buffaloes, both **forelimbs** and **hindlimbs** are evolved for transmission of body weight and locomotion. Therefore, both forelimbs and hindlimbs are built on the same principle. Thus, each limb consists of three segments: (a) proximal segment (thigh/arm); (b) middle segment (leg/forearm); and (c) distal segment (foot/hand).

Each limb is attached to the axial skeleton by a girdle, viz. lower limb by a pelvic girdle and upper limb by a pectoral girdle, respectively.

N.B.

- *Forelimb* should not be confused with the *forearm* which is the middle portion of human upper limb.
- **Girdle** is an integral part of each limb.
  - The **pelvic girdle** is formed by two hip bones, one on each side. They are interconnected anteriorly at pubic symphysis and posteriorly they articulate with sacrum at strong sacroiliac joints.
    It is a complete girdle designed mainly for transmission of weight.
  - The **pectoral girdle** is formed by two scapulae and two clavicles. The scapulae do not articulate posteriorly with axial skeleton by true joints but attached to it by freely mobile scapulothoracic linkages. While the clavicles articulate anteriorly with axial skeleton at small sternoclavicular joints. The scapula is connected to the clavicle by acromioclavicular joint.
    It is an incomplete girdle designed mainly for free movements.
  - Girdles actually function as anchors which attach appendages to the axial skeleton. The girdle bones are therefore a part of appendicular skeleton.

In human beings, due to the evolution of erect posture, the function of weight bearing and locomotion is performed only by the hindlimbs (lower limbs), while upper limbs are spared for prehensile/manipulative activities, such as grasping, holding, and picking (Fig. 1.1).

There are three types of grips: (a) power grip, (b) hook grip, and (c) precision grip. The power and hook grips are primitive in nature, hence found in higher primates. The precision grip is the characteristic of human beings; hence, only humans can properly hold a pen, pencil, needles, instruments, etc. As a result, human beings could make advancements in arts, craft, and technology, of course, with the help of intelligence.

To suit the prehensile activities, the following changes took place in the upper limbs of humans during evolution:

1. Appearance of joints permitting rotatory movements of the forearm, viz. supination and pronation
2. Addition of clavicle to act as a strut for keeping the upper limb away from the body for prehension
3. Rotation of thumb to 90° for opposition
4. Suitable changes for the free mobility of the fingers and hand

N.B.

- The human hand with its digits can perform complex skilled movements under the control of the brain. Hence, man is

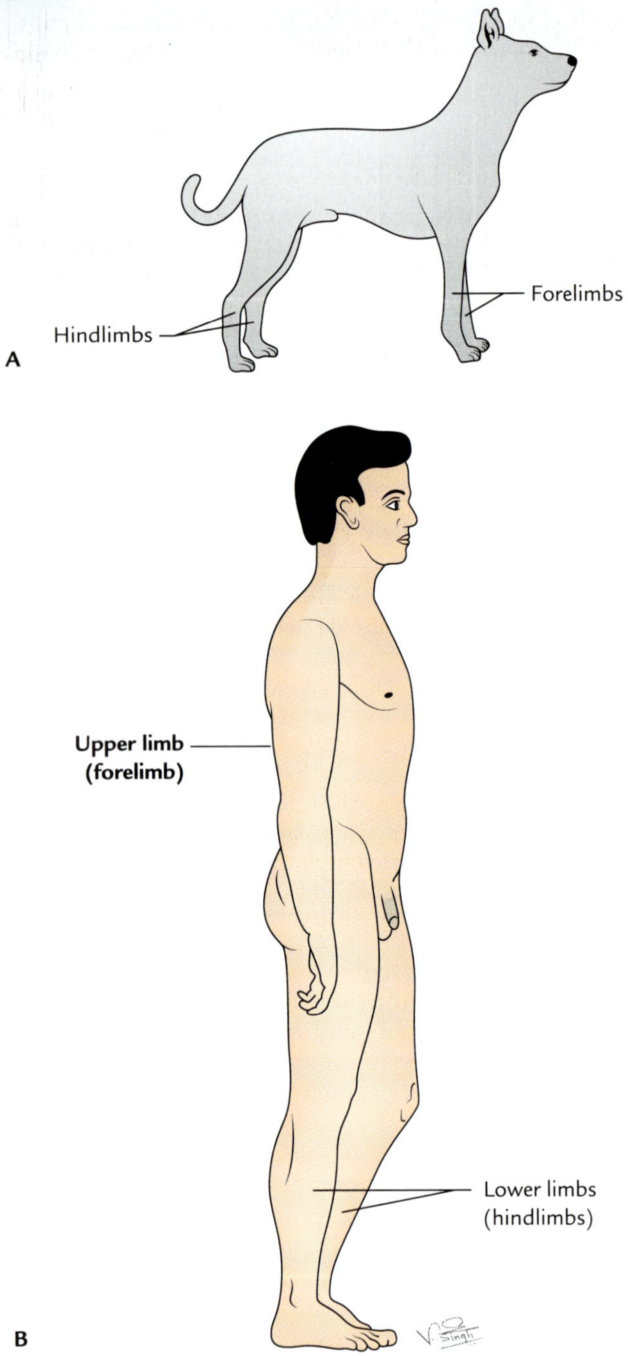

FIG. 1.1 ■ Position of limbs: (**A**) in quadrupeds and (**B**) in humans.

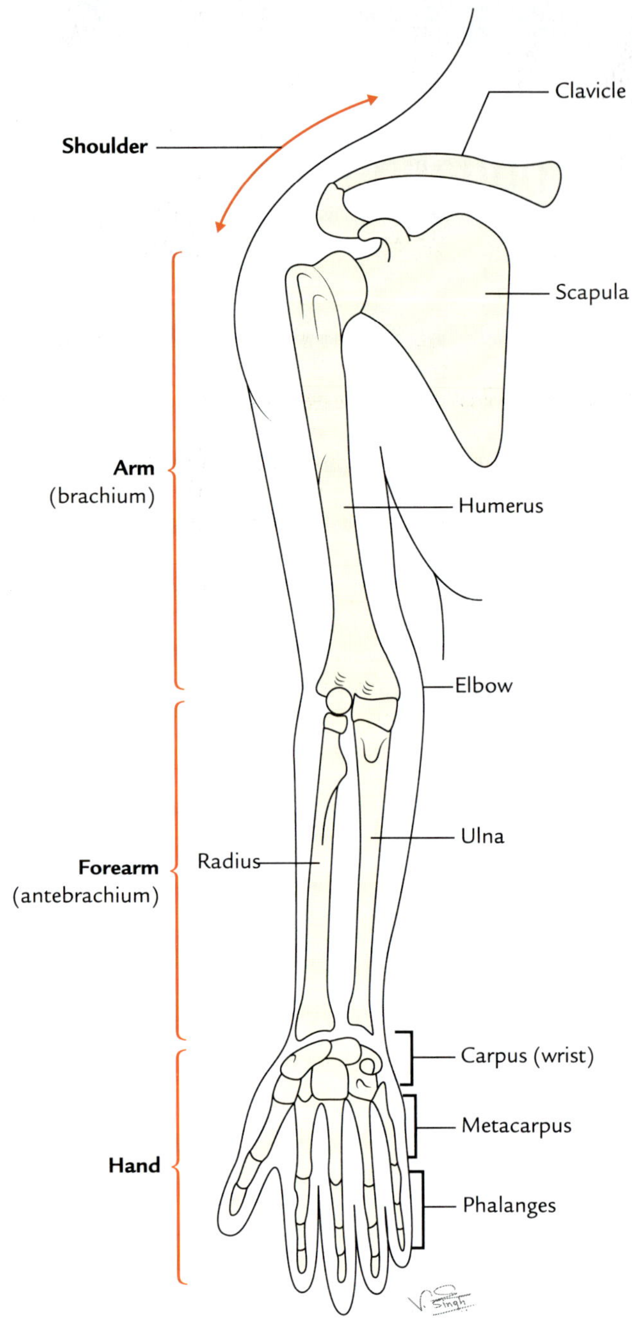

FIG. 1.2 ■ Parts of the upper limb.

considered as the *master mechanic of the animal world*. The disabling effects of an injury to the upper limb, particularly that of a hand, are far more than the extent of an injury. Therefore, a sound understanding of its structure and functions is of great clinical significance—the ultimate aim of treating any ailment of the upper limb is to restore its function.

- Only one small joint **(sternoclavicular joint)** connects the skeleton of the upper limb to the rest of the skeleton of the body.

PARTS OF THE UPPER LIMB

For descriptive purposes, the upper limb is divided into the following four major parts (Fig. 1.2):

1. Shoulder
2. Arm or brachium
3. Forearm or antebrachium
4. Hand or manus

The **shoulder region** includes: (a) axilla or armpit, (b) scapular region or parts around the scapula (shoulder blade), and (c) pectoral or breast region on the front of the chest.

The bones of the shoulder region are the clavicle (collar bone) and the scapula (shoulder blade). They articulate with each other at the acromioclavicular joint and form the shoulder girdle. The shoulder girdle articulates with the rest of the skeleton of the body only at the small sternoclavicular joint.

N.B.

Shoulder girdle/pectoral girdle is formed by scapulae and clavicles. It is incomplete posteriorly and completed anteriorly by manubrium sterni.

The **arm** is the part of the upper limb between the shoulder and elbow (or cubitus). It is the longest segment of the upper limb. The bone of the arm is humerus, which articulates with the scapula at the shoulder joint and upper ends of radius and ulna at the elbow joint.

The **forearm** is the part of the upper limb between the elbow and the wrist. The bones of the forearm are radius and ulna. These bones articulate with humerus at the elbow joint and with each other, forming radio-ulnar joints. Distally they articulate with corpus at radiocarpal joint.

The **hand** (or manus) consists of the following parts: (a) wrist or carpus, (b) hand proper (or metacarpus), and (c) digits (thumb and fingers).

The **wrist** consists of eight carpal bones arranged in two rows, each consisting of four bones. The carpal bones articulate (a) with each other at intercarpal joints, (b) proximally with radius forming radio-carpal/wrist joint, and (c) distally with metacarpal bones at carpometacarpal joints.

The ***hand proper*** consists of five metacarpal bones numbered 1–5 from lateral to medial side in anatomical position. They articulate (a) proximally with the distal row of carpal bones, forming carpometacarpal joints, (b) with each other forming intermetacarpal joints, and (c) distally with proximal phalanges, forming metacarpophalangeal joints.

The ***digits*** are 5 and numbered 1–5 from lateral to medial side. The first digit is called *thumb* and the remaining four digits are *fingers*. Each digit is supported by three short (miniature) long bones—the phalanges—except the thumb, which is supported by only two phalanges. The phalanges form metacarpophalangeal joints with metacarpals and interphalangeal joints with one another. The first carpometacarpal joint has a separate joint cavity; hence, movements of thumb are much freer than that of any digit/finger.

N.B.

The **functional value of the thumb** is immense. For example, in grasping, the functional value of the thumb is equal to other four digits/fingers. Therefore, the loss of the thumb alone is as disabling as the loss of all the four fingers.

The subdivisions, bones, and joints of different parts of the upper limb are summarized in Table 1.1.

COMPARISON AND CONTRAST BETWEEN THE UPPER AND LOWER LIMBS

Both the upper and lower limbs are built on the same basic principle. Each limb is made up of two portions: proximal and distal.

The proximal part is called the *limb girdle* and attaches the limb to the trunk. The distal part is free and consists of proximal, middle, and distal segments, which are referred to as arm, forearm, and hand, respectively, in the upper limb, and thigh, leg, and foot, respectively, in the lower limb. The homologous parts of the upper and lower limbs are enumerated in Table 1.2.

TABLE 1.1 **Parts of the upper limb**

Part	Subdivisions	Bones	Joints
Shoulder region	• Pectoral region • Axilla • Scapular region	• Clavicle • Scapula } Bones of shoulder girdle	• Sternoclavicular • Acromioclavicular • Glenohumeral
Arm	–	Humerus	Shoulder and elbow
Forearm	–	• Radius • Ulna	• Elbow • Radio-ulnar
Hand	• Wrist (carpus)	• Carpal bones (8)	• Wrist/radio-carpal • Intercarpal
	• Hand proper (metacarpus)	• Metacarpal bones (5)	• Carpometacarpal • Intermetacarpal
	• Digits	• Phalanges (14) (Two for thumb and three for each finger)	• Metacarpophalangeal • Proximal and distal interphalangeal

TABLE 1.2 **Homologous parts of the upper and lower limbs**

Upper limb	Lower limb
Shoulder/pectoral girdle	Hip girdle/pelvic girdle
Shoulder joint	Hip joint
Arm	Thigh
Elbow joint	Knee joint
Forearm	Leg
Wrist joint	Ankle joint
Hand (a) Carpus (b) Metacarpus (c) Fingers[a]	Foot (a) Tarsus (b) Metatarsus (c) Toes[a]

[a]The first digit in a hand is termed the ***thumb*** and the first digit in a foot is termed the ***great toe***.

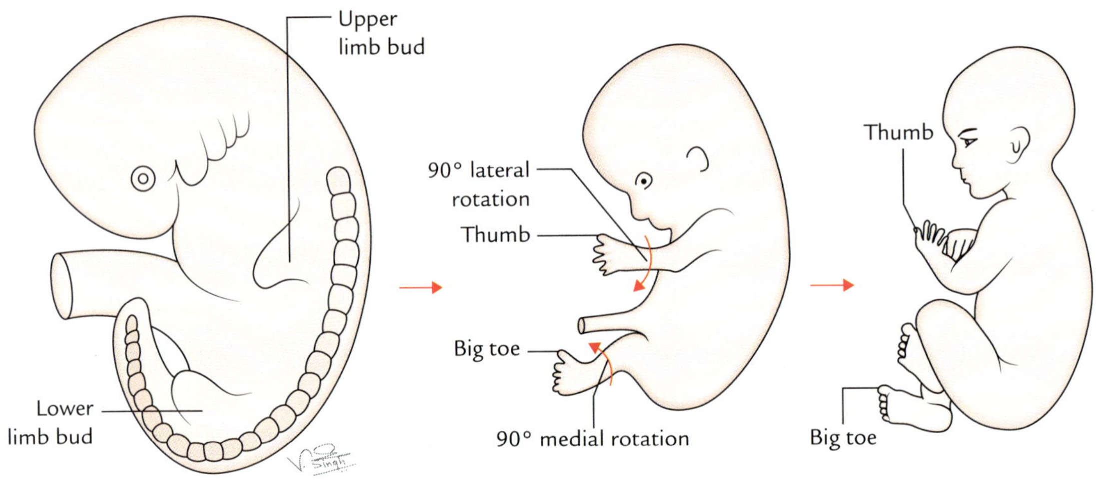

FIG. 1.3 Development of the limbs.

DEVELOPMENT OF LIMBS

A short account of the development of the limbs further makes it easier to understand the differences between the upper and lower limbs (Fig. 1.3).

The development of the upper and lower limbs begins in the fourth week of intrauterine life. A pair of small elevations appears on the ventrolateral aspect of the embryo called *limb buds*. The pair of the upper limb buds appears opposite the lower cervical segments. The pair of the lower limb buds appears three or four days later at the level of lumbar and upper sacral segments. Thus, during an early stage of development, all the four limbs appear as the paired limb buds. First, they are **simple flipper-like appendages** so that the upper and lower limbs are similar in their appearance. Each has dorsal and ventral surfaces, and preaxial and postaxial borders. The **preaxial border** faces towards the head. Later in the development, the ends of the limb buds become expanded and flattened to form the hand and foot plates in which the digits develop. The digits nearest to the preaxial border are the thumb and the big toe in the upper and lower limbs, respectively. The limbs then rotate.

The upper limb buds rotate laterally through 90° so that their preaxial border faces laterally and their extensor surface faces backward.

The lower limb buds rotate medially through 90° so that their preaxial border faces medially and their extensor surface faces forward.

The differences between the upper and lower limbs are listed in Table 1.3.

TRANSMISSION OF FORCE IN THE UPPER LIMB

The pectoral girdle on each side consists of two bones: the clavicle and the scapula; only the clavicle is attached to the rest of skeleton by a small joint—the sternoclavicular joint. The two bones of the girdle are joined together by even a smaller joint, the acromioclavicular joint. The clavicle is attached to the scapula by a strong coracoclavicular ligament (strongest ligament in the upper limb), and the clavicle is anchored to the first costal cartilage by the costoclavicular ligament (Fig. 1.4).

When person falls on an outstretched hand, the forces of impact on the upper limb are transmitted to the axial skeleton

TABLE 1.3 Differences between the upper and lower limbs

	Upper limb	Lower limb
Function	Prehension (i.e. manipulation of objects by grasping)	Locomotion and transmission of weight
Bones	Smaller and weaker	Larger and stronger
Joints	Smaller and less stable	Larger and more stable
Muscles	• Smaller and attached to smaller bony areas • Antigravity muscles less developed	• Larger and attached to larger bony areas • Antigravity muscles more developed
Girdle	Pectoral girdle (a) Made up of two bones: clavicle and scapula (b) No articulation with the vertebral column (c) Articulation with the axial skeleton is very small through sternoclavicular joint	Pelvic girdle (a) Made up of single bone, the hip bone[a] (b) Articulates with vertebral column (c) Articulation with axial skeleton is large, through sacroiliac joint
Preaxial border	Faces laterally	Faces medially

[a]The hip bone essentially consists of three components: **ilium**, **ischium**, and **pubis**, which later fuse to form a single bone.

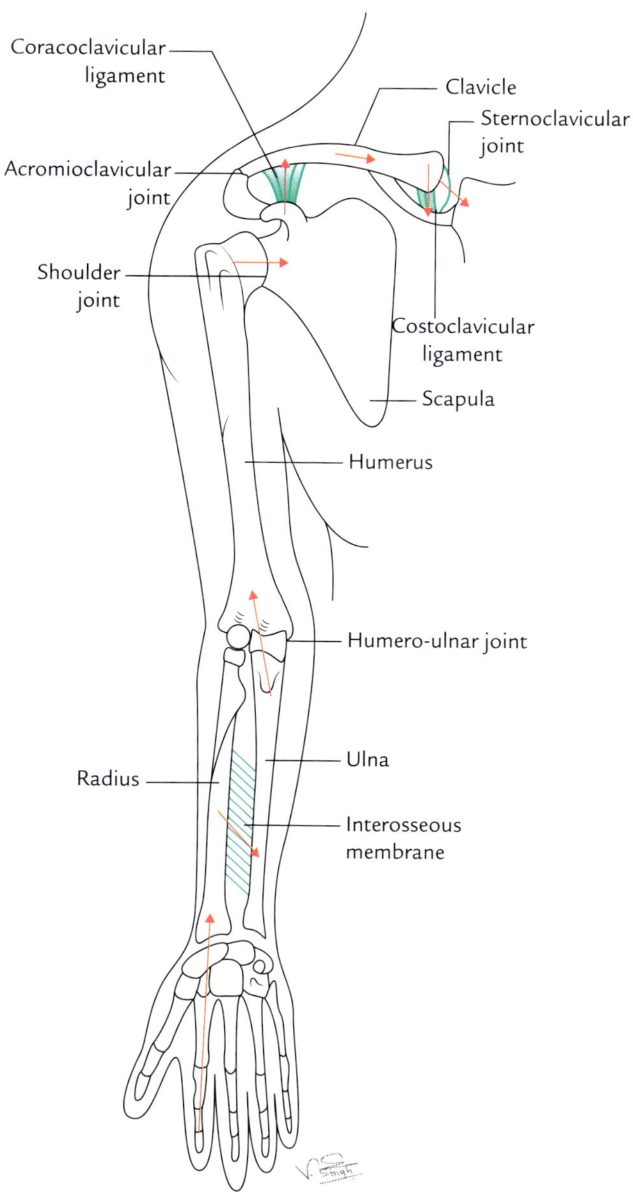

FIG. 1.4 ■ Transmission of force in the upper limb. Lines of force transmission are shown by red arrows.

by the clavicle through the costoclavicular ligament and the sternoclavicular joint. The lines of force transmission in the upper limb are shown in Fig. 1.4 and Flowchart 1.1.

BONES OF THE UPPER LIMB

They are already described with parts of the upper limb (for details, see page 2).

MUSCLES OF THE UPPER LIMB

The muscles of the upper limb include: (a) the muscles that attach the limb and girdle to the body and (b) the muscles of the arm, forearm, and hand. The deltoid muscle covers the shoulder like a hood and is commonly used for intramuscular injections.

The arm and the forearm are invested in the deep fascia like a sleeve and are divided into anterior and posterior compartments by intermuscular septa. The muscles of the anterior and posterior compartments mainly act synergistically to carry out specific functions. The muscles of the anterior compartment are mainly flexors and those of the posterior compartment are extensors.

The muscles of the hand are responsible for its various skilled movements such as grasping.

NERVES OF THE UPPER LIMB

The nerve supply to the upper limb is derived from the brachial plexus (formed by ventral rami of C5–C8 and T1 spinal nerves) (Fig. 1.5). The **five main branches of brachial plexus** are axillary, musculocutaneous, median, ulnar, and radial nerves.

The ***axillary nerve*** supplies the deltoid and teres minor muscles.

The ***musculocutaneous***, ***median***, and ***ulnar nerves*** supply the muscles of anterior (flexor) compartments of the arm and forearm.

The ***radial nerve*** supplies the muscles of the posterior (extensor) compartments of the arm and forearm.

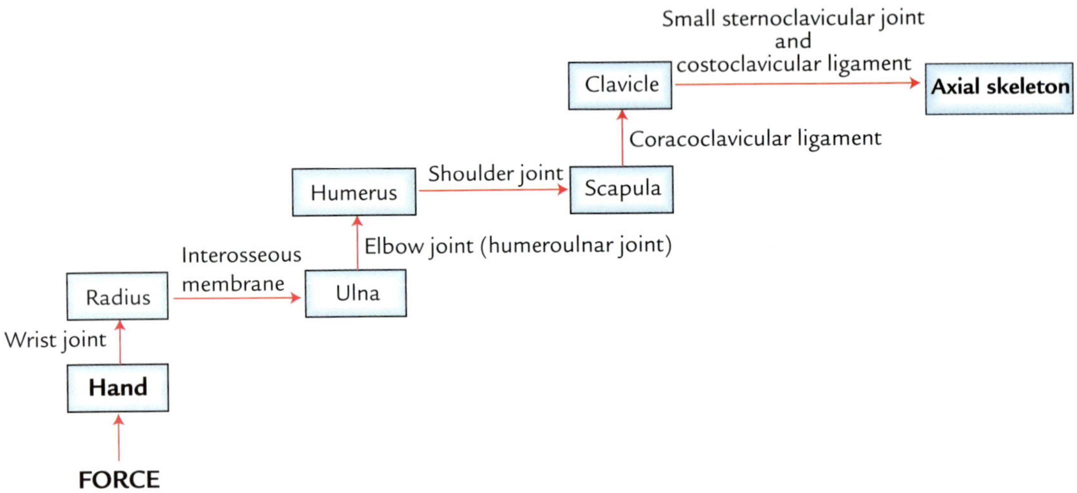

Flowchart 1.1 ■ Lines of force transmission from the upper limb to the axial skeleton.

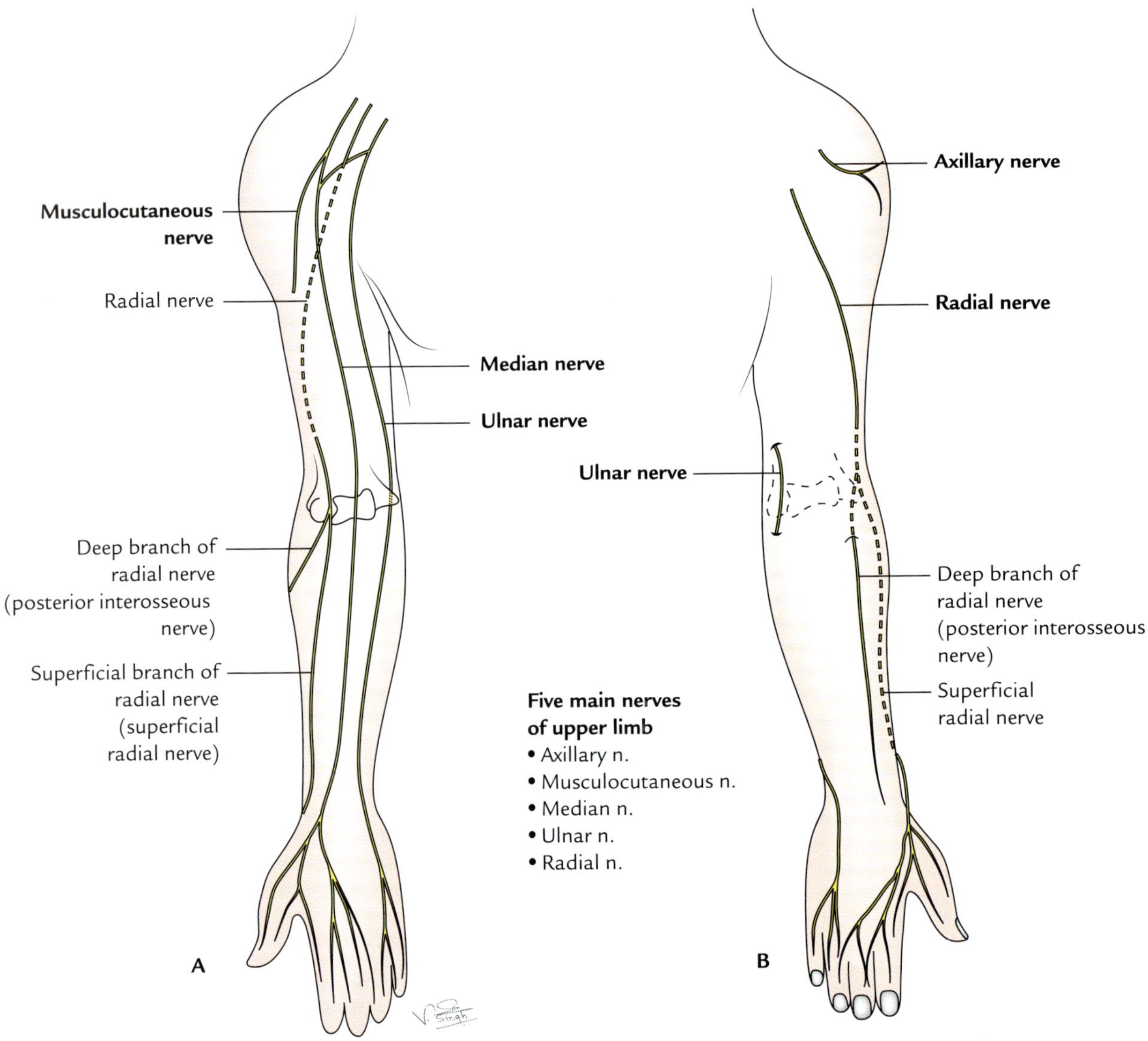

FIG. 1.5 ■ Main nerves of the right upper limb: (**A**) anterior aspect and (**B**) posterior aspect.

N.B.

All the intrinsic muscles of the hand are supplied by the ulnar nerve except muscles of the thenar eminence and first two lumbricals.

ARTERIES OF THE UPPER LIMB

The blood to the upper limb is supplied by four main arteries: **axillary, brachial, radial,** and **ulnar** (Fig. 1.6).

The axillary is the continuation of subclavian artery. At the lower border of the teres major muscle, its name is changed to the brachial artery. The brachial artery continues down the arm and just distal to the elbow joint, it divides into the radial and ulnar arteries, which follow the bones, after which they are named as such. In the hand, the radial artery terminates by forming the deep palmar arch, and the ulnar artery terminates by forming the superficial palmar arch.

The ***axillary artery*** supplies blood to the shoulder region.

The ***brachial artery*** supplies blood to the anterior and posterior compartments of the arm.

The ***radial and ulnar arteries*** supply blood to the lateral and medial parts of the forearm, respectively. They also supply blood to hand through deep and superficial palmar arches.

VEINS OF THE UPPER LIMB

The **deep veins** of the upper limb follow the arteries and run superiorly towards the axilla, where the axillary vein travels superiorly and becomes subclavian vein at the outer border of the first rib. The subclavian vein continues towards the root of the neck where it joins the internal jugular vein to form the brachiocephalic vein. The two brachiocephalic veins (right and left) join each other to form superior vena cava, which drains into the heart.

The **superficial veins** of the upper limb originate from the dorsal venous arch of the hand. The lateral end of the dorsal venous arch forms the *cephalic vein*, which runs along the lateral aspect of the upper limb and terminates into the axillary vein in the axilla. The medial end of the dorsal venous arch forms the *basilic vein*, which ascends along the medial aspect of the upper limb, joins the paired brachial veins to continue as the axillary vein. Anterior to

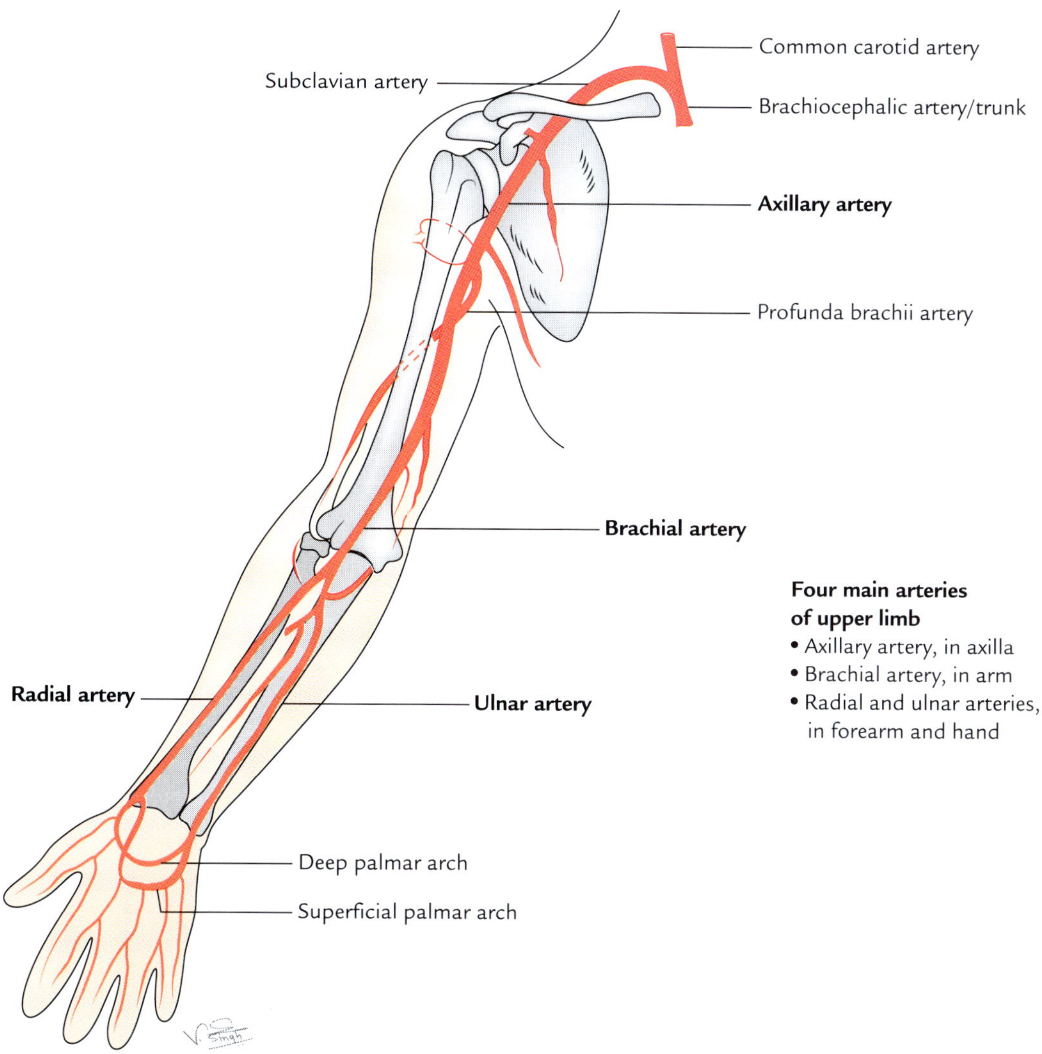

FIG. 1.6 Arteries of the right upper limb.

the hollow of elbow, the cephalic vein is connected to the basilic vein via the median cubital vein.

LYMPHATICS OF THE UPPER LIMB

The lymphatics of the upper limb originate in the hand. The superficial lymph vessels follow the superficial veins. The deep lymph vessels follow the deep arteries (viz. radial, ulnar, and brachial) and pass superiorly to the axilla where they drain into the axillary lymph nodes.

CLINICAL CORRELATION

- **Injuries of the upper limb:** The human upper limb is meant for prehension, that is, grasping, and not for the locomotion and transmission of weight. The mechanism of grasping is provided by the hand with the four fingers flexing against the opposable thumb. The upper limb is, therefore, light built, that is, its bones are smaller and weaker, joints are smaller and less stable, etc. Hence, it is more prone to injuries such as dislocation and fractures.
  - ***Dislocations:*** The common dislocations in the upper limb are the dislocations of the shoulder joint (most commonly dislocated joint in the body), elbow joint, and lunate bone of the hand.
  - ***Fractures:*** The common fractures in the upper limb are the fracture of clavicle (most commonly fractured bone in the body), humerus, radius, and scaphoid. The scaphoid is the most commonly fractured bone of the hand.
  - ***Nerve injuries:*** The common nerve injuries in the upper limb are the injuries of the brachial plexus, median nerve, radial nerve, and ulnar nerve. The compression of the median nerve at wrist is the most common peripheral neuropathy in the body. The three major nerves of the upper limb (e.g. radial, median, and ulnar) have predilection of involvement in leprosy. The ulnar nerve can be easily palpated behind the medial epicondyle of the humerus.
- **Sites for the intramuscular and intravenous injections:**
  - The *intramuscular injection* is most commonly given in the shoulder region in the deltoid muscle.
  - The *intravenous injection* is most commonly given in the superficial veins in front of the elbow and the dorsum of the hand.
- **Sites for feeling arterial pulsations (for details, see pages 189–191):** The arterial pulsation is most commonly felt and auscultated on the medial side of the front of the elbow for recording of blood pressure. The arterial pulse is most commonly felt on the lateral side of the front of the distal forearm for recording the pulse rate.

Golden Facts to Remember

• Most important function of hand	Prehensile activities (i.e. grasping)
• Most important movement of human hand	Opposition of thumb and precision grip
• Only point of bony contact between the upper limb and chest	Sternoclavicular joint
• Part of the upper limb having largest representation in the brain	Hand
• Most important digit of the hand	Thumb
• First bone to ossify in the body	Clavicle
• Most commonly fractured bone in the body	Clavicle
• Most commonly fractured bone of the hand	Scaphoid
• Most commonly compressed peripheral nerve	Median nerve at wrist
• Most commonly fractured metacarpal	Fifth metacarpal
• Most mobile joint in the body	Shoulder joint
• Most commonly dislocated joint in the body	Shoulder joint
• Joint with maximum types of movements in the body	First carpometacarpal joint
• Strongest ligament in the upper limb	Coracoclavicular ligament
• Muscle most commonly used for intramuscular injection	Deltoid
• Most preferred muscle for tendon graft	Palmaris longus
• Artery commonly used for auscultation	Brachial artery in front of the elbow
• Artery commonly used for taking arterial pulse	Radial artery in front of wrist on the lateral side
• Vein commonly used for intravenous injection	Median cubital vein in front of elbow
• Most common fractures in children	Forearm fractures

CHAPTER 2

Bones of the Upper Limb

SPECIFIC LEARNING OBJECTIVES

After studying this chapter, the student should be able to:

- Identity the given bone, its side, important features and keep it in an anatomical position. AN 8.1
- Identify and describe joints formed by a given bone. AN 8.2
- Enumerate the peculiarities of the clavicle. AN 8.3
- Demonstrate important muscle attachment on given bone. AN 8.4
- Identify and name the various bones in an articulated hand. Specify the parts of metacarpals, and phalanges; and enumerate peculiarities of pisiform bone. AN 8.5
- Describe the scaphoid fracture and anatomical basis of its avascular necrosis. AN 8.6
- Give the anatomical basis of the fracture clavicle at the junction of its medial two-thirds and lateral one-third.
- Tell the three common sites of the fracture of the humerus.
- Enumerate the structures attached on: (a) coracoid process of scapula, (b) greater tubercle of the humerus, and (c) posterior border of the ulna.
- Enumerate the carpal bones and tell their ossification.

The study of bones of the upper limb is important to understand the general topography of the upper limb and the attachment of various muscles and ligaments. The students must read the features and attachments of the bones before undertaking the study of the upper limb.

The study of bones also helps to understand the position of various articulations, wide range of the movements executed by the upper limb, and the genesis of various fractures, which are common in the upper limb bones.

Each upper limb contains 32 bones (Fig. 2.1), namely:

- **Scapula**, the shoulder blade (1). } Bones of the pectoral girdle.
- **Clavicle**, the collar bone (1). }
- **Humerus**, the bone of the arm (1).
- **Radius and ulna**, the bones of the forearm (2).

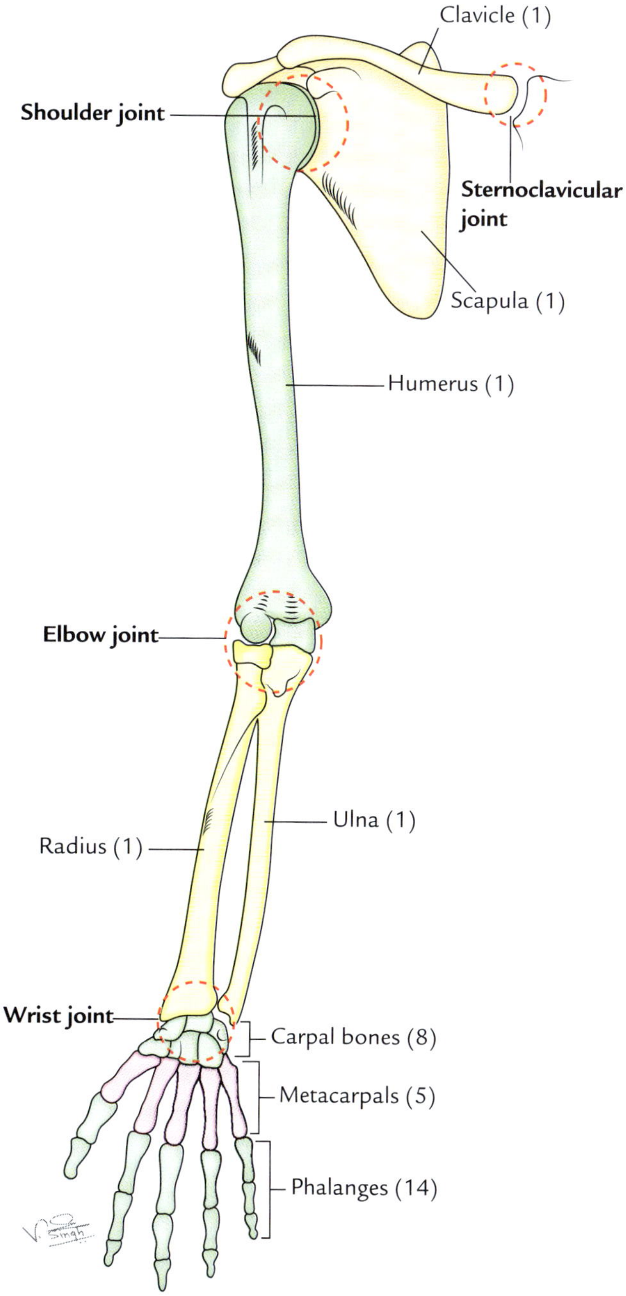

FIG. 2.1 ■ Bones of the upper limb.

- **Carpal bones**, the bones of the wrist (8).
- **Metacarpals**, the bones of the hand (5).
- **Phalanges**, the bones of digits (14).

N.B.

- The hand includes carpus, metacarpus, and digits. Hence, it consists of 27 bones which are arranged in groups as *carpals*, *metacarpals*, and *phalanges*.
- The total number of bones in a human body is 206. Out of which upper limbs only contain 64 bones.

CLAVICLE

AN 8.3

The clavicle (L. clavicle = key) or the collar bone is the long bone, approximately 15 cm (6 in) long with a slight S-shaped curve. It serves as strut between shoulder blade and sternum.

It is located horizontally on the anterior aspect of the body at the junction of the root of the neck and trunk. It articulates medially with the sternum and first rib cartilage and laterally with the acromion process of the scapula. It is subcutaneous and, hence, it can be palpated through its entire extent. It is the only bony attachment between the trunk and the upper limb.

FUNCTIONS

The functions of the clavicle are as follows:

1. It acts as a strut for holding the upper limb far from the trunk so that it can move freely. This allows free swing of the upper limb for various prehensile acts such as holding and catching.
2. It transmits forces from the upper limb to the axial skeleton (sternum).
3. It provides an area for the attachment of muscles.

PECULIARITIES

AN 8.3

The peculiar features of the clavicle are as follows:

1. It is the only long bone that lies horizontally.
2. It has no medullary cavity.
3. It is subcutaneous throughout its extent.
4. It is the first bone to start ossifying [between the fifth and sixth week of intrauterine life (IUL)] and last bone to complete its ossification (at 25 years).
5. It is the only long bone that ossifies by two primary centres.
6. It is the only long bone that ossifies in the membrane except for its medial end, which ossifies in the cartilage (membranocartilaginous ossification) (cf. long bones ossify in the cartilage).
7. It may be pierced through and through by the cutaneous nerve (intermediate supraclavicular nerve).

PARTS

The clavicle consists of three parts: two ends (medial and lateral) and a shaft (Fig. 2.2):

Ends

1. The **lateral (acromial) end** is flattened above downward and articulate with the medial margin of the acromion process.
2. The **medial (sternal) end** is enlarged and quadrilateral. It articulates with the clavicular notch of the manubrium sterni.

Shaft

The **shaft** is curved. Its medial two-thirds is round and convex forward, and its lateral one-third is flattened and concave forward. The inferior surface of the shaft possesses a small longitudinal groove in its middle third.

ANATOMICAL POSITION AND SIDE DETERMINATION

The side of the clavicle can be determined by holding the bone horizontally in such a way that its flattened end is on the lateral side and its enlarged quadrilateral end is on the medial side. The convexity of its medial two-thirds and the concavity of its lateral one-third face forward with the longitudinal groove in the middle third of the shaft facing inferiorly.

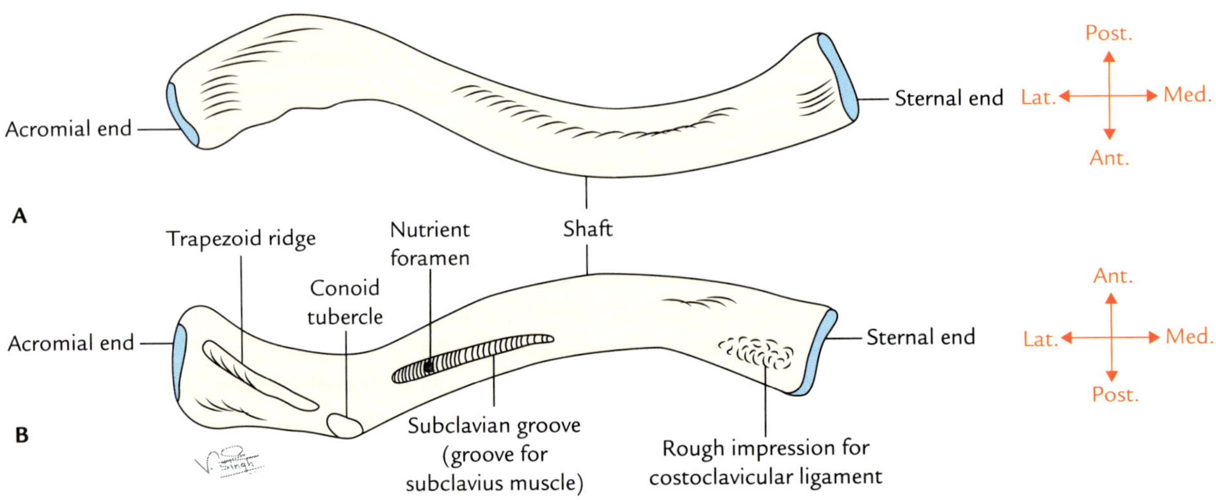

FIG. 2.2 ■ Right clavicle. (**A**) Superior aspect and (**B**) inferior aspect.

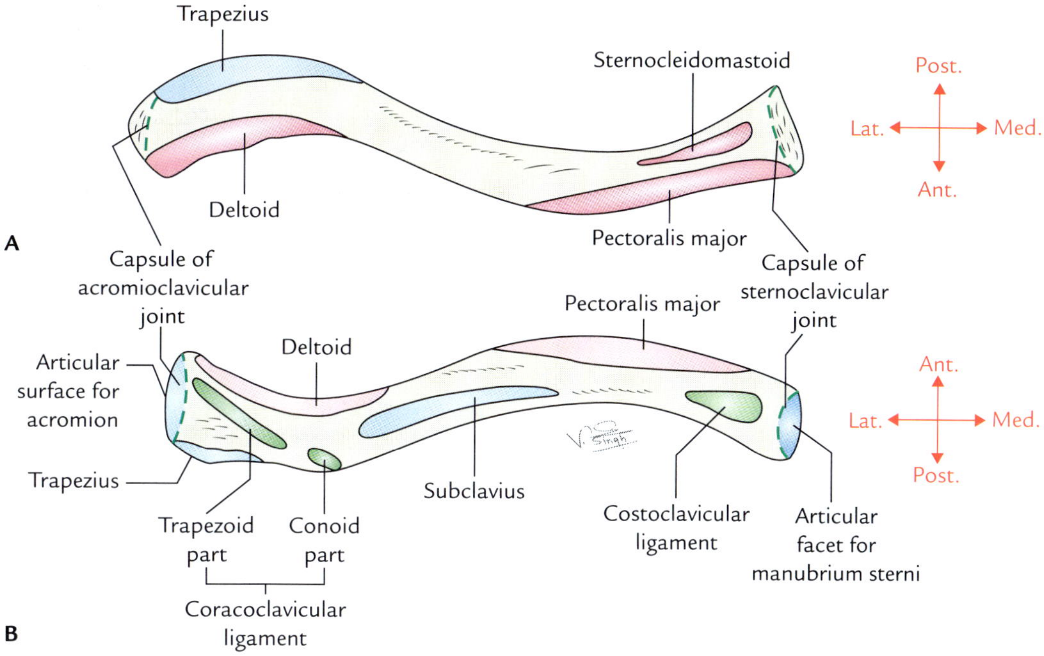

FIG. 2.3 Right clavicle showing attachments of the muscles and ligaments. (**A**) Superior surface and (**B**) inferior surface.

FEATURES AND ATTACHMENTS (FIGS. 2.2 AND 2.3)

Lateral End/Acromial End

It is flattened above downward. An oval facet on this end articulates with the facet on the medial margin of the acromion to form the **acromioclavicular joint**. The lateral end provides attachment to the fibrous capsule of the acromioclavicular joint.

Medial End/Sternal End

The enlarged medial end has a saddle-shaped articular surface that articulates with the clavicular notch of manubrium sterni to form the **sternoclavicular joint**. It provides attachment to the (a) fibrous capsule, (b) articular disc, and (c) interclavicular ligament.

Shaft

The shaft of the clavicle is divided into two parts: lateral one-third and medial two-thirds. The medial two-thirds of the shaft is convex forward and the lateral one-third is concave forward.

Lateral One-Third

It is flattened from above downward. It has two surfaces, that is superior and inferior, and two borders, that is anterior and posterior.

Surfaces

Superior surface: It is subcutaneous between the attachments of deltoid and trapezius.

Inferior surface: It presents a **conoid tubercle** and a **trapezoid ridge**, which provide attachments to conoid and trapezoid parts of the *coracoclavicular ligament*, respectively.

The **conoid tubercle** is located on the inferior surface near the posterior border at the junction of the lateral one-fourth and medial three-fourths of the clavicle. The **trapezoid ridge** extends forward and laterally from the conoid tubercle.

Borders

Anterior border: It is concave forward and gives origin to the deltoid muscle. A small tubercle called the **deltoid tubercle** may be present on this border.

Posterior border: It is convex backward and provides insertion to the trapezius muscle.

Medial Two-Thirds

It is cylindrical in shape and presents four surfaces: anterior, posterior, superior, and inferior.

Anterior surface: It is convex forward and gives origin to the clavicular head of the pectoralis major.

Posterior surface: It is concave backward and gives origin to the sternohyoid muscle near its medial end. The lateral part of this surface forms the anterior boundary of the cervicoaxillary canal and is related to the following structures:

1. Divisions of trunks of the brachial plexus.
2. Third part of the subclavian artery.

Superior surface: The clavicular head of the sternocleidomastoid muscle originates from the medial half of this surface.

Inferior surface: It presents the following features:

1. Costoclavicular ligament is attached to an oval impression at its medial end.
2. *Subclavius muscle* is inserted into the subclavian groove on this surface.
3. *Clavipectoral fascia* is attached to the margins of the subclavian groove.
4. *Nutrient foramen of the clavicle* is located on the lateral end of the subclavian groove.

TABLE 2.1 Muscles and ligaments attached to the clavicle

Muscles	Ligaments
Pectoralis major	Coracoclavicular
Sternocleidomastoid (clavicular head)	Costoclavicular
Deltoid	Interclavicular
Trapezius	
Subclavius	

The muscles and ligaments attached to the clavicle are given in Table 2.1.

CLINICAL CORRELATION

Fracture of the clavicle (Fig. 2.4): The clavicle is one of the most commonly fractured bones in the body. It commonly fractures at the junction of its lateral one-third and medial two-thirds due to fall on the outstretched hand or on the shoulder. It commonly occurs in males in the age group of 15–25 years.

When fracture occurs, the lateral fragment is displaced downward by the weight of the upper limb because the trapezius alone is unable to support the weight of the upper limb. In addition, the lateral fragment is drawn medially by shoulder adductors, namely, teres major, etc. The medial fragment is slightly elevated by the sternocleidomastoid muscle.

The characteristic clinical picture of the patient with the fractured clavicle is that of a man/woman supporting his sagging upper limb with the opposite hand. The fracture at the junction of the lateral one-third and medial two-thirds occurs because it is the weakest site due to:
(a) Two curvatures of the clavicle meet at this site.
(b) Transmission of forces from the scapula to clavicle at this site through the coracoclavicular ligament.

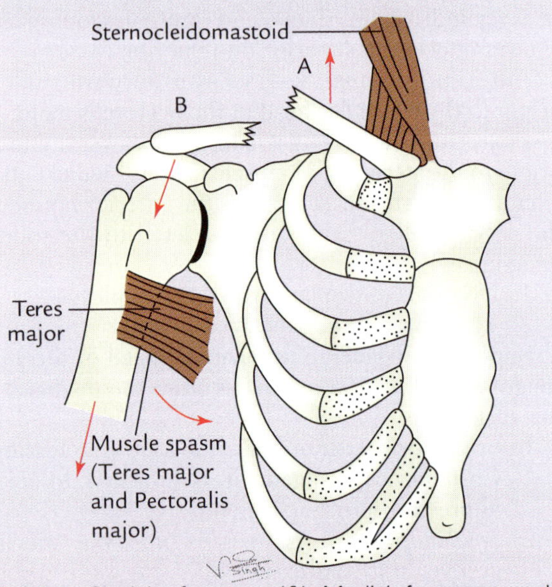

FIG. 2.4 ■ Clavicle fracture. (**A**) Medial fragment and (**B**) lateral fragment. (*Source:* Fig. 2.1, p. 51, *Clinical and Surgical Anatomy*, 2e, Vishram Singh. Copyright Elsevier, 2007. All rights reserved.)

N.B.

- Recently clinicians have found that commonest site of fracture clavicle is in its middle 1/3rd (80%) as it is thinnest part and devoid of muscular and ligamentous attachments. It occurs due to fall on lateral shoulder.
- The clavicle is absent in animals in which the upper limbs are used only for walking and weight transmission, and not for grasping, such as horse.

OSSIFICATION

The ossification of the clavicle is **membranocartilaginous** (Fig. 2.5). It is first bone to begin ossification (5–6 weeks of IUL) and one of the last bone to finish ossification (= 21–25 years of age). Whole of it ossifies in the membrane except its medial end that ossifies in the cartilage. The clavicle begins to ossify before any other bone in the body. It ossifies by four ossification centres: two primary centres for the shaft and two secondary centres, one for each end.

The site of appearance, time of appearance, and time of fusion of various centres is given in Table 2.2.

N.B.

Growing end of the clavicle: The sternal end of the clavicle is its growing end, because epiphysis at this end appears at the age of 19–20 years and unites with the shaft at the age of 21–25 years. It is the last of all the epiphyses in the body to fuse with the shaft. The radiological appearance of this epiphysis in females confirms their bone age for giving the **legal consent to marriage**.

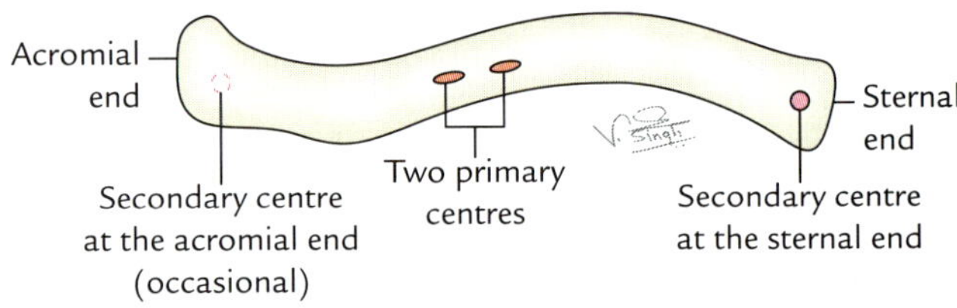

FIG. 2.5 ■ Ossification of the clavicle.

TABLE 2.2 Ossification centres of the clavicle

Site of appearance	Time of appearance	Time of fusion
Two primary centres (medial and lateral) in the shaft	5–6 weeks of intrauterine life (IUL)	Fourth or fifth day after appearance
Secondary centre at sternal end	19–20 years (2 years earlier in female)	21–25 years
Secondary centre at the acromial end (occasional)	20th year	Fuses immediately

CLINICAL CORRELATION

Congenital anomalies:

- **Clavicular dysostosis:** It is a clinical condition in which the medial and lateral parts of the clavicle remain separate due to nonunion of two primary centres of ossification.
- **Cleidocranial dysostosis:** It is a clinical condition characterized by the partial or complete absence of the clavicle due to defective intramembranous ossification. It is often associated with the defective ossification of the skull bones. In this condition, two shoulders can be approximated anteriorly in front of the chest (Fig. 12.3, P. 124, *Textbook of Clinical Embryology*, 3ed. by Vishram Singh).

SCAPULA

The scapula (***Latin:* scapula** = shoulder blade) is a large, flat, triangular bone located on the upper part of the posterolateral aspect of the thorax, against the second to seventh ribs. It forms posterior part of shoulder girdle and provides attachment to about 17 muscles, which helps you to move your shoulders.

PARTS

The scapula is highly mobile bone and consists of four parts: a **body** and **three processes**—spinous, acromion, and coracoid (Fig. 2.6).

N.B.

Some authorities divide the scapula into three parts, namely, *head*, *neck*, and *body*.

The head is thickest lateral angle. The neck is slightly constricted part which surrounds the head. While body of scapula is large triangular major part of bone.

Body

The body is triangular, thin, and translucent. It presents the following features:

1. Two surfaces: (a) costal and (b) dorsal.
2. Three borders: (a) superior, (b) lateral, and (c) medial.
3. Three angles: (a) inferior, (b) superior, and (c) lateral.

The **dorsal surface** presents a shelf-like projection on its upper part called the **spinous process**.

The **lateral angle** is truncated to form an articular surface—the **glenoid cavity**.

The lateral angle is thickened and called the **head of the scapula**, which is connected to the plate-like body by an inconspicuous **neck**.

Processes

There are three processes. These are as follows:

1. Spinous process
2. Acromion process
3. Coracoid process

The **spinous process** is a shelf-like bony projection on the dorsal aspect of the body.

The **acromion process** projects forward almost at the right angle from the lateral end of the spine.

The **coracoid process** is like a bird's beak. It arises from the upper border of the head and bends sharply to project superoanteriorly.

ANATOMICAL POSITION AND SIDE DETERMINATION

The side of the scapula can be determined by holding the scapula in such a way that:

1. The **glenoid cavity** faces laterally, forward, and slightly upward (at an angle of 45° from the coronal plane).
2. The **coracoid process** is directed forward.
3. The shelf-like **spinous process** is directed posteriorly.
4. Inferior angle (apex of the triangular bone) is directed downwards.

FEATURES AND ATTACHMENTS (FIG. 2.7)

Surfaces

Costal surface (subscapular fossa):

1. It is concave and directed medially and forward.
2. It presents three longitudinal ridges, which provide attachment to the intramuscular tendons of the subscapularis muscle.
3. The **subscapularis muscle** (a multipennate muscle) arises from the medial two-thirds of the subscapular fossa/costal surface except near the neck where a *subscapular bursa* intervenes between the neck and the subscapular tendon.
4. The **serratus anterior muscle** is inserted on this surface along the medial border and the inferior angle.

Dorsal surface:

1. The dorsal surface is convex and presents a shelf-like projection called the **spinous process**.
2. The spinous process divides the dorsal surface into supraspinous and infraspinous fossae. The upper, supraspinous fossa is smaller (one-third) and lower, infraspinous fossa is larger (two-thirds).
3. The **spinoglenoid notch** lies between the base of the spine of scapula (to be specific its lateral border) and the dorsal surface of the glenoid process (Fig. 2.7C), the neck of scapula. Through this notch, the supraspinous fossa communicates with the infraspinous fossa and the suprascapular nerve and vessels pass from the supraspinous fossa to the infraspinous fossa.
4. The **supraspinatus muscle** arises from the medial two-thirds of the supraspinous fossa.
5. The **infraspinatus muscle** arises from the medial two-thirds of the infraspinous fossa.
6. The **teres minor muscle** arises from the upper two-thirds of the dorsal surface of the lateral border. This origin is interrupted by the *circumflex scapular artery*.
7. The **teres major muscle** arises from the lower one-third of the dorsal surface of the lateral border and the inferior angle of the scapula.
8. The **latissimus dorsi muscle** also arises from the dorsal surface of the inferior angle by a small slip.

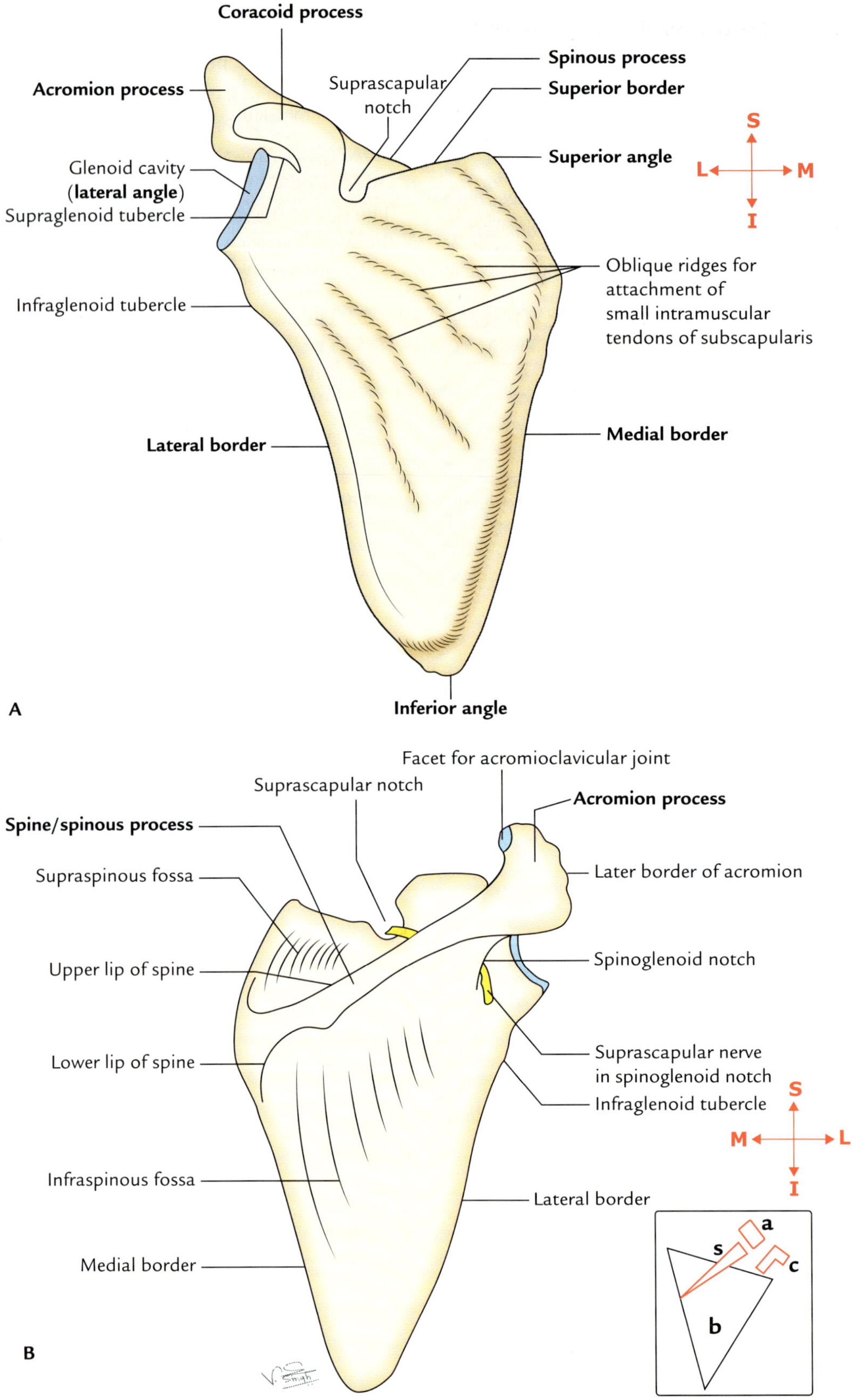

FIG. 2.6 ■ Right scapula. (**A**) Anterior aspect and (**B**) posterior aspect. Figure in the inset on the right side shows parts of scapula: b, body; s, spinous process; a, acromion process; c, coracoid process.

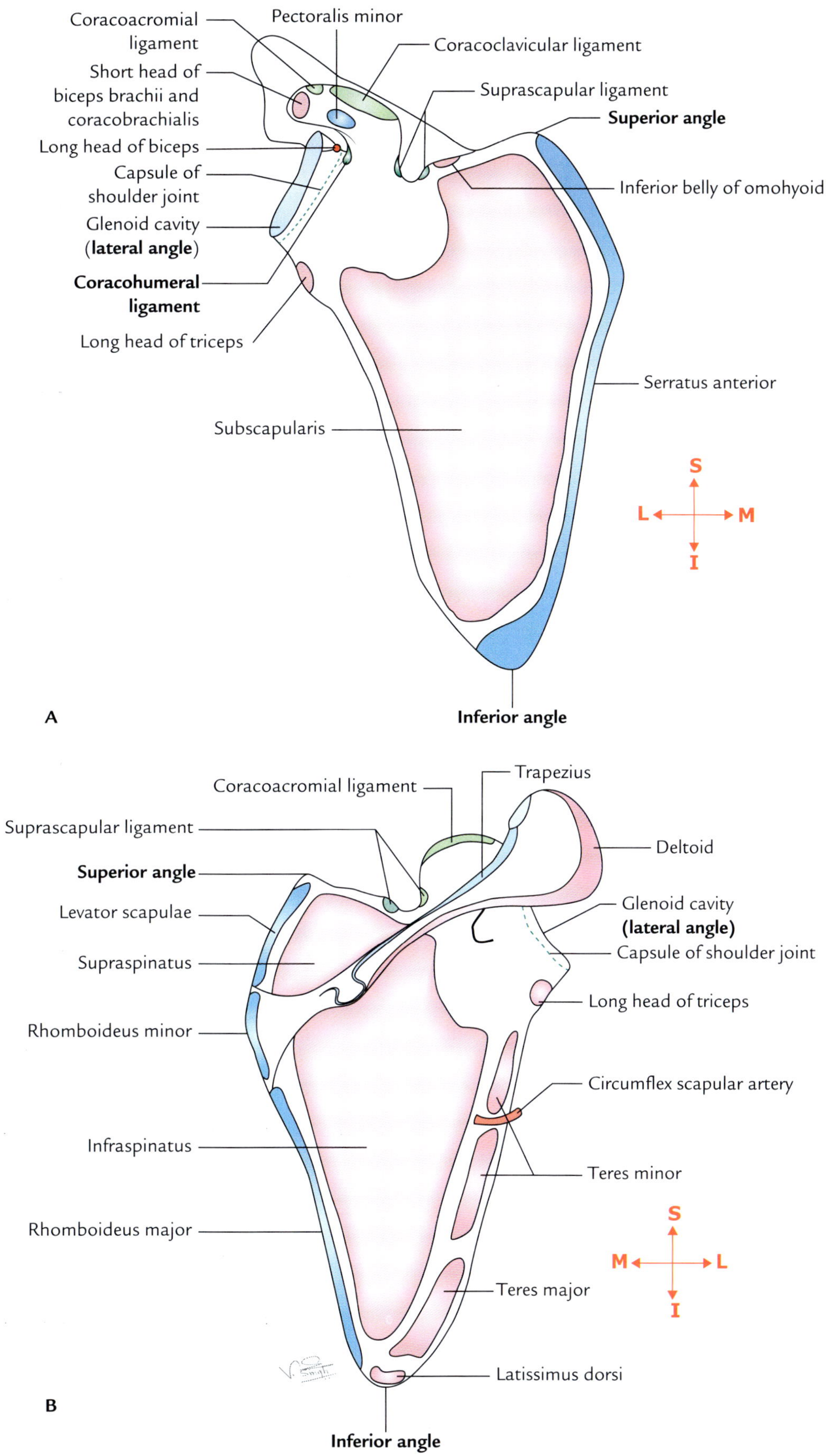

FIG. 2.7 ■ Right scapula showing attachments of the muscles and ligaments. (**A**) Costal surface, (**B**) dorsal surface, and *Continued*

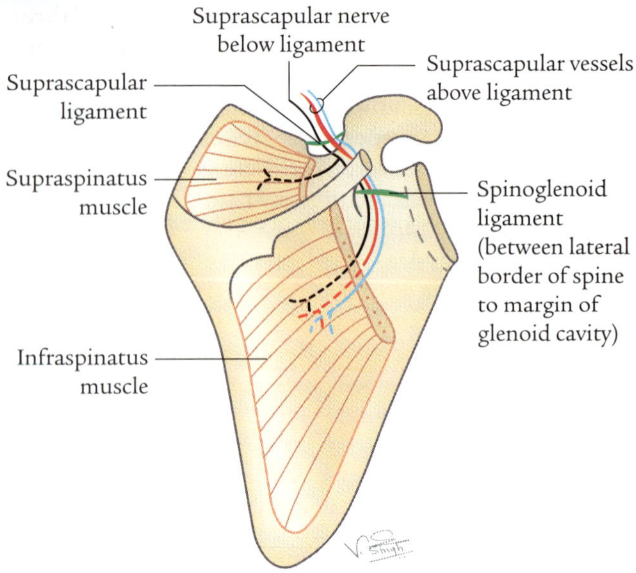

FIG. 2.7, cont'd ■ (**C**) dorsal surface of scapula showing spinoglenoid notch and structures passing through it.

Borders

Superior border:

1. The superior border is the shortest and extends between the superior and lateral angles.
2. The **suprascapular notch** is present on this border near the root of the coracoid process.
3. The suprascapular notch is converted into **suprascapular foramen** by the *superior transverse (suprascapular) ligament.*
4. The suprascapular artery passes above the ligament, and the suprascapular nerve passes below the ligament, through suprascapular foramen. *Mnemonic:* **Air** force flies above the **Navy**, that is **A:** artery is above and **N:** nerve is below the ligament.
5. The **inferior belly of the omohyoid** arises from the superior border near the suprascapular notch.

Lateral border:

1. The **lateral border** is the thickest border and extends from the inferior angle to the glenoid cavity.
2. The **infraglenoid tubercle** is present at its upper end, just below the glenoid cavity.
3. The **long head of the triceps** muscle arises from the infraglenoid tubercle.

N.B.

The lateral border of the scapula is thick because it acts as a fulcrum during the rotation of the scapula.

Medial border (vertebral border):

1. It extends from the superior angle to the inferior angle.
2. It is thin and angled at the root of the spine of the scapula.
3. The **serratus anterior** muscle is inserted on the costal surface of the medial border and the inferior angle.
4. The **levator scapulae muscle** is inserted on the dorsal aspect of the medial border from the superior angle to the root of spine.
5. The **rhomboideus minor muscle** is inserted on the dorsal aspect of the medial border opposite to the root of spine.
6. The **rhomboideus major muscle** is inserted on the dorsal aspect of the medial border from the root of spine to the inferior angle.

Angles

Inferior angle: It lies over the seventh rib or the seventh intercostal space.

Superior angle: It is at the junction of the superior and medial borders, and lies over the second rib.

Lateral angle (head of scapula):

1. It is truncated and bears a pear-shaped articular cavity called the **glenoid cavity** that articulates with the head of the humerus to form the *glenohumeral (shoulder) joint*.
2. A fibrocartilaginous rim, the **glenoid labrum** is attached to the margins of the glenoid cavity to deepen its concavity.
3. The **capsule of the shoulder joint** is attached to the margins of the glenoid cavity, proximal to the attachment of the glenoid labrum.
4. The **long head of the biceps brachii** arises from the supraglenoid tubercle. This origin is intracapsular.

Processes

Spinous process (spine of scapula):

1. It is a triangular shelf-like bony projection, attached to the dorsal surface of the scapula at the junction of its upper one-third and lower two-thirds.
2. It divides the dorsal surface of the scapula into two parts: upper supraspinous fossa and lower infraspinous fossa.
3. The spine has two surfaces—(a) superior and (b) inferior, and three borders—(a) anterior, (b) posterior, and (c) lateral.

Surfaces

(a) The *superior surface of spine* forms the lower boundary of the supraspinous fossa and gives origin to supraspinatus.

(b) The *inferior surface of spine* forms the upper limit of the infraspinous fossa and gives origin to infraspinatus.

Borders

(a) The *anterior border of spine* is attached to the dorsal surface of the scapula.

(b) The *lateral border of spine* bounds the **spinoglenoid notch** through which the suprascapular nerve and vessels pass from the supraspinous fossa to infraspinous fossa.

(c) The *posterior border of spine* is also called the **crest of spine**. Trapezius is inserted to the upper lip of the crest of spine, while the posterior fibres of the deltoid take origin from its lower lip.

Acromion process (acromion):

1. It projects forward almost at the right angle from the lateral end of spine and overhangs the glenoid cavity.
2. Its superior surface is subcutaneous.
3. It has a tip, two borders (medial and lateral), and two surfaces (superior and inferior).
4. The medial and lateral borders of the acromion continue with the upper and lower lips of the crest of the spine of scapula, respectively.
5. Its superior surface is rough and subcutaneous.
6. Its inferior surface is smooth and related to the **subacromial bursa**.
7. The medial border of the acromion provides insertion to the trapezius muscle. Near the tip, the medial border presents a circular facet that articulates with the lateral end of the clavicle to form the acromioclavicular joint.
8. The lateral border of the acromion gives origin to the intermediate fibres of the deltoid muscle.
9. The coracoacromial ligament is attached to the tip of the acromion.
10. The acromial angle is at the junction of the lateral border of the acromion and the lower border of the crest of the spine of scapula.

Coracoid process:

1. It arises from the upper part of the head of scapula and bent sharply so as to project forward and slightly laterally.
2. The coracoid process provides attachment to **three muscles**—short head of the biceps brachii, coracobrachialis, and pectoralis minor—and **three ligaments**—coracoacromial, coracoclavicular, and coracohumeral.
3. The *short head of biceps brachii* and *coracobrachialis* arise from its tip by a common tendon.
4. The *pectoralis minor* muscle is inserted on the medial border of the upper surface.
5. The *coracoacromial ligament* is attached to its lateral border.
6. The *conoid part of the coracoclavicular ligament* is attached to its knuckle.
7. The *trapezoid part of the coracoclavicular ligament* is attached to a ridge on its superior aspect between the pectoralis minor muscle and coracoacromial ligament.
8. The *coracohumeral ligament* is attached to its root adjacent to the glenoid cavity.

N.B.

- In living individuals, the tip of the coracoid process can be palpated 2.5 cm below the junction of the lateral one-fourth and the medial three-fourths of the clavicle.
- In reptiles, the coracoid process is a separate bone, but in humans, it is attached to the scapula and, thus, it represents *atavistic epiphysis*.

OSSIFICATION

The ossification of the scapula is membranocartilaginous. Body is formed by membranous ossification while other parts are formed by cartilaginous ossification. The scapula is ossified by **eight centres**—one primary and seven secondary (Fig. 2.8).

The *primary centre* appears in the body.

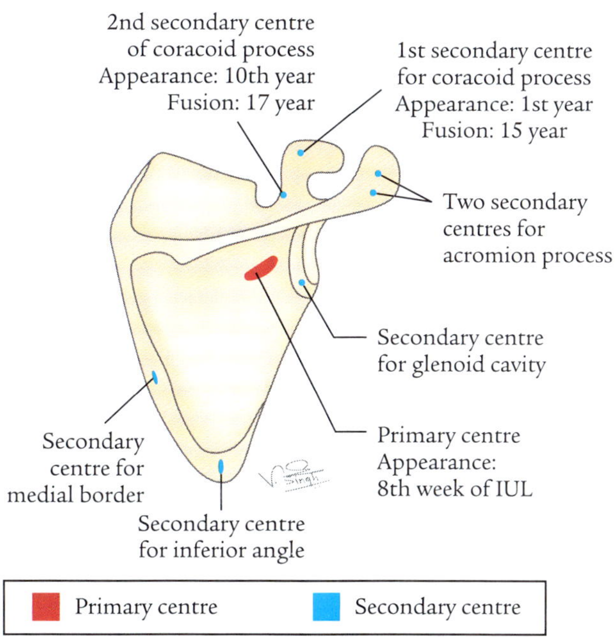

FIG. 2.8 Ossification of scapula.

The *secondary centres* appear as follows:

1. Two centres appear in the coracoid process – one in middle of process, and other in the root of process (subcoracoid centre).
2. Two centres appear in the acromion process.
3. One centre appears each in the (a) medial border, (b) inferior angle, and (c) in the lower part of the rim of the glenoid cavity.

The primary centre in the body appears near glenoid cavity during eighth week of IUL. The first secondary centre in the middle of coracoid process appear in the first year of postnatal life, and fuses at the age of 15 years. Second coracoid centre appears in the root of coracoid process during 10th year and fuses at the age of 17 years.

All other secondary centres appear at about puberty and fuse by the 20th year.

N.B.

The *first coracoid centre* represents the *precoracoid element* and the *second coracoid (subcoracoid) centre* represents the *coracoid proper* of the reptilian girdle.

CLINICAL CORRELATION

Sprengel's deformity of the scapula (congenital high scapula): The scapula develops in the neck region during IUL and then migrates downward to its adult position (i.e. upper part of the back of the chest). Failure of descent leads to *Sprengel's deformity of the scapula*.

HUMERUS

The humerus is the long bone of the arm. It is the longest and strongest bone of the upper limb, which extends from shoulder to the elbow.

PARTS

It consists of three parts: upper rounded end, lower flattened end, and long middle shaft (Fig. 2.9).

Upper End

The upper end presents the following five features:

1. Head
2. Neck
3. Greater tubercle
4. Lesser tubercle
5. Intertubercular sulcus

The head is smooth and rounded, and forms less than half of a sphere. It is directed medially backward and upward. It articulates with the glenoid cavity of the scapula to form the glenohumeral (shoulder) joint.

Lower End

The lower end presents the following seven features:

1. **Capitulum**, a lateral rounded convex projection.
2. **Trochlea**, a medial pulley-shaped structure.
3. **Radial fossa**, a small fossa above the capitulum.
4. **Coronoid fossa**, a small fossa above the trochlea.
5. **Medial epicondyle**, a prominent projection on the medial side.
6. **Lateral epicondyle**, a prominent projection on the lateral side but less than the medial epicondyle.
7. **Olecranon fossa**, a large, deep hollow on the posterior aspect above the trochlea.

Shaft

The shaft is a long part of bone extending between its upper and lower ends. It is cylindrical in the upper half and flattened anteroposteriorly in the lower half.

ANATOMICAL POSITION AND SIDE DETERMINATION

The side of the humerus can be determined by holding it vertically in such a way that:

1. The **rounded head** at the upper end faces medially, backward, and upward.
2. The lesser tubercle, greater tubercle, and vertical groove (intertubercular groove) at the upper end faces anteriorly.
3. The **olecranon fossa** on the lower flattened end faces posteriorly.

FEATURES AND ATTACHMENTS (FIG. 2.10)

Upper End Head

1. It is smooth, rounded, and forms one-third of a sphere.
2. It is covered by an articular hyaline cartilage, which is thicker in the centre and thinner at the periphery.

Neck

The humerus has three necks:

Anatomical neck:

1. It is constriction at the margins of the rounded head.
2. It provides attachment to the capsular ligament of the shoulder joint, except *superiorly* where the capsule is deficient, for the passage of the tendon of the long head of the biceps brachii, *medially* the capsule extends down from the anatomical neck to the shaft for about 1–2 cm.

Surgical neck:

1. It is short constriction in the upper end of the shaft below the greater and lesser tubercles/below the epiphyseal line.
2. It is related to the axillary nerve and posterior and anterior circumflex humeral vessels.
3. It is the most important feature of the proximal end of the humerus because it is weaker than the more proximal regions of the bone; hence, it is one of the sites where the humerus commonly fractures, leading to the damage of associated nerves and vessels.

Morphological neck:

1. It is the junction between diaphysis and epiphysis.
2. It is represented by an epiphyseal line in the adult bone.
3. It is a true junction of the head with the shaft.

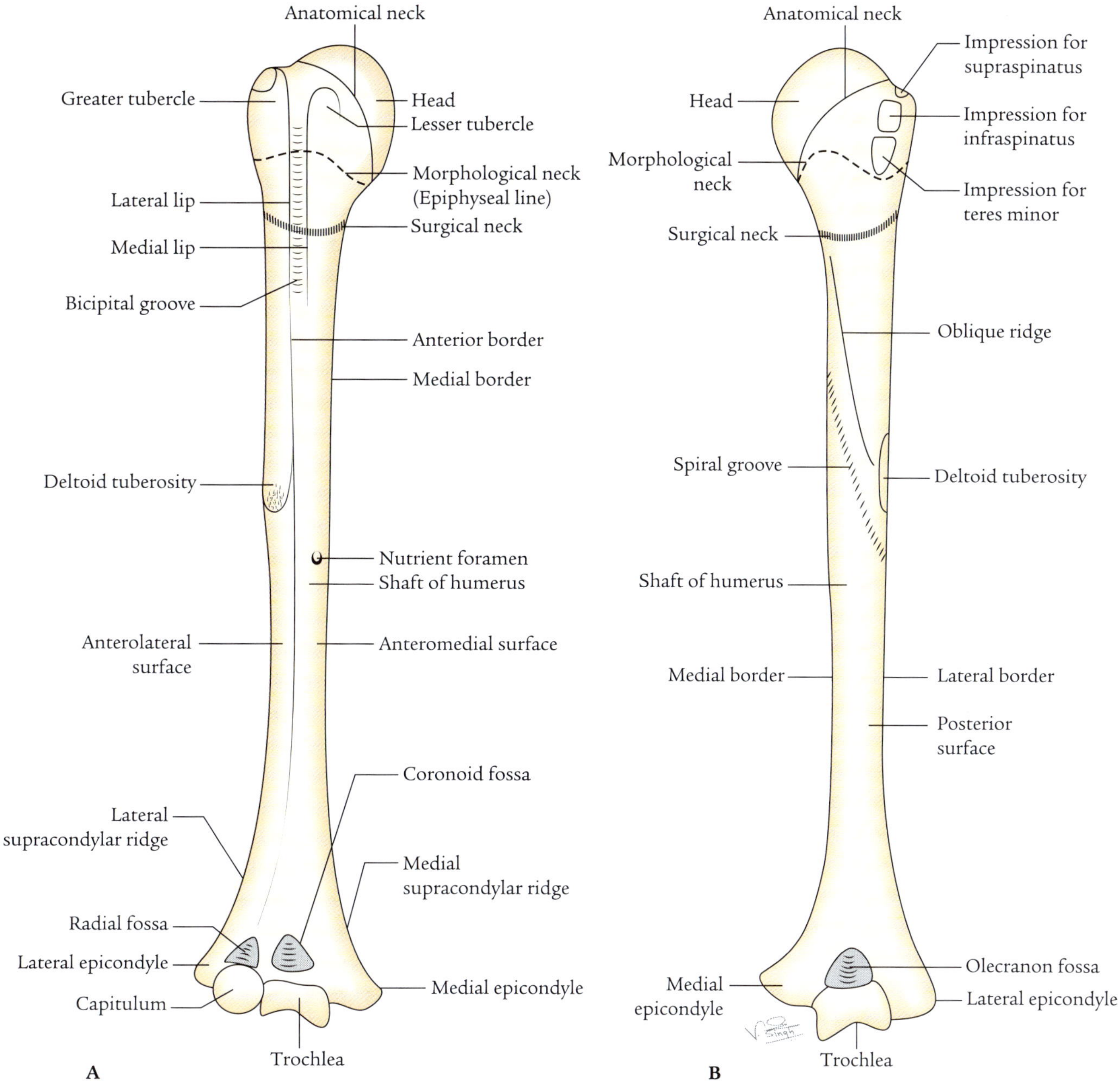

FIG. 2.9 ■ Right humerus. (**A**) Anterior view and (**B**) posterior view.

Greater Tubercle

1. It is the most lateral part of the proximal end of humerus.
2. Its posterosuperior aspect bears three flattened facet-like impressions: upper, middle, and lower, which provide attachment to *supraspinatus, infraspinatus*, and *teres minor muscles*, respectively.

Mnemonic: **SIT** (**s**upraspinatus, **i**nfraspinatus, **t**eres minor).

Lesser Tubercle

1. It is small elevation on the front of the upper end of the humerus, just above the surgical neck.
2. It provides attachment to the *subscapularis muscle*.

Intertubercular Sulcus/Bicipital Groove

1. It is a vertical groove between lesser and greater tubercles.
2. It contains (a) the long head of biceps, enclosed in the synovial sheath and (b) the ascending branch of the anterior circumflex humeral artery.
3. Three muscles are attached in the region of this groove:
   (a) Pectoralis major on the lateral lip of the groove.
   (b) Teres major on the medial lip of the groove.
   (c) Latissimus dorsi in the floor of the groove.

Mnemonic: Lady between **2** *Majors*. The **'L'** of lady stands for **l**atissimus dorsi and **'2 M'** stands for the pectoralis **m**ajor and teres **m**ajor.

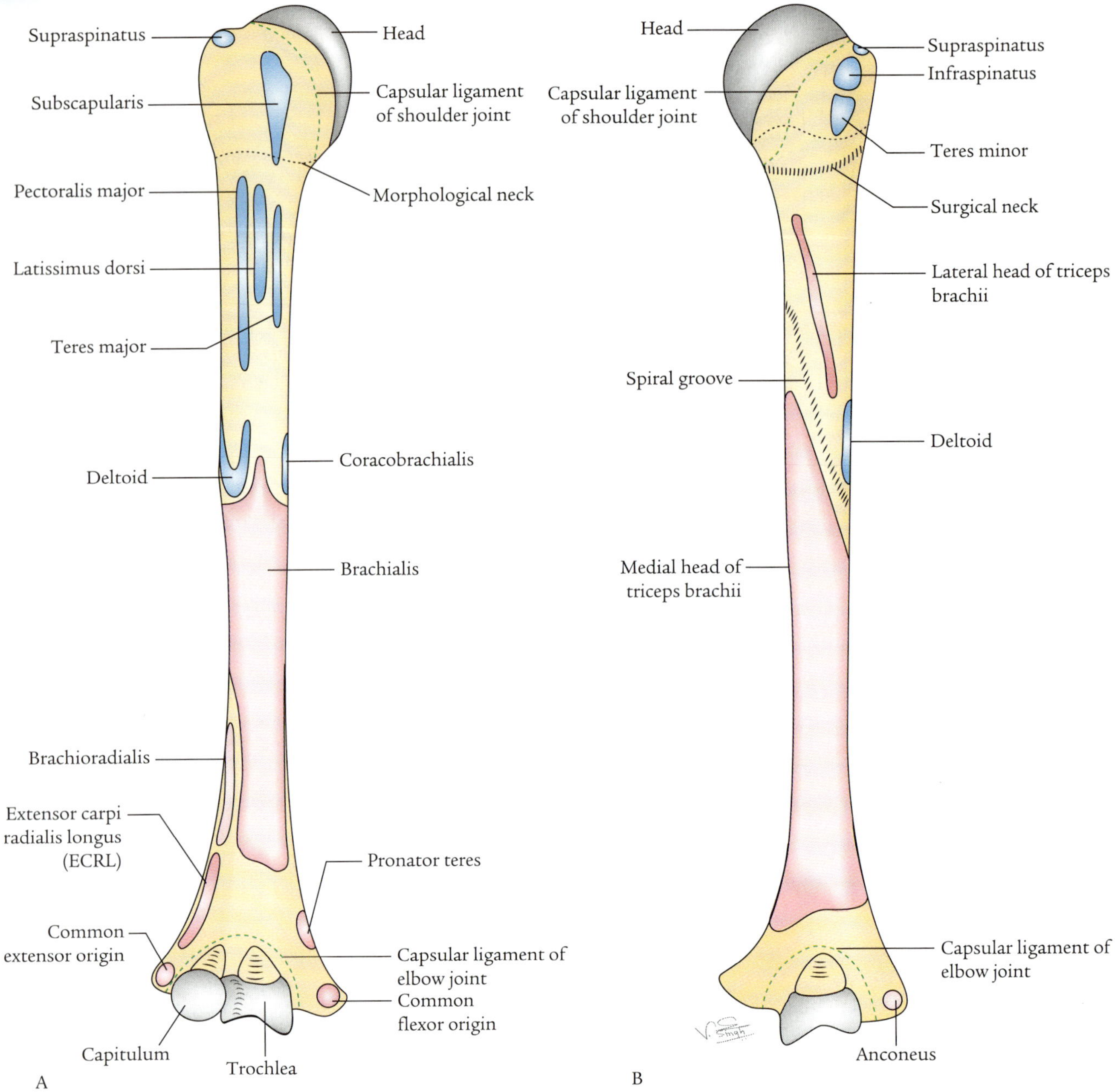

FIG. 2.10 ■ Right humerus showing attachments of the muscles and ligaments. (**A**) Anterior aspect and (**B**) posterior aspect.

Shaft

The upper part of the shaft is cylindrical and its lower part is triangular in cross section. It has three borders and three surfaces.

Borders

Anterior border: It starts from the lateral lip of the intertubercular sulcus and extends down to the anterior margin of the deltoid tuberosity and becomes smooth and rounded in the lower half, where it ends in the radial fossa.

Medial border:

1. It extends from the medial lip of the intertubercular sulcus down to the medial epicondyle. Its lower part is sharp and called the medial supracondylar ridge. This ridge provides attachment to the medial intermuscular septum.
2. A rough strip on the middle of this border provides insertion to the coracobrachialis muscle.
3. A narrow area above the medial epicondyle provides origin to the humeral head of the pronator teres.

Lateral border:

1. Its upper part is indistinct while its lower part is prominent where it forms the **lateral supracondylar ridge**. Above the lateral supracondylar ridge, it is ill defined but traceable to the posterior part of the greater tubercle.

2. About its middle, this border is crossed by the radial groove from behind.
3. The lower part of this border, lateral supracondylar ridge, provides attachment to the lateral intermuscular septum, brachioradialis and ext. carpi radialis longus.

Surfaces

Anterolateral surface:

1. It lies between the anterior and lateral borders.
2. A little above the middle, this surface presents a characteristic V-shaped tuberosity—the **deltoid tuberosity** which provides insertion to the deltoid muscle.

Anteromedial surface:

1. It lies between the anterior and medial borders.
2. The upper part of this surface forms the floor of the intertubercular sulcus.
3. About its middle and close to the medial border, it presents a nutrient foramen directed downward.

Posterior surface:

1. It lies between the medial and lateral borders.
2. In the upper one-third of this surface, there is an oblique ridge directed downward and laterally. This ridge provides origin to the lateral head of the triceps brachii.
3. Below and medial to the ridge is the radial/spiral groove, which lodges the radial nerve and profunda brachii vessels.
4. The entire posterior surface below the spiral groove provides origin to the medial head of the triceps brachii.

Lower End

1. It is flattened from before backward and expanded from side to side.
2. The capitulum (rounded convex projection laterally) articulates with the head of the radius.
3. The trochlea (pulley-shaped projection medially) articulates with the trochlear notch of the ulna.
4. The ulnar nerve is related to the posterior surface of the medial epicondyle.
5. The anterior surface of the medial epicondyle provides an area for the common flexor origin of the superficial flexors of the forearm.
6. The anterolateral part of the lateral epicondyle provides an area for the common extensor origin.
7. The posterior surface of the lateral epicondyle gives origin to the anconeus muscle.
8. The coronoid process of the ulna fits into the *coronoid fossa* (above the trochlea) during full flexion of the elbow.
9. The head of the radius fits into the *radial fossa* (above capitulum) during full flexion of the elbow.
10. The olecranon process of the ulna fits into the *olecranon fossa* (on posterior aspect above the trochlea) during full extension of the elbow.
11. The capsule of the elbow joint is attached above the coronoid and radial fossae anteriorly and above the olecranon fossa posteriorly.

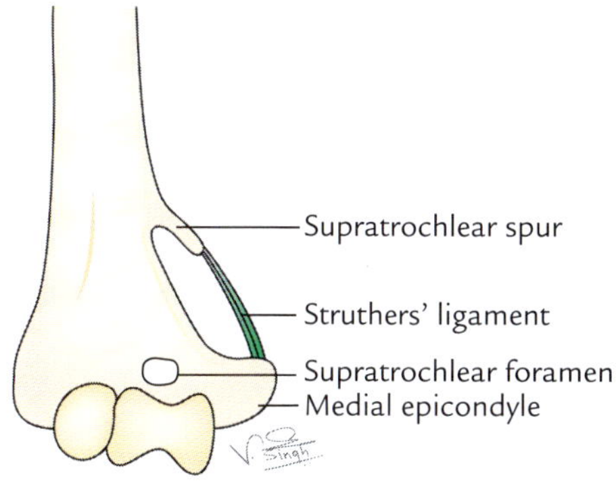

FIG. 2.11 Supratrochlear spur. (*Source:* Fig. 17.1, p. 154, *Anatomy for Excellence: Must Know Facts*, 2e, Vishram Singh. Copyright Elsevier, 2013. All rights reserved.)

N.B.

- *Supratrochlear process* (Fig. 2.11): It is a small hook-like bony process that may sometimes arise from the anteromedial surface, about 5 cm above the lower end of the humerus. A fibrous band called *Struthers' ligament* stretches from it to the medial epicondyle. In such cases, the brachial artery along with the median nerve deviates from their normal course and pass under the Struthers' ligament and may get compressed.
- Sometimes a bony bar separating the coronoid and olecranon fossae is perforated and forms '*supratrochlear foramen*'.
- *The angle of humeral torsion*: It is an angle formed by the superimposition of the long axis of the upper and lower articular surfaces of the humerus.

CLINICAL CORRELATION

- **Nerves directly related to the humerus:** The three nerves (axillary, radial, and ulnar) are closely related to the back of the humerus as follows (Fig. 2.12):
  (a) ***A***xillary nerve around the surgical neck.
  (b) ***R***adial nerve in the radial/spiral groove.
  (c) ***U***lnar nerve behind the medial epicondyle.

Mnemonic: **A**unty **R**eacts **U**nnecessarily.

Therefore, these nerves are often involved in the fracture of the humerus at the above sites:

- **Common sites of the fracture of the humerus:** These are (a) surgical neck, (b) midshaft, and (c) supracondylar region.
  (a) **Fracture surgical neck of humerus:** It is most frequently fractured site, of humerus, especially in elderly over 65 years of age due to osteoporosis.
  (b) **Midshaft fracture of humerus:** It occurs in 3% cases due to fall or high energy injuries, *viz.* motor vehicle collisions, etc. In older people, it occurs due to weakening of bone from osteoporosis.
  (c) **Supracondylar fracture of the humerus** (Fig. 2.13): It is caused by a fall on the outstretched hand and commonly occurs in the young age. Clinically, it presents as a backward displacement of the lower fragment with an unduly prominent elbow; however, the three bony points of the elbow (*viz. medial epicondyle, lateral epicondyle*, and *olecranon process*) still form the usual *equilateral triangle* because the olecranon process

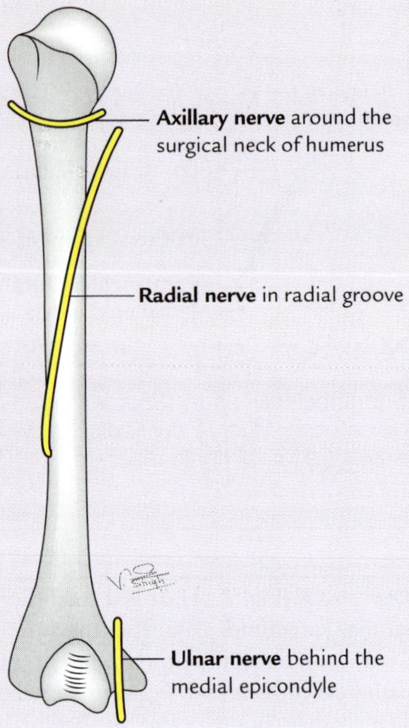

FIG. 2.12 ■ Three nerves closely related to the back of the humerus.

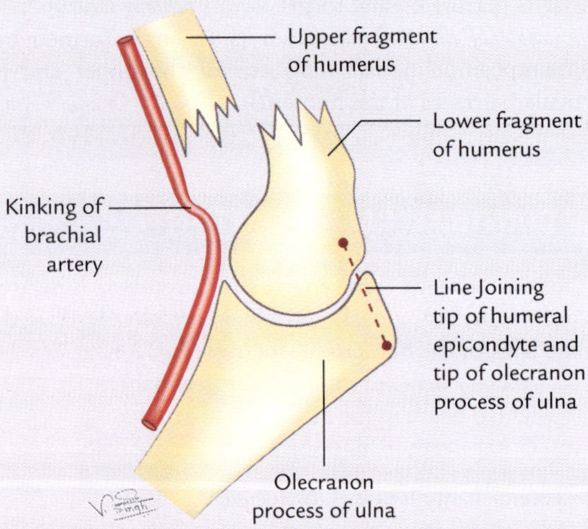

FIG. 2.13 ■ Supracondylar fracture of the humerus. (*Source:* Fig. 2.2(B): (C), p. 52, *Clinical and Surgical Anatomy*, Vishram Singh, 2e. Copyright Elsevier, 2007. All rights reserved.)

always moves with the lower fragment (for details see Fig. 10.9, p. 133). This fracture may cause injury to the median nerve and occlusion of brachial artery.

The injury to the brachial artery may cause **Volkmann's ischaemic contracture** and myositis ossificans. The occlusion of brachial artery causes ischaemia of anterior compartment of forearm, leading to increased pressure and swelling within it. This results in shortening of muscles (contracture) due to hypoxia.

Median nerve is most commonly involved in the supracondylar fracture of the humerus.

N.B.

Nonunion of the fracture of the humerus is common, if fracture occurs at the junction of its upper one-third and middle one-third due to poor blood supply.

OSSIFICATION

The humerus is formed by cartilaginous ossification by one primary and seven secondary centres. These are as follows:

1. One primary centre for the shaft.
2. Three secondary centres for the upper end.
3. Four secondary centres for the lower end.

The site of appearance, time of appearance, and time of fusion of these centres are given in Table 2.3.

CLINICAL CORRELATION

The separate centre for the medial epicondyle and its late union with the shaft may be mistaken for the *fracture of medial epicondyle of the humerus*.

RADIUS

There are two bones in the forearm, radius and ulna (Fig. 2.14). The **radius** is the lateral bone of the forearm and is homologous to the medial bone of the leg, the tibia.

The radius is relatively shorter than ulna, but it is larger and weight-bearing bone of the forearm. The

TABLE 2.3 **Ossification centres of the humerus**

Site of appearance	Time of appearance		Time of fusion
Mid shaft: One centre	8th week of IUL		
Upper end: Three centres			
• Head	1st year	Fuse together during 7th year to form one compound upper epiphysis	Joins with the shaft 20th year
• Greater tubercle	3rd year		
• Lesser tubercle	5th year		
Lower end: Four centres			
• Capitulum and lateral flange of trochlea	2nd year	Fuse together during 14th year to form large compound lower epiphysis	Joins with the shaft 16th–17th year
• Medial part of trochlea	10th year		
• Lateral epicondyle	12th year		
• Medial epicondyle (appears separately)	6th year (form a separate small lower epiphysis)		18th year

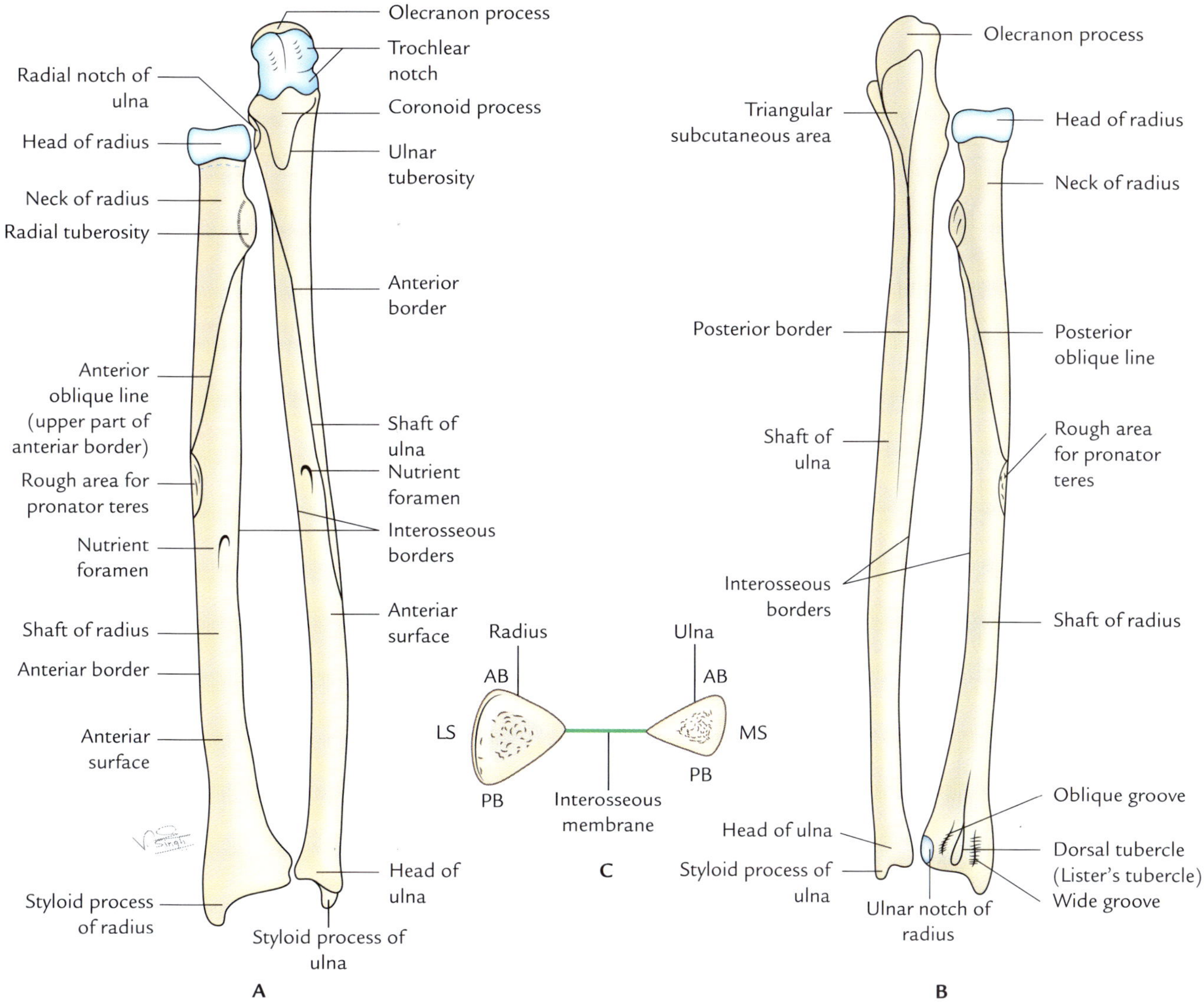

FIG. 2.14 Right radius and ulna. (**A**) Anterior view, (**B**) posterior view, and (**C**) transverse section through radius and ulna (anterior view) showing interosseous membrane, joining the interosseous borders of two bones (AB = anterior border, PB = posterior border, LS = lateral surface, MS = medial surface).

radius and ulna are joined together by a fibrous interosseous membrane (Fig. 10.13, page 134).

PARTS

The radius is a long bone and consists of three parts: upper end, shaft, and lower end (Fig. 2.14).

Upper End

The **upper end** presents the head, neck, and radial tuberosity. The head is disc shaped and articulates above with the capitulum of the humerus. The neck is constricted part below the head. The radial tuberosity is just below the medial part of the neck. It has smooth anterior part and rough posterior part.

Shaft

The **long shaft** extends between the upper and lower ends and presents a lateral convexity. It widens rapidly towards the distal end and is concave anteriorly in its distal part. Its sharpest interosseous border is located on the medial side.

Lower End

The **lower end** is the widest part and presents five surfaces. The lateral surface projects distally as the *styloid process*. The dorsal surface presents a palpable dorsal tubercle (*Lister's tubercle*), which is limited medially by an oblique groove.

ANATOMICAL POSITION AND SIDE DETERMINATION

The side of the radius can be determined by keeping the bone vertically in such a way that:

1. The **narrow disc-shaped end** (head) is directed upward.
2. The **sharpest border** (**interosseous border**) of the shaft is kept medially.
3. The **styloid process** at the lower end is directed laterally and prominent tubercle (*Lister's tubercle*) at the lower end faces dorsally.
4. The **convexity of the shaft** faces laterally, and the concave anterior surface of shaft faces anteriorly.

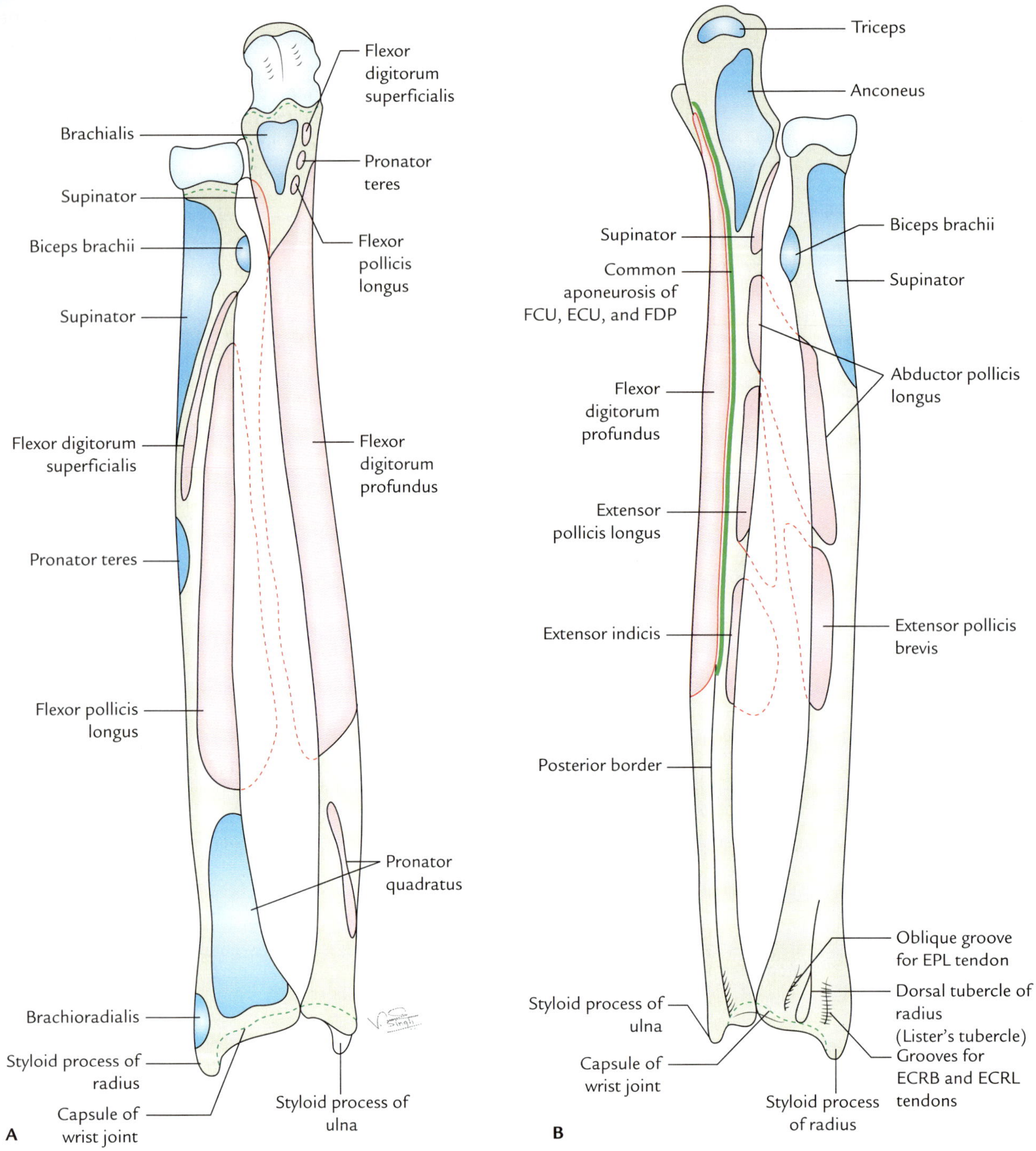

FIG. 2.15 ■ Radius and ulna of the right side showing attachments of the muscles and ligaments. (**A**) Anterior aspect, (**B**) posterior aspect (FCU = flexor carpi ulnaris, ECU = extensor carpi ulnaris, FDP = flexor digitorum profundus, EPL = extensor pollicis longus, ECRB = extensor carpi radialis brevis, ECRL = extensor carpi radialis longus).

FEATURES AND ATTACHMENTS (FIG. 2.15)

Upper End

Head

1. It is shaped like a disc and in living, it is covered with an articular hyaline cartilage.
2. It articulates superiorly with the capitulum to form *humeroradial articulation*.
3. The circumference of the head is smooth and articulates medially with the radial notch of the ulna, rest of it is encircled by the *annular ligament* (Fig. 2.15).

Neck

1. It is the constricted part just below the head and is embraced by the lower part of the annular ligament.
2. The **quadrate ligament** is attached to the medial side of the neck.

Radial Tuberosity

1. The biceps tendon is inserted to its rough, posterior part.
2. A small synovial bursa covers its smooth anterior part and separates it from the biceps tendon.

Shaft

The shaft has three borders and three surfaces.

Borders

Anterior border:

1. It starts below the anterolateral part of radial tuberosity and runs downward and laterally to the styloid process.
2. The upper part of this border is called the **anterior oblique line** and the lower part forms the sharp lateral border of the anterior surface.
3. Its anterior oblique line gives origin to the radial head of the flexor digitorum superficialis (FDS).

Posterior border:

1. It is well defined only in its middle third of the shaft.
2. Above it runs upward and medially to the radial tuberosity and forms the **posterior oblique line**.

Medial (interosseous) border:

1. It is the sharpest border.
2. It extends above up to radial tuberosity and below its lower part forms the posterior margin of the small triangular area on the medial side of the lower end of the bone.
3. *Interosseous membrane* is attached to its lower three-fourths.

Surfaces

Anterior surface:

1. It is concave and lies between the anterior and interosseous borders.
2. *Flexor pollicis longus* originates from its upper two-fourths.
3. *Pronator quadratus* is inserted on its lower one-fourth.
4. *Nutrient foramen* is present a little above the middle of this surface in its upper part. The nutrient canal is directed upward. The nutrient artery for the radius is a branch from the anterior interosseous artery.

Posterior surface:

1. It lies between the interosseous and posterior borders.
2. *Abductor pollicis longus* (APL) arises from the middle one-third of this surface.
3. *Extensor pollicis brevis* (EPB) arises from the lower part of this surface.

Lateral surface:

1. It lies between the anterior and posterior borders.
2. *Supinator* is inserted on the widened upper one-third of this surface.
3. *Pronator teres* is inserted on the rough area in the most convex middle part of this surface.

Lower End

The lower end is the widest part of the bone and has five surfaces.

Anterior surface: The anterior surface presents a thick ridge that provides attachment to the *palmar radiocarpal ligament of the wrist joint*.

Posterior surface: The posterior surface presents the *dorsal tubercle of the Lister* lateral to the groove for the tendon of the *extensor pollicis longus*. It also presents grooves for other extensor tendons.

The groove lateral to the Lister's tubercle is traversed by the tendons of *extensor carpi radialis longus* (ECRL) and *extensor carpi radialis brevis* (ECRB). Through the groove medial to groove for *extensor pollicis longus* passes the tendons of the extensor digitorum and extensor indicis.

Medial surface: The medial surface presents the ulnar notch for articulation with the head of the ulna. The *articular disc of the inferior radioulnar joint* is attached to the lower margin of the ulnar notch.

Lateral surface: The lateral surface projects downward as the styloid process and is related to the tendons of the *APL* and *EPB*. The *brachioradialis* is inserted to the base of the styloid process and the radial collateral ligament of the wrist joint is attached to the tip of the styloid process.

Inferior surface: The inferior (distal) surface presents a lateral triangular area for articulation with the scaphoid and a medial quadrangular area for articulation with the lateral part of the lunate.

CLINICAL CORRELATION

Common fractures of radius: The radius is a **weight-bearing bone** of the forearm; hence, fractures of the radius are more common than those of the ulna.

(a) **Fracture head of radius**, characteristically occur due to falling on an outstretched hand. The radial head is forced into capitulum to fracture.

(b) **In the fracture shaft of the radius**, with the *fracture line* below the insertion of biceps and above the insertion of the pronator teres, the upper fragment is supinated by the supinator and the lower fragment is pronated by the pronator teres.

(c) **Colles' fracture (fracture distal end of radius)**: It is most common fracture of radius (90%). It occurs due to fall on outstretched and in older people due to osteoporosis. The distal fragment is displaced backward and upward, and wrist shows a typical *dinner fork deformity*. The reverse of Colles' fracture is called ***Smith's fracture*** (Fig. 2.16). It occurs due to fall on back of hand and distal fragment is displaced anteriorly.

N.B.

- The radius is most commonly fractured bone in people over 50 years of age. It is often fractured as a result of a fall on outstretched hand.
- **Fracture of the styloid process** of the radius is termed ***'Chauffeur's fracture'***.

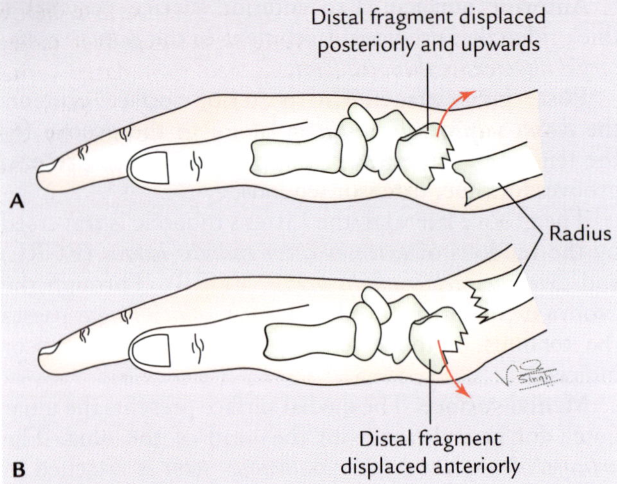

FIG. 2.16 ■ Fracture at the distal end of the radius. (**A**) Colles' fracture with dinner-fork deformity and (**B**) Smith's fracture. (*Source:* Fig. 2.3, p. 53, *Clinical and Surgical Anatomy,* 2e, Vishram Singh. Copyright, 2007. All rights reserved.)

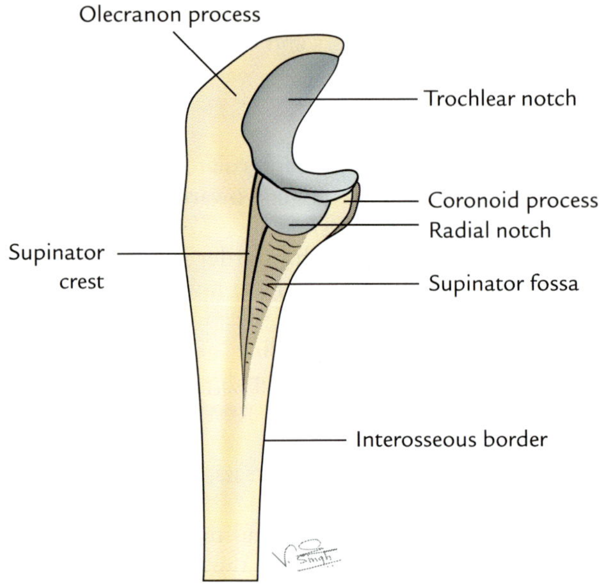

FIG. 2.17 ■ Lateral view of the upper end of ulna.

OSSIFICATION

The radius ossifies from the following three centres:

1. One primary centre appears in the mid-shaft during the eighth week of IUL.
2. Two secondary centres, one for each end:
   (a) Centre for the lower end appears at the age of the first year.
   (b) Centre for the upper end appears during the fifth year.
3. The upper epiphysis fuses at the age of 12 years.
4. The lower epiphysis fuses at the age of 20 years.

CLINICAL CORRELATION

Madelung deformity: It is a congenital anomaly of the radius that presents the following clinical features:

- The anterior bowing of the distal end of the radius due to an abnormal growth of distal epiphysis.
- It occurs between 10 and 14 years of age.
- There is premature disappearance of the distal epiphyseal line.
- There may be subluxation or dislocation of the distal end of the ulna due to the defective development of distal radial epiphysis.

ULNA

The **ulna** is the medial bone of the forearm and is homologous to the lateral bone of the leg—the *fibula*. It is thin and longer than radius and lies parallel to it. The ulna acts as stabilizing bone with radius pivoting to produce movements. It has upper expanded end which possesses a large notch and narrow rounded lower end. So this bone looks like a ***pipe wrench***.

PARTS

The ulna is a long bone and consists of three parts: **upper end**, **lower end**, and **shaft** (Fig. 2.14).

Upper End

The **upper end** is expanded and hook like with the concavity of the hook facing forward. The concavity of the upper end (**trochlear notch**) lies between the large olecranon process above and the small coronoid process below.

Shaft

The **long shaft** extends between the upper and lower ends. Its thickness diminishes progressively from above downward throughout its length. *The lateral border (interosseous border) is sharp crest like.*

Lower End

The **lower end** is slightly rounded and called *head*. A small bony projection from distal end of ulna is called *styloid process*. The styloid process is posteromedial to the head.

N.B.

The ulna looks like a **pipe wrench** with the olecranon process resembling the *upper jaw*, the coronoid process, the *lower jaw*, and the trochlear notch the *mouth of the wrench* (Fig. 2.17).

ANATOMICAL POSITION AND SIDE DETERMINATION

The side of the ulna can be determined by keeping the bone vertically in such a way that:

1. The **broad hook-like end** is directed upward.
2. The **sharp crest-like interosseous border** of the shaft is directed laterally.
3. The **concavity** of the hook-like upper end and the coronoid process are facing forward.

FEATURES AND ATTACHMENTS (FIG. 2.15)

Upper End

The **upper end** has two processes: coronoid and olecranon, and two notches: trochlear and radial.

Processes

Olecranon process: It projects upward from the upper end and bends forward at its summit like a beak. It has the following five surfaces:

1. Upper surface:
   (a) Its rough posterior two-thirds provides insertion to the *triceps brachii*.
   (b) *Capsular ligament of the elbow joint* is attached anteriorly near its margins.
   (c) A synovial bursa lies between the tendon of the triceps and capsular ligament.
2. **Anterior surface:** It is smooth and forms the upper part of the trochlear notch.
3. Posterior surface:
   (a) It forms a subcutaneous triangular area.
   (b) A synovial bursa (**subcutaneous olecranon bursa**) lies between the posterior surface and skin.
4. **Medial surface:** Its upper part provides attachments to three structures: (a) ulnar head of the flexor carpi ulnaris (origin), (b) posterior, and (c) oblique bands of the ulnar collateral ligament.
5. **Lateral surface:** It is smooth and continues as a posterior surface of the shaft.

Coronoid process: It is bracket-like projection from the front of the upper end of the ulna below the olecranon process. It has four surfaces: superior, anterior, medial, and lateral.

1. **Superior surface:** It is smooth and forms the lower part of the trochlear notch.
2. **Anterior surface:** It is triangular in shape.
   (a) Its lower corner presents an ulnar tuberosity.
   (b) Brachialis muscle is inserted to the whole of the anterior surface, including ulnar tuberosity.
   (c) The medial margin of the anterior surface is sharp and has a tubercle at its upper end called the **sublime tubercle**. The medial margin provides attachment to the following structures from proximal to distal:
      (i) Anterior band of the ulnar collateral ligament.
      (ii) Oblique band of the ulnar collateral ligament.
      (iii) Humeroulnar head of the flexor digitorum superficialis.
      (iv) Ulnar head of the pronator teres.
      (v) Ulnar head of the flexor pollicis longus.
3. **Medial surface:** It gives origin to the flexor digitorum profundus.
4. **Lateral surface** (Fig. 2.17)**:** The upper part of this surface possesses a radial notch for articulation with the head of the radius.
   (a) The *annular ligament* is attached to the anterior and posterior margins of the radial notch.
   (b) The lower part of the lateral surface below the radial notch has a depressed area called **supinator fossa** that accommodates radial tuberosity during supination and pronation.
   (c) **Supinator fossa** is bounded behind by the supinator crest. Supinator crest and adjoining part of the supinator fossa give origin to the *supinator muscle*.

Notches (Articular Surfaces)

Trochlear notch

1. It is C-shaped (semilunar) and articulates with the trochlea of the humerus.
2. It has a nonarticular strip at the junction of its olecranon and coronoid parts.
3. Its superior, medial, and anterior margins provide attachment to the capsule of the elbow joint.

Radial notch

It articulates with the head of the radius to form the superior radioulnar joint.

Shaft

It has three borders—lateral, anterior, and posterior—and three surfaces—anterior, medial, and posterior.

Borders

Lateral (interosseous) border:

1. It is sharpest and is continuous above with the supinator crest.
2. It is ill defined below.
3. *Interosseous membrane* is attached to this border except for its upper part.

Anterior border:

1. It extends from the medial side of the ulnar tuberosity to the base of the styloid process.
2. It is thick and round.
3. It upper three-fourths gives origin to the *flexor digitorum profundus*.

Posterior border:

1. It starts from the apex of the triangular subcutaneous area on the back of the olecranon process and descends to the styloid process.
2. It is subcutaneous throughout and hence can be palpated along its entire length.
3. It provides attachment to three muscles by a common aponeurosis. The muscles are as follows:
   (a) Flexor digitorum profundus.
   (b) Flexor carpi ulnaris.
   (c) Extensor carpi ulnaris.

Surfaces

Anterior surface:

1. It lies between the anterior and interosseous borders.
2. The *flexor digitorum profundus* arises from its upper three-fourths.
3. The *pronator quadratus* arises from an oblique ridge on the lower one-fourth of this surface.

4. The *nutrient foramen* is located a little above the middle of this surface and is directed upward.

Medial surface:

1. It lies between the anterior and posterior borders.
2. The *flexor digitorum profundus* arises from the upper two-thirds of this surface.

Posterior surface:

1. It lies between the posterior and interosseous borders.
2. It is divided into the smaller upper part and large lower part by an oblique line, which starts at the junction of the upper and middle third of the posterior border and runs towards the posterior edge of the radial notch.
3. Area above the oblique line receives insertion of the *anconeus muscle.*
4. Area below the oblique line is divided into the larger medial and smaller lateral parts by a faint vertical line. The lateral part provides attachment to three muscles from proximal to distal as follows:
   (a) APL in the upper one-fourth.
   (b) Extensor pollicis longus in the middle one-fourth.
   (c) Extensor indicis in the next one-fourth.
   (d) The distal one-fourth is devoid of any attachments.

Lower End

The lower end consists of the head and styloid process.

Head

1. It presents a convex articular surface on its lateral side for articulation with the ulnar notch of the radius to form the **inferior radioulnar joint**.
2. Its inferior surface is smooth and separated from the wrist joint by an articular disc of the inferior **radioulnar joint**.

Styloid Process

1. It projects downward from the posteromedial aspect of the head of the ulna.
2. Its tip provides attachment to the medial collateral ligament of the wrist joint.
3. The apex of the triangular articular disc is attached to the depression between the head and base of the styloid process.
4. The **tendon of the extensor carpi ulnaris** lies in the groove between the back of the head of the ulna and styloid process.

N.B.

The styloid process is subcutaneous and may be felt in living individual slightly distal to the head when the forearm is pronated.

CLINICAL CORRELATION

- Ulna stabilizes the forearm by gripping the lower end of the humerus by its trochlear notch and provides foundation for the radius to produce supination and pronation at the superior and inferior radioulnar joints.
- Fracture of olecranon process is fairly common and occurs due to direct fall on the point of elbow.
- The fracture of the upper third of the shaft of the ulna with the dislocation of the radial head at the superior radioulnar joint is called ***Monteggia fracture dislocation.***
- The fracture of the lower third of the shaft of the radius associated with the dislocation of the inferior radioulnar joint is called ***Galeazzi fracture dislocation.***
- A fracture of the shaft of the ulna due to direct injury when a night watchman reflexly raises his forearm to ward off the blow of the stick is termed *night-stick fracture*.

OSSIFICATION

The ulna ossifies from the three main centres: one primary centre for the shaft and two secondary centres, one each for the lower end and the upper end.

Primary centre:

It appears in the midshaft during the *eighth week of IUL.*

Secondary centres:

Upper end

Appearance: 9 years on top of the olecranon process.
Fusion: 16–17 years.

Lower end (middle of the head)

Appearance: 6 years.
Fusion: 18–20 years.

N.B.

Distal part of the olecranon process is formed as an upward extension of the shaft.

The differences between radius and ulna are given in Table 2.4.

TABLE 2.4 Differences between radius and ulna—the two bones of forearm

Radius	Ulna
• Present on lateral side of the forearm	• Present on medial side of the forearm
• Larger but slightly shorter	• Smaller but slightly longer
• Weight-bearing bone	• Stabilizing bone
• Upper end is smaller and discoidal in shape	• Upper end is large, expanded and possesses a notch
• Lower end is larger and expanded	• Lower end is smaller and rounded
• Upper end is called head	• Lower end is called head

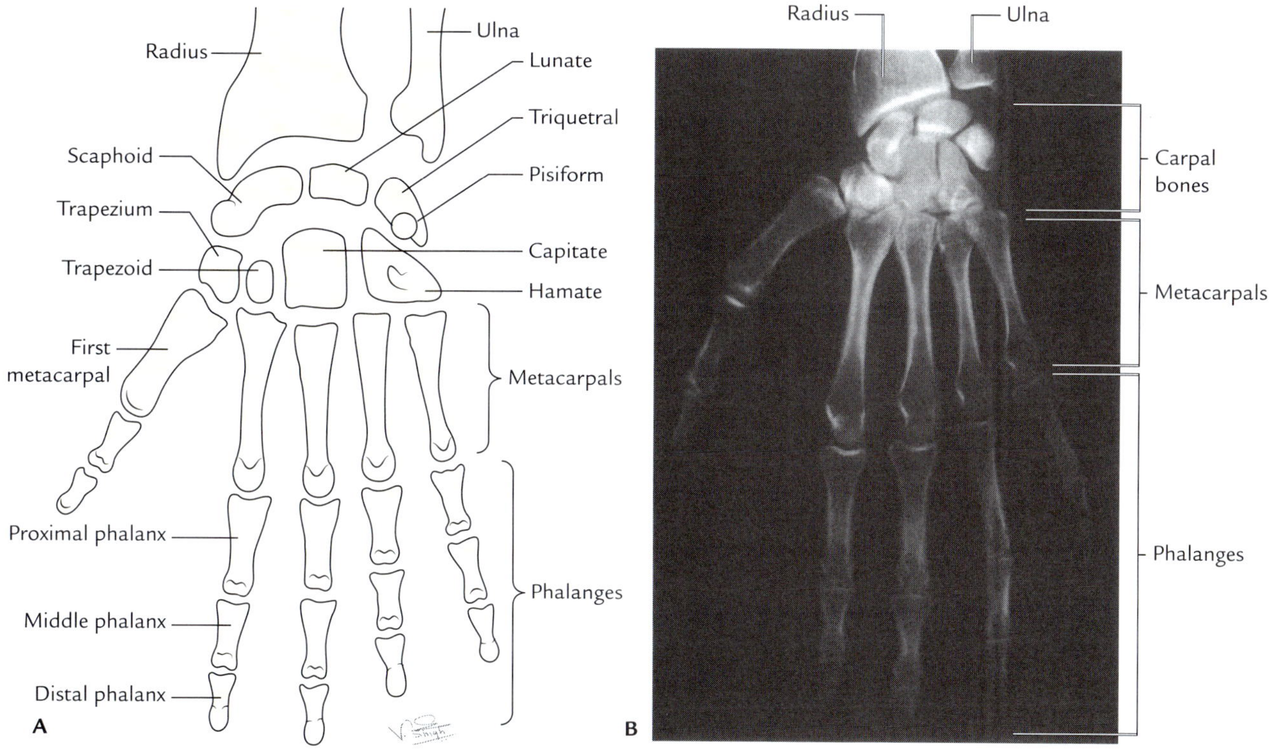

FIG. 2.18 ■ Bones in the articulated hand. **AN 8.5** (**A**) Schematic diagram and (**B**) as seen in radiographs. **AN 13.5** (*Source:* Fig. 7.91B, p. 710, *Gray's Anatomy for Students,* Richard L Drake, Wayne Vogl, Adam WM Mitchell.

CARPAL BONES **AN 8.5, AN 13.5**

The carpus (Greek: Karpos = wrist) consists of the eight carpal bones (Fig. 2.18), which are arranged in two rows: proximal and distal. Each row consists of four bones.

The **proximal row** of carpal bones consists of the following bones from the lateral to medial side:

1. **S**caphoid
2. **L**unate
3. **T**riquetral
4. **P**isiform

The **distal row** of carpal bones consists of the following bones from the lateral to medial side:

1. **T**rapezium
2. **T**rapezoid
3. **C**apitate
4. **H**amate

Mnemonic: **S**he **L**ooks **T**oo **P**retty. **T**ry **T**o **C**atch **H**er.

IDENTIFICATION OF INDIVIDUAL CARPAL BONES

The individual carpal bones can be identified by looking at their shape and few other features. These are given in Table 2.5.

N.B.

Morphology: Carpus of primitive tetrapods consists of three bones in the proximal row, five bones in the distal row, and an '*Os centrale*' between the two rows.

The pisiform bone is usually regarded as a sesamoid bone developed in the tendon of flexor carpi ulnaris, but some authorities regard it as a displaced '*Os centrale*'.

TABLE 2.5 **Identification of the carpal bones**

Carpal bone	Identifying features
1. Scaphoid	– Boat shaped – Has constriction (neck) – Has tubercle on the distal part of its palmar surface
2. Lunate	Half-moon shaped/crescentic
3. Triquetral	– Pyramidal in shape – Oval facet on the distal part of its palmar surface for articulation with pisiform
4. Pisiform	– Pea shaped/pea like – Oval facet on the proximal part of its dorsal surface
5. Trapezium	– Quadrilateral in shape – Has groove and crest (tubercle) on its palmar surface
6. Trapezoid	– Small shoe shaped – Smallest bone of second row
7. Capitate	– Largest carpal bone – Has rounded head on its proximal surface
8. Hamate	– Wedge shaped – Hook-like process projects from the distal part of its palmar surface

CLINICAL CORRELATION **AN 8.6**

- **Scaphoid fracture (Figs. 2.19 and 2.20):** Fracture of the scaphoid is the *most common fracture of carpus* (60%–70%) and usually occurs due to fall on the outstretched hand. Fracture occurs at the narrow waist of the scaphoid.

Clinically, it presents as tenderness in the anatomical snuff-box. Blood vessels mostly enter the scaphoid through its both ends. But in 10%–15% cases, all the blood vessels supplying the proximal segment enter it through its distal pole. Under this condition, when the waist of the scaphoid is fractured, the proximal segment is deprived of blood supply and may undergo **avascular necrosis** (Fig. 2.20).

N.B.

Fracture scaphoid is often misdiagnosed as **sprained wrist**.

- **Dislocation of lunate:** Lunate is the most commonly dislocated bone of carpus. It occurs due to fall on acutely dorsiflexed hand. If it undergoes necrosis due to lack of blood supply it causes **Kienböck's disease**.

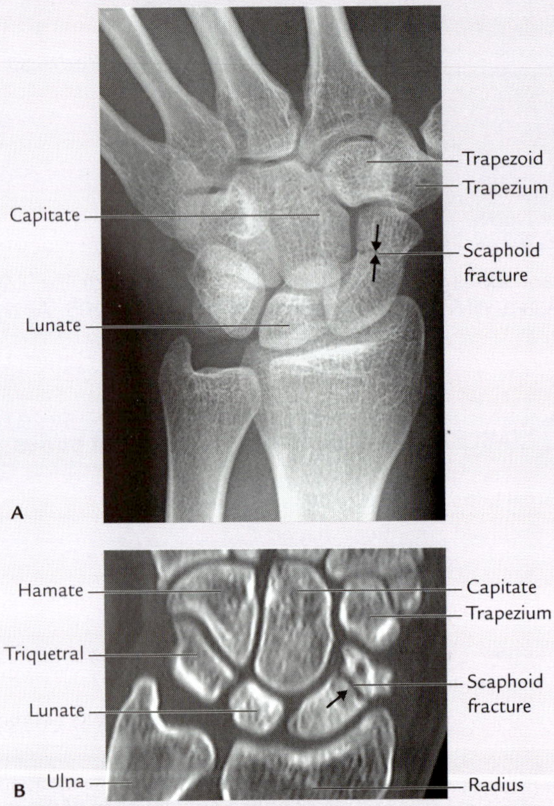

FIG. 2.19 ■ Fracture of scaphoid bone (arrow). (**A**) In the radiograph of the hand (AP view) and (**B**) CT scan of the wrist. (*Source:* Fig. 5.6, p. 131, *Integrated Anatomy,* David J.A. Heylings, Roy A.J. Spence, Barry E. Kelly. Copyright Elsevier Limited, 2007. All rights reserved.)

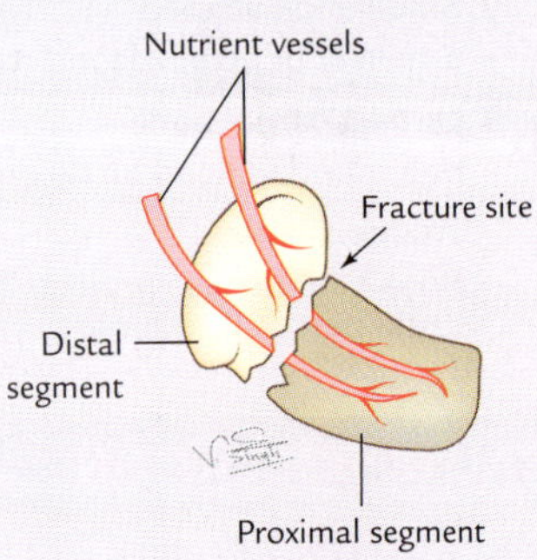

FIG. 2.20 ■ Fracture of scaphoid bone showing avascular necrosis of proximal segment.

OSSIFICATION

The carpal bones are cartilaginous at birth. Each carpal bone ossifies by one centre and all these centres appear after birth.

The centres appear as follows:

Bone	Time of appearance
Capitate	Second month
Hamate	End of the third month
Triquetral	Third year
Lunate Scaphoid Trapezium Trapezoid	Fourth year in females and fifth year in males
Pisiform	12th year in males, 9th to 11th year in females

The spiral sequence of the ossification of the carpal bones and approximate ages in years is given in Fig. 2.21.

N.B.

The capitate is the first bone to ossify and pisiform is the last bone to ossify.

Peculiarities of pisiform bone:
- Is sesamoid bone in tendon of FCU.
- Is smallest carpal bone.
- Is pea shaped.
- Is last carpal bone to ossify.

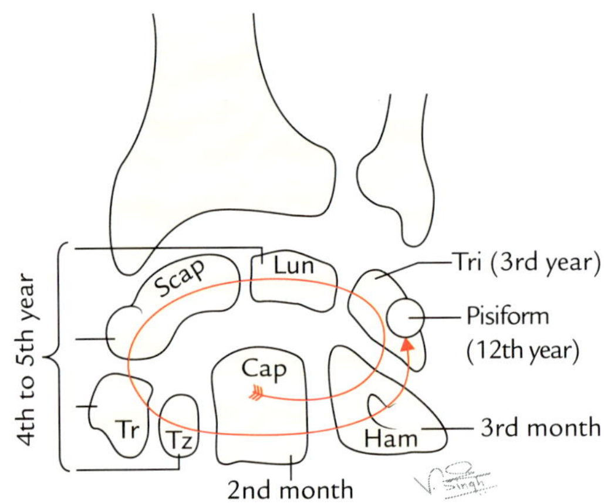

FIG. 2.21 ■ Ossification of the carpal bones (Scap = scaphoid, Lun = lunate, Tri = triquetral, Tr = trapezium, Tz = trapezoid, Cap = capitate, Ham = hamate).

CLINICAL CORRELATION

The knowledge of ossification of carpal bones is important in determining the bone age of the child.

The pisiform bone was palpated in earlier days in some parts of India to see the level of maturity in girls, before sending them to in-laws house.

METACARPAL BONES

The metacarpus consists of five metacarpal bones. They are conventionally numbered 1–5 from the lateral (radial) to medial (ulnar) side.

PARTS

Each metacarpal is a miniature long bone and consists of three parts: (a) head, (b) shaft, and (c) base.

Head

The **head** is at the distal end and rounded.

Shaft

The **shaft** extends between the head and base. It is concave on the palmar aspect and on sides. Its dorsal surface presents a triangular area in its distal part.

Base

The **base** is the proximal end and expanded.

PECULIARITIES OF THE FIRST METACARPAL

1. It is the shortest and stoutest metacarpal.
2. It is rotated medially through 90° so that its dorsal surface faces laterally.
3. Its base possesses a concavo-convex (saddle-shaped) articular surface for articulation with trapezium.
4. The head is less convex and broader than other metacarpals.
5. The sesamoid bones glide on the radial and ulnar corners of the palmar aspect of head and produces impressions of gliding.
6. Its base does not articulate with any other metacarpal.
7. It has epiphysis at its proximal end unlike other metacarpals, which have epiphysis at their distal end.

FUNCTIONAL SIGNIFICANCE OF METACARPUS

The metacarpals also form arches of hand which allows fingertips and thumb to be brought together to make a fist. For details, see page 166.

OSSIFICATION

Each metacarpal bone ossifies by two centres: one primary centre for the shaft and one secondary centre for the head.

N.B.

The secondary centre of the first metacarpal bone appears at its base.

The time of appearance of the centres and their fusion is given in the box below:

Centre	Time of appearance	Fusion
Primary centre for shaft	Ninth week of IUL	
Secondary centre for the head of the second, third, fourth, and fifth metacarpals	2 years	16 years
Secondary centre for the base for the first metacarpal	2 years	18 years

CLINICAL CORRELATION AN 8.6

- **Bennet's fracture:** It is an oblique fracture of the base of the anterior part of the first metacarpal on ulnar side. It is intraarticular and may be associated with subluxation or dislocation of metacarpal. Thumb cannot be opposed and fist cannot be made. It is most common fracture of thumb (Fig. 2.22).
- **Boxer's fracture** (Fig. 2.23): It is the fracture of the neck of metacarpal and most commonly involves the neck of the fifth metacarpal.

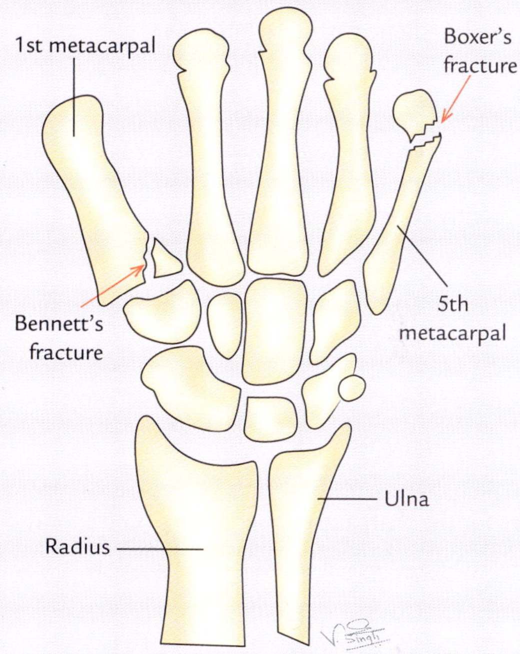

FIG. 2.22 Bennett's and boxer's fractures.

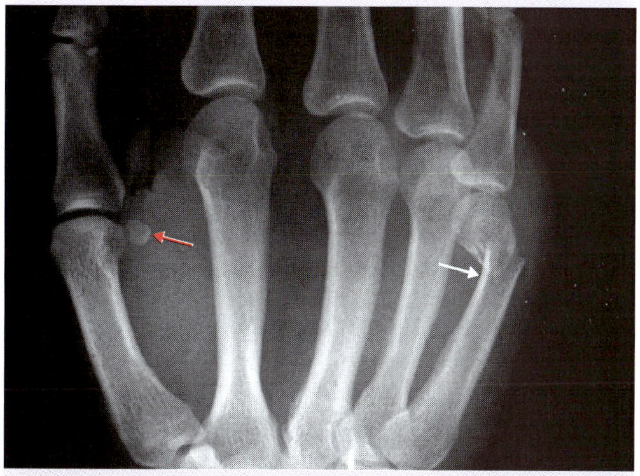

FIG. 2.23 An X-ray of the hand showing boxer's fracture—neck of the fifth metacarpal (arrow). Red arrow shows sesamoid bone in relation to the first metacarpal. (*Source:* Fig. 5.8, p. 131, *Integrated Anatomy*, David J.A. Heylings, Roy A.J. Spence, Barry E. Kelly. Copyright Elsevier Limited, 2007.)

PHALANGES

There are 14 phalanges in each hand: two in the thumb and three in each finger.

PARTS AND FEATURES

Each phalanx is a short long bone and has three parts: (a) base (proximal end), (b) head (distal end), and (c) shaft (extending between the two ends).

Base

1. The bases of proximal phalanges have a concave oval facet for articulation with the heads of metacarpals.
2. The bases of middle and distal phalanges possess pulley-shaped articular surfaces.

Shaft

1. The shaft tapers towards the head.
2. The dorsal surface is convex from side to side.
3. The palmar surface is flat from side to side but gently concave in the long axis.

Head

1. The heads of the proximal and middle phalanges are pulley shaped.
2. The heads of distal phalanges are nonarticular and have rough horseshoe-shaped tuberosity.

OSSIFICATION

Each phalanx ossifies by the two centres: one primary centre for the shaft and one secondary centre for the base.

Their time of appearance is as follows:

Primary Centres

For proximal phalanx: 10th week of IUL.
For middle phalanx: 12th week of IUL.
For distal phalanx: 8th week of IUL.

Secondary Centres

Appearance: 2 years.
Fusion: 16 years.

CLINICAL CORRELATION

Distal phalanx fracture: Distal phalanx of middle finger is most commonly fractured, usually due to crush injury. Clinically it presents as painful and swollen fingertip.

An *undisplaced fracture of the phalanx* can be treated satisfactorily by strapping the fractured finger with the neighbouring finger.

This is called as '**buddy finger splint**'.

N.B.

Sesamoid bones:

The ***sesamoid bones in the region of the hand*** are found on the following sites:

(a) Sesamoid bone in the distal part of tendon of the flexor carpi ulnaris called pisiform.
(b) Two sesamoid bones on the palmar surface of the head of the first metacarpal.
(c) Sesamoid bone in the capsule of the interphalangeal (IP) joint of the thumb (in 75% cases).
(d) Sesamoid bone on the ulnar side of the capsule of the MCP joint of the little finger (in 75% cases).

Sesamoid bones act as pulleys providing a smooth surface for tendons to slide over to transmit muscular forces efficiently.

The sesamoid bones related to the head of the first metacarpal bones are generally noticed in the X-ray of the hand (Fig. 2.23, red arrow).

Golden Facts to Remember

• Most commonly fractured bone in the body	Clavicle
• Most important feature of the proximal end of the humerus	Surgical neck
• Commonest site of the fracture clavicle	Junction of its lateral one-third and medial two-thirds
• Strongest ligament of the upper limb	Coracoclavicular ligament
• Thickest border of the scapula	Lateral border
• Commonest fracture of the humerus	Supracondylar/ supraepicondylar fracture
• Most commonly injured nerve in supracondylar fracture of the humerus	Median nerve
• Most common site of the fracture of radius	Fracture of distal end of radius 2.5 cm proximal to the wrist (Colles' fracture)
• Wrist bones (bones of carpus)	Eight carpal bones
• Most commonly fractured carpal bone	Scaphoid
• Most commonly dislocated carpal bone	Lunate
• Largest carpal bone	Capitate
• First carpal bone to ossify	Capitate
• Shortest and stoutest metacarpal	First metacarpal
• Most common fracture of thumb	Bennet's fracture
• Most common fracture of little finger	Boxer's fracture
• Longest metacarpal	Third metacarpal
• All metacarpals have epiphysis at their distal end (i.e. head) except	First metacarpal, which has epiphysis at its proximal end (i.e. base)

CLINICAL CASE STUDY

A 55-year-old individual sustained a severe blow on his right flexed elbow. He developed pain and swelling in the elbow region. He was taken to an orthopaedic surgeon who on examination found that the three bony points (olecranon, medial epicondyle, and lateral epicondyle) in the elbow region were forming an equilateral triangle. He suspected a fracture and advised the X-ray of the elbow region. The X-ray revealed the **supraepicondylar/supracondylar fracture of the humerus**.

QUESTIONS

1. What are the three common sites of the fracture of the shaft of the humerus? Name the nerves related to these sites.
2. Why the triangular relation of three bony points is not disturbed in the supracondylar fracture of the humerus?
3. Which is the most commonly injured nerve in the supracondylar fracture of the humerus?
4. On clinical examination, how will you differentiate the supracondylar fracture of the humerus from the posterior dislocation of the elbow?

ANSWERS

1. *Sites:* (a) surgical neck, (b) midshaft, and (c) supracondylar. *Nerves:* (a) axillary nerve, (b) radial nerve, and (c) median nerve.
2. In the flexed elbow, the three bony points of the elbow (olecranon, medial, and lateral epicondyles) form an **equilateral triangle/isosceles triangle**. It is not disturbed in supracondylar fracture because the line of fracture lies above these points.
3. Median nerve.
4. In the supracondylar fracture of the humerus, the triangular relationship of three bony points in the elbow region is not disturbed (*vide supra*), but in the posterior dislocation of the elbow, it is disturbed because the olecranon shifts posterosuperiorly.

CHAPTER 3

Pectoral Region

SPECIFIC LEARNING OBJECTIVES

After studying this chapter, the student should be able to:

- Identify and demonstrate the surface landmarks in the pectoral region. AN 13.6
- Describe the development of breast. AN 9.3
- Describe the location, extent, deep relations, structure, age changes, blood supply, lymphatic drainage, microanatomy and applied anatomy of breast. AN 9.2
- Give the origin, insertion, nerve supply, and actions of pectoralis major and pectoralis minor muscles. AN 9.1
- Give the anatomical basis of: (a) spread of cancer breast, (b) winging of scapula, (c) free mobility of normal breast, and (d) Krukenberg's tumour.
- Enumerate: (a) structures piercing clavipectoral fascia and (b) structures lying deep to mammary gland.
- Describe the attachments of serratus anterior muscle with action. AN 10.11

The pectoral region is the upper part of anterior region of the thorax (chest). The important structures present in this region are:

1. Muscles that connect the upper limb with the anterolateral chest wall.
2. Breasts (mammary glands) that secrete milk (in female).

SURFACE LANDMARKS AN 13.6

The following landmarks can be felt on the surface of the body in this region (Fig. 3.1):

1. **Clavicle:** Being subcutaneous in location, it is palpable along its whole length at the junction of the root of the neck and front of the chest.
2. **Suprasternal notch (jugular notch):** It is a palpable notch at the upper border of manubrium sterni between the medial ends of two clavicles.
3. **Sternal angle (angle of Louis):** It is felt as a transverse ridge about 5 cm below the suprasternal notch. It marks the junction of manubrium and the body of the sternum. On either side, the costal cartilage of second rib articulates with the sternum at this level. *The sternal angle, thus, serves as a useful landmark to identify the second rib and subsequently helps in counting down the other ribs.*
4. **Infraclavicular fossa:** It is a triangular depression below the junction of middle and lateral third of the clavicle.
5. **Coracoid process:** The tip of the coracoid process is felt in the infraclavicular fossa, 2.5 cm below the clavicle.
6. **Acromion process:** A bony process felt at the top of shoulder.
7. **Nipple:** It is the most important surface feature of the pectoral region. Its position varies considerably in the female. But in the male, it usually lies in the fourth intercostal space just medial to the midclavicular line.

LINES OF ORIENTATION (Fig. 15.1, page 193)

The following lines are often used to describe the surface features on the anterior chest wall:

1. **Midsternal line:** It runs vertically downward in the median plane on the front of the sternum.
2. **Midclavicular line:** It runs vertically downward from the midpoint of the clavicle to the midinguinal point.
3. **Anterior axillary line:** It runs vertically downward from the anterior axillary fold.
4. **Midaxillary line:** It runs vertically downward from a point located midway between the anterior and posterior axillary folds.
5. **Posterior axillary line:** It runs vertically downward from the posterior axillary fold.

CUTANEOUS INNERVATION

The skin of the pectoral region is supplied by the following cutaneous nerves (Fig. 3.2):

1. The skin above the horizontal line drawn at the level of the sternal angle is supplied by the supraclavicular nerves (C3 and C4).
2. The skin below this horizontal line is supplied by the anterior and lateral cutaneous branches of the second to sixth intercostal nerves (T2–T6).

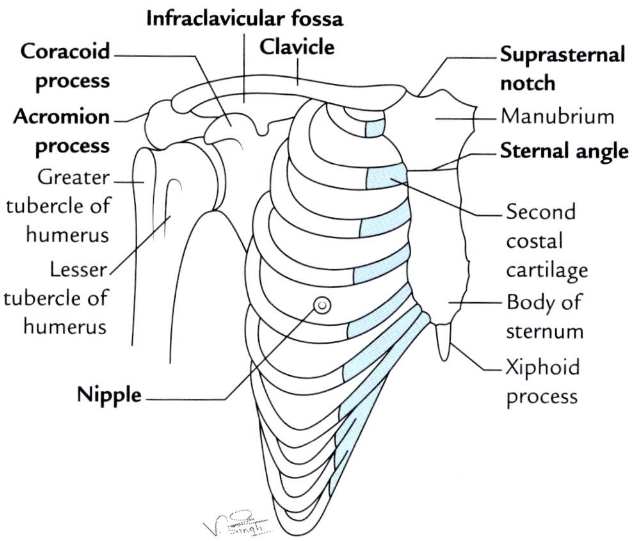

FIG. 3.1 ■ Skeletal framework and surface landmarks of the pectoral region.

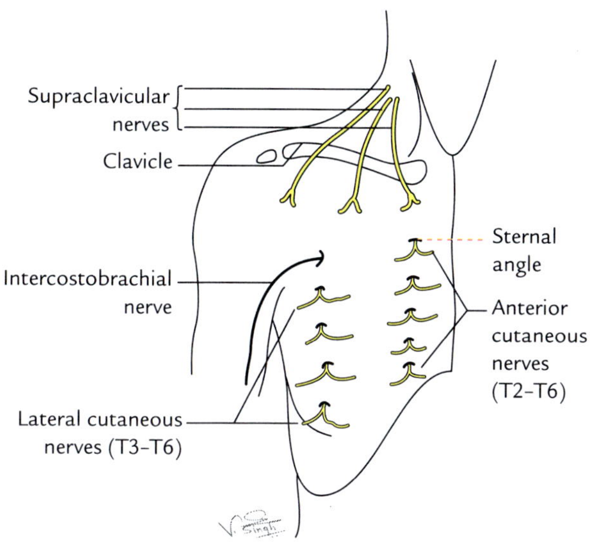

FIG. 3.2 ■ Cutaneous nerves of the pectoral region.

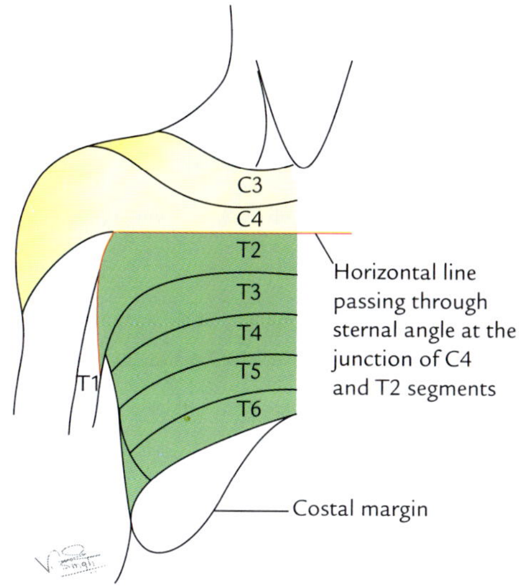

FIG. 3.3 ■ Dermatomes in the pectoral region.

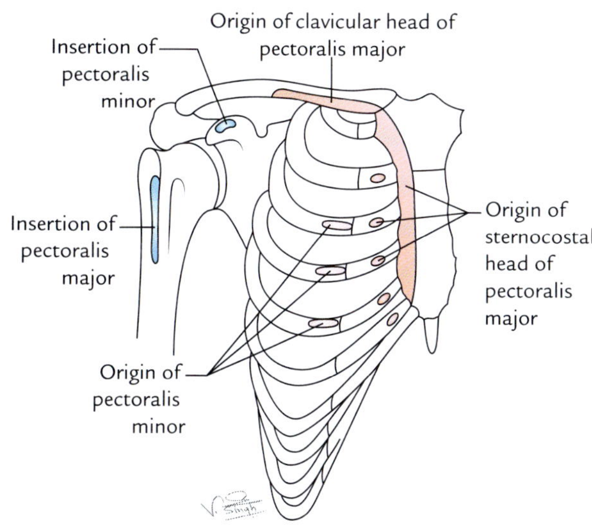

FIG. 3.4 ■ Bony attachments of the pectoralis major and minor muscles.

DERMATOMES

A dermatome is an area of skin supplied by a single spinal nerve. The pectoral regions supplied by C3 to C4 and T2 to T6 spinal nerves hence has seven dermatomes (Fig. 3.3).

N.B.

The area supplied by the C4 spinal segment meets directly to the area supplied by the T2 spinal segment at a horizontal line passing through sternal angle (Fig. 3.3). This is because the nerves derived from intervening C5 to T1 spinal segments form *brachial plexus* to supply the upper limb.

MUSCLES **AN 9.1, AN 13.7**

The muscles of the pectoral region are:

1. Pectoralis major
2. Pectoralis minor
3. Subclavius
4. Serratus anterior*

PECTORALIS MAJOR

It is the largest muscle of the pectoral region (Figs. 3.4 and 3.5).

Origin

Pectoralis major muscle is a thin, fan-shaped muscle and arises by two heads, *viz.*

1. Small clavicular head
2. Large sternocostal head

Clavicular head: It arises from the medial half of the anterior aspect of the clavicle.

Sternocostal head: It arises from the (a) lateral half of the anterior surface of the sternum, up to sixth costal cartilage,

*The serratus anterior is a thin muscular sheet overlying the lateral aspect of chest wall, hence; it is not a muscle of pectoral region but grouped with pectoral muscles for convenience of study and surgical significance.

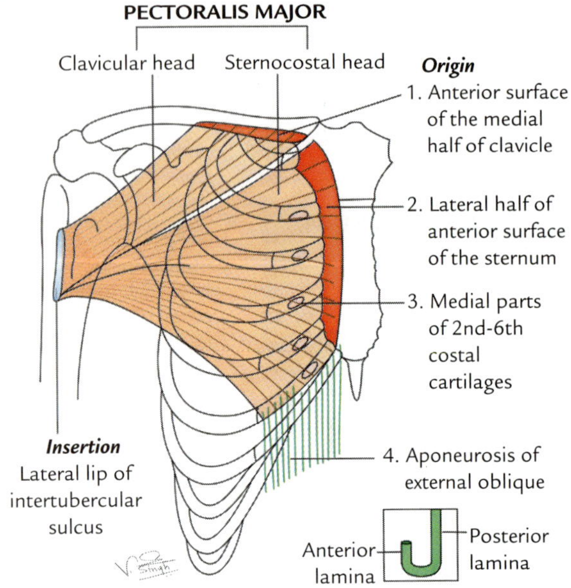

FIG. 3.5 ■ Origin and insertion of the pectoralis major muscle. Figure in the inset shows bilaminar tendon of insertion.

(b) medial parts of second to sixth costal cartilages, and (c) aponeurosis of the external oblique muscle of the abdomen.

Insertion

Pectoralis major is inserted by a U-shaped (bilaminar) tendon on to the lateral lip of the bicipital groove. The **anterior lamina** of the tendon is formed by the clavicular fibres, while the posterior lamina is formed by sternocostal and aponeurotic fibres. The two laminae are continuous with each other inferiorly. The anterior lamina is thick and short as compared to the posterior lamina that is thin and long (Fig. 3.5, inset).

The lower sternal and abdominal aponeurotic fibres in their course to insertion are twisted around the lower border of the same muscle in such a way that fibres, which are lowest are inserted highest.

This twisting of these fibres forms the rounded anterior axillary fold.

Nerve Supply

Nerve supply is by lateral (C5–C7) and medial pectoral (C8 and T1) nerves.

N.B.

- The *pectoralis major* and *pectoralis minor muscles* are the only muscles of the upper limb, which are *supplied by all five spinal segments that form the brachial plexus*.
- Occasionally, a vertical sheet of muscle fibres extending from the root of the neck to the upper part of the abdomen passes superficial to the medial part of the pectoralis major. It is termed ***rectus sternalis/sternalis muscle***.

Actions

- When acting as a whole (i.e. when two heads acting together) it causes adduction and medial rotation of humerus against resistance.
- The *clavicular head* flexes the arm against resistance, whereas the *sternocostal head* adducts the arm against resistance.

Clinical Testing

AN 13.7

- On lifting a heavy rod, the clavicular head becomes prominent and when one attempts to depress the rod, the sternocostal head becomes prominent.
- On pressing the fists against each other whole muscle becomes prominent.

CLINICAL CORRELATION

Congenital anomaly of the pectoralis major: Occasionally, a part of the pectoralis major, usually the sternocostal part, is absent at birth in children with **Poland syndrome.** This causes weakness in adduction and medial rotation of the arm.

PECTORALIS MINOR

It is the small triangular muscle that lies deep to the pectoralis major muscle (Figs. 3.4 and 3.6).

Origin

It arises from the third, fourth, and fifth ribs, near their costal cartilages.

Insertion

It is inserted by a short, thick tendon into the medial border and upper surface of the coracoid process of the scapula.

Nerve Supply

Nerve supply is by medial and lateral pectoral nerves.

Actions

1. Assists the serratus anterior in drawing the scapula forward (*protraction*) for punching action.
2. Depresses the point of shoulder.
3. Acts as an accessory muscle of respiration, during forced inspiration.

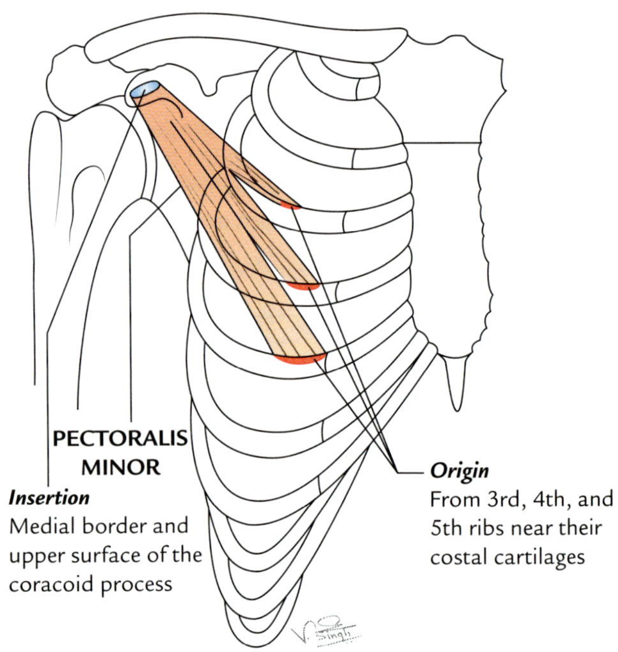

FIG. 3.6 ■ Origin and insertion of the pectoralis minor muscle.

N.B.

- The **pectoralis minor** is considered as the '**key muscle**' of axilla because it crosses in front of the axillary artery and, thus, used to divide this artery into three parts.
- The origin of the pectoralis minor is variable. It may be prefixed (i.e. arises from the second to fifth ribs) or postfixed (i.e. arises from the fourth to sixth ribs).
- Rarely some fibres of the pectoralis minor separate and pass from the first rib to the coracoid process to constitute what is called the *pectoralis minimus muscle*.

SUBCLAVIUS

It is the small-rounded muscle that lies horizontally inferior to the clavicle (Fig. 3.7).

Origin

It arises from the first rib at the costochondral junction.

Insertion

Subclavius is inserted into the subclavian groove on the inferior surface (middle-third) of the clavicle.

Nerve Supply

It is by nerve to subclavius, which arises from the upper trunk of the brachial plexus.

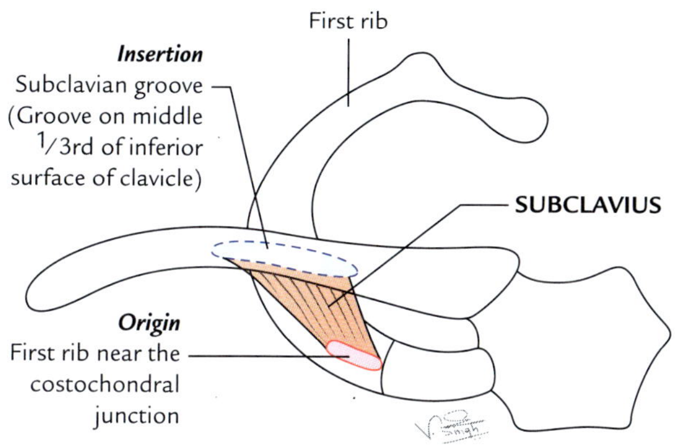

FIG. 3.7 ■ Origin and insertion of the subclavius muscle.

Actions

The subclavius stabilizes the clavicle by pulling it inferiorly and medially, during movement at the shoulder joint.

CLINICAL CORRELATION

The **subclavian vessels and divisions of the brachial plexus** pass behind the middle one-third of the shaft of the clavicle separated from it only by a small **subclavius muscle** that provides protection to these structures. The fractures of the clavicle are common. Rarely subclavian vessels are torn by fragments of the fractured clavicle that may lead even to death. For example, this was a *cause of death of Sir Robert Peel, the prime minister of U.K. during 1834–1835 and 1841–1846 following a fall from the back of a horse.*

SERRATUS ANTERIOR

AN 10.11

The serratus anterior (Fig. 3.8) is a broad sheet of muscle that clothes the side wall of upper thorax. *Thus, strictly speaking, it is not a muscle of the pectoral region. But, for convenience, it is described with the muscles of the pectoral region.*

Origin

It arises by a series of eight digitations from upper eight ribs. The first digitation arises from the first and second ribs, whereas all other digitations arise from their corresponding ribs.

N.B.

Lower four digitations (i.e. fifth to eighth) interdigitate with those of external oblique muscle.

Insertion

It is inserted into the costal surface of the scapula along its medial border. (The **first digitation** is inserted into the superior angle, **next two digitations** into the medial border, and the **lower five digitations** into the inferior angle of the scapula.)

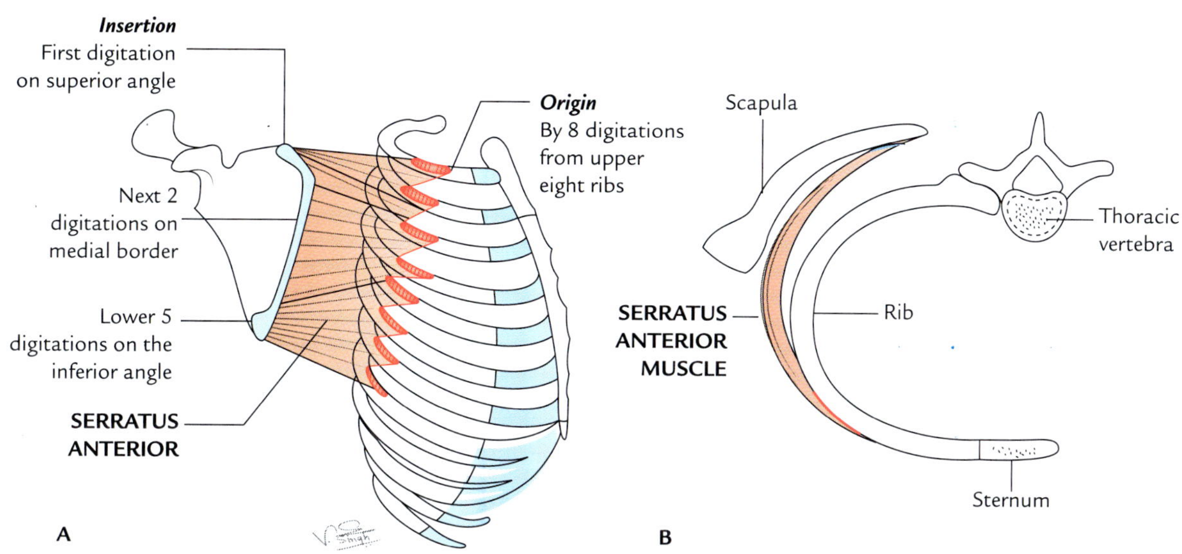

FIG. 3.8 ■ Serratus anterior muscle: (**A**) origin and insertion and (**B**) horizontal section through axilla showing the relationship with the thoracic wall.

Nerve Supply

It is by long thoracic nerve/nerve to serratus anterior (C5–C7).

Actions

1. It is a powerful protractor of the scapula. It along with pectoralis minor muscle, pulls the scapula forward around the chest wall to protract the upper limb for pushing and punching movements as required during boxing. Hence, the serratus anterior is also called **boxer's muscle**.
2. It keeps the medial/vertebral border of the scapula in firm contact with the chest wall.
3. Its lower four or five digitations along with the lower part of the trapezius rotate the scapula laterally and upward during the overhead abduction of the arm.

Clinical Testing **AN 13.7**

When a protracted hand is pushed against the resistance, the muscular digitations of serratus anterior can be seen or felt on the side of rib cage.

N.B.

Long thoracic nerve: It arises in the neck form C5, C6 and C7 roots of brachial plexus, passes down behind clavicle and superficial to 1st and 2nd ribs. It continues to descend longitudinally along the side of thoracic wall, in mid-axillary line on the superficial surface of the serratus anterior muscle which it innervates by giving branches to individual slips. Due to its long and relatively superficial course, it is susceptible to damage.

CLINICAL CORRELATION

Paralysis of the serratus anterior: The paralysis of the serratus anterior muscle following an injury to the *long thoracic nerve* by a stab injury or during the removal of the breast tumour leads to the following effects:

(a) Protraction of the scapula for punching is weakened.
(b) Inferior angle and medial border of the scapula become unduly prominent particularly when the patient pushes his hands against the wall, producing a clinical condition called ***winging of the scapula*** (Fig. 3.9).

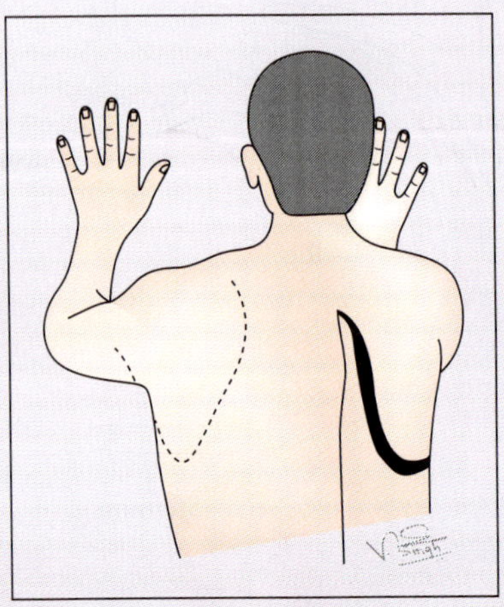

FIG. 3.9 Winging of the right scapula.

FASCIAE

PECTORAL FASCIA

It is the deep fascia covering the anterior aspect of the pectoralis major muscle. It is thin and anchored firmly to the muscle by numerous fasciculi.

Extent

1. **Superiorly,** it is attached to the clavicle.
2. **Inferiorly,** it is continuous with the fascia of the anterior abdominal wall.
3. **Superolaterally,** it passes over the deltopectoral groove to become continuous with the fascia covering the deltoid muscle.
4. **Inferolaterally,** it curves round the inferolateral border of the pectoralis major to become continuous with the axillary fascia. The axillary fascia is a dense fibrous sheet that extends across the base of the axilla.

CLAVIPECTORAL FASCIA

The clavipectoral fascia (Fig. 3.10) is a strong fascial sheet deep to the clavicular head of the pectoralis major muscle, filling the space between the clavicle and the pectoralis minor muscle.

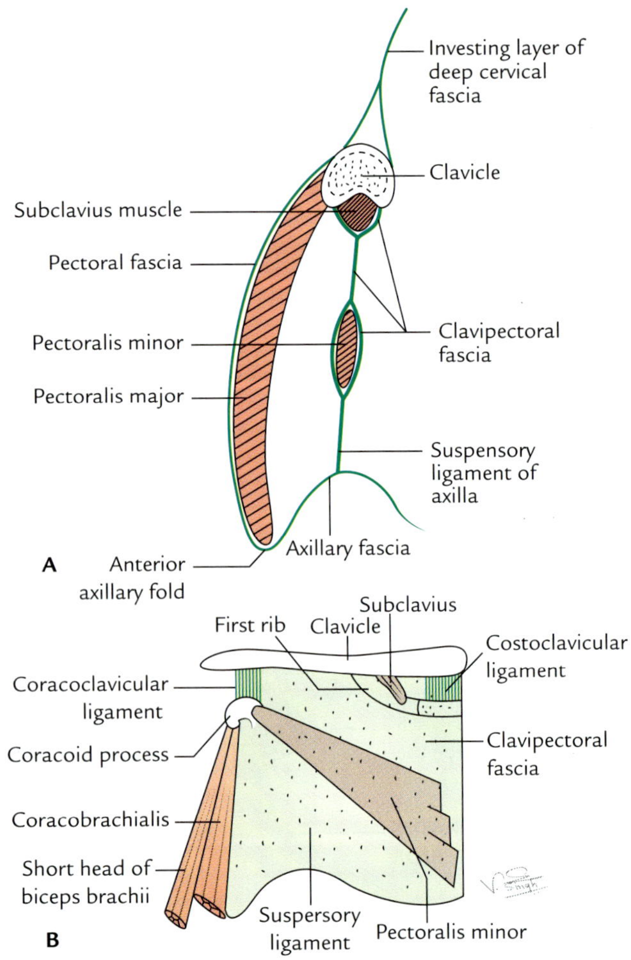

FIG. 3.10 Clavipectoral fascia: (**A**) as seen in the sagittal section of the anterior axillary wall and (**B**) as seen from the front.

Extent

1. **Vertically,** it extends from the clavicle above to the axillary fascia below. Its upper part splits into two laminae to enclose the subclavius muscle. The posterior lamina becomes continuous with the investing layer of the deep cervical fascia and gets fused with the axillary sheath. The anterior lamina gets attached to the clavicle.
   Its lower part splits to enclose the pectoralis minor muscle. Below this muscle, it extends downward as the **suspensory ligament of axilla**, which is attached to the dome of the axillary fascia. The suspensory ligament keeps the dome of axillary fascia pulled up, thus maintaining the concavity of the axilla.
2. **Medially,** clavipectoral fascia is attached to the first rib and costoclavicular ligament and blends with the external intercostal membrane of the upper two intercostal spaces.
3. **Laterally,** it is attached to the coracoid process and blends with the coracoclavicular ligament. The thick upper part of the fascia extending from the first rib near the costochondral junction to the coracoid process is called the **costocoracoid ligament**.

N.B.

The clavipectoral fascia encloses two muscles: subclavius and pectoralis minor.

Structures Piercing the Clavipectoral Fascia

These are as follows (Fig. 3.11):

1. Lateral pectoral nerve.
2. Thoracoacromial artery/acromiothoracic artery.
3. Lymphatics from the breast to the apical group of the axillary lymph nodes.
4. Cephalic vein. The first two structures pass outward, whereas the last two structures pass inward.
   Mnemonic: **CLAP**.
   Cephalic vein,
   Lymphatics,
   Acromiothoracic artery,
   Pectoral nerve (lateral).

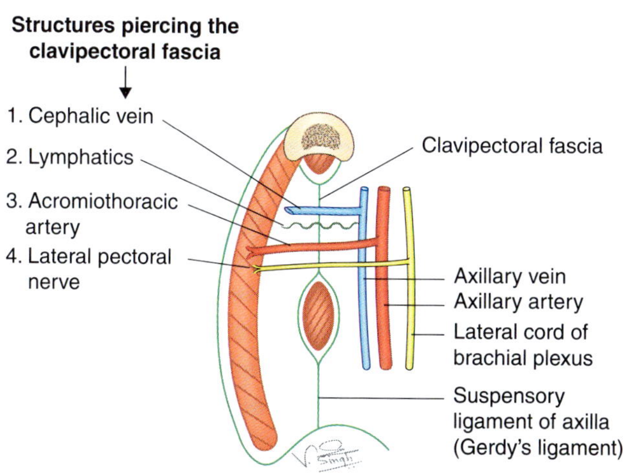

FIG. 3.11 ■ Structures piercing the clavipectoral fascia. (*Source:* Fig. 1.9, p. 11, *Selective Anatomy Prep Manual for Undergraduates*, Vol. I, Vishram Singh. Copyright Elsevier 2014. All rights reserved.)

BREAST (MAMMARY GLAND) AN 9.2

The breast (mammary gland) is the most important structure present in the pectoral region. It is a modified apocrine sweat gland present in the superficial fascia of the pectoral region. The breast is found in both male and female. However, it remains rudimentary in male throughout life but develops well in female at puberty to form hemispheric bulge. On rare occasions, the breasts of males become enlarged; this condition is called **gynaecomastia.** *In females, it forms an accessory sex organ of the female reproductive system and provides milk to the newborn baby.* Primary purpose of breasts in female is to nourish infants. The anatomy of breast is of great surgical importance and, therefore, needs to be studied in detail.

The adult female breast is described in the following text.

LOCATION

The breast is located in the superficial fascia of the pectoral region sitting atop the pectoralis major (pec = chest muscle) (Fig. 3.12). A small extension of breast tissue from its superolateral part (**axillary tail of Spence**), pierces the deep fascia and extends into the axilla (Fig. 3.13). The aperture in the deep fascia through which axillary tail passes into the axilla is called the **foramen of Langer**. The *axillary tail is the site of a high percentage of breast tumour.*

SHAPE AND EXTENT

Shape (Fig. 3.12)
Hemispherical bulge.

Extent (Fig. 3.12)

1. **Vertically,** it extends from the second rib to the sixth rib.
2. **Horizontally,** it extends from the lateral border of the sternum to the midaxillary line.

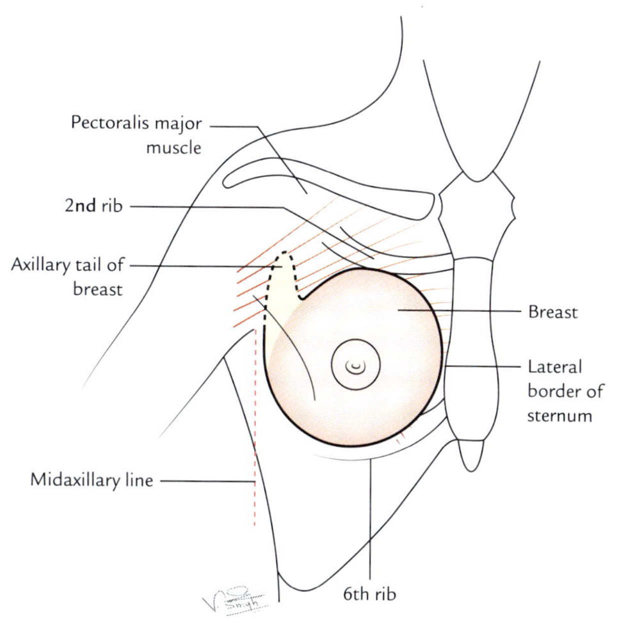

FIG. 3.12 ■ Location and extent of the breast.

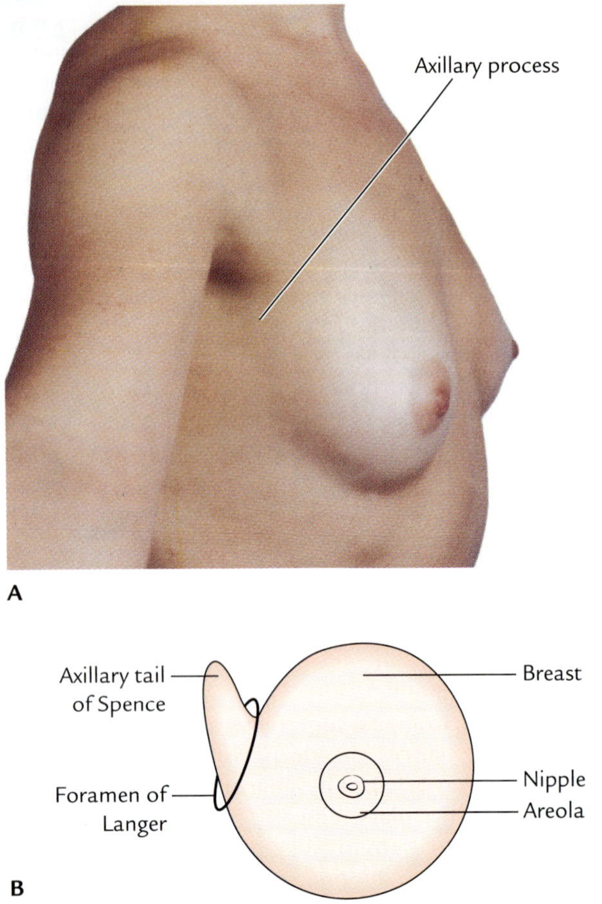

FIG. 3.13 ■ Axillary tail of the breast (of Spence) (**A**) as seen in lateral view of chest wall of a woman. (*Source:* Fig. 3.98B, Page 232, Gray's Anatomy for Students, Third edition, Richard L Drake, Wayne Vogl, Adam WM Mitchell. Copyright Elsevier Inc. 2005. All rights reserved.) (**B**) Schematic diagram to show its passage through the foramen of Langer.

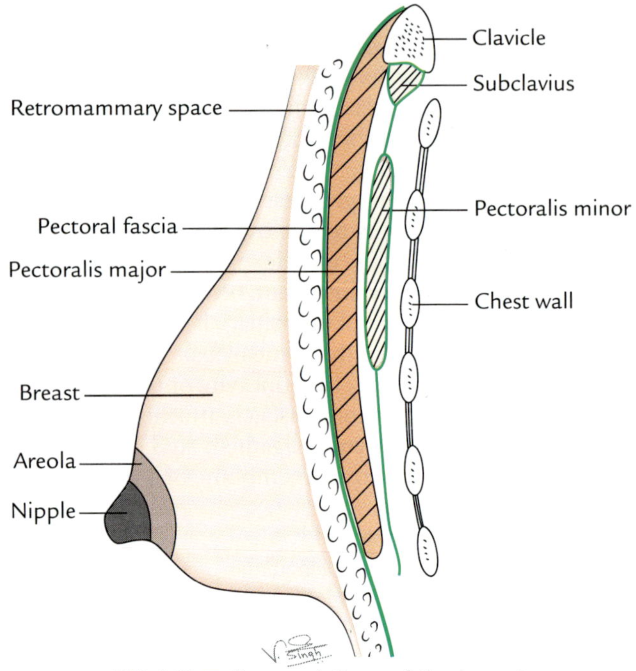

FIG. 3.14 ■ Deep relations of the breast.

N.B.

Despite individual variations in the size of breast, the extent of its base remains fairly constant, *viz.*, from the sternal edge to the midaxillary line and from the second to sixth ribs.

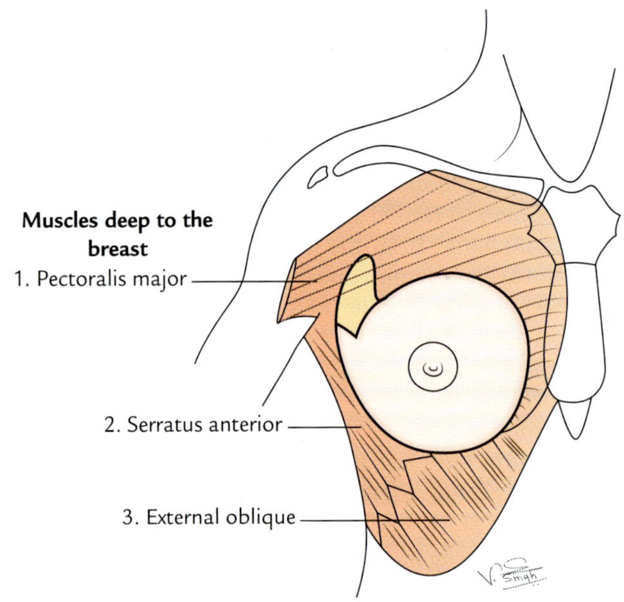

FIG. 3.15 ■ Muscles lying deep to the breast.

RELATIONS

The deep aspect of breast is related to the following structures from superficial to deep:

1. **Pectoral fascia,** the deep fascia covering the anterior aspect of the pectoralis major (Fig. 3.14).
2. **Three muscles**—pectoralis major, serratus anterior, and external oblique (Fig. 3.15).

N.B.

The breast is separated from the *pectoral fascia* by a space (retromammary space), which is filled with loose areolar tissue. Due to the presence of loose areolar tissue, deep to the breast, the breast can be moved freely up and down and from side to side over the pectoral fascia.

STRUCTURE

The breast consists of the following three components (Fig. 3.16):

1. Skin
2. Stroma
3. Parenchyma/glandular tissue/mammary gland proper

Skin: It is the covering for the breast and presents the following features:

1. **Nipple** (Fig. 3.17): It is a conical projection below the centre of the breast, usually at the level of the fourth intercostal space. It contains smooth muscle fibres, which can make the nipple stiff and erect or flatten it. Being richly innervated by sensory nerve endings, the

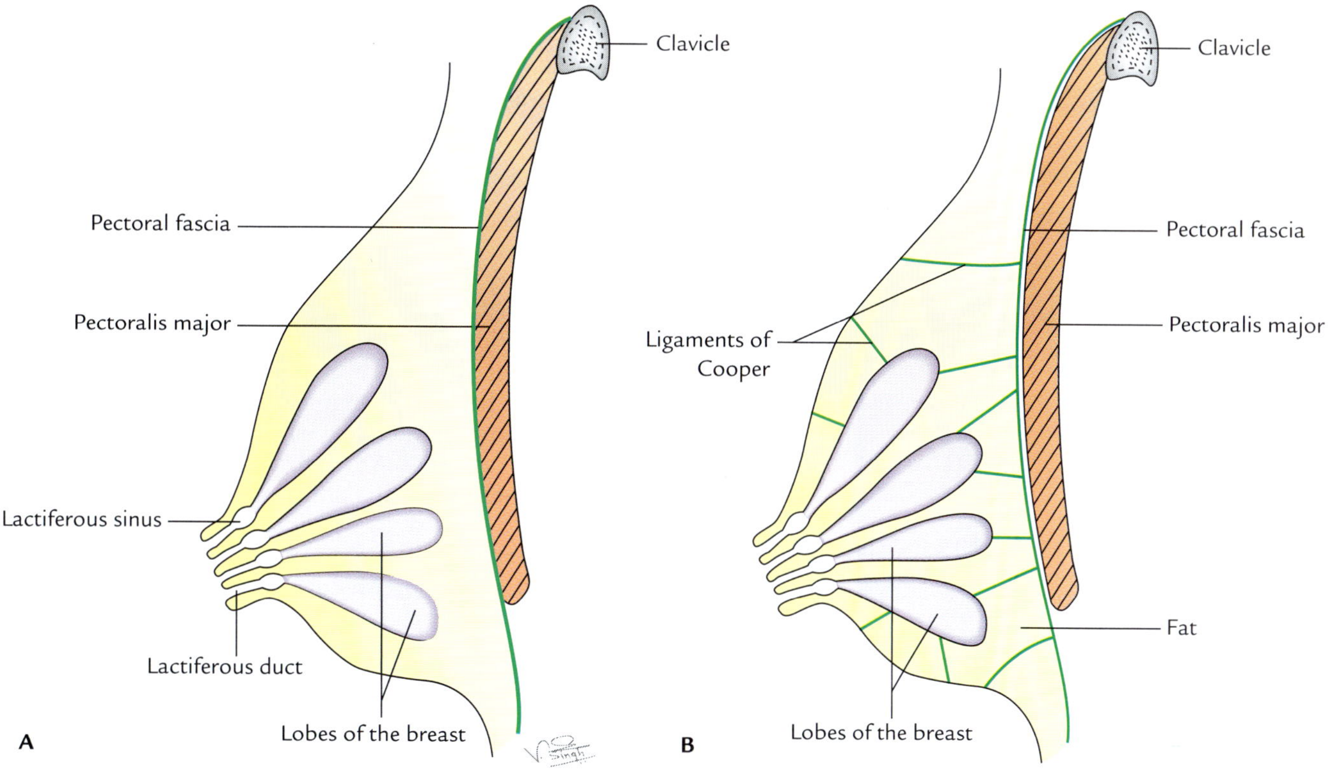

FIG. 3.16 ■ Structure of the breast: (**A**) parenchyma (lobes of the breast) and (**B**) stroma of the breast (suspensory ligaments of Cooper and fat).

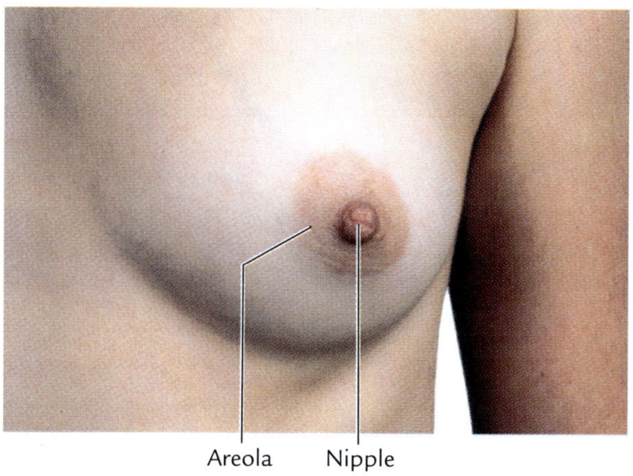

FIG. 3.17 ■ Natural view of nipple and surrounding areola of female breast. (*Source:* Fig. 3.98A, Page 232, Gray's Anatomy for Students, Third edition, Richard L Drake, Wayne Vogl, Adam WM Mitchell. Copyright Elsevier Inc. 2005. All rights reserved.)

nipple is the most sensitive part of the breast to tactile stimulation and become erect during sexual arousal.

2. **Areola** (Fig. 3.17): It is the circular area of pigmented skin surrounding the base of the nipple. It contains a large number of modified sebaceous glands, particularly at its outer margin. The glands produce oily secretion, which lubricates the nipple and areola, and thus prevents them from drying and cracking. The colour of the areola and nipple varies with the complexion of the woman. During pregnancy, the areola becomes darker and enlarged.

N.B.

The sebaceous glands in the areola are enlarged during pregnancy and appear as small nodular elevations called **Montgomery's tubercles**.

Stroma: The stroma of the breast consists of connective tissue and fat. It forms the supporting framework of the breast.

The connective tissue condenses to form fibrous strands/septa, called **suspensory ligaments of Cooper**.

The suspensory ligaments of Cooper are arranged in a radial fashion. They connect the dermis of the overlying skin to the ducts of the breast and pectoral fascia. The ligaments of the Cooper maintain the protuberance of the breast. Their atrophy due to ageing makes the breast pendulous in old age.

The fat forms the most of the bulk of the breast. It is distributed all over the breast except beneath the areola and the nipple.

Parenchyma: The parenchyma/glandular tissue of the breast secretes milk to feed the newborn baby. It consists of about **15–20 lobes** arranged in a radial fashion like the spokes of a wheel and converge towards the nipple. Each lobe is divided into lobules that consist of a cluster of acini. Each lobe is drained by a **lactiferous duct**. The ducts from different lobes converge towards the nipple and open at its summit. Near its termination, each duct expands into a **lactiferous sinus** that serves as a reservoir of milk during lactation (Fig. 3.18).

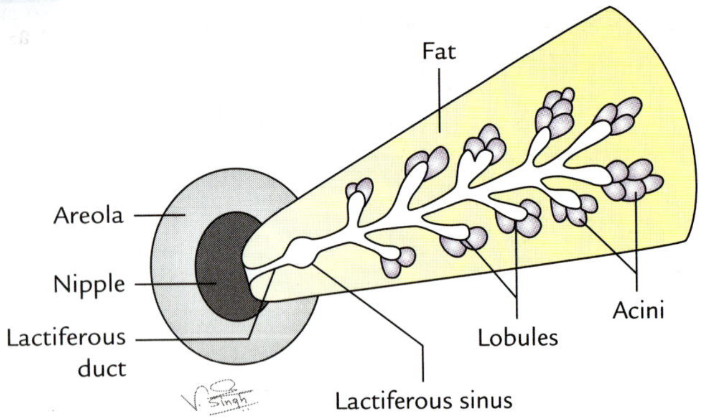

FIG. 3.18 ■ Structure of the lobe of the mammary gland.

N.B.

Male breast resembles a rudimentary female breast. It is devoid of lobes and lobules. Its small nipple and areola lie over the fourth intercostal space.

ARTERIAL SUPPLY

The breast is highly vascular. It is supplied by the following arteries (Fig. 3.19):

1. **Internal thoracic (mammary) artery,** through its perforating branches, which pierce the second, third, and fourth intercostal spaces
2. ***Lateral thoracic artery***, a branch of axillary artery
3. **Posterior intercostal arteries** through their lateral branches
4. **Pectoral branch** of thoracoacromial artery
5. Superior thoracic artery

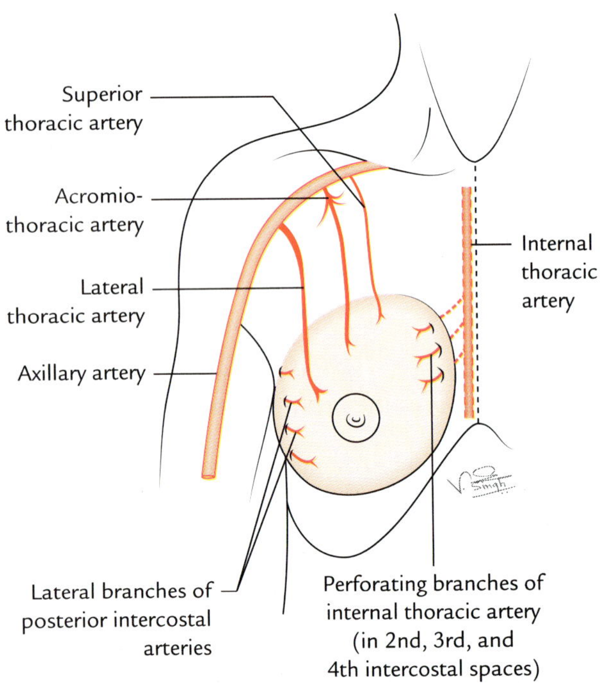

FIG. 3.19 ■ Arterial supply of the breast.

N.B.

Blood supply of the breast is mainly derived from the lateral thoracic artery.

VENOUS DRAINAGE

The venous drainage of the breast takes place by the following veins:

1. Axillary vein
2. Internal thoracic vein
3. Posterior intercostal veins

The veins follow the arteries. First, they converge towards the base of the nipple where they form an anastomotic venous circle (venous plexus of Haller). From there, they run into superficial and deep sets.

The **superficial veins** drain into the internal thoracic vein.

The **deep veins** drain into the internal thoracic, axillary, and posterior intercostal veins.

Apart from lymph vessels, the cancer breast can also spread through segmental veins. Here, it is important to know that veins draining the breast communicates with vertebral venous plexus.

CLINICAL CORRELATION

Metastasis of the breast cancer to the brain: It occurs through the following venous route:

Cancer cells from the breast → posterior intercostal veins → vertebral venous plexus → intracranial dural venous sinuses → brain.

NERVE SUPPLY

The nerve supply of the breast is primarily somatosensory. It is derived from the second to sixth intercostal nerves through their anterior and lateral cutaneous branches.

These nerves provide sensory innervation to the skin and carry autonomic fibres to the smooth muscle and blood vessels of the breast.

The sensory nerve endings in the nipple and areola play an important role in stimulating the release of milk from the mammary gland in response to suckling by the infant.

N.B.

The secretion of milk from the breast is not under neural control but is enabled by the ***prolactin hormone*** secreted by the pituitary gland.

LYMPHATIC DRAINAGE

The knowledge of the lymphatic drainage of the breast is of great significance to surgeons because the carcinoma of the breast spreads mostly through lymphatics. For better understanding (a) lymph nodes and (b) lymphatics draining the breast are described in detail in the following text.

Lymph Nodes Draining the Breast (Fig. 3.20)

The lymph from the breast is drained into the following group of lymph nodes:

1. **Axillary lymph nodes** lying in the axilla and divided into five groups: (a) anterior/pectoral, (b) posterior, (c) central, (d) lateral , and (e) apical (for details, see page 53).
2. **Internal mammary nodes** lying along the internal thoracic vessels.
3. **Supraclavicular nodes** lying above the clavicle.
4. **Posterior intercostal nodes** lying in the posterior parts of intercostal spaces in front of the head of the ribs.
5. **Cephalic (deltopectoral) nodes** lying in the deltopectoral groove.

N.B.

In addition to the aforementioned nodes, the lymph from the breast also drains into subdiaphragmatic and subperitoneal lymph plexuses.

Lymphatics Draining the Breast

The lymphatics draining the breast are divided into two groups: (a) superficial and (b) deep.

Superficial lymphatics drain the skin of the breast except that of the nipple and areola.

Deep lymphatics drain the parenchyma of the breast, and the skin of the nipple and areola. A plexus of lymph vessels deep to the areola is called the **subareolar plexus of Sappey** (Fig. 3.21). The subareolar plexus and most of the lymph from the breast drain into the anterior group of axillary lymph nodes.

The superficial lymphatics of the breast of one side communicate with those of the opposite side. Consequently, the unilateral malignancy may become bilateral.

The **lymphatic drainage from the breast** occurs as follows (Fig. 3.22):

1. The lymph from lateral quadrants of the breast is drained into the *anterior axillary* or *pectoral group of lymph nodes*. These lymph nodes are situated deep to the lower border of the pectoralis minor.
2. The lymph from medial quadrants is drained into *internal mammary (parasternal) lymph nodes* situated along the internal mammary artery. Some lymphatics may go to the internal mammary lymph nodes of the opposite side.
3. A few lymph vessels from the lower lateral quadrant of the breast follow the posterior intercostal arteries and drain into *posterior intercostal nodes* located along the course of these arteries.
4. The few lymph vessels from the lower medial quadrant of the breast cross costal margin, pierce the linea alba and communicate with *subdiaphragmatic* and *subperitoneal lymph plexuses*.
5. The lymph vessels from the deep surface of the breast pierce pectoralis major and clavipectoral fascia to drain into the *apical group of axillary lymph nodes* (Fig. 3.23).

N.B.

About 75% of the lymph from the breast is drained into axillary nodes, 20% into internal mammary lymph nodes, and 5% into the posterior intercostal lymph nodes.

Among the axillary lymph nodes, most of the lymph drains into the anterior axillary nodes, and the remaining into posterior and apical groups. The lymph from anterior, posterior and lateral groups first goes to the central group, and then through them into the supraclavicular lymph nodes.

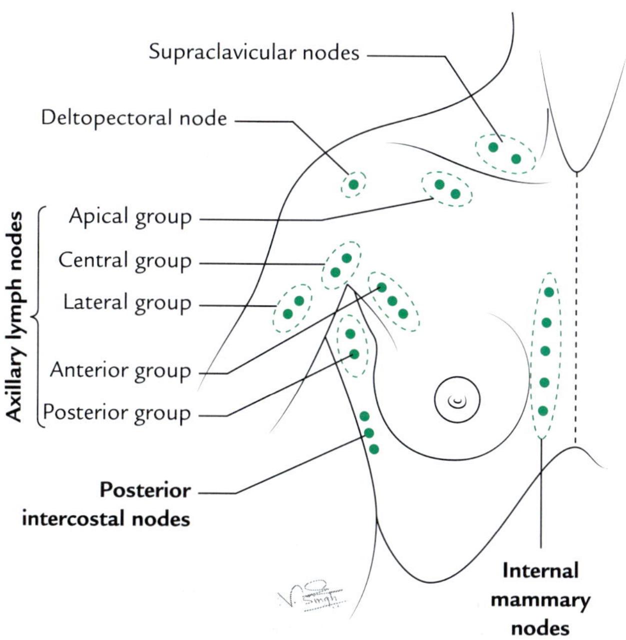

FIG. 3.20 ■ Lymph nodes draining the breast.

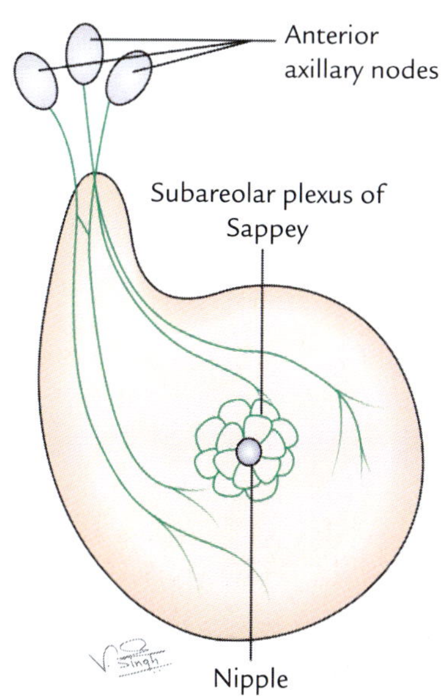

FIG. 3.21 ■ Subareolar plexus of Sappey.

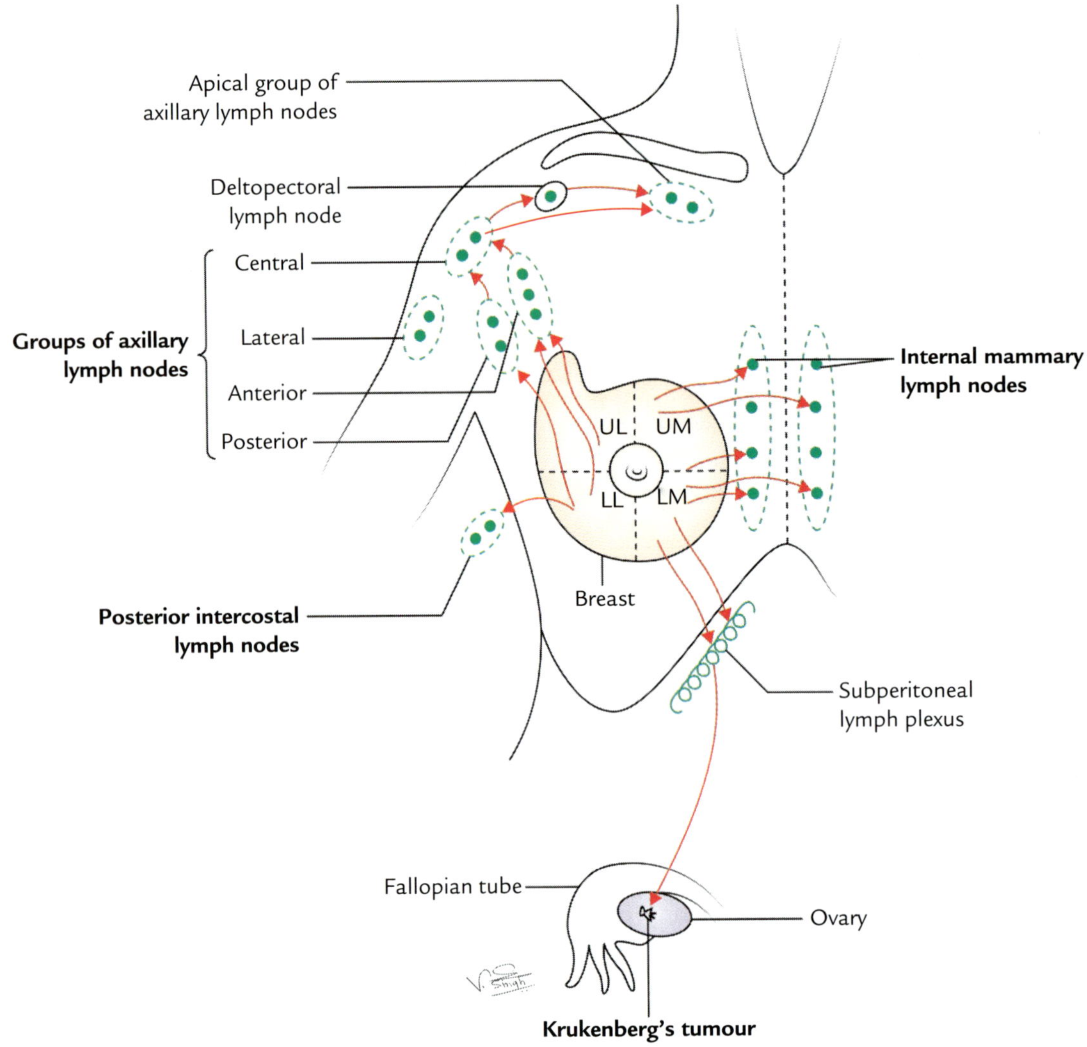

FIG. 3.22 ■ Mode of the lymphatic drainage of the breast (UL = upper lateral quadrant, LL = lower lateral quadrant, UM = upper medial quadrant, and LM = lower medial quadrant).

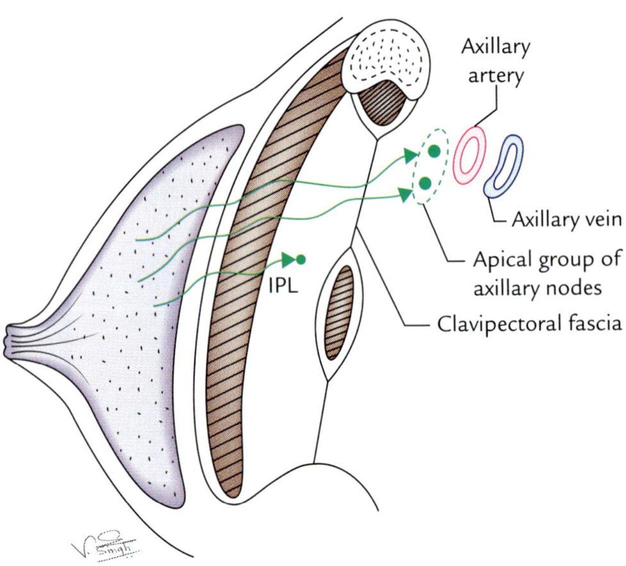

FIG. 3.23 ■ Direct pathway of deep lymphatics of the breast through pectoralis major and clavipectoral fascia to the apical group of axillary nodes (IPL=interpectoral lymph node).

CLINICAL CORRELATION

- **Breast cancer (carcinoma of the breast):** It is the most common cancer in females. It arises from the epithelial cells lining the **lactiferous** ducts or **acini of lobules.** In about 60% cases, it occurs in the upper lateral quadrant and commonly affects females between 40 and 60 years of age.

  Clinically, it presents as a very serious problem with the following **signs and symptoms:**

  (a) *Presence of a painless hard lump.*

  (b) *Breast becomes fixed and immobile*, due to infiltration of suspensory ligaments by cancer cells.

  (c) *Retraction of skin*, due to infiltration of suspensory ligaments by cancer cells.

  (d) *Retraction of nipple* due to infiltration and fibrosis of lactiferous ducts.

  (e) *Peau d'orange appearance of the skin* (i.e. skin giving rise to appearance like that of the skin of an orange) because pits of hair follicles appear to be retracted beneath the level of skin due to the obstruction of superficial lymphatics.

- **Metastasis:** The knowledge of the lymphatic drainage of the breast is of great clinical importance due to a high percentage of occurrence of cancer in the breast and its subsequent dissemination of cancer cells (metastasis) along the lymph vessels to the regional lymph nodes.

Some lymph vessels from the inferomedial quadrant of the breast communicate with the *subperitoneal lymph plexus* and carry cancer cells to it. From here, cancer cells migrate transcoelomically and get deposited on the ovary, producing a secondary tumour in the ovary called *Krukenberg's tumour*.

- **Early detection of breast cancer:** Breast cancer is a serious and often a fatal disease in women. The **mammography** (Fig. 3.24) and **regular self-examination of the breast** (Fig. 3.25) help in the early detection of the breast cancer and its effective treatment.
- **Mammography**
  It is an X-ray examination of breast to detect cancer. The mammogram is the X-ray picture of breast (Fig. 3.24). It is looked by doctors to look for early signs of breast cancer, viz. *characteristic masses or microcalcifications*.
- ***Self-examination of the breast***
  The **six steps of the breast self-examination** are as follows (Fig. 3.25):
  1. Stand in front of a long mirror and inspect both breasts for any discharge from the nipples, puckering, or dimpling of the skin. Now, look for any change in shape or contour of the breasts.
  2. Clasp hands behind your head and press hands forward.
  3. Press hands firmly on the hips and bow slightly forward.
  4. During shower raise your one arm and use the fingers of the other hand to palpate the breast in a circular fashion from periphery to the nipple for unusual lump or mass under the skin.
  5. Gently squeeze the nipple and look for any discharge. Do similar examination on the other side.
  6. Steps 4 and 5 should be repeated in the lying down position. In this position, the breasts are flattened, which makes it easier to palpate them.

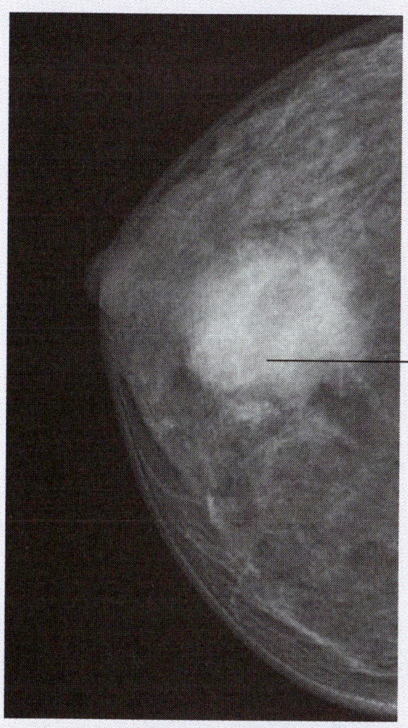

FIG. 3.24 Mammogram depicting carcinoma. (*Courtesy:* Dr. Sunil Upadhyay, Radio-oncologist, London, UK.)

Treatment

Surgical treatment of breast cancer is in the form of ***lumpectomy*** and ***mastectomy***.

- ***Lumpectomy*** is the removal of only tumour.
- ***Mastectomy*** is the removal of one or both breasts.

In classical operation of *radical mastectomy*, the whole breast is removed along with the axillary lymph nodes, pectoralis major, and minor muscles.

DEVELOPMENT OF THE BREAST

AN 9.3

The breast develops from an ectodermal thickening called **milk line/ridge (of Schultz)** (Fig. 3.26). This line appears in a young embryo as early as in the fourth week and extends from axilla to the groin. In lower animals, several mammary glands develop along this line. But in human beings, this ridge disappears except for its small part in the pectoral region. Here it thickens, becomes depressed, and gives off 15–20 solid cords, which grow in the underlying mesenchyme and proliferate to form lobes of the gland. At birth, the depressed ectodermal thickening is raised to form the nipple. The stroma of the breast develops from the surrounding mesoderm.

MICROSCOPIC STRUCTURE OF BREAST

The microscopic anatomy of breast differs in resting and lactating phases of breast.

In resting phase, lobules and ducts are not well defined but have abundant connective tissue and fat.

On the other hand, the lactating breast has well-developed glandular tissue but less connective tissue and fat.

AGE CHANGES IN BREAST

AN 9.2

With age there is decrease in fat and glandular tissue of breast. The connective tissue that supports the breast becomes less elastic. Many of these changes occur due to decrease in oestrogen level of blood at menopause. As a result of these changes, *in old women breasts become smaller, loose and sag*.

CLINICAL CORRELATION

Developmental anomalies of the breast: The following developmental anomalies of the breasts are encountered during clinical practice:

- ***Polythelia/supernumerary nipple:*** It appears along the milk ridge and is often mistaken for moles.
- ***Retracted nipple/inverted nipple:*** It occurs if the nipple fails to develop from the ectodermal pit. In this condition, suckling of an infant cannot take place and the nipple is prone to infection.
- ***Polymastia:*** The development of more than one breast along the milk line.
- ***Gynaecomastia:*** The development of the breast in a male, mainly at puberty. Usually, it is bilateral and thought to occur due to hormonal imbalance.

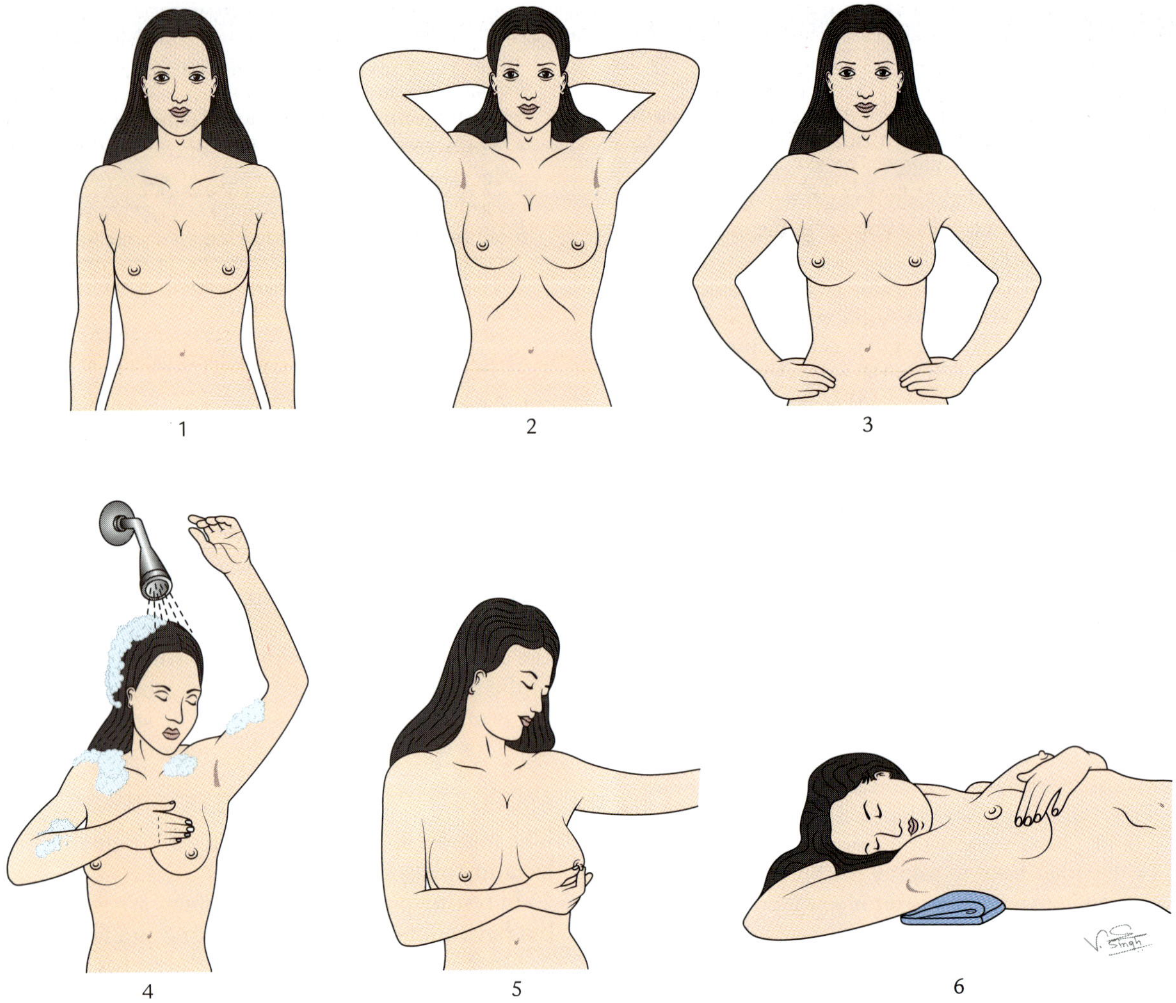

FIG. 3.25 ■ Steps of the self-examination of the breast.

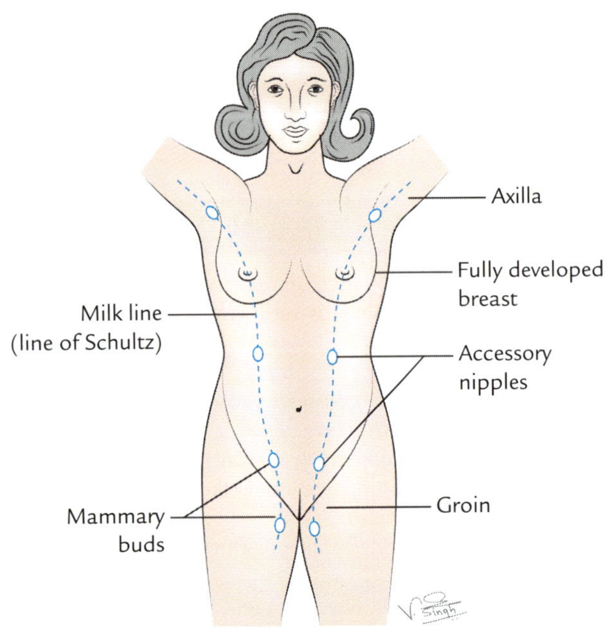

FIG. 3.26 ■ Development of the breast. Note the extent of the milk line and possible positions of accessory nipples.

Golden Facts to Remember

• Most important structure of the pectoral region in a female	Breast
• Largest muscle of the pectoral region	Pectoralis major
• Key muscle of the pectoral region	Pectoralis minor
• Most of the lymph from the breast (75%) is drained into	Axillary lymph nodes, mainly into anterior nodes
• Subareolar plexus of Sappey	Plexus of lymph vessels deep to the areola, which drains into the anterior axillary lymph nodes
• Rotter's lymph nodes	Interpectoral lymph nodes
• Most common site of the breast cancer	Upper and outer quadrants of the breast
• Main artery supplying the breast	Lateral thoracic artery

CLINICAL CASE STUDY

A 55-year-old female complained to her family physician of hard painless lump in the upper and outer portion of her right breast. The examination of the breast revealed the *peau d'orange* appearance of the skin, loss of mobility of the breast, and retraction of the nipple. The examination of axilla revealed the enlargement of axillary lymph nodes. The X-ray of the vertebral column revealed an irregular shadow in the vertebral bodies of T6 and T7 vertebrae. **She was diagnosed as a case of the breast cancer**.

QUESTIONS

1. What do you understand of **lump in the breast**? What are its common causes?
2. Mention the anatomical basis of the *peau d'orange* appearance of skin, retraction of the nipple, and loss of mobility of the breast.
3. Name the three muscles lying deep to the base of the breast.
4. What is the venous route of the spread of breast cancer?
5. What is the most common site of the breast cancer?

ANSWERS

1. Any abnormal mass or thickening of the breast tissue is called **lump in the breast**. Lump in the breast may occur due to **fibroadenoma** (a benign tumour of the breast, which is usually a firm solitary mass that is mobile beneath the skin) or **breast cancer** (a malignant tumour of the breast, which is adherent to underlying tissue and immobile).
2. The **peau d'orange appearance of skin** (i.e. skin like orange peel) is due to the retraction of pits of hair follicles beneath the oedematous skin following the retraction of ligaments of Cooper. The condition is due to the blockage of lymphatics draining the skin, leading to the stagnation of lymph and oedema of skin.

   Retraction of the nipple occurs due to the infiltration of lactiferous ducts by the cancer cells and their subsequent fibrosis.
3. Pectoralis major, serratus anterior, and aponeurosis of the external oblique muscle of the abdomen.
4. Cancer cells of the breast → posterior intercostal veins → vertebral venous plexus → vertebral bodies (also see, page 42).
5. Upper and outer quadrants of the breast.

CHAPTER 4

Axilla (Armpit)

SPECIFIC LEARNING OBJECTIVES

After studying this chapter, the student should be able to:

- Identify and describe the boundaries and contents of axilla. AN 10.1
- Identify, describe, and demonstrate the origin, extent, course, parts, relations, and branches of axillary artery, and tributaries of axillary vein. AN 10.2
- Describe the location, formation, components, relations, and branches of the brachial plexus. AN 10.3
- Describe the course and relations of terminal branches of brachial plexus. AN 10.3
- Describe the anatomical groups of axillary lymph nodes and specify their area of drainage. AN 10.4
- Explain variations in formation of brachial plexus. AN 10.5
- Give the anatomical basis of: (a) Erb's paralysis and (b) Klumpke's analysis. AN 10.6
- Explain the anatomical basis of enlarged axillary lymph nodes. AN 10.7
- Describe the arterial anastomosis around scapula.
- Write short notes on: (a) axillary artery, (b) axillary vein, and (c) cervicoaxillary canal.

The **axilla** or **armpit** is a pyramidal space under shoulder between the upper arm and the side of the chest wall, bounded in front and behind by axillary folds (Fig. 4.1). It contains the brachial plexus, axillary vessels, and lymph nodes embedded in the fibrofatty tissue. It also acts as a funnel-shaped tunnel for neurovascular structures to pass from the root of the neck to the upper limb and vice versa. Groups of lymph nodes within it drain the upper limb and the breast. The study of the axilla is clinically important because axillary lymph nodes are often enlarged and, hence, routinely palpated during the physical examination of the patient. Abscess in this region is also common.

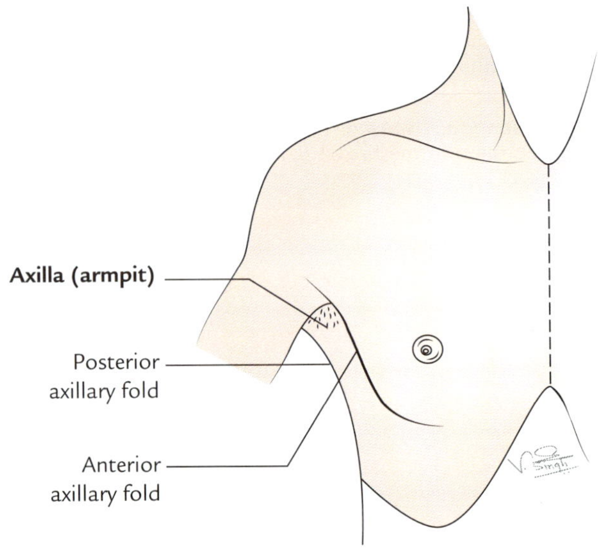

FIG. 4.1 ■ Location of the axilla.

N.B.

The anterior axillary fold is musculocutaneous ridge formed by the lateral edge of the pectoralis major, and the posterior axillary fold is a musculocutaneous ridge formed by the latissimus dorsi and teres major.

BOUNDARIES AN 10.1

The axilla resembles a truncated four-sided pyramid and presents an **apex**, a **base** and **four walls (anterior, posterior, medial, and lateral)** (Fig. 4.2). It is disposed obliquely in such a way that its apex is directed upward and medially towards the root of neck and base is directed downward.

- **Apex/cervicoaxillary canal:** It is a passageway between the neck and the axilla. It is directed upward and medially into the root of the neck and corresponds to the triangular space bounded in front by the clavicle, behind by the upper border of the scapula and medially by the outer border of the first rib (Fig. 4.3). The axillary artery and brachial plexus enter the axilla from the neck through this gap; hence, it is also termed the **cervicoaxillary**

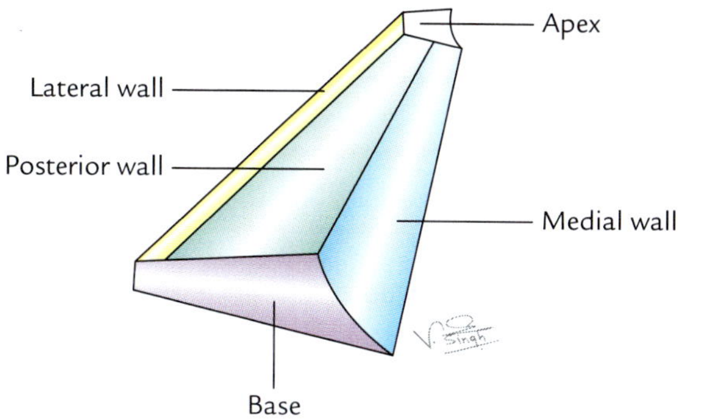

FIG. 4.2 Boundaries of the axilla (note the anterior wall is not seen).

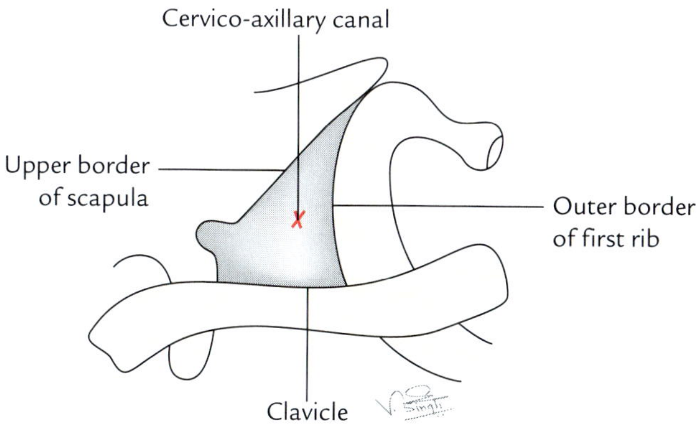

FIG. 4.3 Boundaries of the cervicoaxillary canal (apex of the axilla).

canal. The axillary vein enters the neck from the axilla through this canal (Fig. 4.4).

- **Base/floor:** *It is at the lower end of the axilla* and directed downward. It is formed by the axillary fascia. The base corresponds to the hollow bounded in front by the *anterior axillary fold*, formed by the lower border of the pectoralis major muscle, behind by the *posterior axillary fold*, formed by the tendon of latissimus dorsi and teres major muscles, and medially by the lateral aspect of the chest wall.

N.B.

The perpendicular line dropped from a point midway between the anterior and posterior axillary folds is called the *midaxillary line*—an important surface landmark.

- **Anterior wall:** It is formed by the pectoralis major, subclavius, and pectoralis minor muscles.
- **Posterior wall:** It is formed by the subscapularis muscle above and latissimus dorsi and teres major muscles below.
- **Medial wall:** It is formed by the upper four or five ribs and corresponding intercostal spaces covered by the serratus anterior muscle.
- **Lateral wall:** It is formed by the tendon of long head of biceps brachii in the bicipital groove of humerus, coracobrachialis and short head of biceps brachii. The lateral wall is extremely narrow because the anterior and posterior walls of the axilla converge at this site.

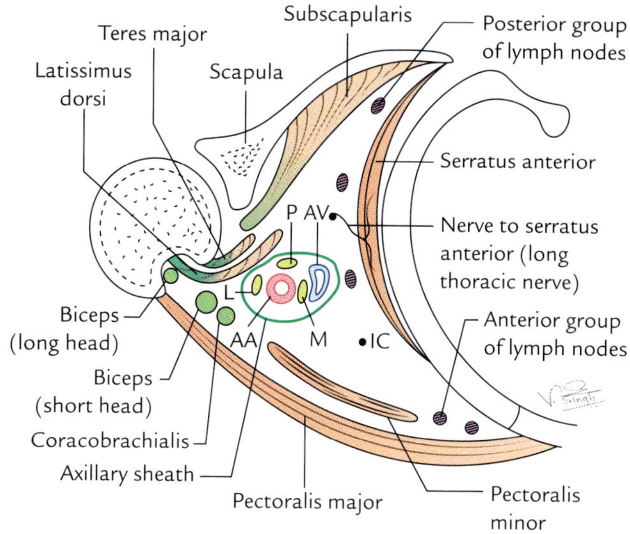

FIG. 4.4 Boundaries and contents of the axilla as seen in a horizontal section (AV = axillary vein, AA = axillary artery, P = posterior cord, L = lateral cord, M = medial cord, IC = intercostobrachial nerve).

N.B.

The smoothness of the anterior and posterior axillary folds is due to the twisting of the sternoaponeurotic part of the pectoralis major muscle around the upper fibers of this muscle and the twisting of the latissimus dorsi muscle around the teres major muscle, respectively.

CONTENTS OF THE AXILLA — AN 10.2

The contents of the axilla are as follows:

1. Axillary artery and its branches.
2. Axillary vein and its tributaries.
3. Cords of the brachial plexus (i.e. infraclavicular part of brachial plexus).
4. Axillary lymph nodes.
5. Fibrofatty tissue.
6. Axillary tail of breast.
7. Long thoracic and intercostobrachial nerves.

N.B.

The **neurovascular structures in the axilla** are normally protected by the arm on the side of the body and the cushioning matrix—the axillary fat, but they are vulnerable to injury when the arm is abducted.

FURTHER DETAILS

1. AXILLARY ARTERY — AN 10.2

The axillary artery (Fig. 4.5) is the main artery of the upper limb. It begins at the outer border of the first rib

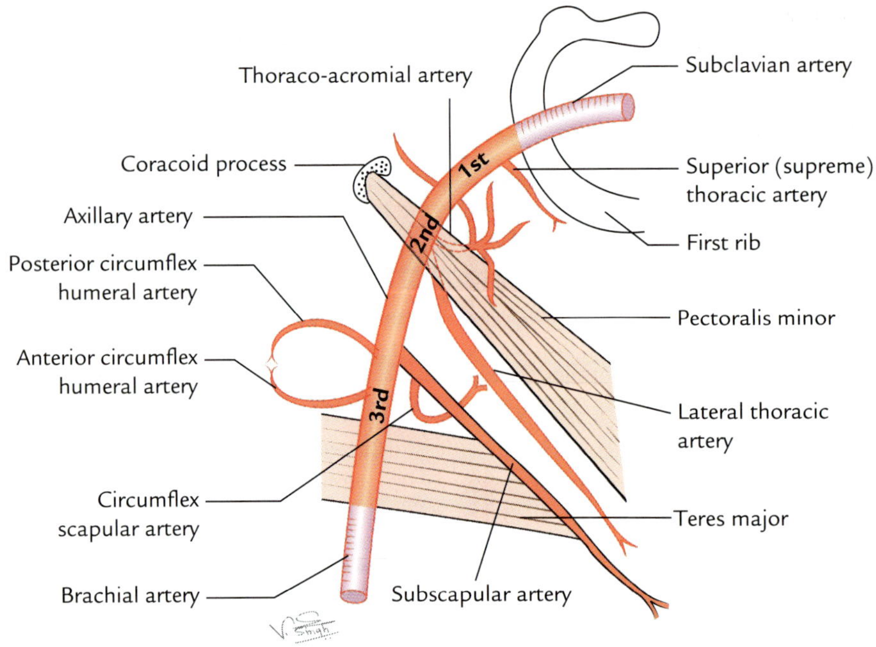

FIG. 4.5 ■ Course and branches of the axillary artery. (Extent: from outer border of first rib to lower border of teres major muscle.)

as the continuation of the subclavian artery and ends by becoming the brachial artery at the lower border of teres major. In axilla, it runs from its apex to the base lying nearer to the anterior wall than the posterior wall. During its course through axilla, it is crossed on its superficial aspect by the pectoralis minor muscle, which divides it into three parts. The axillary vein is medial to the artery, and the cords of the brachial plexus are arranged around the second part of the artery (i.e. part deep to the pectoralis minor), the lateral cord being lateral, the medial cord medial, and the posterior cord being posterior.

Parts

The axillary artery is divided into the following three parts by the pectoralis minor (Fig. 4.5):

1. **First part,** superior (or proximal) to the muscle.
2. **Second part,** posterior (or deep) to the muscle.
3. **Third part,** inferior (or distal) to the muscle.

Relations

The axillary vein lies medial to the axillary artery throughout its course, but the relationship of cords of brachial plexus and their branches are different for each of the three parts of the artery (Fig. 4.6). The relations of the three parts of the axillary artery are given in Table 4.1.

Branches of the Axillary Artery

The axillary artery gives six branches: **one branch from the first part, two branches from the second part, and three branches from the third part** (Fig. 4.5). Most of these branches go to and supply walls of the axilla.

A. From the First Part

Superior thoracic artery, a very small branch, arises near the subclavius, passes between the pectoralis major and minor muscles, and supplies these muscles and medial wall of the axilla.

B. From the Second Part

1. **Thoracoacromial artery (acromiothoracic artery)** emerges at the upper border of the pectoralis minor, pierces clavipectoral fascia and soon breaks up into four branches: (a) *pectoral branch*, (b) *deltoid branch*, (c) *acromial branch*, and (d) *clavicular branch*. These branches radiate at a right angle to each other. The **pectoral branch** supplies pectoral muscles, **deltoid branch** runs in the deltopectoral groove, **acromial branch** ends by joining anastomosis over the acromion, and **clavicular branch** supplies sternoclavicular joint and subclavius.
2. **Lateral thoracic artery** emerges at and runs along the inferior border of the pectoralis minor, supplying the branches to pectoralis major, pectoralis minor, and serratus anterior muscles. In females, the lateral thoracic artery is large and provides important supply to the breast through its lateral mammary branches.

C. From the Third Part

1. **Subscapular artery,** the *largest branch of axillary artery*, runs along the lower border of the subscapularis and ends near the inferior angle of the scapula. It gives a large branch, the *circumflex scapular artery*, which passes through the upper triangular intermuscular space, winds round the lateral border of scapula to enter infraspinous fossa. In addition, it gives numerous small branches.
2. **Anterior circumflex humeral artery,** a small branch, passes in front of the surgical neck of humerus and anastomoses with the posterior circumflex humeral artery to form an arterial circle around

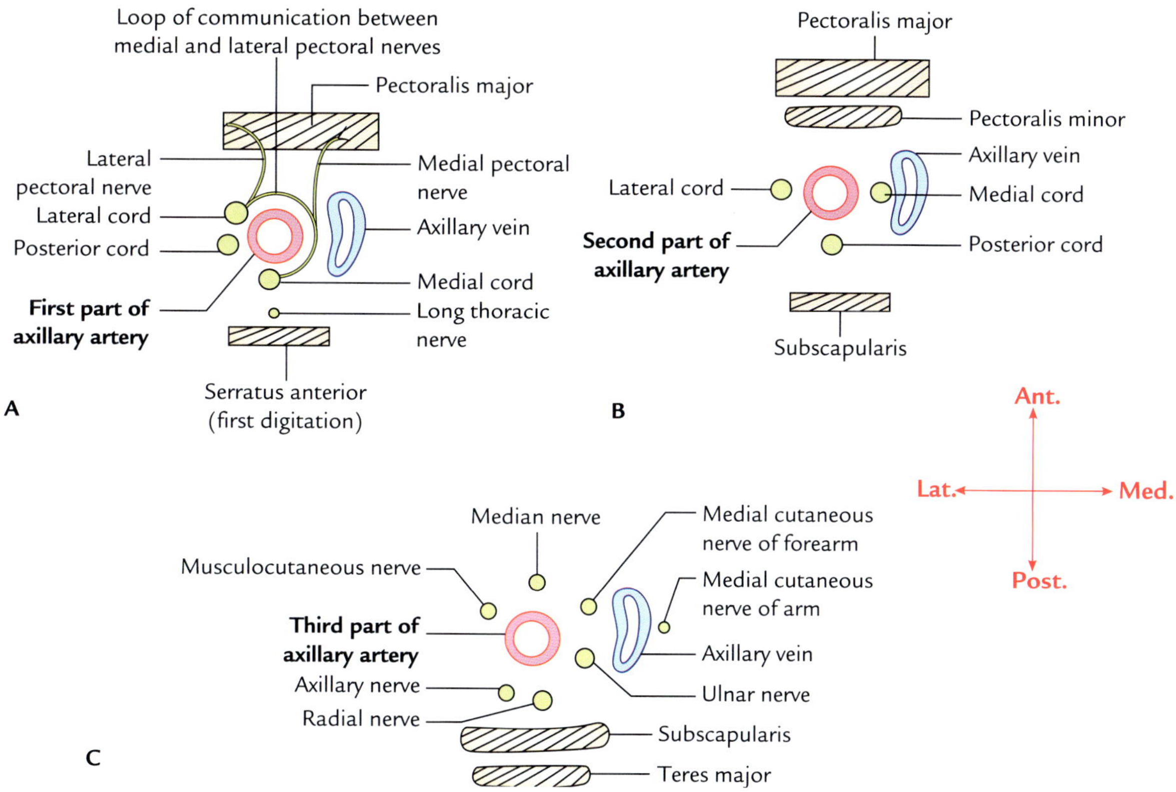

FIG. 4.6 Relations of the axillary artery. (**A**) First part, (**B**) second part, and (**C**) third part.

TABLE 4.1 Relations of the axillary artery (Fig. 4.6)

Part	Anterior	Posterior	Medial	Lateral
First part	• Pectoralis major (clavicular part) • Loop of communication between the lateral and medial pectoral nerves	• Medial cord of the brachial plexus • Long thoracic nerve • Serratus anterior (first digitation)	Axillary vein	Lateral and posterior cords of the brachial plexus
Second part	• Pectoralis minor • Pectoralis major	• Posterior cord of the brachial plexus • Subscapularis	• Medial cord of the brachial plexus • Axillary vein	Lateral cord of the brachial plexus
Third part	• Median nerve • Pectoralis major	• Radial nerve • Axillary nerve • Subscapularis (in the upper part) • Teres major (in the lower part)	• Axillary vein • Medial cutaneous nerve of the forearm • Ulnar nerve	Musculocutaneous nerve

the surgical neck of humerus. It gives an *ascending branch*, which runs upward into the intertubercular sulcus of humerus to supply the head of the humerus and shoulder joint.

3. **Posterior circumflex humeral artery,** larger than the anterior circumflex humeral artery, passes backward, along with the axillary nerve through the quadrangular intermuscular space, crosses the posterior aspect of the surgical neck of humerus to anastomose with the anterior circumflex humeral artery. It supplies the deltoid muscle and shoulder joint.

Branches of the axillary artery are summarized in Table 4.2.

Arterial Anastomosis Around Scapula (Scapular Anastomosis) AN 10.9

The arterial anastomosis around scapula is principally formed between the branches of the first part of the subclavian and the third part of the axillary arteries (Fig. 4.7).

The scapular anastomosis takes place at two sites: around the body of the scapula and over the acromion process of the scapula.

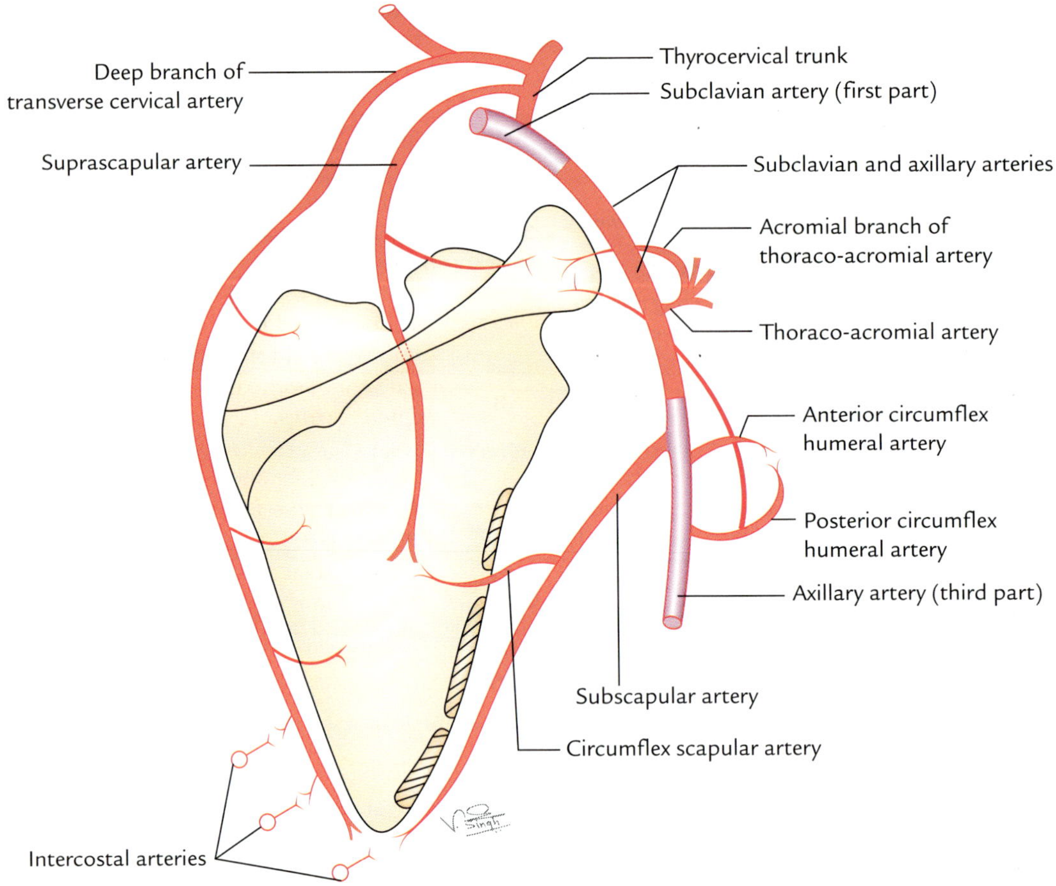

FIG. 4.7 ■ Anastomosis around the scapula (scapular anastomosis).

TABLE 4.2 Branches of the axillary artery

Parts of axillary artery	Branches
First part	• Superior thoracic artery
Second part	• Acromiothoracic artery (Thoracoacromial artery) • Lateral thoracic artery
Third part	• Subscapular artery • Anterior circumflex humeral artery • Posterior circumflex humeral artery

Mnemonic: **S-AL-SAP.**

1. Around the body of the scapula: It occurs between the
   (a) *suprascapular artery*, a branch of the thyrocervical trunk from the first part of the subclavian artery,
   (b) *circumflex scapular artery*, a branch of the subscapular artery from the third part of the axillary artery, and
   (c) deep branch of the transverse cervical artery, a branch of the thyrocervical trunk.
2. Over the acromion process: It occurs between the
   (a) acromial branch of the thoracoacromial artery,
   (b) acromial branch of the suprascapular artery, and
   (c) acromial branch of the posterior circumflex humeral artery.

CLINICAL CORRELATION

- **Collateral circulation through scapular anastomosis:** If the subclavian and axillary arteries are blocked anywhere between the first part of the subclavian artery and the third part of the axillary artery, the scapular anastomosis serves as a potential pathway (collateral circulation) between the first part of the subclavian artery and the third part of the axillary artery, to ensure the adequate circulation to the upper limb.
- **Axillary artery pulsations and compression:**
  - Axillary artery pulsations can be felt in the lower part of the lateral wall of the axilla.
  - Axillary artery can be effectively compressed against the lower part of the lateral wall of the axilla to control the bleeding from distal part of the upper limb.

2. AXILLARY VEIN

AN 10.2

The axillary vein is formed at the lower border of the teres major muscle by the union of the *basilic vein* and *venae comitantes of the brachial artery* (Fig. 4.8). It runs upward along the medial side of the axillary artery and ends at the outer border of the first rib by becoming the subclavian vein.

Tributaries

The tributaries of the axillary vein are as follows:

1. Veins, which correspond to the branches of the axillary artery, namely, the lateral thoracic vein and the subscapular vein.

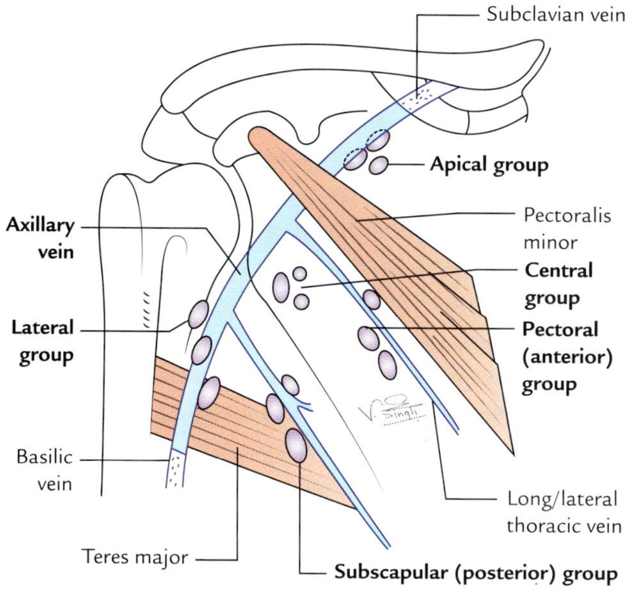

FIG. 4.8 Axillary vein and lymph nodes.

2. Cephalic vein, which joins it after piercing the clavipectoral fascia.

N.B.

There is no or very thin axillary sheath around the axillary vein; hence, it can freely expand during increased venous return.

CLINICAL CORRELATION

Spontaneous thrombosis of the axillary vein: Occasionally, a muscular band—the *axillary arch*—overlies the vein. It may compress the vein, following excessive and unaccustomed movements of the arm at the shoulder joint and cause spontaneous thrombosis of the axillary vein.

3. CORDS OF BRACHIAL PLEXUS

The cords of brachial plexus are described on page 54.

4. AXILLARY LYMPH NODES

AN 10.4

The axillary lymph nodes (Fig. 4.8) are scattered in the fibrofatty tissue of the axilla. Their number varies between 20 and 30. They are divided into the following five groups:

a. **Anterior or pectoral group:** They lie along the lateral thoracic vein at the lower border of the pectoralis minor. They receive the lymph from the upper half of the trunk anteriorly and from the major part of the breast. The axillary tail of Spence is in actual contact with these lymph nodes. Therefore, cancer involving the axillary tail of the breast may be misdiagnosed as an enlarged lymph node.
b. **Posterior or subscapular group:** They lie on the posterior axillary fold along the subscapular vein. They receive the lymph from the upper half of the trunk posteriorly, and from the axillary tail of the breast.
c. **Lateral group:** They lie along the upper part of the humerus in relation to the axillary vein. They drain the lymph from the upper limb.
d. **Central group:** They are situated in the upper part of the axilla. They receive the lymph from the other groups and drain into the apical group (vide infra). The intercostobrachial nerve passes among these nodes. Therefore, the enlargement of these nodes such as in cancer may compress this nerve, causing pain in the area of distribution of this nerve, that is, along the inner border of the arm.
e. **Apical group:** They are 5 to 6 in number and situated partly posterior to upper portion of pectoralis minor muscle and partly above the upper border of this muscle at the apex of the axilla along the axillary vein.

   They are of great clinical importance because they receive lymph directly from the upper and outer parts of the breast and indirectly from the rest of the breast through the central group of axillary nodes. Although these lymph nodes are located very deeply, they can be palpated by pushing the fingers of one hand into the apex of axilla from below and fingers of the other hand behind the clavicle from above.

N.B.

The axillary lymph nodes are also described in terms of levels at which they are situated, *viz.*

- **Level I nodes:** They lie lateral to the lower border of the pectoralis minor muscle.
- **Level II nodes:** They lie deep to the pectoralis minor muscle.
- **Level III nodes:** They lie medial to the upper border of the pectoralis minor muscle.

The lymph nodes first receive the lymph from the area of the breast involved in cancer and are termed *sentinel lymph nodes*. These are usually the level I lymph nodes. The **sentinel nodes** are confirmed by injecting a radioactive substance into the affected area of the breast.

5. FIBROFATTY TISSUE OF AXILLA

It acts as packing material of structures passing through axilla. In block dissection of axillary lymph nodes, it should be carefully removed to prevent inadvertent damage of **long thoracic nerve, thoracodorsal nerve, intercostobrachial nerve,** etc. Also see clinical box on page 54.

6. AXILLARY TAIL OF SPENCE

It is an extension of breast tissue from its upper lateral quadrant into axilla through an opening in the deep fascia called foramen of Langer (for details see page 39).

7. LONG THORACIC NERVE (IN AXILLA)

It arises from C5 to C7 roots and descends in axilla posterior to brachial plexus to innervate the serratus anterior muscle which anchors the scapula to the chest wall.

8. INTERCOSTOBRACHIAL NERVE (IN AXILLA)

It arises from lateral cutaneous branch of second intercostal nerve. Then runs through axilla and innervates the skin of axilla and upper medial aspect of arm. If damaged during axillary dissection, it causes *intercostobrachial nerve syndrome* which leads to fairly constant paraesthesia and burning pain in the area innervated by it.

CLINICAL CORRELATION

- **Enlargement of axillary lymph nodes:** The axillary lymph nodes are enlarged due to infection or other inflammatory process of upper limb and other, drainage areas, *viz.* breast wall of thorax and upper abdominal wall above umbilicus.
- **Palpation of axillary lymph nodes:** *The palpation of axillary lymph nodes* is part of the clinical examination of the breast due to their involvement in breast cancer.
- **Axillary clearance of lymph nodes:** In breast cancer surgery, axillary lymph nodes are sometimes cleared. While doing this procedure utmost care should be taken to avoid inadvertent damage of **long thoracic, thoracodorsal** and **intercostobrachial nerves** to avoid postoperative complications, *viz.* winging of scapula, pain and paraesthesia in the region, etc.
- **Axillary abscess:** *An abscess in the axilla arises from the infection and suppuration of the axillary lymph* nodes. The abscess may grow to a considerable size before the patient feels pain. The pus of the axillary abscess may track up into the neck or down into the arm if it enters into the axillary sheath or between the pectoral muscles if it breaks through the clavipectoral fascia.

  The axillary abscess is drained by giving an incision in the floor (base) of the axilla, for it being the most dependent part, midway between the anterior and posterior axillary folds nearer to the medial wall to avoid injury to the main vessels running along the anterior, posterior, and lateral walls of the axilla.
- **Boils in the axillary region:** The boils are small swollen painful red bumps, which occur due to the infection of hair follicles and sebaceous glands. The boils are common in the axillary region because this region has abundant axillary hair. As the hair are associated with hair follicles and sebaceous glands.

BRACHIAL PLEXUS

AN 10.3

The brachial plexus is the plexus of nerves formed by the **anterior primary rami** of lower four cervical and the first thoracic (i.e. C5–C8, and T1) spinal nerves and provides sensory and motor innervation of the upper limb.

N.B. AN 10.5

Variations in formation of brachial plexus: These are prefixed and postfixed brachial plexuses.

If the contribution from C4 is large and that from T1 is insignificant, it is called the ***prefixed brachial plexus***. On the other hand, if the contribution from T2 is large and that from C5 is insignificant, it is termed the ***postfixed brachial plexus***.

COMPONENTS

The brachial plexus consists of four components: (a) *roots*, (b) *trunks*, (c) *divisions*, and (d) *cords* (Fig. 4.9). The roots and trunks are located in the neck, divisions behind the clavicle, and the cords in the axilla.

Roots

The roots (*five*) consist of the anterior primary rami of the C5–T1 spinal nerves. They are located in the neck, deep to the scalenus anterior muscle.

Trunks

The trunks (*three*) are formed as follows:
The C5 and C6 roots join to form the *upper trunk*, the C7 root alone forms the *middle trunk*, and C8 and T1 roots join to form the *lower trunk*. They lie in the neck occupying the cleft between the scalenus medius behind and the scalenus anterior in front.

Divisions (Six)

Each trunk divides into anterior and posterior divisions. They lie behind the clavicle.

Cords

The cords (*three*) are formed as follows: the anterior divisions of the upper and middle trunks unite to form the *lateral cord* and the anterior division of the lower trunk continues as the *medial cord*. The posterior divisions of the three trunks unite to form the *posterior cord*.

BRANCHES (FIG. 4.10)

A. From Roots (Fig. 4.10)

1. *Long thoracic nerve/nerve of Bell* (C5–C7) which supplies serratus anterior muscle, responsible for protraction and overhead abduction of arm. For details see page 38.
2. *Dorsal scapular nerve (C5)* which supplies the rhomboids and levator scapulae. For details see page 64.

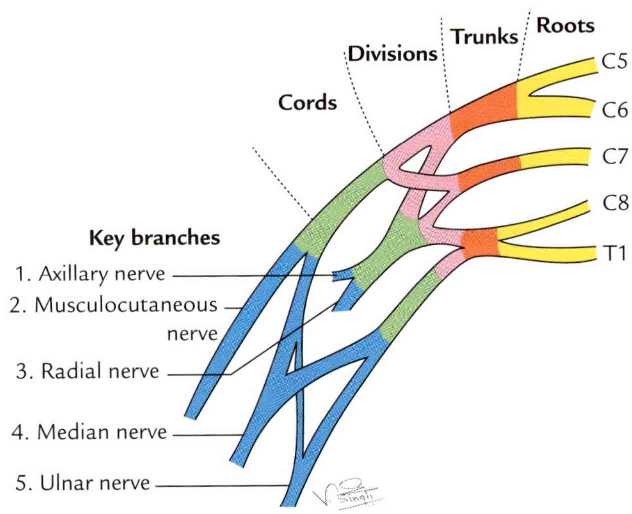

FIG. 4.9 ■ Components and key branches of the brachial plexus.

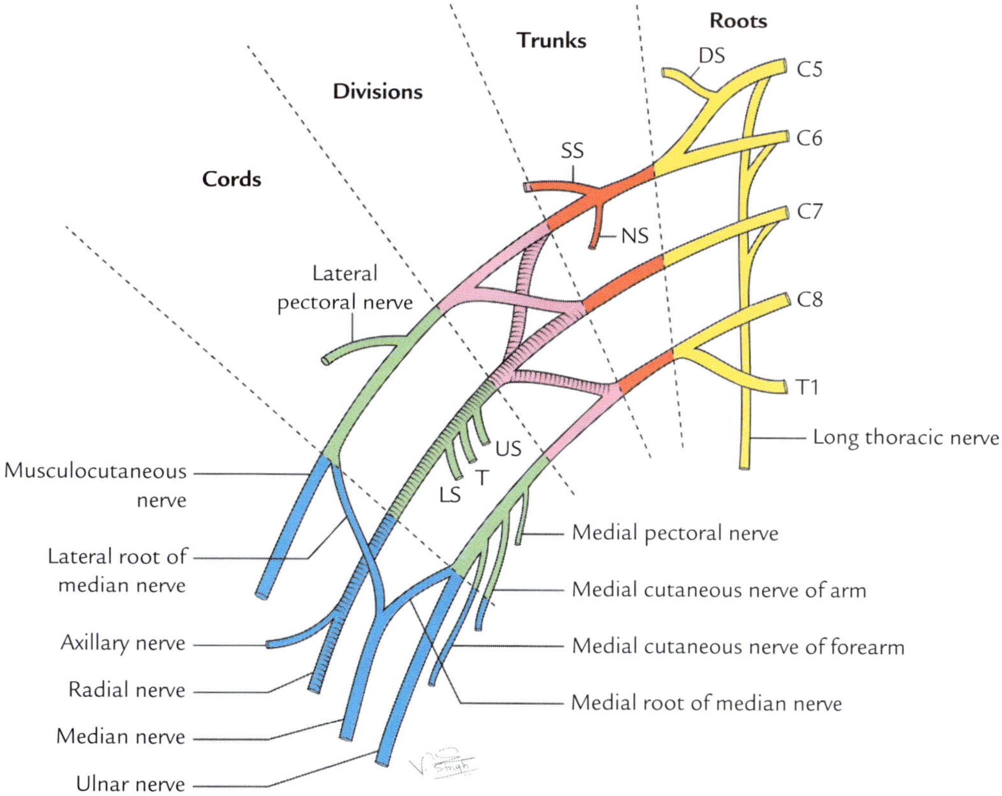

FIG. 4.10 Brachial plexus and its branches (SS = suprascapular nerve, NS = nerve to subclavius, US = upper subscapular nerve, LS = lower subscapular nerve, T = thoracodorsal nerve, DS = dorsal scapular nerve).

In addition to the *long thoracic nerve* and *dorsal scapular nerve*, branches are given by the roots to supply scalene muscles and longus colli (C5–C8), and there is contribution to the phrenic nerve (C5) which supplies diaphragm.

B. From Trunks: Only the Upper Trunk Gives Branches; Fig. 4.10

These are two in number as under:

1. *Suprascapular nerve (C5 and C6)* supplies supraspinatus and infraspinatus muscles.
2. *Nerve to subclavius (C5 and C6)* supplies a small subclavius muscle underneath clavicle.

Erb's point (Fig. 4.11)***:*** It is the region of the upper trunk of the brachial plexus where six nerves meet as follows: fifth and sixth cervical roots join to form the upper trunk, which gives off two nerves—suprascapular and nerve to subclavius—and then divides into anterior and posterior divisions.

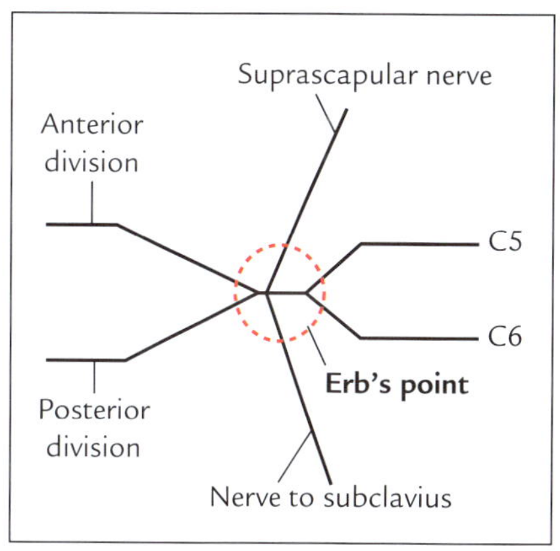

FIG. 4.11 Erb's point.

N.B.

The branches arising from the roots and trunks are the **supraclavicular branches** of the brachial plexus.

C. From Cords (Fig. 4.10)

1. From the lateral cord
   (a) **L**ateral pectoral nerve (C5–C7).
   (b) **L**ateral root of the median nerve (C5–C7).
   (c) **M**usculocutaneous nerve (C5–C7).
   Mnemonic: **LLM.**
2. From the medial cord
   (a) **M**edial pectoral nerve (C8 and T1).
   (b) **M**edial cutaneous nerve of the arm (C8 and T1).
   (c) **M**edial cutaneous nerve of the forearm (C8 and T1).
   (d) **U**lnar nerve (C7, C8, and T1).
   (e) **M**edial root of the median nerve (C8 and T1).
   Mnemonic: **M**ake **M**any **M**oves **U**sing **M**uscles.
3. From the posterior cord
   (a) **R**adial nerve (C5–C8 and T1).
   (b) **A**xillary nerve (C5 and C6).

(c) Thoracodorsal nerve/nerve to latissimus dorsi (C6–C8).
(d) Upper **S**ubscapular nerve (C5 and C6).
(e) Lower **S**ubscapular nerve (C5 and C6).
Mnemonic: **RATS** or **STAR**

The cords of brachial plexus are described in the following text.

Branches of Lateral Cord

1. **Lateral pectoral nerve** supplies both pectoralis major and minor muscles.
2. **Lateral root of median nerve** joins medial root of median nerve to form **median nerve**. The median nerve is one of three main nerves of the upper limb. It is described in detail on page 99.
3. **Musculocutaneous nerve** is the nerve of muscles on the front of arm, hence, described in detail on page 98–100.

Branches of Medial Cord

1. **Medial pectoral nerve** supplies both pectoralis minor and pectoralis major muscles.
2. **Medial cutaneous nerve of arm** provides sensory innervation to the medial side of the arm. Note: It is the smallest and most medial branch of brachial plexus.
3. **Medial cutaneous nerve of forearm** provides sensory innervation to the medial side of forearm.
4. **Ulnar nerve** is one of the main nerves of upper limb. It is described in detail on page 99.
5. **Medial root median nerve** joins lateral root of median to form median nerve.

Branches of Posterior Cord

1. **Upper subscapular nerve** supplies subscapular muscle.
2. **Nerve to latissimus dorsi**/thoracodorsal nerve supplies latissimus dorsi muscle.

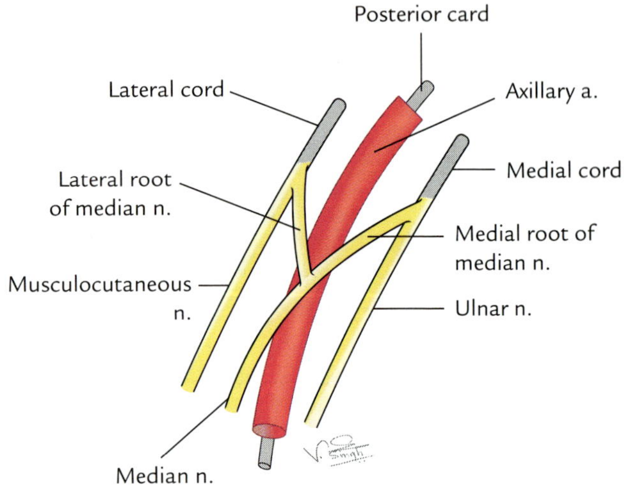

FIG. 4.12 ■ **'M'** of brachial plexus. Also note the relationship of brachial plexus to axillary artery.

3. **Lower subscapular nerve** supplies subscapularis and teres major muscles.
4. **Axillary nerve** supplies deltoid and teres minor muscles.
5. **Radial nerve** is the largest of three main nerves of the upper limb. For details see Chapter 13.

N.B.

'M' of brachial plexus (Fig. 4.12): The lateral root of lateral cord and medial root of medial cord join to form median nerve. All these together form a shape of letter 'M' usually superficial to axillary artery. The three arms of 'M' in brachial plexus represents
a. Musculocutaneous nerve
b. Median nerve
c. Ulnar nerve

CLINICAL CORRELATION AN10.6

- **Lesions of the brachial plexus:** For understanding the effects of the lesions of the brachial plexus, the student will find it helpful to know the spinal segments which control the various movements of the upper limb:
  - *Adduction of the shoulder* is controlled by the C5 segment.
  - *Abduction of the shoulder* is controlled by the C6 and C7 segments.
  - *Flexion of the elbow* is controlled by the C5 and C6 segments.
  - *Extension of the elbow* is controlled by the C6 and C7 segments.
  - *Flexion of the wrist and fingers* is controlled by the C8 and T1 segments.

The important lesions of the brachial plexus are as follows:

(a) ***Erb's paralysis (upper plexus injury)***: It is caused by the excessive increase in the angle between the head and the shoulder, which may occur by fall from the back of a horse and landing on the shoulder or traction of the arm during the birth of a child (Fig. 4.13). This involves upper trunk (C5 and C6 roots) and leads to a typical deformity of the limb called *policeman's tip hand/porter's tip hand/waiter's tip hand.* In this deformity, the arm hangs by the side, adducted and medially rotated, and the forearm is extended and pronated (Fig. 4.14). The detailed account of the clinical features of Erb's paralysis is as follows:
  - *Adduction of the arm* due to the paralysis deltoid muscle.
  - *Medial rotation of the arm* due to paralysis supraspinatus, infraspinatus, and teres minor muscles.
  - *Extension of the elbow* due to the paralysis of biceps brachii.
  - *Pronation of the forearm* due to the paralysis of biceps brachii.
  - Loss of sensation (minimal) along the outer aspect of arm due to involvement of roots of C5, C6 spinal nerves.

(b) ***Klumpke's paralysis (lower plexus injury)***: It is caused by the hyperabduction of the arm, which may occur when one falls on an outstretched hand or an arm is pulled into machinery or during delivery (extended arm in a breech presentation) (Fig. 4.15). The nerve roots involved in this injury are C8 and T1 and sometimes C7. The clinical features of Klumpke's paralysis are as follows:
  - *Claw hand* due to the paralysis of the flexors of the wrist and fingers (C6–C8), and all intrinsic muscles of the hand (C8 and T1).

- Loss of sensations along the medial border of the forearm and hand (T1).
- *Horner's syndrome* (characterized by partial ptosis, miosis, anhydrosis, and enophthalmos) due to the involvement of sympathetic fibres supplying the head and neck, which leave the spinal cord through T1.

N.B.

Horner's syndrome occurs only if T1 is injured proximal to white ramus communicates to the first thoracic sympathetic ganglion.

The important features of Erb's and Klumpke's paralysis are enumerated in Table 4.3.

- **Surgical approach to axilla:** The axilla is approached surgically through the skin of the floor of the axilla for the excision of axillary lymph nodes to treat breast cancer. The structures at risk during this procedure are: (a) intercostobrachial nerve, (b) long thoracic nerve, (c) thoracodorsal nerve, and (d) thoracodorsal artery. Efforts should be made to safeguard the aforementioned structures.

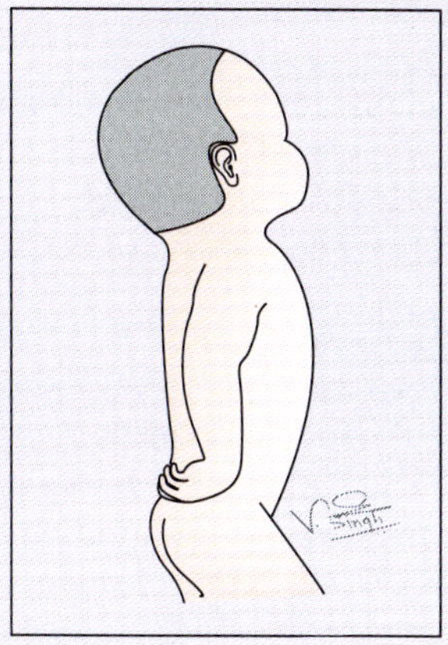

FIG. 4.14 Policeman receiving a tip position of the upper limb in Erb's paralysis.

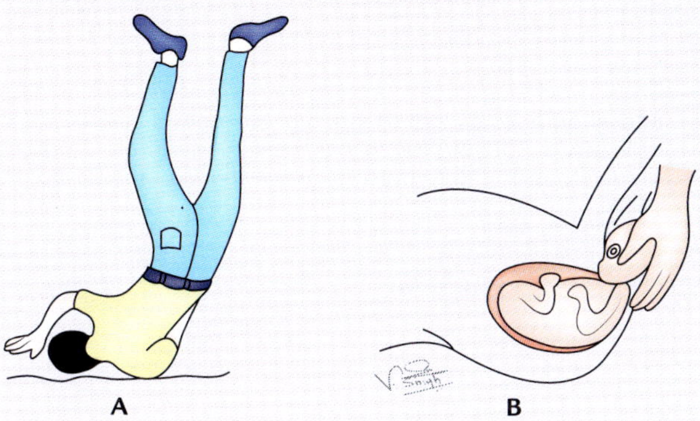

FIG. 4.13 Injury of the upper brachial plexus leading to the excessive increase in the angle between the head and shoulder. (**A**) Fall from the height and landing on a shoulder and (**B**) traction of the arm and the hyperextension of the neck.

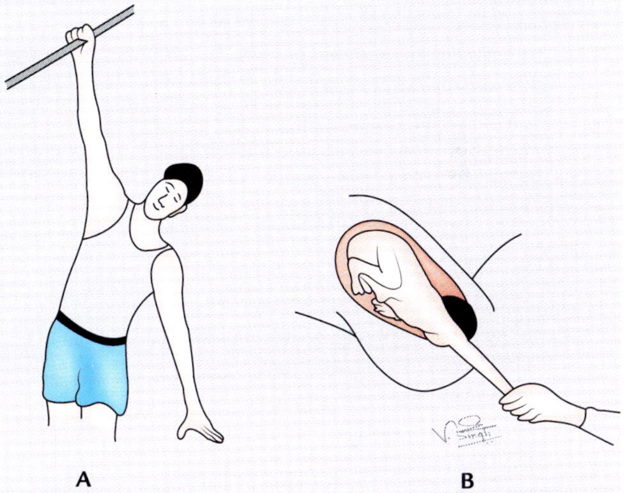

FIG. 4.15 Injury of the lower brachial plexus leading to the excessive increase in the angle between the trunk and shoulder. (**A**) Sudden upward pull of the arm and (**B**) arm pulled during delivery.

TABLE 4.3 **Features of Erb's and Klumpke's paralysis**

	Erb's paralysis	Klumpke's paralysis
Nerve roots involved	C5 and C6	C8 and T1
Muscles paralyzed	Deltoid, supraspinatus, infraspinatus, biceps brachii, brachialis, brachioradialis, supinator, and extensor carpi radialis longus	All intrinsic muscles of the hand
Position of the upper limb/hand	Policeman's tip/porter's tip/waiter's tip position	Claw hand
Sensory loss (sometimes)	Along the outer aspect of the arm	Along the medial border of the forearm and hand
Autonomic signs	Absent	Present (Horner's syndrome)

Golden Facts to Remember

• Most dependent part of the axilla	Floor of the axilla
• Axillary lymph node group receiving most of the lymph from the breast	Anterior or pectoral group
• Largest branch of the brachial plexus	Radial nerve
• Kuntz's nerve	Communicating branch between the T1 and T2 nerves, which carry sympathetic fibres from the third thoracic ganglion to the upper limb via the T2 nerve
• Cervicoaxillary canal	Apex of the axilla through which the axillary artery and brachial plexus enter the axilla from the root of the neck
• Five key nerves of the upper limb (terminal branches of brachial plexus)	(a) Radial nerve (b) Median nerve (c) Ulnar nerve (d) Axillary nerve (e) Musculocutaneous nerve
• Largest branch of axillary artery	Subscapular artery

CLINICAL CASE STUDY

A baby boy was delivered in a hospital by an obstetrician by pulling the baby's head using forceps (*forceps delivery*). Two weeks later, the parents took the baby to the paediatrician for check-up. While examining the baby, the paediatrician found that the baby's right arm was medially rotated and adducted, while his forearm was extended and pronated. He also noticed sensory loss on the lateral aspect of the right upper limb. He was diagnosed as a case of **Erb's paralysis**.

Questions

1. Name the position of the upper limb of the baby observed by the paediatrician.
2. Name the clinical condition responsible for this position of upper limb.
3. Name the site of lesion and the cause that produced this condition.
4. What is the cause of sensory loss in the upper limb?

Answers

1. Policeman's tip hand/Porter's tip hand.
2. Erb's paralysis.
3. Erb's point due to the excessive separation of the neck and shoulder caused by pulling the baby's head during delivery.
4. Involvement of the ventral root of the C5 and C6 spinal nerves.

Back of the Body and Scapular Region

CHAPTER 5

SPECIFIC LEARNING OBJECTIVES

After studying this chapter, the student should be able to:

- Describe the origin, insertion, nerve supply, and actions of trapezius and latissimus dorsi muscles. AN 10.8
- The mid-point on the lateral aspect of deltoid region is preferred site for intramuscular injection. Give its anatomical basis.
- Explain the anatomical basis of injury to axillary nerve during intramuscular injections in deltoid muscle. AN 10.13
- Write a short note on: (a) triangle of auscultation and (b) rotator cuff/musculotendinous cuff. AN 10.9
- Describe the boundaries and structures passing through the quadrangular, upper, and lower triangular subscapular spaces.
- Describe and identify the deltoid and rotator cuff muscles. AN 10.10

The superficial structures on the back of the body are studied with the upper limb because the shoulder girdle is attached posteriorly with the axial skeleton by a number of muscles. These muscles are called **posterior axio-appendicular muscles**. They play an important role in the movements of the scapula. Further removal of the scapula in malignant disease (e.g. *fibrosarcoma*) requires detailed knowledge of the muscles, nerves, and vessels on the back.

SURFACE LANDMARKS (FIG. 5.1) AN 13.6

1. **Scapula (shoulder blade)** is the most important surface landmark on the back. It is placed at a tangent on the posterolateral aspect of the rib cage. Vertically, it extends from second to seventh rib. Although it is thickly covered by the muscles, still most of its outline can be felt in the living individual:
   (a) *Acromion process* can be easily felt at the top of the shoulder.
   (b) *Crest of the spine of the scapula* runs medially and slightly downwards from the acromion to the medial border of the scapula, hence it can be easily palpated by finger drawn along it.
   (c) *Medial border* can be traced upwards to the superior angle and downwards to *the inferior angle. The superior angle of the scapula lies opposite the spine of T2 vertebra, the root of the spine lies at the level of T3 vertebra and the inferior angle* of the scapula lies at the level of T7 vertebra.

N.B.

The scapula is freely mobile as about 15 muscles are attached to its processes and fossae. The two scapulae are drawn apart when the arms are folded across the chest. The medial borders of the two scapulae are close to the midline when shoulders are drawn back.

2. **Eighth rib** is palpable, immediately inferior to the inferior angle of the scapula. The lower ribs can be counted from it.
3. **Twelfth rib** can be palpated if it projects beyond the lateral margin of the erector spinae muscle, about 3 cm above the iliac crest.
4. **Iliac crest** is felt as a curved bony ridge below the waist. When traced forwards and backwards, it ends as *anterior* and *posterior superior iliac spines*, respectively. The posterior superior iliac spine may be felt in shallow dimple of skin above the buttock, about 5 cm from the median line.
5. **Sacrum**—the back of sacrum lies between the right and left dimples (vide supra) and its spines can be palpated in the median plane.
6. **Coccyx** is a slightly movable bone and may be felt deep between the buttocks in the *natal cleft*.
7. **Spines of vertebrae** lie in the median furrow of the back and may be felt. The spine of seventh cervical vertebra (*vertebra prominens*) is readily felt at the root of the neck at the lower end of nuchal furrow. The approximate levels of other spines are given in Table 5.1.
8. **External occipital protuberance and superior nuchal lines**—the *external occipital protuberance* is a bony projection felt in the midline on the back of the head. The curved bony ridge extending laterally on each side from external occipital protuberance is the

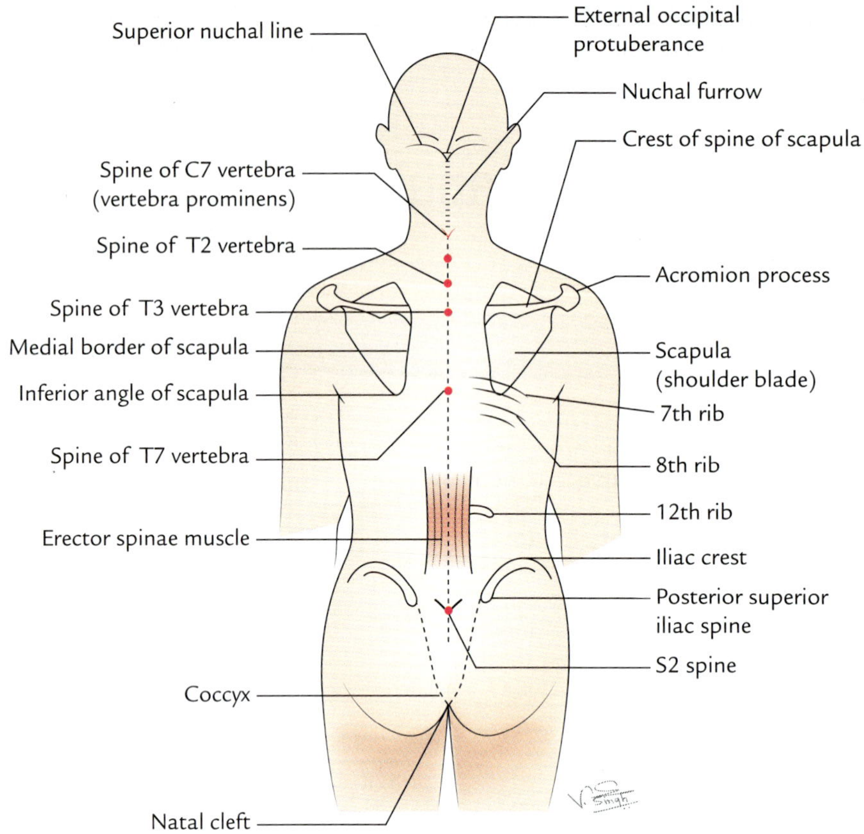

FIG. 5.1 ■ Surface landmarks on the back of the body.

superior nuchal line. These bony features demarcate the junction between the head and neck posteriorly.

9. **Nuchal groove/furrow** is the median furrow, which extends from external occipital protuberance to the spine of C7 vertebra.
10. **Ligamentum nuchae** is the median fibrous partition on the back of neck, which extends from external occipital protuberance to the spine of C7 vertebra and separates the short cervical spines from the skin.

TABLE 5.1 Approximate levels of some spines on the back of the body

Vertebral spine	Level
T2	Superior angle of the scapula
T3	Where crest of spine of the scapula meets its medial border
T7	Inferior angle of the scapula
L4	Highest point of iliac crest
S2	Posterior-superior iliac spine

CUTANEOUS NERVES (FIG. 5.2)

The cutaneous nerves on the back are derived from the posterior rami of the spinal nerves. Each primary ramus divides into medial and lateral branches:

1. Up to T6, the cutaneous innervation is provided by medial branches, which emerge close to the median plane.

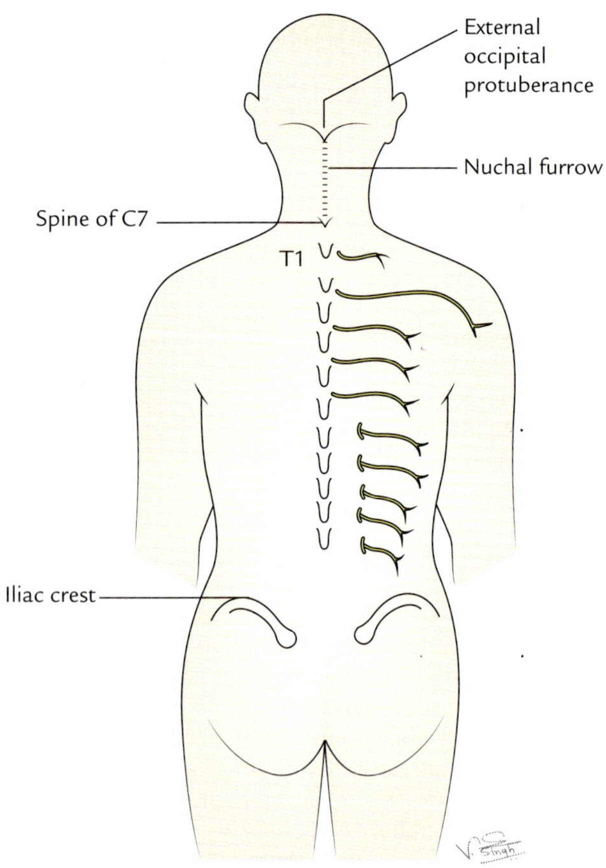

FIG. 5.2 ■ Cutaneous nerves of the back.

2. Below T6, the cutaneous innervation is provided by lateral branches, which emerge in line with the lateral edge of the erector spinae muscle.

The cutaneous branches of upper three lumbar nerves emerge a short distance above the iliac crest and turn down over it to supply the skin of the gluteal region.

N.B.

The posterior rami of C1, C7, C8, L4, and L5 do not give any cutaneous branches.

CUTANEOUS ARTERIES

The arteries which accompany the cutaneous nerves on the back of body in the thoracic and lumbar regions are the dorsal branches of the posterior intercostal and lumbar arteries, respectively.

POSTERIOR AXIO-APPENDICULAR MUSCLES (MUSCLES CONNECTING SCAPULA WITH THE VERTEBRAL COLUMN)

The muscles that attach the scapula to the back of the trunk (vertebral column) are arranged in two layers (two in the superficial layer and three in the deep layer).

1. Superficial layer of the muscles (Fig. 5.3)
   (a) Trapezius
   (b) Latissimus dorsi
2. Deep layer of the muscles
   (a) Levator scapulae
   (b) Rhomboideus major
   (c) Rhomboideus minor

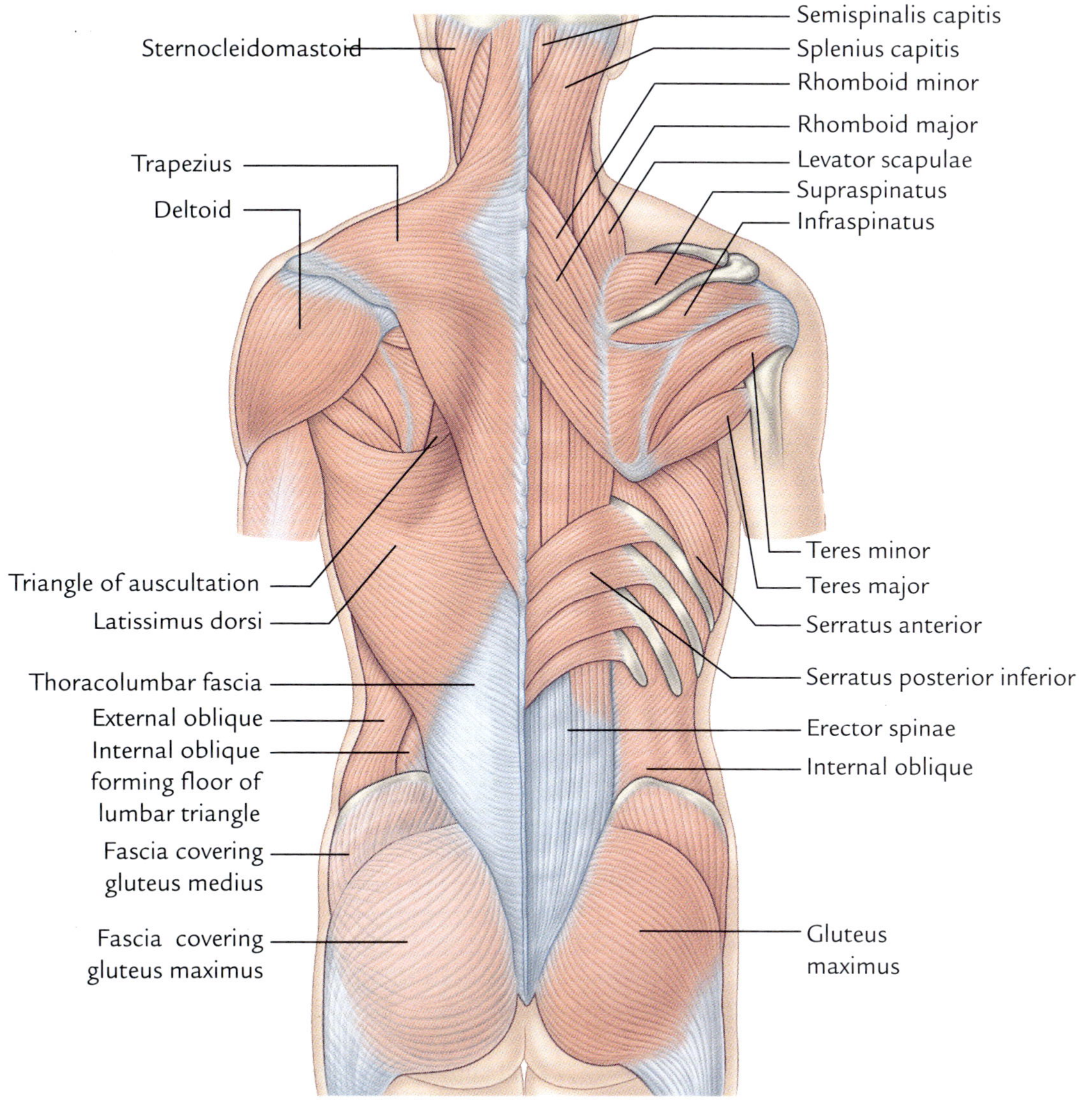

FIG. 5.3 Superficial muscles of the back. (*Source: Gray's Anatomy: The Anatomical Basis of Clinical Practice*, Forty Second edition: Susan Standring, Fig. 46.71, Elsevier Ltd. 2021.)

SUPERFICIAL POSTERIOR AXIO-APPENDICULAR MUSCLES

Trapezius Muscle (Fig. 5.4) AN 10.8

The trapezius is a flat triangular muscle on the back of the neck and the thorax. The muscles of two sides lie side by side in the midline and together form a diamond shape/trapezoid shape, hence the name trapezius.

Origin

It arises from:

(a) medial third of the superior nuchal line,
(b) external occipital protuberance,
(c) ligamentum nuchae,
(d) spine of seventh cervical vertebra, and
(e) spines of all thoracic vertebrae.

Insertion

The insertion occurs as follows:

1. The **superior fibres** runs downwards and laterally to be inserted on to the posterior border of the lateral third of the clavicle.
2. The **middle fibres** proceed horizontally to be inserted on to the medial margin of the acromion and upper lip of the crest of the spine of the scapula.

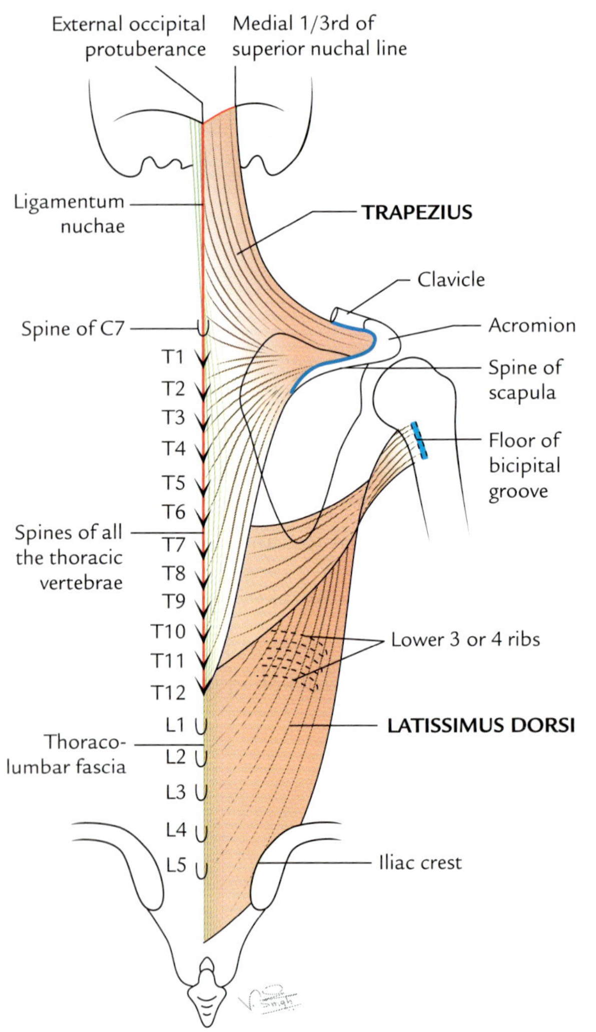

FIG. 5.4 ■ Origin and insertion of the trapezius and latissimus dorsi muscles.

3. The **lower fibres** pass upward and laterally into an aponeurosis to be inserted on to the deltoid tubercle—at apex of a triangular area at the medial end of spine.

Nerve supply

It is by:

(a) spinal part of the accessory nerve (provides motor supply), and
(b) ventral rami of C3 and C4 (carry proprioceptive sensations).

Actions

1. The upper fibres of trapezius along with levator scapulae elevate the scapula as in ***shrugging the shoulder.***
2. The middle fibres of trapezius along with rhomboids retract the scapula as in *bracing back the shoulder.*
3. The lower fibres of trapezius depress the medial part of the spine of the scapula.
4. Acting with serratus anterior, the trapezius rotates the scapula upwards so that the arm can be abducted beyond 90°.

Clinical testing AN 13.7

Palpate the trapezius while the shoulder is shrugged against the resistance. Inability to shrug (to raise) the shoulder is suggestive of muscle weakness.

Latissimus Dorsi (Latissimus = Widest, Dorsi = Back; Fig. 5.4) AN 10.8

The latissimus dorsi is a wide, flat, triangular muscle on the back (lumbar region and lower thorax). It is mostly superficial except a small portion, covered posteriorly by the lower part of trapezius.

Origin

It arises from:

(a) spines of lower six thoracic vertebrae anterior to the trapezius, by tendinous fibres,
(b) posterior lamina of thoraco-lumbar fascia (by which it is attached to the spines of lumbar and sacral vertebrae) by tendinous fibres,
(c) outer lip of the posterior part of the iliac crest by muscular slips,
(d) lower three or four ribs by fleshy slips,
(e) dorsal surface of inferior angle of the scapula.

Insertion

From its extensive origin, the fibres pass laterally with different degrees of obliquity (the upper fibres are nearly horizontal, the middle are oblique, and lower are almost vertical) to form a sheet that overlaps the inferior angle of the scapula. This sheet curves around the inferolateral border of the teres major to gain its anterior surface. Here it ends as flattened tendon, which is inserted into the floor of intertubercular sulcus (bicipital groove) of the humerus.

The latissimus dorsi and teres major together form the **posterior axillary fold**.

Nerve supply

The latissimus dorsi is supplied by *thoraco-dorsal nerve* (C6, C7, and C8) from the posterior cord of the brachial plexus.

Actions

1. Latissimus dorsi is active in adduction, extension, and rotation, especially medial rotation of the humerus.
2. It pulls up the trunk upwards and forwards during climbing. This action is in conjunction with the pectoralis major muscle.
3. It assists backward swinging of the arm during walking.
4. It takes part in all violent expiratory efforts.

N.B.

Because of its attachment on the ilium and sacrum, the latissimus dorsi is able to elevate the pelvis if the arms are stabilized. This action occurs when the arms are stabilized on crutch-handles. This is a very good example of '*reversal of muscle action*' where proximal attachment (i.e. *origin*) pulls the distal attachment (i.e. *insertion*).

Clinical testing

AN 13.7

The posterior axillary fold becomes accentuated when a 90° abducted arm is adducted against the resistance or when patient coughs violently.

CLINICAL CORRELATION

- **Musculocutaneous flap of latissimus dorsi:** The latissimus dorsi is supplied by a *single dominant vascular pedicle* formed by the *thoraco-dorsal artery*, a continuation of the subscapular artery. This artery and its accompanying venae comitantes and *thoraco-dorsal nerve* descend in the posterior wall of axilla and enter the costal surface of the muscle at a single neuro-vascular hilum about 1–4 cm medial to the lateral border of the muscle. The presence of single dominant vascular pedicle provides the anatomical basis for raising the muscle alone, or along with the overlying skin in the form of *musculocutaneous flap*. The musculocutaneous flap of latissimus dorsi is often used in reconstructing a breast following mastectomy.
- **Conditioning of latissimus dorsi to act as a cardiac muscle:** The latissimus dorsi if conditioned with pulsated electrical impulses, starts functioning like a cardiac muscle, that is it will be nonfatigable and use oxygen at a steady pace. Thus following conditioning, the latissimus dorsi can be used as an autotransplant to repair a surgically removed portion of heart. The procedure involves detaching the latissimus dorsi from its vertebral origin keeping the neurovascular pedicle intact and slipping it into the pericardial cavity, where it is wrapped around the heart like a towel. A pacemaker is required to provide the continuous rhythmic contractions.

DEEP POSTERIOR AXIO-APPENDICULAR MUSCLES (FIG. 5.5)

Levator Scapulae

Origin

The levator scapula is a slender muscle. It arises by tendinous slips from

(a) transverse processes of atlas and axis vertebrae, and
(b) posterior tubercles of the transverse processes of the third and fourth cervical vertebrae.

Insertion

The four discrete slips of the muscles fibres descend diagonally towards the scapula to be inserted on to the upper part of its medial border between superior angle and the triangular smooth surface at the medial end of the scapular spine.

Nerve supply

The levator scapulae is innervated by:

(a) direct branches of C3 and C4 spinal nerves, and
(b) C5 spinal nerve through the dorsal scapular nerve.

Action

The levator scapulae elevate and steady the scapula during movements of the arm.

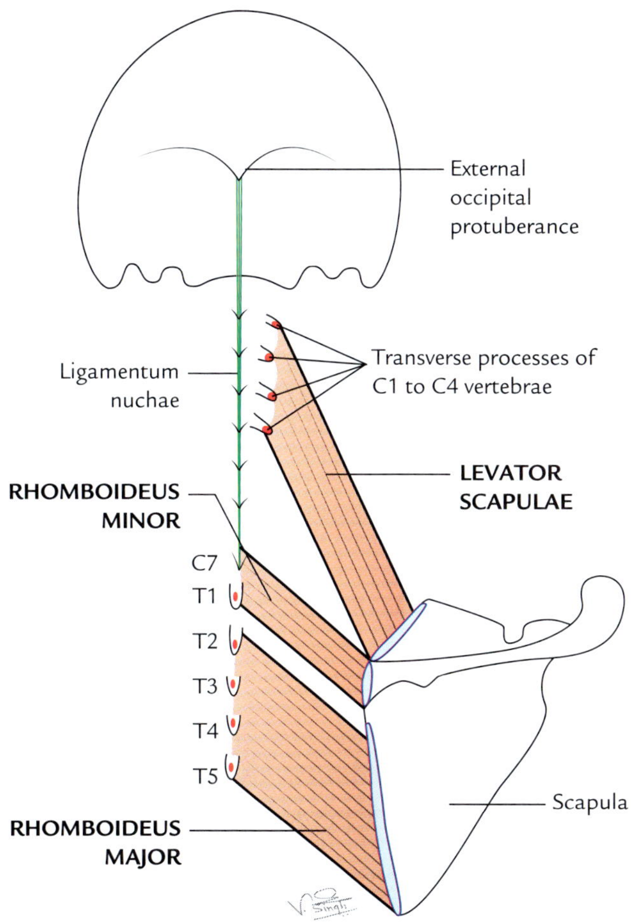

FIG. 5.5 Origin and insertion of the levator scapulae rhomboideus major and rhomboideus minor muscles.

Rhomboideus Minor

Origin

The rhomboideus minor is a thick cylindrical muscle, which arises from:

(a) lower part of the ligamentum nuchae, and
(b) spines of the seventh cervical and first thoracic vertebrae.

Insertion

It is inserted on to the base of triangular area at the root of the spine of the scapula.

Rhomboideus Major

Origin

The thin flat rhomboideus major muscle is about two times wider than the rhomboideus minor. It arises from spine of T2, T3, T4, and T5 vertebrae and intervening supraspinous ligaments.

Insertion

The fibres run downwards and laterally to be inserted on the medial border of the scapula between the root of the spine and inferior angle of the scapula.

Nerve supply of the rhomboids

Both the rhomboideus major and minor are supplied by the dorsal scapular nerve (C5).

Actions of the rhomboids

Both the rhomboideus major and minor retract the scapula as in squaring the shoulders.

Clinical testing of the rhomboids

The rhomboids can be palpated along the medial borders of the scapulae deep to trapezius on bracing the shoulder back against the resistance.

Dorsal scapular nerve (nerve to rhomboids)

The dorsal scapular nerve arises from C5 spinal nerve in the root of neck. The nerve pierces the scalenus medius and comes to lie on the anterior surface of the levator scapulae in the posterior triangle of the neck. Here it is accompanied by deep branch of the transverse cervical artery (or dorsal scapular artery). Then the dorsal scapular nerve and artery descend to the back along the anterior surface of the levator scapulae. [Note: The spinal accessory nerve and superficial branch of the transverse cervical artery runs on the posterior surface of the levator scapulae (Fig. 5.6)].

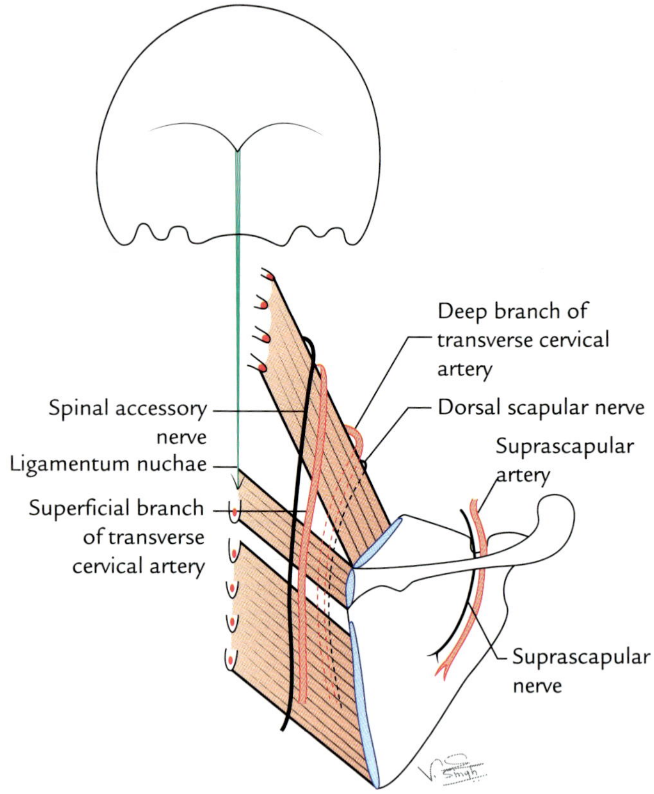

FIG. 5.6 ■ Nerves and vessels related to deep posterior axio-appendicular muscles.

CLINICAL CORRELATION AN 10.9

Triangle of auscultation (Fig. 5.7): It is small triangular gap in the musculature on the back of the thorax near the inferior angle of the scapula. Its boundaries are:

- Superior horizontal border of the latissimus dorsi.
- Medial border of the scapula.
- Inferolateral border of the trapezius.

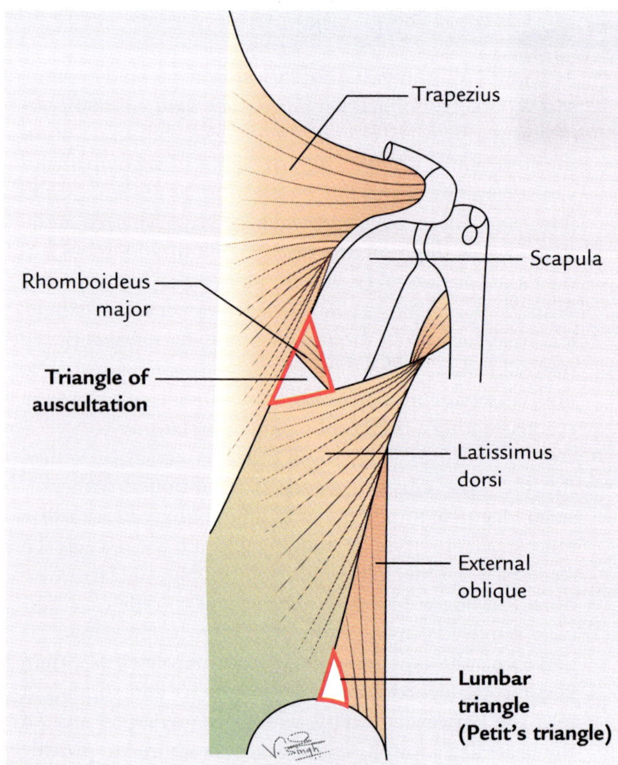

FIG. 5.7 ■ Triangle of auscultation.

The floor *of this triangle* is formed by, sixth and seventh ribs and the sixth intercostal space.

The upper part of the lower lobe of the lung lies deep to this triangle. When the scapulae are drawn anteriorly by folding the arm across the chest and the trunk is flexed, this triangle enlarges and becomes more subcutaneous. Now the lower lobe of the lung can be auscultated by putting the stethoscope in this region.

The sounds are not muffled by the muscles of back in this area.

The origin, insertion, nerve supply, and actions of the muscles, which connect scapula with the vertebral column are summarized in Table 5.2.

SCAPULAR REGION

The **scapular region includes** parts/structures around the scapula. The following text deals with the scapulohumeral muscles, intermuscular spaces in the subscapular region, nerve and vessels and anastomosis around the scapula.

SCAPULOHUMERAL MUSCLES

The **scapulohumeral muscles** are relatively short muscles, which pass from scapula to the humerus and act on the glenohumeral joint (shoulder joint proper). They are also called **intrinsic shoulder muscles**. There are six in number as follows:

1. Deltoid
2. Supraspinatus
3. Infraspinatus
4. Teres minor
5. Teres major
6. Subscapularis

Deltoid (Fig. 5.8) AN 10.10

The deltoid is a '*three-in-one muscle*'. It is thick, powerful, and curved triangular muscle covering the shoulder and forming its rounded contour. The deltoid is shaped like the inverted Greek letter Delta (δ), hence its name deltoid. The deltoid muscle is divided into three parts: (a) anterior unipennate part, (b) posterior unipennate part, and (c) middle multipennate part.

Origin

The deltoid has a V-shaped origin from the subcutaneous bony arch formed by (a) lateral one-third of clavicle, (b) acromion process, and (c) crest of spine of the scapula. The details are as under:

1. The *anterior unipennate part*—arises from the upper surface and anterior border of the lateral third of the clavicle.
2. The *middle multipennate part*—arises from the lateral margin and upper surface of the acromion.
3. The *posterior unipennate part*—arises from the lower lip of the crest of the spine of the scapula.

TABLE 5.2 Origin, insertion, nerve supply, and actions of the muscles connecting scapula with the vertebral column

Muscle	Origin	Insertion	Nerve supply	Actions
Trapezius	• Medial one-third of superior nuchal line • Ligamentum nuchae • External occipital protuberance • Spines of C7–T12 vertebrae	• Lateral one-third of clavicle • Medial margin of acromion • Superior margin of crest of spine of the scapula	• Spinal accessory (motor) • C3, C4 spinal nerves (proprioceptive)	• Upper fibres elevates the scapula • Middle fibres retract the scapula • Lower fibres depress the scapula
Latissimus dorsi	• Spines of T7–T12 vertebrae • Thoraco-lumbar fascia • Iliac crest • Lower three or four ribs • Inferior angle of the scapula	Floor of intertubercular sulcus of the humerus	Thoraco-dorsal nerve (C6, C7, C8)	• Adduction • Extension and medial rotation of the arm • Raises body towards arm as in climbing
Levator scapulae	Transverse processes of C1–C4 vertebrae	Medial border of the scapula between the superior angle and root of spine	• Dorsal scapular nerve (C5) • C3 and C4 spinal nerves (proprioceptive)	Elevation and medial rotation of the scapula and tilts its glenoid cavity inferiorly
Rhomboideus minor	• Lower part of the ligamentum nuchae • Spines of C7 and T1 vertebrae	Base of triangular area at the root of spine of the scapula	Dorsal scapular nerve (C5)	Retraction and elevation of the scapula
Rhomboideus major	Spines of T2–T5 vertebrae	Medial border of the scapula from root of spine to the inferior angle	Dorsal scapular nerve (C5)	Retraction, medial rotation, and elevation of the scapula

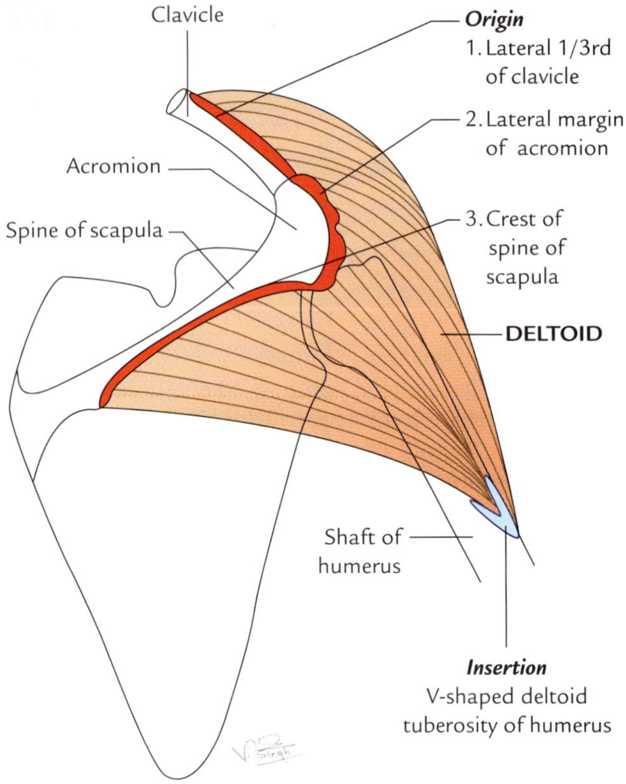

FIG. 5.8 ■ Origin and insertion of the deltoid muscle.

Insertion

The fibres converge inferiorly to form a short thick tendon, which is inserted onto the V-shaped deltoid tuberosity/tubercle on the lateral aspect of the midshaft of the humerus.

N.B.

The fibres of multipennate middle part arise from four septa that are attached above to the acromion. These fibres converge onto the three septa of insertion, which are attached to the deltoid tuberosity. Due to multipennate arrangement, the middle acromial part of the deltoid is the strongest part (Fig. 5.9).

Nerve supply

The deltoid is supplied by the axillary nerve (C5 and C6).

Actions

1. The anterior (clavicular) fibres are flexors and medial rotators of the arm.
2. The posterior (spinous) fibres are the extensors and lateral rotators of the arm.
3. The middle (acromial) fibres are the strong abductor of the arm from 15° to 90°.

Middle (acromial) fibres cannot abduct the arm from 0° to 15° when the arm is by the side of body because its vertical pull corresponds to the long axis of the arm.

N.B.

The deltoid muscle is like three muscles in one: the anterior fibres flex the arm, middle fibres abduct the arm, and posterior fibres extend the arm.

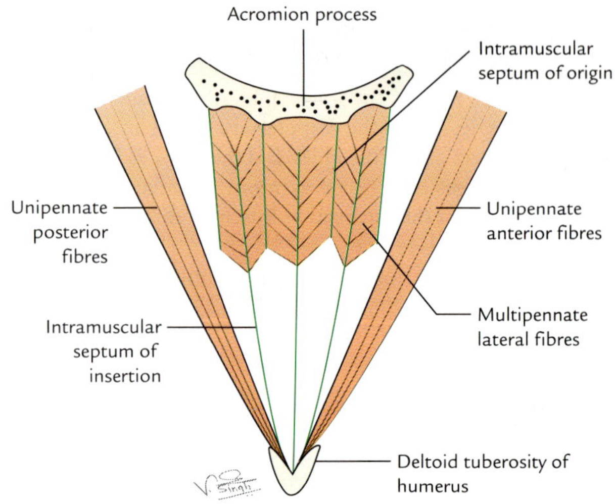

FIG. 5.9 ■ Architecture of the deltoid muscle.

Clinical testing

The deltoid can be easily seen and felt to contract when the arm is abducted against resistance.

CLINICAL CORRELATION AN 10.13

Anatomical basis of injury to axillary nerve during intramuscular injection in deltoid (Fig. 5.10): The intramuscular injections should be given in the thick middle part on the lateral aspect of deltoid, 2.5–5 cm below the acromion process. To locate this area, lay three fingers across the deltoid muscle, below the acromion process. This is essential to avoid injury to the axillary nerve, which winds around the surgical neck of the humerus deep to deltoid muscle.

If intramuscular injection is given in the lower part of deltoid, the axillary nerve may be damaged.

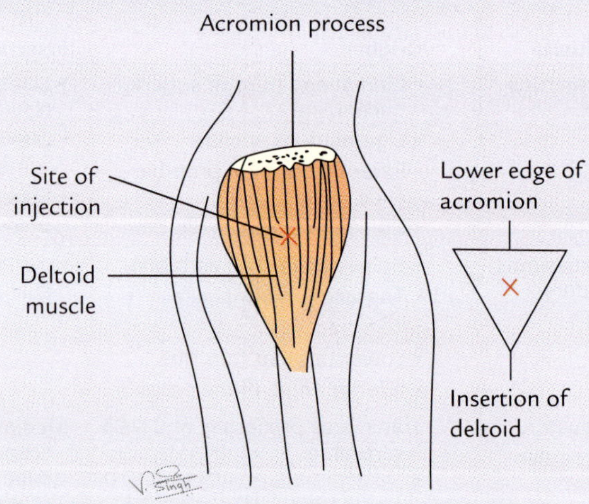

FIG. 5.10 ■ The site for intramuscular injection in the deltoid muscle. The injection is given in the center of a triangle (figure on the right side), formed by the lower edge of the acromion and insertion of the deltoid muscle.

N.B.

Earlier it was thought that the intramuscular injection is given in the **upper and outer quadrant of the deltoid region**.

Structures under cover of deltoid

- **Bones:** Upper end of the humerus and coracoid process.
- **Joints and ligaments:** Shoulder (glenohumeral) joint and coracoacromial ligament.
- **Bursae around the shoulder joint:** Subscapular, subacromial/subdeltoid, and infraspinatus (Fig. 6.6).
- **Muscles:**
  (a) Insertions of pectoralis minor, pectoralis major, teres major, latissimus dorsi, subscapularis, supraspinatus, infraspinatus, and teres minor.
  (b) Origins of long head of biceps, short head of biceps, coracobrachialis, long and lateral heads of triceps.
- **Vessels:** Anterior and posterior circumflex humeral artery and vein.
- **Nerves:** Axillary nerve.
- **Spaces:** Quadrangular and triangular subscapular intermuscular spaces (Fig. 5.16).

Supraspinatus (Fig. 5.11)

Origin

Supraspinatus arises from medial two-thirds of the supraspinous fossa of the scapula.

Insertion

The fibres pass forward and converge under the acromion, into a tendon, which crosses above the shoulder joint and is inserted on to the superior facet on the greater tubercle of the humerus.

Nerve supply

Supraspinatus is supplied by the *suprascapular nerve* (C5 and C6).

Actions

Supraspinatus initiates the abduction of shoulder. It is responsible for first 15° of abduction of the shoulder and thus assists the deltoid in carrying abduction thereafter, that is from 15° to 90°.

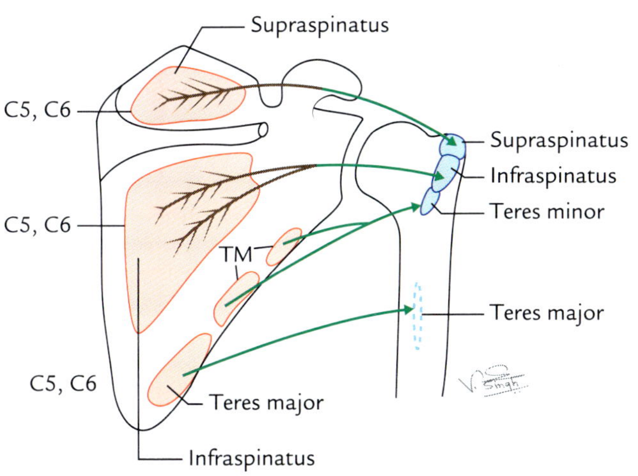

FIG. 5.11 Origin and insertion of the supraspinatus, infraspinatus, teres minor, and teres major muscles (TM = teres minor).

Clinical testing

The supraspinatus can be palpated deep to the trapezius and above the spine of the scapula when the arm is abducted against the resistance.

> **CLINICAL CORRELATION**
>
> **Rupture of supraspinatus tendon:** It is a common soft tissue injury in the shoulder region. The patient with ruptured supraspinatus tendon when asked to raise his hand above the head on the affected side, he will first tilt his body on the affected side so that arm swings away from the body leading to an initial abduction of 15° or he will slightly (about 15°) raise the affected arm by the hand of the healthy side-a common '*trick-device*' learned by the patients with ruptured supraspinatus tendon.

Infraspinatus (Fig. 5.11)

It is a thick triangular muscle, which occupies most of the infraspinous fossa.

Origin

It arises from the medial two-thirds of the fossa by tendinous fibres from ridges on its surface.

Insertion

Its fibres converge to form a tendon, which passes across the posterior aspect of the shoulder joint to be inserted on to the middle facet of the greater tubercle of the humerus.

Nerve supply

Infraspinatus is supplied by the *suprascapular nerve* (C5 and C6).

Action

Infraspinatus is the lateral rotator of the humerus.

Clinical testing

The infraspinatus can be palpated inferior to the spine of the scapula when the arm is laterally rotated against the resistance.

Teres Minor (Fig. 5.11)

Origin

This narrow elongated muscle arises from posterior aspect of the lateral border of the scapula.

Insertion

The fibres run upwards and laterally across the shoulder joint to be inserted on to the lower facet of the greater tubercle of the humerus.

Nerve supply

Teres minor is supplied by a branch of the axillary nerve (C5 and C6). The *nerve to teres minor possesses a pseudoganglion.*

Actions

Teres minor acts as a lateral rotator and weak adductor of the humerus.

Teres Major (Fig. 5.11)

Origin

This thick flat muscle arises from the oval area on the dorsal surface of the inferior angle and adjoining lateral border of the scapula.

Insertion

The fibres run upwards and laterally, and end in a flat tendon, which is inserted on to the medial lip of the intertubercular sulcus of the humerus.

Nerve supply

Teres major is supplied by the *lower subscapular nerve* (C5 and C6).

Action

Teres major acts as a medial rotator of the arm.

Subscapularis (Fig. 5.12)

It is a bulky triangular muscle, which fills the subscapular fossa.

Origin

Subscapularis arises from (a) medial two-thirds of the costal surface of the scapula and (b) tendinous intramuscular septa attached to the ridges on the bone.

Insertion

The fibres converge laterally into a broad tendon, which passes in front of the capsule of glenohumeral joint to be inserted on to the lesser tubercle of the humerus. The tendon is separated from the neck of the scapula by a large **subscapular bursa,** which generally communicates with the synovial cavity of the shoulder joint.

Nerve supply

The subscapularis is supplied by the *upper and lower subscapular nerves* (C5, C6).

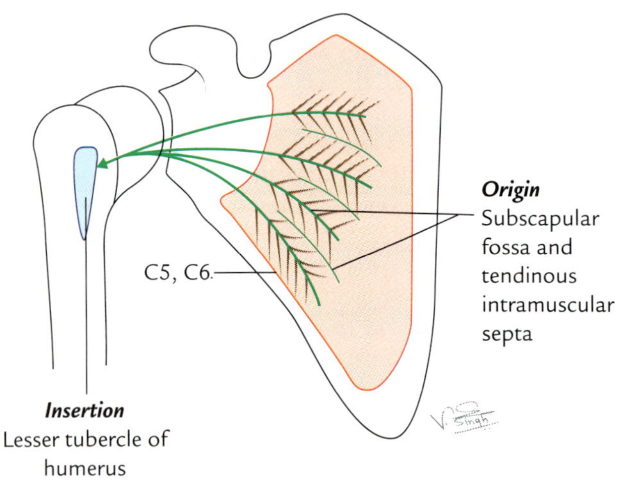

FIG. 5.12 ■ Origin and insertion of the subscapularis muscle.

Actions

Subscapularis is the medial rotator of the humerus. Together with supraspinatus, infraspinatus, and teres minor, it stabilizes the head of the humerus in glenoid fossa during shoulder movements.

The origin, insertion, nerve supply, and actions of the scapulohumeral muscles are described in Table 5.3.

ROTATOR CUFF MUSCLES **AN 10.10**

The four of scapulohumeral muscles, viz. supraspinatus infraspinatus, teres minor, and subscapularis (often referred to as *SITS muscles*) are called **rotator cuff muscles** for they form **musculotendinous/rotator cuff around the glenohumeral joint**.

Mnemonic: **SITS** muscles:

Supraspinatus
Infraspinatus
Teres minor
Subscapularis

} Anticlockwise from top to bottom

The SITS muscles are so referred in reference to the first letter of their names.

ROTATOR CUFF (MUSCULOTENDINOUS CUFF)

The rotator cuff (Fig. 5.13) is the name given to the tendons of supraspinatus, infraspinatus, teres minor, and subscapularis which are fused with each other and the underlying capsule of the glenohumeral joint. Tendon of supraspinatus fuse superiorly, tendons of infraspinatus and teres minor fuse posteriorly, and that of subscapularis fuse anteriorly.

This cuff plays an important role in stabilizing the shoulder joint during its movements. *The primary function of rotator cuff muscles is to grasp the relatively large head of humerus and hold it against the smaller, shallow glenoid cavity* (Fig. 6.8).

MOVEMENTS OF THE SCAPULA (FIG. 5.14)

The scapula is able to glide freely on the posterior chest wall because of the loose connective tissue between the serratus anterior and the chest wall.

The movements of scapula are produced by the muscles that attach it to the trunk and indirectly by the muscles passing from trunk to the humerus when the glenohumeral joint is fixed.

All the movements of scapula occurring on the chest wall (**scapulothoracic linkage**) involves concomitant movements at sternoclavicular and acromioclavicular joints.

The various movements of the scapula are as follows:

1. Protraction
2. Retraction
3. Elevation
4. Depression
5. Rotation (lateral and medial)

Protraction In this movement, scapula moves forwards on the chest wall. It is produced by **serratus anterior**

TABLE 5.3 Origin, insertion, nerve supply, and actions of the scapulohumeral muscles

Muscle	Origin	Insertion	Nerve supply	Actions
Deltoid (a) Clavicular part—unipennate (b) Acromial part—multipennate (c) Spinous part—unipennate	• Anterior aspect of lateral one-third of clavicle • Lateral border of acromion • Lower lip of the spine of scapula	Deltoid tuberosity of humerus	Axillary nerve (C5, C6)	• Flexion and medial rotation by the anterior fibres • Abduction (15°–90°) of the arm by middle fibres • Extension and lateral rotation of the arm by posterior fibres
Supraspinatus (multipennate)	• Medial two-thirds of the supraspinous fossa of scapula	Superior facet of greater tubercle of the humerus	Suprascapular nerve (C5, C6)	Initiates abduction of the arm and carries it up to 15°
Infraspinatus (multipennate)	• Medial two-thirds of the infraspinous fossa of scapula	Middle facet of greater tubercle of the humerus	Suprascapular nerve (C5, C6)	Lateral rotation of the arm
Teres minor	Upper two-thirds of the dorsal aspect of the lateral border of scapula	Inferior facet of greater tubercle of the humerus	Axillary nerve (C5, C6)	Lateral rotation of the arm
Teres major	Inferior one-third of the dorsal aspect of the lateral border and inferior angle of scapula	Medial lip of the intertubercular sulcus of the humerus	Lower subscapular nerve (C5, C6)	Adduction and medial rotation of the arm
Subscapularis (multipennate)	• Medial two-thirds of the subscapular fossa	Lesser tubercle of the humerus	Upper and lower subscapular nerves (C5, C6, C7)	• Adduction and medial rotation of the arm • Helps to hold the humeral head in glenoid cavity

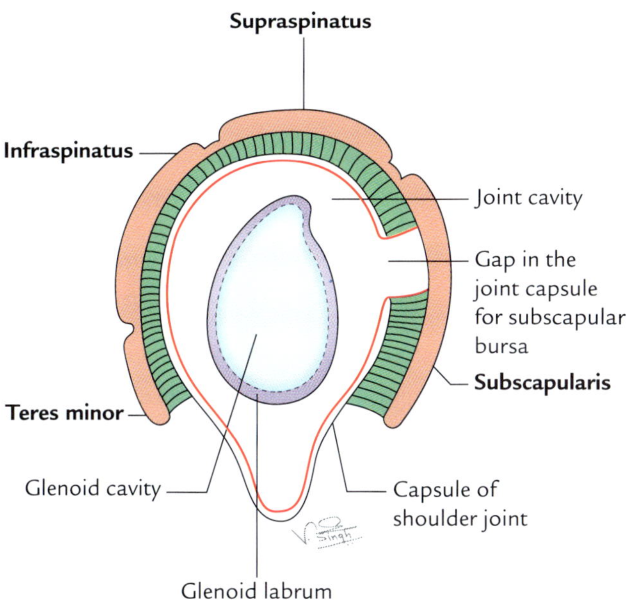

FIG. 5.13 Musculotendinous cuff (rotator cuff). Note the location of rotator cuff muscles.

assisted by the pectoralis minor muscle. Protraction is required for punching (e.g. boxing), pushing, and reaching forwards.

Retraction In this movement, the scapulae are drawn backwards towards the median plane in bracing back of the shoulders. It is produced by middle fibres of trapezius and rhomboids.

Elevation The scapula is elevated, as in shrugging, by simultaneous contraction of the levator scapulae and upper fibres of the trapezius.

Depression The scapula is depressed by simultaneous contraction of the pectoralis minor, lower fibres of trapezius, and latissimus dorsi.

Rotation The rotation of scapula takes place around the horizontal axis passing through the middle of the spine of scapula and sternoclavicular joint.

1. **Medial rotation** is brought about by simultaneous contraction of levator scapulae, rhomboids, and latissimus dorsi. The gravity (e.g. weight of the upper limb) plays a key role in this movement.
2. **Lateral rotation** is brought about by the *trapezius* (its upper fibres raise the acromion process and its lower fibres depress the medial end of the spine of the scapula) and *serratus anterior* (its lower five digitations pull the inferior angle of the scapula forwards and laterally). The lateral rotation of the scapula tilts its glenoid cavity upwards—which is essential for abduction of the upper limb above 90°.

The movements of scapula and the muscles which produce them are summarized in Table 5.4 and Fig. 5.14.

SUBSCAPULAR SPACES (INTERMUSCULAR SPACES IN THE SCAPULAR REGION; FIG. 5.15)

These are quadrangular (one) and triangular (two) intermuscular spaces in the scapular region, which are clearly seen from behind after reflecting the posterior part of the deltoid. The knowledge of these spaces is essential during surgery in the shoulder region.

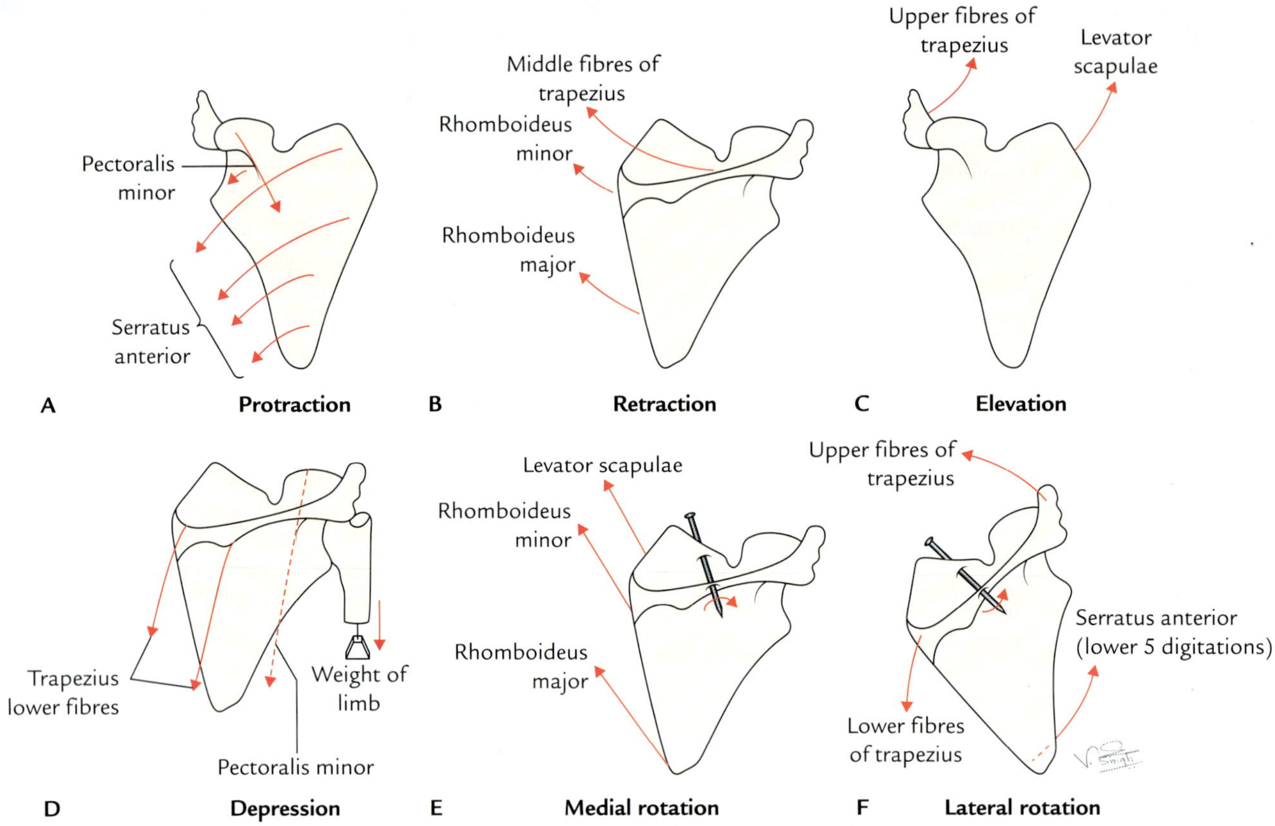

FIG. 5.14 ■ Movements of the scapula (A–F).

TABLE 5.4 Movements of the scapula and the muscles producing them

Movement of scapula	Muscles producing the movements
Protraction	• Serratus anterior • Pectoralis minor (assists)
Retraction	• Trapezius (middle fibres) • Rhomboideus minor • Rhomboideus major
Elevation	• Trapezius (upper fibres) • Levator scapulae
Depression	• Pectoralis minor • Trapezius (lower fibres) • Latissimus dorsi • Weight of the upper limb
Medial rotation[a]	• Levator scapulae • Rhomboideus minor • Rhomboideus major
Lateral rotation	• Trapezius (upper and lower fibres) • Serratus anterior (lower five digitations)

[a]The gravity (e.g. weight of the upper limb) plays a major part in medial rotation of the scapula.

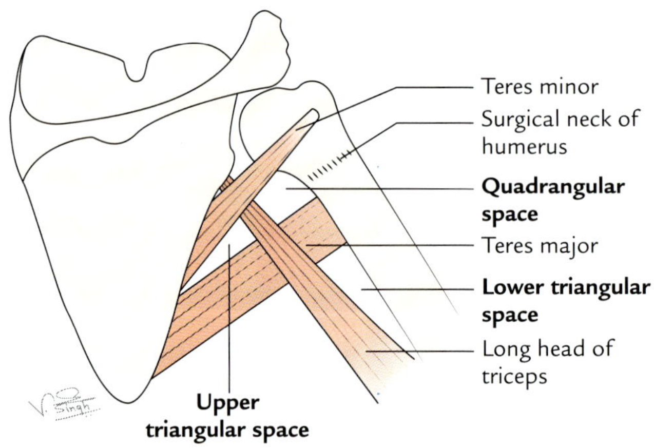

FIG. 5.15 ■ Intermuscular spaces of the subscapular region (subscapular spaces).

QUADRANGULAR SPACE (FIG. 5.15)

Boundaries

Superior:
- Teres minor (posteriorly)
- Subscapularis (anteriorly)
- Capsule of shoulder joint between the above two muscles

Inferior: Teres major

Medial: Long head of the triceps

Lateral: Surgical neck of the humerus

Structures passing through this space (Fig. 5.16)
- Axillary nerve
- Posterior circumflex humeral artery and vein

UPPER TRIANGULAR SPACE (FIG. 5.15)

Boundaries

Superior:	Teres minor
Lateral:	Long head of triceps
Inferior:	Teres major

Structure passing through this space (Fig. 5.16): Circumflex scapular artery (this artery interrupts the origin of teres minor to reach the infraspinous fossa).

LOWER TRIANGULAR SPACE (FIG. 5.15)

Boundaries

Medial:	Long head of triceps
Lateral:	Shaft of humerus
Superior:	Teres major

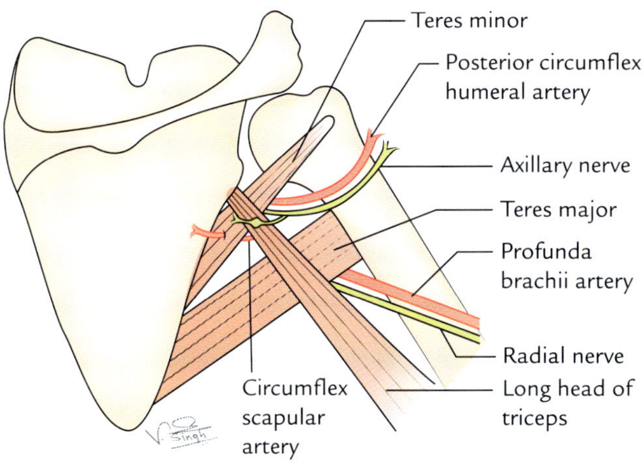

FIG. 5.16 Intermuscular spaces of the scapular region (subscapular spaces) and structures passing through them.

Structures passing through this space (Fig. 5.16)
- Radial nerve
- Profunda brachii artery and vein

NERVES AND VESSELS

AXILLARY NERVE (FIG. 5.17)

The study of axillary nerve is very important because it supplies the deltoid muscle which is the chief abductor of shoulder joint. Further, it is commonly injured in shoulder dislocation and fracture surgical neck of humerus (a constricted upper part of humeral shaft below tuberosities).

The axillary nerve (C5, C6) arises from the posterior cord of the brachial plexus as its smaller terminal branch near the lower border of the subscapularis in axilla. It runs backwards on subscapularis to pass through the quadrangular space along with the posterior circumflex humeral artery. Here it is intimately related to the medial aspect of the surgical neck of the humerus immediately inferior to the capsule of the shoulder joint (glenohumeral joint). The nerve gives an *articular branch* to the shoulder joint, and then runs laterally to divide into the anterior and posterior divisions/branches, deep to deltoid.

The *posterior branch* supplies teres minor and posterior part of the deltoid. It then continues over the posterior border of the deltoid as *upper lateral cutaneous nerve* of the arm and supplies the skin over the lower half of the deltoid. The nerve to teres minor possesses a '*pseudoganglion*'.

The *anterior branch* continues horizontally between the deltoid and surgical neck of the humerus with posterior circumflex humeral vessels. It supplies deltoid and sends a few branches through it to innervate the overlying skin.

CLINICAL CORRELATION

Injury of the axillary nerve: The axillary nerve is at risk of damage in inferior dislocation of the shoulder joint and in fractures of the surgical neck of the humerus because of its close relation to these structures (Fig. 6.2B). The

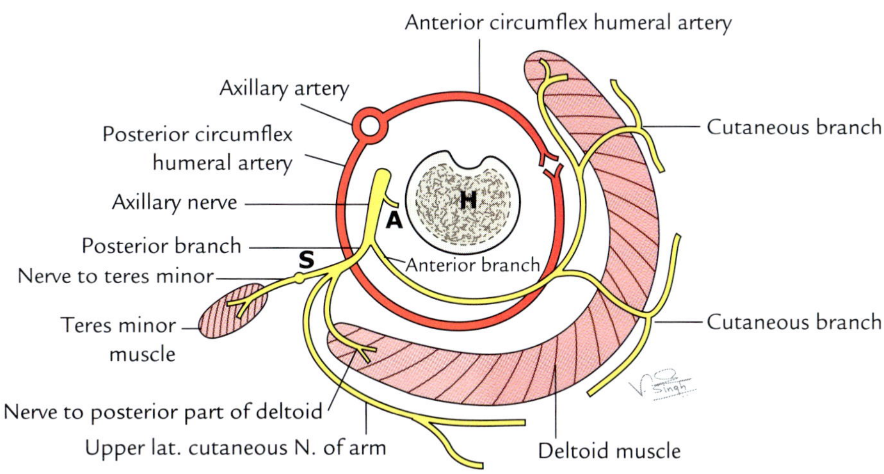

FIG. 5.17 Axillary nerve as seen in the horizontal section of deltoid region at the level of surgical neck of the humerus (H = surgical neck of humerus; A = articular branch to shoulder joint; S = pseudoganglion).

damage of axillary nerve presents the following clinical features:

- *Impaired abduction of the shoulder*—due to paralysis of the deltoid and teres minor muscles.
- *Loss of sensations over the lower half of the deltoid ('regimental badge' area of the sensory loss)*—due to involvement of the upper lateral cutaneous nerve of the arm.
- *Loss of shoulder contour with prominence of greater tubercle of the humerus*—due to wasting of the deltoid muscle.

CIRCUMFLEX HUMERAL ARTERIES

These arteries arise from the third part of the axillary artery and together form a circular anastomosis around the surgical neck of the humerus.

ARTERIAL ANASTOMOSIS AROUND THE SCAPULA

This anastomosis is clinically important because it ensures adequate arterial supply to scapula and provides a subsidiary route through which the blood can pass from the first part of the subclavian artery to the third part of the axillary artery when either the subclavian artery or axillary artery is blocked between these two sites (for details see Chapter 4, pages 51 and 52).

Golden Facts to Remember

• Only muscle that suspends the pectoral girdle from the cranium	Trapezius
• Widest muscle on the back of the body	Latissimus dorsi
• Climbing muscles	Latissimus dorsi and pectoralis major
• Largest cutaneous nerve on the back of shoulder region	T2 which lies across the spine of the scapula
• Rotator cuff muscles	• Subscapularis • Supraspinatus • Infraspinatus • Teres minor
• All the rotator cuff muscles are the rotators of the humerus *except*	Supraspinatus
• Tendon most commonly torn in rotator cuff injury	Tendon of supraspinatus
• Best site for hearing lung sounds on the back of chest	Triangle of auscultation
• Three in one muscle	Deltoid
• Chief abductor of arm	Deltoid
• Strongest part of deltoid	Middle multipennate acromial part
• Muscle responsible for rounded shoulder contour	Deltoid

CLINICAL CASE STUDY

A 45-year-old man, a chronic user of crutch went to his family physician and complained that he had noticed loss of shoulder contour on the right side during the last 2 months. He also told that he feels no sensations in this region and could see the bony projection at the upper end. On examination, the physician found that patient could not abduct his arm up to the 90° and there was a loss of skin sensation over the lower half of the deltoid muscle. He could also notice the prominence of greater tubercle of the humerus. He was diagnosed as a case of **axillary nerve injury**.

Questions

1. Mention the origin and root value of axillary nerve.
2. What are the three common causes of axillary nerve injury?
3. Mention the cause of loss of skin sensation over the lower half of the deltoid.
4. What is the cause of loss of shoulder contour and prominence of greater tubercle of humerus?
5. Name the muscles supplied by the axillary nerve.

Answers

1. The axillary nerve arises from the posterior cord of the brachial plexus (C5 and C6).
2. Axillary nerve can be injured: (a) by the pressure of a badly adjusted crutch, pressurising upwards, into the armpit, (b) by inferior dislocation of the shoulder joint, (c) by fracture surgical neck of humerus, and (d) by the intramuscular injection.
3. Due to involvement of the upper lateral cutaneous nerve of the arm.
4. Due to wasting of the deltoid muscle.
5. Deltoid and teres minor.

Shoulder Joint Complex (Joints of Shoulder Girdle)

CHAPTER 6

SPECIFIC LEARNING OBJECTIVES

After studying this chapter, the student should be able to:

- Describe the shoulder joint (glenohumeral joint) under following headings: (a) type, (b) articular surfaces, (c) capsule, (d) synovial membrane, (e) ligaments, (f) relations, (g) movements and muscles producing them, (h) blood supply, (i) nerve supply, and (j) clinical anatomy. AN 10.12
- Describe sternoclavicular and acromioclavicular joints. AN 13.4
- Give the anatomical basis of: (a) dislocation of shoulder joint, (b) Dawbarn's sign, (c) frozen shoulder, and (d) subacromial bursitis.
- Write short notes on: (a) coracoacromial arch, (b) subacromial/subdeltoid bursa, and (c) scapulohumeral rhythm.

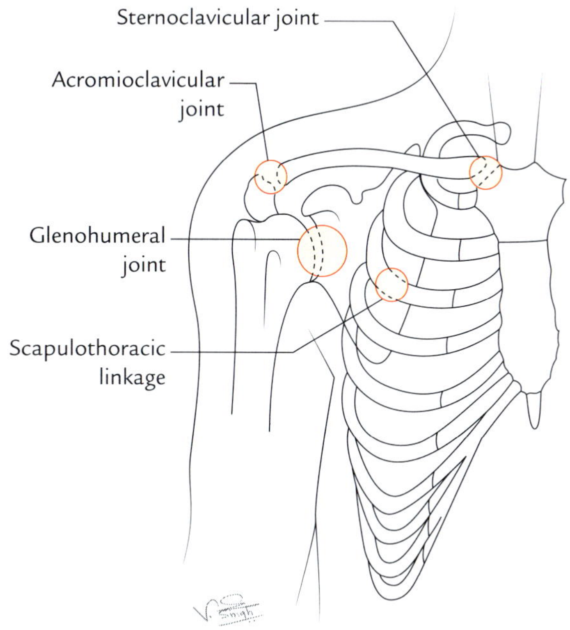

FIG. 6.1 ■ Articulations of the shoulder complex (joints of the shoulder girdle).

The **'shoulder joint complex'** consists of four basic articulations, namely (Fig. 6.1):

1. Glenohumeral joint,
2. Acromioclavicular joint,
3. Sternoclavicular joint,
4. Scapulothoracic articulation/scapulothoracic linkage (functional linkage between the scapula and thorax)/floating joint.

Normal function of the shoulder girdle requires smooth coordination of movements on all these joints. The impairment of any one of these joints leads to functional defect of the whole complex.

The main function of the shoulder in man is to enable him to place his hand where he wishes to in a coordinated and controlled manner.

From weight-bearing forelimb of a quadruped to a freely mobile upper limb in human beings, substantial phylogenetic changes have occurred in the shoulder girdle. In human beings, shoulder girdle has sacrificed stability for mobility, which is responsible for most of the pathological changes that take place in it.

The **glenohumeral** joint is the primary articulation of the shoulder girdle and generally termed shoulder joint by the clinicians. It is quite commonly affected by disease hence it needs to be described in detail.

SHOULDER JOINT (GLENOHUMERAL JOINT) AN 10.12

It is a joint between the head of humerus and glenoid cavity of the scapula.

The shoulder joint is the most movable joint of the body and consequently one of the least stable. It is most common joint to dislocate and to undergo recurrent dislocations. Therefore, the students must study it very thoroughly.

TYPE

The shoulder joint is a ball-and-socket type of synovial joint (Fig. 6.2).

ARTICULAR SURFACES (FIG. 6.2)

The shoulder joint is formed by articulation of large round **head of humerus** with the relatively shallow

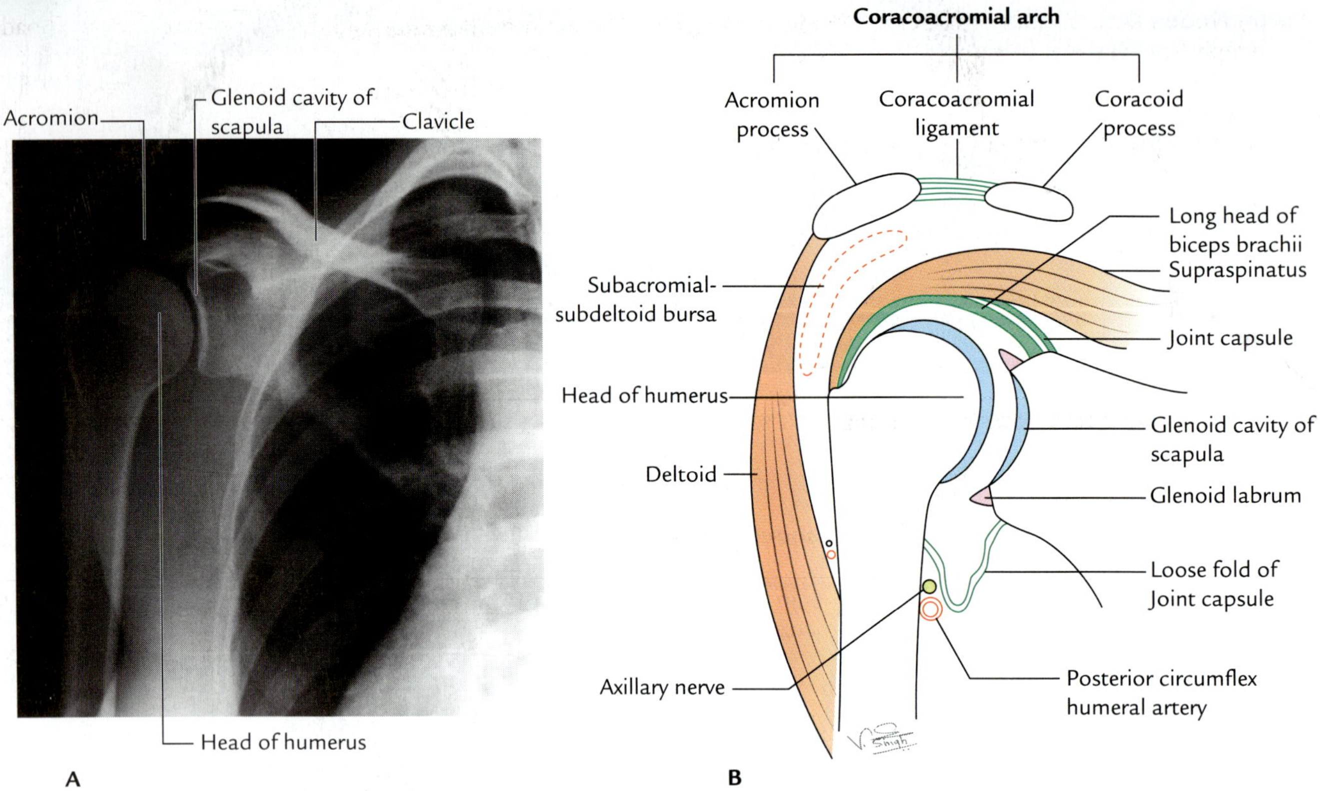

FIG. 6.2 ■ Shoulder joint: (**A**) a radiograph showing articular surfaces and (**B**) coronal section. (*Source*: Fig. 7.25, Page 628, *Gray's Anatomy for Students,* Richard L Drake, Wayne Vogl, Adam WM Mitchell. Copyright Elsevier Inc. 2005. All rights reserved.)

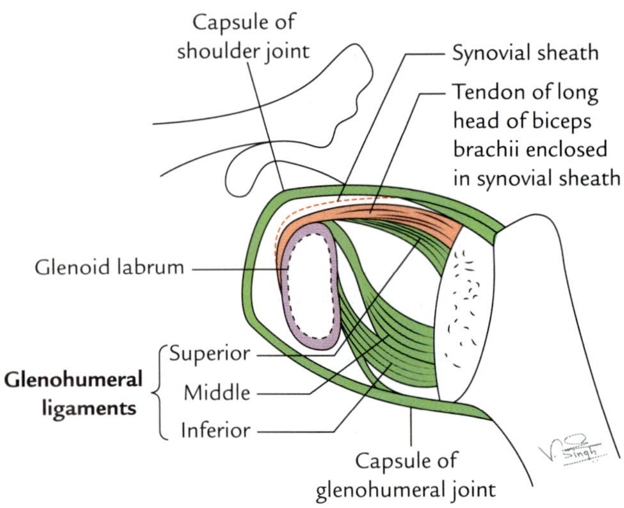

FIG. 6.3 ■ Interior of the shoulder joint exposed from behind to show the glenohumeral ligaments.

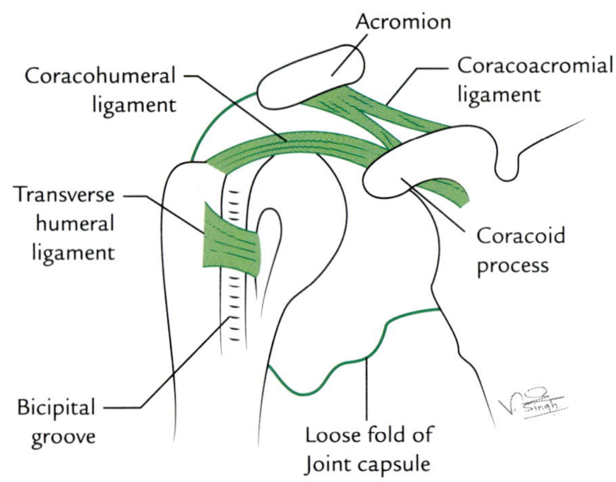

FIG. 6.4 ■ Coracoacromial, coracohumeral, and transverse humeral ligaments as seen from the anterior aspect.

glenoid cavity of the scapula. The glenoid cavity is deepened slightly but effectively by the fibrocartilaginous ring called **glenoid labrum.**

JOINT CAPSULE (CAPSULAR LIGAMENT)

The thin fibrous layer of the joint capsule surrounds the glenohumeral joint (Fig. 6.2B). It is attached medially to the margins of the glenoid cavity beyond the glenoid labrum and laterally to the anatomical neck of the humerus, except inferiorly where it extends downwards 1.5 cm or more on the surgical neck of the humerus. Medially the attachment extends beyond the supraglenoid tubercle thus enclosing the long head of biceps brachii within the joint cavity.

The capsule remains lax to allow the mobility of shoulder joint, hence that of upper limb. For stability it relies on ligaments and muscles tendons which surround it and form rotator-cuff. The anterior aspect of capsule thickens on its inner aspect for three special **glenohumeral ligaments.** The coracoacromial arch acts as secondary socket for head of the humerus which is further strengthened by long head of biceps brachii which runs intracapsularly and form a dome-shaped arch over humeral head (Fig. 6.2B) to prevent its upward displacement.

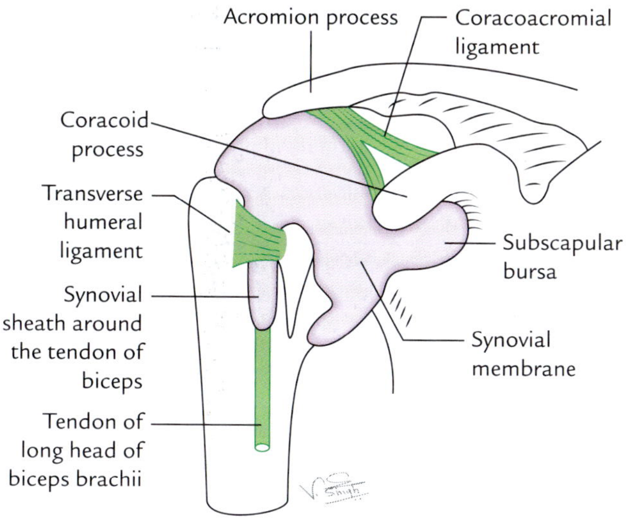

FIG. 6.5 Synovial membrane lining the interior of shoulder joint and its extensions.

SYNOVIAL MEMBRANE (FIG. 6.5)

The **synovial membrane** lines the inner surface of the joint capsule and reflects from it to the glenoid labrum and humerus as far as the articular margin of the head. The synovial cavity of the joint presents the following features:

(a) It forms tubular sheath around the tendon of long head of biceps brachii where it lies in the bicipital groove of the humerus.
(b) It communicates with subscapular and infraspinatus bursae, around the joint.

Thus there are three apertures in the joint capsule:

(a) An opening between the tubercles of the humerus for the passage of tendon of long head of biceps brachii.
(b) An opening situated anteriorly inferior to the coracoid process to allow communication between the synovial cavity and subscapular bursa.
(c) An opening situated posteriorly to allow communication between synovial cavity and infraspinatus bursa.

LIGAMENTS (FIGS. 6.3 AND 6.4)

These are as under:

1. **Glenohumeral ligaments:** There are three thickenings on the inner aspect of the anterior part of the fibrous capsule; to strengthen it. These are called *superior, middle*, and *inferior glenohumeral ligaments*. Hence, they are visible only from interior of the joint. They play different roles in the stability of head of humerus, depending on arm position and degree of rotation, viz. *superior* in adduction, *middle* in external rotation and *inferior* in abduction and external rotation.

   A defect exists between superior and middle glenohumeral ligaments, which acquire importance in the **anterior dislocation of the shoulder joint**.
2. **Coracohumeral ligament:** It is a strong band of fibrous tissue that passes from the base of the coracoid process to the anterior aspect of the greater tubercle of the humerus.
3. **Transverse humeral ligament:** It is a broad fibrous band, which bridges the bicipital groove between the greater and lesser tubercles. This ligament converts the groove into a canal that provides passage to the tendon of long head of biceps surrounded by a synovial sheath.

Accessory Ligaments (Fig. 6.2B)

The accessory ligaments of the shoulder joint are as follows:

1. **Coracoacromial ligament:** It extends between coracoid and acromion processes. It protects the superior aspect of the joint.
2. **Coracoacromial arch:** The coracoacromial arch in a way acts as an accessory ligament. It is formed by coracoid process, acromion process, and coracoacromial ligament between them. This osseoligamentous structure forms a protective arch for the head of humerus above and prevents its superior displacement above the glenoid cavity. The **supraspinatus muscle** passes under this arch and lies deep to the deltoid where its tendon blends with the joint capsule. The large **subacromial bursa** lies between the arch superiorly and tendon of supraspinatus and greater tubercle of humerus inferiorly. This facilitates the movement of supraspinatus tendon.

BURSAE RELATED TO THE SHOULDER JOINT

Several bursae are related to the shoulder joint but the important ones are as follows (Fig. 6.6):

1. **Subscapular bursa** (Fig. 6.6)**:** It lies between the tendon of subscapularis and the anterior aspect of the neck of the scapula; and protects the tendon from friction against the neck. This bursa usually communicates with the joint cavity.
2. **Subacromial bursa** (Fig. 6.7)**:** It lies between the coracoacromial ligament and acromion process above, and supraspinatus tendon and joint capsule below. It continues downwards beneath the deltoid, hence it is also referred to as **subdeltoid bursa**. It is the *largest synovial bursa in the body* and facilitates the movements of supraspinatus tendon under the coracoacromial arch. It is also called *subacromial-subdeltoid bursa*.
3. **Infraspinatus bursa:** It lies between the tendon of infraspinatus and posterolateral aspect of the joint capsule. It may sometime communicate with the joint cavity.

N.B.

The bursae around the shoulder joint are clinically important as some of them communicate with synovial cavity of the joint. Consequently, opening a bursa may mean entering into the cavity of the joint.

RELATIONS OF THE SHOULDER JOINT (FIG. 6.6)

The shoulder joint is related:

Superiorly: to coracoacromial arch, subacromial bursa, supraspinatus muscle, and deltoid muscle.

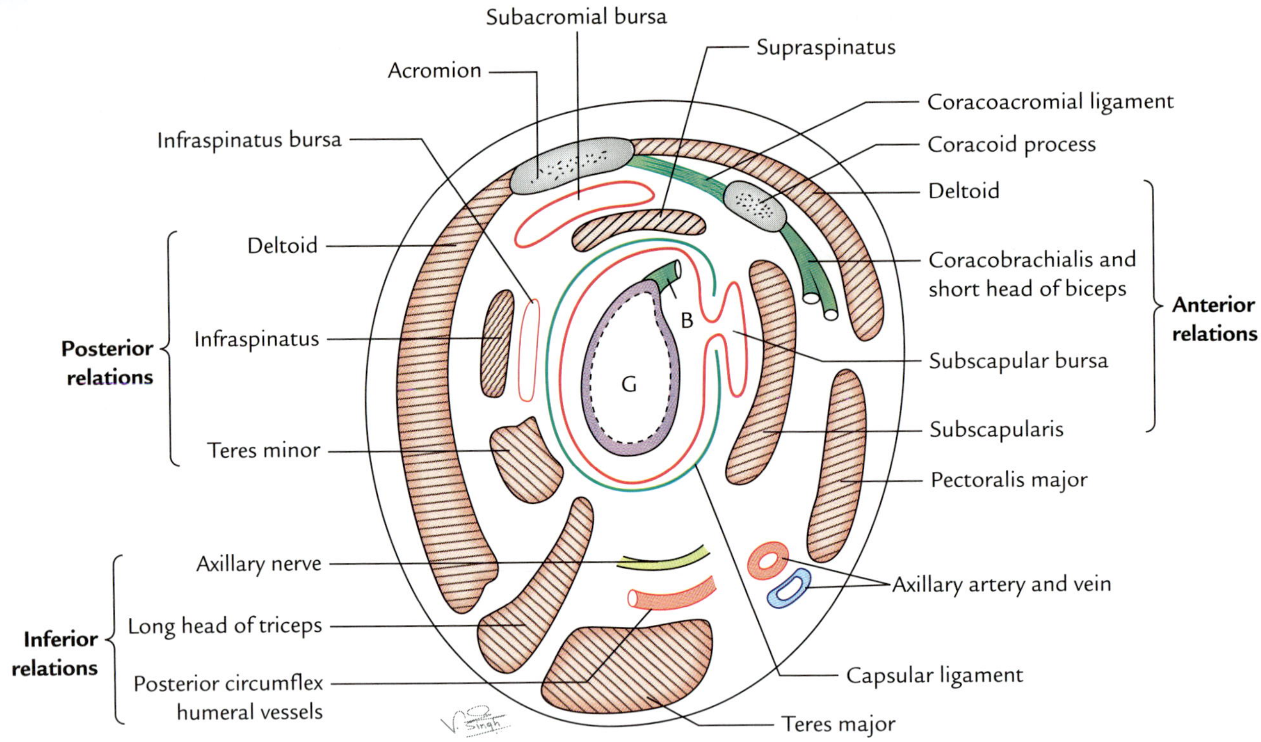

FIG. 6.6 ■ Relations of the shoulder joint as seen in sagittal section (G = glenoid fossa, B = long head of biceps).

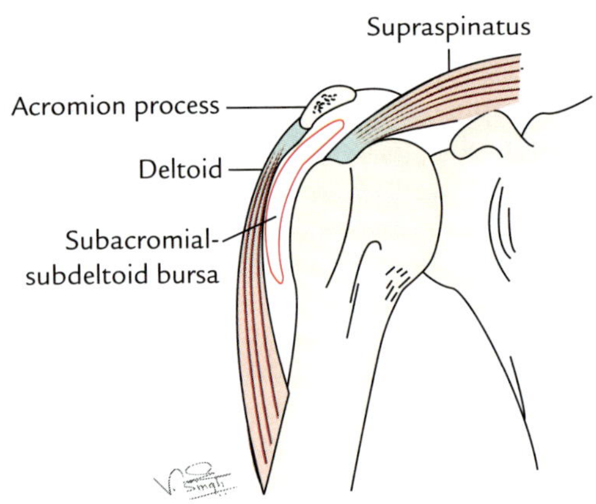

FIG. 6.7 ■ Subacromial/subdeltoid bursa. (*Source:* Fig. 2.6, Page 57, *Clinical and Surgical Anatomy*, 2e, Vishram Singh. Copyright Elsevier 2007. All rights reserved.)

Inferiorly: to long head of triceps, axillary nerve and posterior circumflex humeral vessels.

Anteriorly: to subscapularis, subscapular bursa, coracobrachialis, short head of biceps brachii, and deltoid.

Posteriorly: to infraspinatus, teres minor, and deltoid.

ARTERIAL SUPPLY

The glenohumeral joint is supplied by the following arteries:

1. Anterior and posterior circumflex humeral arteries.
2. Suprascapular artery.
3. Subscapular artery.

NERVE SUPPLY

The glenohumeral joint is supplied by the following nerves:

1. Axillary nerve.
2. Suprascapular nerve.
3. Musculocutaneous nerve.

FACTORS PROVIDING STABILITY TO THE SHOULDER JOINT

The factors providing stability to the joint are as follows:

1. Rotator cuff (musculotendinous cuff).
2. Coracoacromial arch.
3. Long head of biceps tendon.
4. Glenoid labrum.

The **rotator cuff/musculotendinous cuff** is formed by the blending together of the tendons of subscapularis, supraspinatus, infraspinatus, and teres minor around the joint capsule (for details see Chapter 5, page 68).

The *tone of rotator cuff muscles* grasp the head of humerus like a hand-grip, and pull it medially to hold it against the smaller and shallow glenoid cavity. It also helps the head of humerus rotating against the glenoid fossa during joint motion, which is what the term *rotator* refers to (Fig. 6.8).

The **coracoacromial arch** forms the **secondary socket of the glenohumeral joint** and protects the joint from above and prevents the upward dislocation of the head of humerus.

The **long head of biceps brachii** passes above the head of humerus (intracapsular course), hence prevents its upward displacement.

The **glenoid labrum** provides protection by deepening the shallow glenoid cavity.

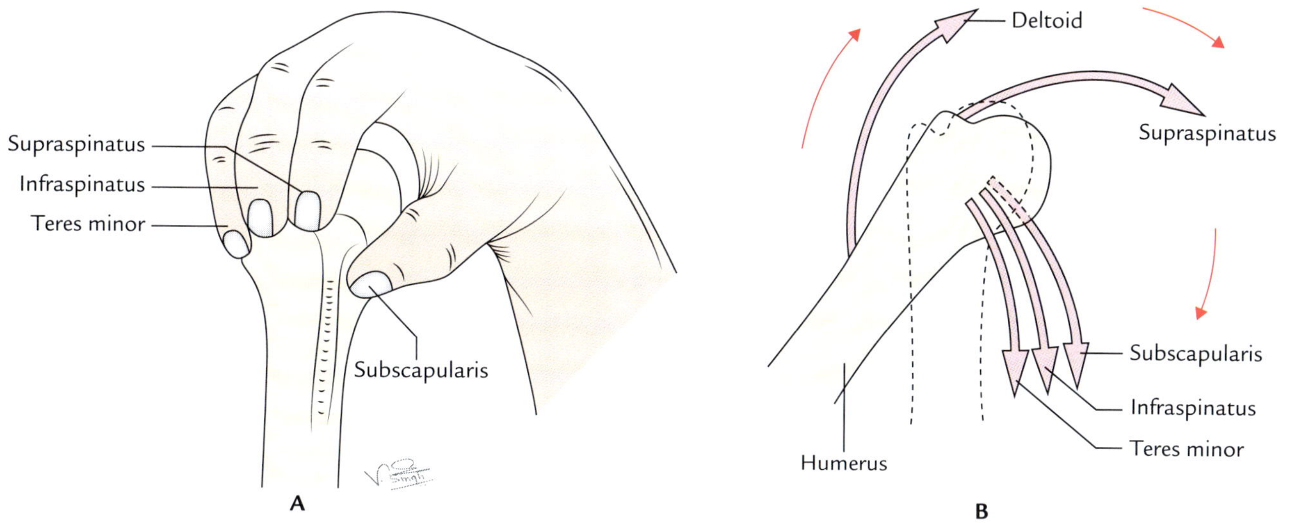

FIG. 6.8 ■ Action of the rotator cuff muscles: (**A**) they grasp and pull the relatively large head of the humerus medially to hold it against the smaller and shallow glenoid cavity; (**B**) combined function of the rotator cuff muscles and deltoid.

MOVEMENTS OF THE SHOULDER JOINT (FIGS. 6.9 AND 6.10)

The shoulder joint has more freedom of mobility than any other joint in the body, due to the following factors:

1. Laxity of joint capsule.
2. Articulation between relatively large humeral head and smaller and shallow glenoid cavity.

The glenohumeral joint permits four groups of movements:

1. Flexion and extension.
2. Abduction and adduction.
3. Medial and lateral rotation.
4. Circumduction.

The movements of shoulder joint occur in all the three planes and around all the three axes:

- The **flexion** and **extension**/hyperextension occur in sagittal plane around the frontal axis.
- The **abduction** and **adduction** occur in frontal plane around the sagittal axis.
- The **medial** and **lateral rotation** occur in transverse plane around the vertical axis.
- The circumduction is really only a combination of all above movements.

N.B.

Plane of the glenohumeral joint: The scapula does not lie in the coronal plane but is so oriented that its glenoid cavity faces forwards and laterally, therefore the plane of this joint lies obliquely at about 45° to the sagittal plane. The movements of shoulder joint are, therefore, described in relation to this plane.

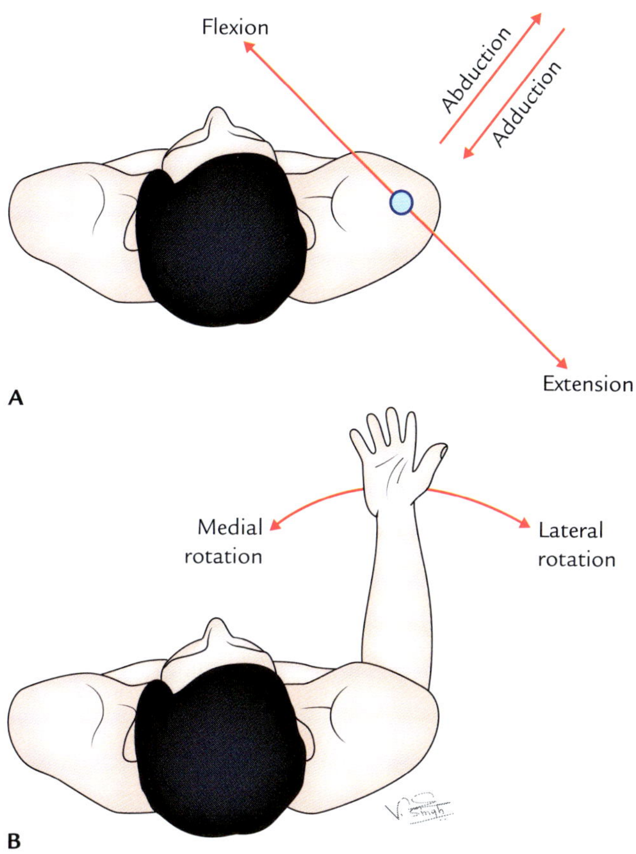

FIG. 6.9 ■ Planes of movements of the shoulder joint: (**A**) planes of flexion and extension, and abduction and adduction; (**B**) plane of medial and lateral rotation.

The details are as under:

1. **Flexion and extension:** During flexion, the arm moves forwards and medially, and during extension it moves backwards and laterally. These movements take place parallel to the plane of glenoid cavity (i.e. midway between the coronal and sagittal planes).
2. **Abduction and adduction:** During abduction, the arm moves anterolaterally away from the trunk and during adduction the arm moves posteromedially

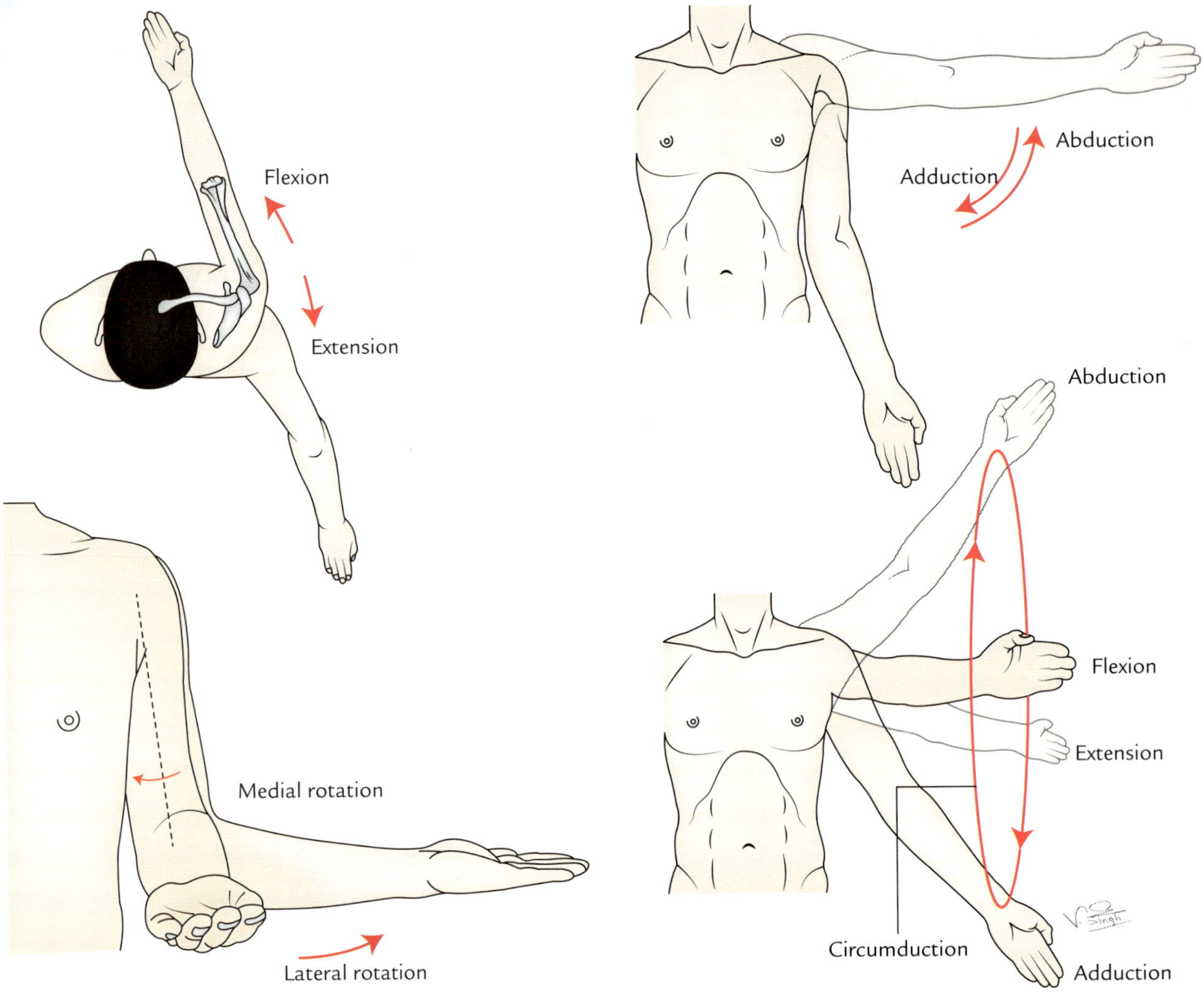

FIG. 6.10 ■ Movements of the shoulder joint. (*Source*: Fig. 7.4, Page 611, *Gray's Anatomy for Students*, Richard L Drake, Wayne Vogl, Adam WM Mitchell. Copyright Elsevier Inc. 2005. All rights reserved.)

towards the trunk. These movements occur at right angle to the plane of flexion and extension (i.e. in the plane of the body of the scapula).

3. **Medial and lateral rotation:** These movements are best demonstrated in midflexed elbow. In this position, the hand moves medially in medial rotation and laterally in lateral rotation.
4. **Circumduction:** The circumduction at glenohumeral joint is an orderly sequence of flexion, abduction, extension, and adduction or the reverse. During this movement the upper limb moves along a circle.

The muscles producing the various movements at the shoulder joint are listed in Table 6.1.

Mechanism of Abduction

The abduction at shoulder is a complex movement, hence student must understand it.

The total range of abduction is 180° called overhead abduction. Abduction up to 90° occurs at the glenohumeral joint. Abduction from 90° to 120° can occur only if the humerus is rotated laterally. Abduction from 120° to 180° can occur if the scapula rotates forwards on the chest wall.

The detailed analysis is as under:

1. The articular surface of the head of humerus permits elevation of arm only up to 90°, because when the upper end of humerus is elevated to 90° its greater tubercle impinges upon the under surface of the acromion and can only be released by lateral rotation of the arm.
2. Therefore, the arm rotates laterally and carries abduction up to 120°.
3. Abduction above 120° can occur only if scapula rotates. So that the scapula rotates forwards on the chest wall.

N.B.

- The humerus and scapula move in the ratio of 2:1 during abduction, that is for every 15° elevation, the humerus moves 10° and scapula moves 5°.
- During early and terminal stages of elevation, the sternoclavicular and acromioclavicular joints move maximum, respectively.

TABLE 6.1 **Movements at the shoulder joint and muscles producing them**

Movements	Main muscles (prime movers)	Accessory muscles (synergists)
Flexion	• Pectoralis major (clavicular part) • Deltoid (anterior fibres)	• Biceps brachii (short head) • Coracobrachialis • Sternocostal head of pectoralis major
Extension	• Deltoid (posterior fibres) • Latissimus dorsi	• Teres major • Long head of triceps
Adduction	• Pectoralis major (sternocostal part) • Latissimus dorsi	• Teres major • Coracobrachialis • Short head of biceps • Long head of triceps
Abduction	• Deltoid (middle/lateral fibres) • Supraspinatus	• Serratus anterior • Upper and lower fibres of trapezius
Medial rotation	• Subscapularis	• Pectoralis major • Latissimus dorsi • Deltoid (anterior fibres) • Teres major
Lateral rotation	• Deltoid (posterior fibres)	• Infraspinatus • Teres minor

Range of Motion (ROM) of Various Movements

During clinical examination, the knowledge of range of motion of various movements is very important. It is given in the box below:

Movements	Range of motion
• Flexion	90°
• Extension	45°
• Abduction	180°
• Adduction	45°
• Lateral rotation	45°
• Medial rotation	55°

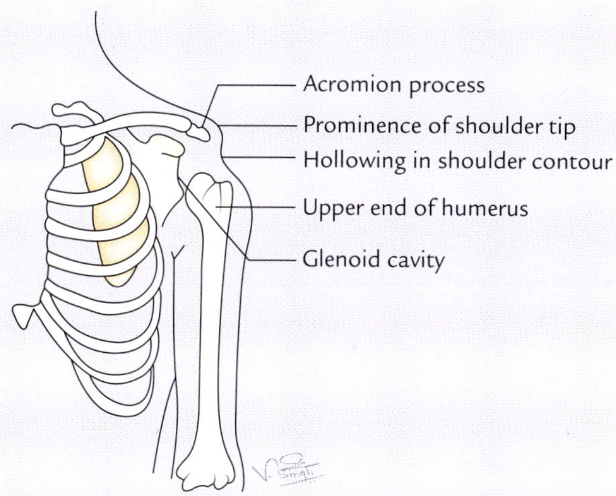

FIG. 6.11 Dislocation of the shoulder joint. Note the changes in the contour of shoulder.

CLINICAL CORRELATION

- **Dislocation of the shoulder joint:** It is quite common due to disproportionate sizes of its articular surfaces. Only 1/3rd of humeral head comes in contact with glenoid fossa. Hence, head of humerus often pops out of the shallow glenoid fossa.

  Types: There are three types of shoulder dislocations:
  1. **Anterior (forward) dislocation:** It is the most common type of dislocation (70%). In this the head of humerus moves forward in front of glenoid fossa. It is usually caused by a blow to the abducted, externally rotated and extended arm, viz. blocking a basketball shot.
  2. **Posterior (backward) dislocation:** It is less common type of dislocation (3%). In this head of humerus moves behind and above the glenoid cavity. It is caused by anteriorly directed shoulder trauma, viz. grabbing the dashboard in motor vehicle collision.
  3. **Inferior dislocation (luxatio erecta):** In this head of humerus is pushed down and out of the socket toward the arm pit. The arm is abducted above the head, permanently. It frequently occurs when patient falls and suddenly grasp on to an object above the head resulting in hyperabduction.

     This type of injury is rare.

  Further, inferiorly the joint is supported by inferior glenohumeral ligament and long head of triceps. It often injures the axillary nerve because of its close relation to the inferior part of the joint capsule.

  Clinically, it presents as (Fig. 6.11):

  (a) Hollow in rounded contour of the shoulder
  (b) Prominence of shoulder tip

N.B.

Earlier it was though that the dislocation of shoulder joint mostly occurs inferiorly because the joint is least supported on this aspect.

- **Frozen shoulder (adhesive capsulitis):** It is a clinical condition characterized by pain and uniform limitation of all movements of the shoulder joint, though there are no radiological changes in the joint. It occurs due to shrinkage of the joint capsule, hence the name *adhesive capsulitis*. This condition is generally seen in individuals of 40–60 years of age.
- **Rotator cuff disorders:** The most common disorders of rotator cuff include *calcific supraspinatus tendinitis* and *subacromial bursitis*. The rotator cuff injuries represent overall the most common cause of shoulder pain. The rotator cuff is commonly injured during repetitive use of the upper limb above the horizontal level (e.g. in throwing sports, swimming, and weight lifting). The deposition of calcium in the supraspinatus tendon is common. The calcium deposition irritates the overlying subacromial bursa causing *subacromial bursitis*. Consequently, when the arm is abducted the inflamed bursa is caught between tendon and acromion – the *subacromial impingement*, which causes severe pain. In most people, pain occurs during 60°–120° of abduction (*painful arc syndrome*). The rotator cuff disorders usually occur in males after 50 years of age.
  The pain due to *subacromial bursitis* is elicited when the deltoid is pressed just below the acromion, when the arm is adducted. The pain cannot be elicited by the pressure on the same point when the arm is abducted because the bursa slips/disappears under the acromion process (**Dawbarn's sign**).
- **Aspiration of shoulder joint (arthrocentesis).** In this synovial fluid is aspirated and analysed to differentiate inflammatory arthritis from noninflammatory arthritis. In anterior approach, the needle is inserted medial to humeral head and lateral to coracoid process (Fig. 6.12).
- **Exclusion of shoulder joint disease.** The common symptoms and signs of shoulder disease are: shoulder pain, tenderness, joint stiffness, decrease range of movement, cracking sound in joint, etc. During routine examination, the shoulder joint disease is excluded if the patient can raise his arms above head and bring down the palms together.

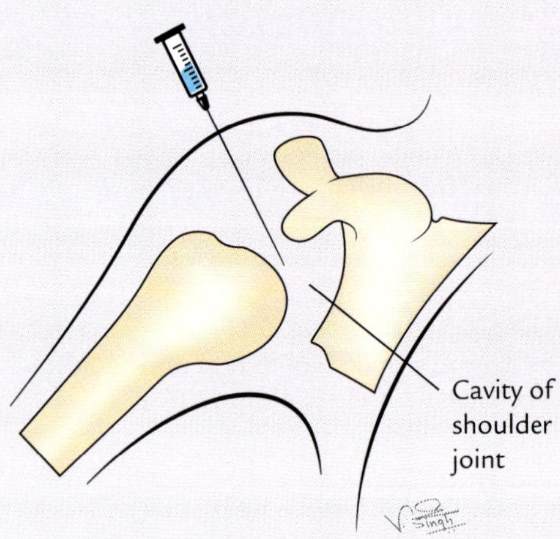

FIG. 6.12 ■ Site of aspiration (arthrocentesis of shoulder joint).

ACROMIOCLAVICULAR JOINT (FIG. 6.13)

TYPE

It is a **plane type of the synovial joint** between the lateral end of the clavicle and acromion process of the scapula. The acromioclavicular joint is located about 2.5 cm medial to the point of the shoulder.

Articular Surfaces

These are small facets present on the lateral end of clavicle and the medial margin of the acromion process of the scapula. The articular surfaces are covered with fibrocartilage. The joint cavity is subdivided by an incomplete wedge-shaped articular disc.

Joint Capsule

It is thin, lax fibrous sac attached to the margins of articular surfaces.

Ligaments

These are acromioclavicular and coracoclavicular ligaments.

1. **Acromioclavicular ligament:** It is a fibrous band that extends from acromion to the clavicle. It strengthens the acromioclavicular joint superiorly.
2. **Coracoclavicular ligament:** It lies a little away from the joint itself but plays an important role in maintaining the integrity of the joint.

The coracoclavicular ligament consists of two parts: (a) conoid and (b) trapezoid, which are united posteriorly and often separated by a bursa.

- *The conoid ligament* is an inverted cone-shaped fibrous band. The apex is attached to the root of the coracoid process just lateral to the scapular notch and base is attached to the conoid tubercle on the inferior surface of the clavicle.
- *The trapezoid ligament* is a horizontal fibrous band that stretches from upper surface of the coracoid process to the trapezoid line on the inferior surface of lateral end of the clavicle.

N.B.

The *coracoclavicular ligament* is largely responsible for suspending the weight of the scapula and upper limb from clavicle.

The coracoclavicular ligament is the strongest ligament of the upper limb.

Movements

The acromioclavicular joint permits the rotation of acromion of scapula at the acromial end of the clavicle. These movements are associated with movements of scapula at the scapulothoracic joint/linkage.

STERNOCLAVICULAR JOINT (FIG. 6.13) AN 13.4

TYPE

The sternoclavicular joint is a saddle type of the synovial joint because its articular surfaces are reciprocally concavoconvex.

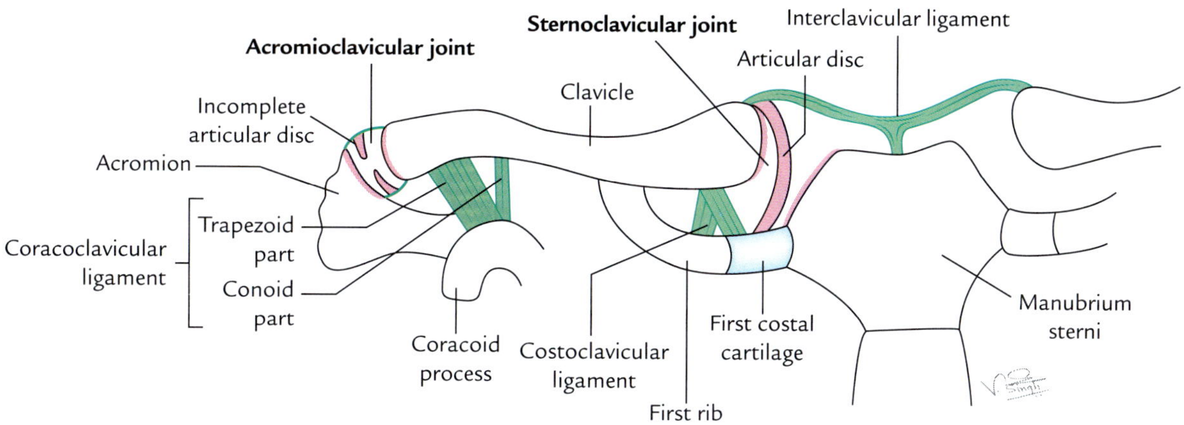

FIG. 6.13 ■ Sternoclavicular and acromioclavicular joints.

Articular Surfaces

The *rounded sternal end of clavicle* articulates with the shallow socket at the superolateral angle of the manubrium sterni *(clavicular notch of manubrium sterni)* and adjacent part of the first costal cartilage. The medial end of clavicle rises higher than the manubrium, hence it poorly fits into its shallow socket. But a strong thick articular disc of fibrocartilage attached superiorly to the clavicle and first costal cartilage inferiorly prevents the displacement of the medial end of the clavicle.

The articular surface of clavicle is convex from above downwards and slightly concave from front to back. The articular surface of sternum is reciprocally curved. The articular surfaces are covered with fibrocartilage.

N.B.

(a) Sternoclavicular joint is also called a *compound joint* because of involvement of three skeletal elements, viz., clavicular notch of manubrium, medial end of clavicle, and upper surface of first costal cartilage.
(b) Sternoclavicular joint is also called *complex joint* because its articular surfaces are covered by fibrocartilage and its cavity is divided into two parts by intraarticular disc.
(c) Sternoclavicular joint is also called *synovial joint* because its cavity is lined by a synovial membrane.

Articular Capsule

The joint capsule is attached to the margins of the articular surfaces including the periphery of the articular disc. The synovial membrane lines the internal surface of the fibrous joint capsule, extending to the edges of the articular disc.

Ligaments

1. **Anterior and posterior sternoclavicular ligaments:** They reinforce the joint capsule anteriorly and posteriorly. The posterior ligament is weaker than the anterior ligament.
2. **Interclavicular ligament:** It is T-shaped and connects the sternal ends of two clavicles and strengthens the joint capsule superiorly. In between, it is attached to the superior border of the suprasternal notch.
3. **Costoclavicular ligament (Rhomboid ligament):** It anchors the inferior surface of the sternal end of clavicle to the first rib and adjoining part of its cartilage.

CLINICAL CORRELATION

- **Dislocation of the sternoclavicular joint:** It is rare because the sternoclavicular (SC) joint is extremely strong. However, dislocation of this joint in people below 25 years of age may result from fractures through the epiphyseal plate because epiphysis at the sternal end of clavicle does not unite until 23–25 years of age. The medial end is usually dislocated anteriorly. Backward dislocation is prevented by the costoclavicular ligament.
- **Transmission of weight of the upper limb:** The weight of the upper limb is transmitted from scapula to the clavicle through *coracoclavicular ligament*, and then from clavicle to sternum through *sternoclavicular joint*. Some of the weight is transmitted to the first rib through *costoclavicular ligament* (Fig. 1.4).
- **Dislocation of the acromioclavicular joint:** It may occur following a severe blow on the superolateral part of the shoulder. In severe form, both acromioclavicular and coracoclavicular ligaments are torn. Consequently the shoulder separates from the clavicle and falls because of the weight of the limb. The acromioclavicular joint dislocation is often termed as *shoulder separation*.

Movements

The sternoclavicular joint allows the movements of pectoral girdle. This joint is critical to the movement of the clavicle.

SCAPULOTHORACIC ARTICULATION/LINKAGE

The **scapulothoracic articulation** is not a true articulation (also called floating joint) but a functional linkage between the ventral aspect of the scapula and lateral aspect of the thoracic wall. The linkage is provided by serratus anterior muscle. The movements of scapula around the chest wall are facilitated by the presence of loose areolar tissue between the serratus anterior and subscapularis muscles.

TABLE 6.2 Types of articulations in various components of shoulder joint complex

Component	Type of articulation
1. Shoulder joint (glenohumeral joint)	Ball and socket type of synovial joint
2. Acromioclavicular joint	Plane type of synovial joint
3. Sternoclavicular joint	Saddle type of synovial joint (also called compound/ complex joint)
4. Scapulothoracic joint	Functional joint (i.e. not a true articulation)

Types of articulations in various components of shoulder joint are given in Table 6.2.

SCAPULOHUMERAL RHYTHM

Most of the movements at the shoulder involve the movements of humerus and scapula simultaneously and not successively.

According to older concept, abduction of shoulder up to 90° occurs at the **glenohumeral/scapulohumeral** joint and beyond 90° the movement is essentially an upward rotation of the scapula.

But recently it has been established beyond doubt by fluoroscopic studies that there is rotation of scapula even from the initial stages of abduction at the shoulder. Thus there is rhythm between the scapular and humeral movements called ***scapulohumeral rhythm***. In abduction, there is 1° of lateral rotation of scapula for every 2° of movement at the scapulohumeral joint. The paralysis of muscles, which interferes with this rhythm seriously affects the movements of the shoulder.

Golden Facts to Remember

• Primary articulation of shoulder girdle	Glenohumeral joint
• Most freely mobile joint in the body • Most commonly dislocated joint in the body • Most common joint to undergo recurrent dislocation • Most commonly surgically approached joint	Shoulder joint
• Commonest dislocation of the shoulder joint	Anterior dislocation
• Largest synovial bursa in the body	Subacromial/ subdeltoid bursa
• Most important factor to provide stability to the shoulder joint • Guardian of the shoulder joint	Musculotendinous cuff/rotator cuff
• Most common cause of the shoulder pain	Disorders of the rotator cuff
• Chief anchor of the acromioclavicular joint	Coracoclavicular ligament
• Chief anchor of the sternoclavicular joint	Articular disc
• Strongest ligament of the upper limb	Coracoclavicular ligament
• Type of sternoclavicular joint	Synovial (saddle/ compound/ complex type)

CLINICAL CASE STUDY

A 54-year-old executive officer fell down from the stairs. He was feeling severe pain in his right shoulder. He was taken to the emergency OPD. On examination, the doctors observed that the officer was sitting on the stool with right arm by the side of his body and he was supporting his right elbow with his left hand. The inspection of right shoulder revealed loss of its normal rounded contour and loss of skin sensations in the lower half of the deltoid region. Any attempt to perform active or passive movement was stopped by severe pain in shoulder. **He was diagnosed as a case of dislocation of right shoulder joint**.

Questions

1. Why shoulder joint is commonly dislocated?
2. What is the most common type of shoulder dislocation?
3. What is the cause of loss of normal rounded contour of the shoulder?
4. What is the cause for loss of skin sensation in the lower half of the deltoid region?

Answers

1. Because of the disproportionate size of articular surfaces and lax joint capsule.
2. Inferior (commonly called *anterior dislocation* by the clinicians).
3. (a) Paralysis of deltoid muscle and (b) pull of pectoralis major and subscapularis muscles displacing the upper end of humerus medially.
4. Injury to the axillary nerve.

CHAPTER 7

Innervation, Venous Drainage, and Lymphatic Drainage of the Upper Limb

SPECIFIC LEARNING OBJECTIVES

After studying this chapter, the student should be able to:

- Describe the dermatomes of upper limb. AN 13.2
- Describe the veins of upper limb. AN 13.1
- Describe the lymphatic drainage of the upper limb. AN 13.1
- Describe the beginning, course, and termination of cephalic and basilic veins.
- Write short notes on: (a) segmental innervation of upper limb and (b) median cubital vein.
- Give the anatomical basis of: (a) median cubital vein is most preferred vein for venepuncture, viz. intravenous infusion or injections and (b) basilic vein is preferred for cardiac catheterization.
- Describe the anatomical basis of venepuncture of cubital veins. AN 11.3

INNERVATION

CUTANEOUS INNERVATION

The knowledge of cutaneous innervation is essential during physical examination of the patient. The sensory testing of skin of the upper limb is performed whenever a damage of nerves arising from C3 to T2 spinal segments is suspected. Light touch and pin-prick are the main sensations tested routinely, but the temperature, two-point discrimination, and vibration are also tested in special cases. The area of anaesthesia and paraesthesia are mapped out and matched with the dermatomal distribution. In compression of nerve roots of spinal nerves arising from C3 to T2 spinal segments due to spondylitis, pain is referred to the respective dermatomes.

CUTANEOUS NERVES OF THE UPPER LIMB AN 13.1

The cutaneous nerves of the upper limb are derived from the ventral rami of spinal nerves derived from C3 to T2 spinal segments. These nerves are derived from the ventral rami because the upper limb buds develop from ventral half of the body opposite the C3-T2 spinal segments. During dissection, the cutaneous nerves are seen to arise from three sources, *viz.*

1. Cervical plexus.
2. Brachial plexus.
3. Intercostobrachial nerve.

The cutaneous nerves carry sensations of pain, touch, temperature, and pressure. In addition, they carry sympathetic fibres, which supply sweat glands, dermal arterioles, and arrector pili muscles. The effect of sympathetic stimulation on skin, therefore, is sudomotor, vasomotor, and pilomotor, respectively. The area of skin supplied by a single spinal nerve/segment is termed '**dermatome**'. *The cutaneous nerves contain fibres from more than one spinal nerve and each spinal nerve provides fibres to more than one cutaneous nerve. As a result, skin areas supplied by the cutaneous nerves do not correspond with dermatomes.*

CUTANEOUS NERVES SUPPLYING DIFFERENT REGIONS OF THE UPPER LIMB (FIG. 7.1)

These are as follows:

1. Pectoral region:
   Above the second rib, this region is supplied by the supraclavicular nerves (C3, C4) and below the second rib by the intercostal nerves (T2-T6).
2. Axilla:
   The skin of the armpit is supplied by:
   (a) intercostobrachial nerve (T2) and
   (b) small branches from T3.
3. Shoulder:
   a) Upper half of the deltoid region is supplied by the **lateral supraclavicular nerve** (C3, C4).
   b) Lower half of the deltoid region is supplied by the **upper lateral cutaneous nerve** of the arm, which is a cutaneous branch of the axillary nerve.
4. Arm (brachium):
   (a) *Upper medial part* of the arm is supplied by the **intercostobrachial nerve** (T2) derived from second intercostal.
   (b) *Lower medial part* of the arm is supplied by the **medial cutaneous nerve of the arm** (T1) from medial cord of the brachial plexus.

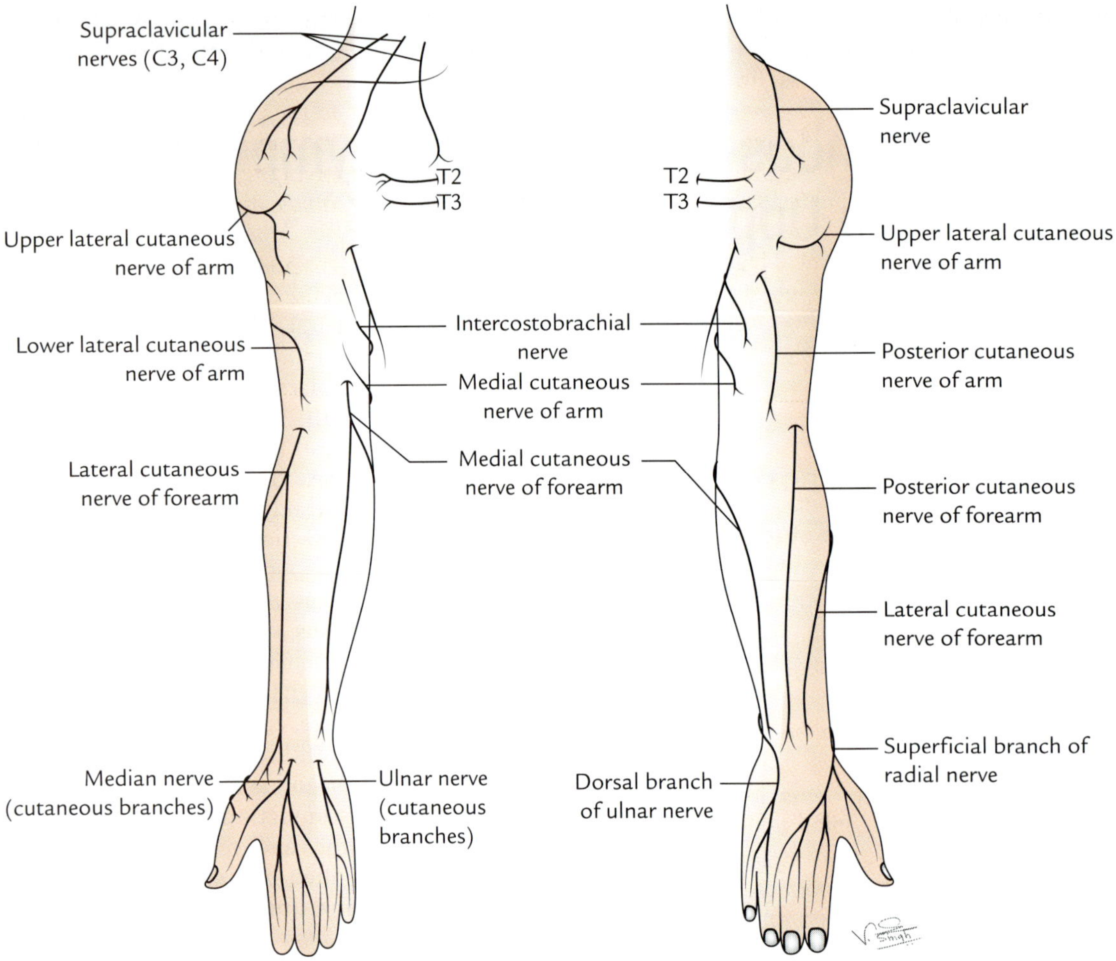

FIG. 7.1 ■ Cutaneous innervation of the upper limb.

(c) *Upper lateral half* of the arm is supplied by the **upper lateral cutaneous nerve of the arm** from axillary nerve.

(d) *Lower lateral half* of the arm is supplied by the **lower lateral cutaneous nerve** of the arm (C5, C6) from radial nerve.

(e) *Posterior aspect* of the arm is supplied by the **posterior cutaneous nerve** of the arm (C5) from radial nerve.

FOREARM (ANTEBRACHIUM)

It is supplied by *medial, lateral,* and *posterior cutaneous nerves* derived from the medial, lateral, and posterior cords of the brachial plexus, respectively.

- *Medial side* of the forearm is supplied by the **medial cutaneous nerve** of the forearm (C8, T1) from the medial cord of the brachial plexus. It becomes cutaneous halfway down the arm along the basilic vein.
- *Lateral side* of the forearm is supplied by the **lateral cutaneous nerve of the forearm (C5, C6)** from musculocutaneous nerve a branch from the lateral cord of the brachial plexus. It is the continuation of the musculocutaneous nerve. It emerges at the lateral border of the biceps and divides into anterior and posterior branches.
- *Posterior side* of the forearm is supplied by the **posterior cutaneous nerve** of the forearm (C6, C7, C8) from radial nerve, a branch from the posterior cord of the brachial plexus. It runs down the posterior aspect of forearm up to the wrist.

HAND

1. Palm of the hand
   (a) Lateral two-thirds of the palm is supplied by the palmar cutaneous branch of the median nerve.
   (b) Medial one-third of the palm is supplied by the palmar cutaneous branch of the ulnar nerve.
2. Dorsum of the hand
   (a) *Lateral two-thirds of the dorsum of hand* is supplied by the superficial terminal branch of the radial nerve (superficial radial nerve).
   (b) *Medial one-third of the dorsum of hand* is supplied by the dorsal branch/posterior cutaneous branch of the ulnar nerve.

DIGITS

1. Palmar aspects of the lateral 31/2 digits and their dorsal aspects up to distal half of the middle phalanges including nail beds are supplied by the digital branches of *median nerve*.

2. Palmar aspects of the medial 11/2 digit and their dorsal aspects up to distal half of the middle phalanges by the palmar digital branches of the *ulnar nerve*.
3. Dorsal aspects of the lateral 31/2 digits up to proximal half of their middle phalanges are supplied by the digital branches of the *radial nerve* except the nail beds.
4. Dorsal aspects of the medial 11/2 digit up to their middle phalanges are supplied by the digital branches of the *ulnar nerve*.

DERMATOMES OF THE UPPER LIMB (FIGS. 7.2 AND 7.3) AN 13.2

As already mentioned, **the area of the skin supplied by a single spinal nerve is** called **dermatome**.

In the trunk, the arrangement of dermatomes is simple (typical) because spinal nerves supplying it do not form plexuses and are arranged segmentally. A **typical dermatome** extends on the side of the trunk from the anterior median line to the posterior median line.

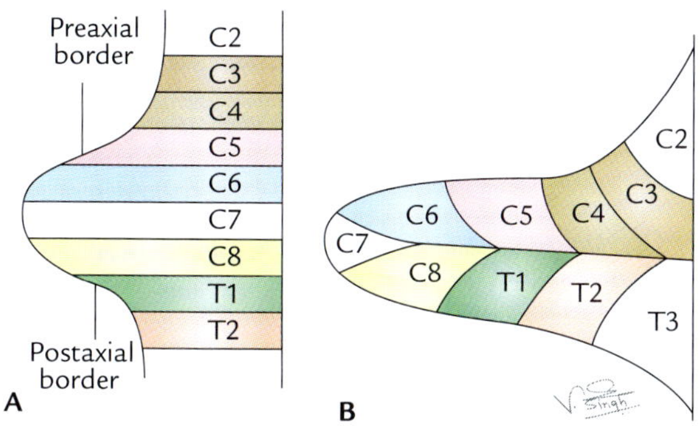

FIG. 7.2 ■ Arrangement of dermatomes in the developing upper limb: (**A**) simple dermatomal pattern to begin with C5 supplying the preaxial strip and T1 the postaxial strip; (**B**) definitive dermatomal pattern of the upper limb bud.

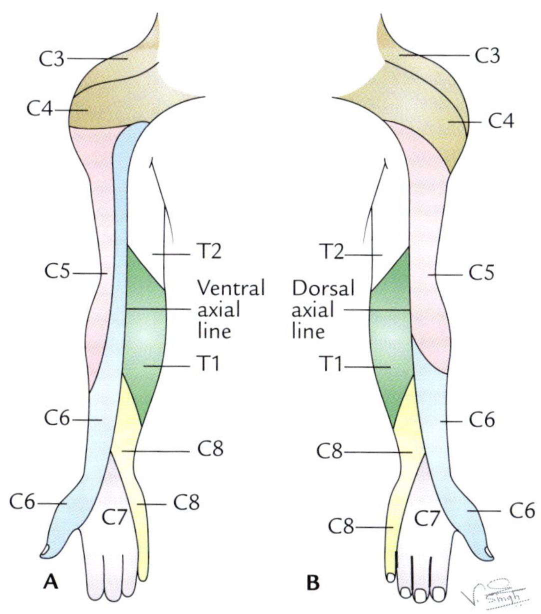

FIG. 7.3 ■ Dermatomes of the upper limb: (A) anterior aspect and (B) posterior aspect. Nipple not shown.

In the limbs, the arrangement of dermatomes is complicated because of the rotation of the limbs during their development. It becomes further complicated because spinal nerves supplying them form plexuses. (For details, see ***Chapter 5 of Textbook of Clinical Neuroanatomy, 4ed*** by Vishram Singh.) During development, before rotation each limb has preaxial and postaxial borders with former being directed towards the head. The digits along the preaxial border are thumb in the upper limb and big toe in the lower limb. During rotation of the limbs, the upper limb rotates laterally. As a result its preaxial border and thumb lie on the lateral side. The lower limb rotates medially. Therefore, its preaxial border and big toe lie on the medial side. Consequently the dermatomes are arranged consecutively downwards on the lateral side of the upper limb and upwards on the medial side of the upper limb.

To be very precise, the dermatomes of the upper limb are arranged in a numerical sequence as follows:

1. From the shoulder to the thumb, along the preaxial border by C3-C6 spinal segments.
2. From the thumb to the little finger by C6-C8 spinal segments.
3. From the little finger to the axilla along the postaxial border by C8-T2 spinal segments.

The segmental innervation is summarized in Table 7.1 and Fig. 7.3.

CLINICAL CORRELATION

Significance of dermatome: As discussed in the beginning, the understanding of dermatomal arrangement of upper limb is clinically important because the physicians commonly test the integrity of spinal cord segments from C3 to T2 by performing the sensory examination for touch, pain, and temperature. This is so because the sensory loss of the skin following injuries to the cord conforms to the dermatome.

TABLE 7.1 Segmental innervations of the upper limb

Area	Segment
Nipple	T4
Tip of the shoulder	C4
Lateral side of the arm	C5
Lateral side of the forearm	C6
Thumb	C6
Hand and middle 3 digits	C7
Little finger	C8
Medial side of the forearm	C8
Medial side of the arm	T1
Axilla	T2

N.B.

Overlapping of adjacent dermatomes: The students must remember that there is varying degrees of overlapping of adjacent dermatomes. Consequently, the area of sensory loss following a damage to the cord segments is always less than the area of distribution of the dermatomes.

MOTOR INNERVATION (MYOTOMES)

The embryological muscle mass and muscles derived from it are innervated by a single segment of spinal cord or spinal nerve is called *myotome*.

Most of the muscles of upper limb are made of more than one myotome hence innervated by multiple spinal segments. Hence multiple spinal segments are involved in producing movements of the upper limb. The details are described with the individual muscles.

N.B.

The intrinsic muscles of hand are derived from single myotome (T1).

VENOUS DRAINAGE OF THE UPPER LIMB AN 13.1

They drain the deoxygenated blood from hand, forearm, and arm. The veins draining the upper limb, as elsewhere in the body, are divided into two sets/groups (a) superficial and (b) deep. Both groups of veins are interconnected with one another.

The **superficial veins** are located in the superficial fascia and are easily accessible. Being easily accessible, they are frequently used by the clinicians for venepuncture.

The **deep veins** lie deep to deep fascia and run through muscles and accompany arteries as *venae comitantes.*

SUPERFICIAL VEINS

INTRODUCTION

The knowledge of superficial veins of upper limb is of utmost importance in medical practice as they are commonly used for venepuncture for giving intravenous injections and taking out blood for performing various clinical tests.

GENERAL FEATURES

Superficial veins have the following **general features**:

1. They lie in the superficial fascia (subcutaneous fascia).
2. They have a tendency to run away from the pressure points, hence they are absent in the palm (fist area), along the ulnar border of the forearm, and back of the elbow (supporting border of upper limb). For this reason, they course spirally from posterior to anterior surface of upper limb.
3. They join to form two major superficial veins, one runs along the **preaxial/cephalic border** and the other **along the postaxial/caudal border of the limb**. The preaxial vein (**cephalic vein**) is longer than the postaxial vein (**basilic vein**), but the postaxial **basilic** vein drains more efficiently. The load of long cephalic vein is greatly relieved as a good amount of its blood is transferred to the efficient basilic vein by the **median cubital vein** (communicating channel). Both cephalic and basilic veins originate from *dorsal venous arch/network* on the dorsum of the hand (Figs. 7.4 and 7.5).

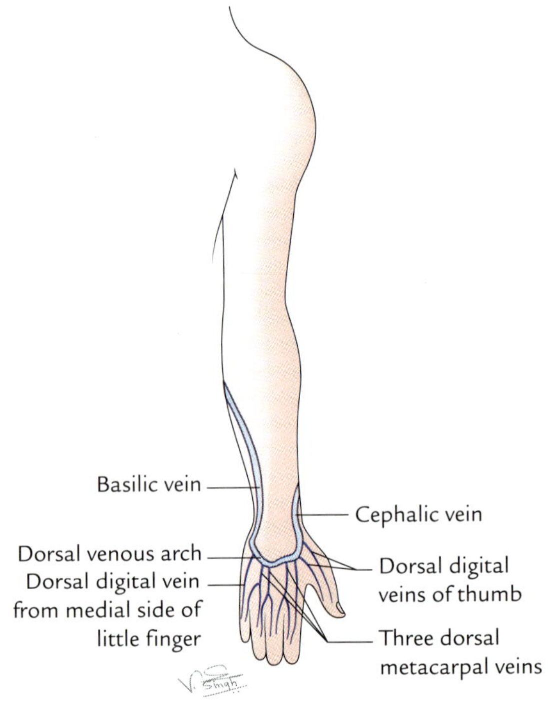

FIG. 7.4 ■ Dorsal venous arch and initial parts of the course of cephalic and basilic veins.

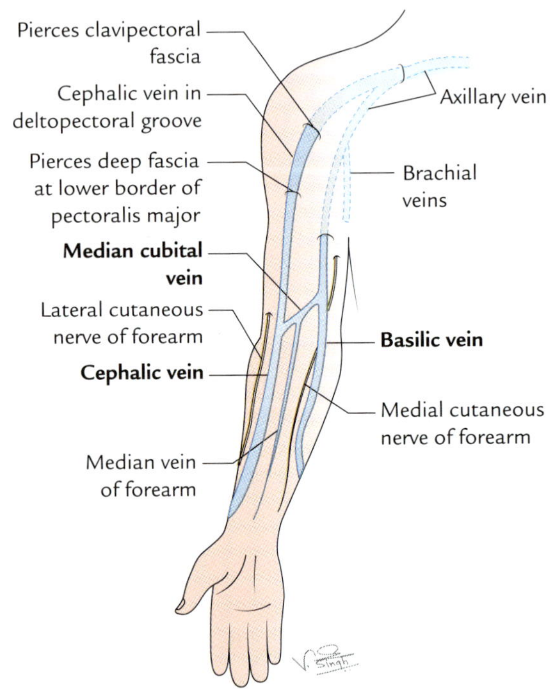

FIG. 7.5 ■ Cephalic and basilic veins.

4. The superficial veins are accompanied by the cutaneous nerves and superficial lymphatics.

Listing of veins

The superficial veins comprise:

1. Dorsal venous arch
2. Cephalic vein
3. Basilic vein
4. Median cubital vein
5. Median vein of forearm

Dorsal Venous Arch (Fig. 7.4)

The dorsal venous arch is a network of veins on the dorsum of hand. It presents irregular arrangement of veins usually with its transverse element, which lies 2–3 cm proximal to the heads of metacarpals.

Tributaries

The tributaries of dorsal venous arch are:

1. Three dorsal metacarpal veins.
2. A dorsal digital vein from the medial side of little finger.
3. A dorsal digital vein from the lateral side of index finger.
4. Two dorsal digital veins of the thumb.
5. Veins draining palm of hand. These are (a) veins that pass around the margins of the hand and (b) perforating veins, which pass dorsally through the interosseous spaces.

The dorsal venous arch drains into cephalic and basilic veins—the efferent vessels of dorsal venous arch.

N.B.

The pressure on the palm during gripping does not hamper the venous return of the palm, rather it facilities the return because venous blood from the palm is drained into dorsal venous arch.

Cephalic Vein (Figs. 7.4 and 7.5)

The cephalic vein (**preaxial vein of upper limb**) begins as the continuation of lateral end of the dorsal venous arch. **It is homologous to great saphenous vein of lower limb.**

It *crosses through the roof of anatomical snuff box*, ascends on the radial border of the forearm, continues upwards in front of elbow along the lateral border of biceps, pierces the deep fascia at the lower border of the pectoralis major, runs in cleft between the deltoid and pectoralis major (deltopectoral groove) up to the infraclavicular fossa, where it pierces the clavipectoral fascia and drains into the axillary vein.

N.B.

- At elbow, greater amount of blood from the cephalic vein is shunted into the basilic vein through *median cubital vein.*
- Cephalic vein is accompanied by the *lateral cutaneous nerve of the forearm.*
- An *accessory cephalic vein* from back of the forearm (occasional) ends in the cephalic vein below the elbow.
- Cephalic vein is the *preaxial vein of the upper limb* and corresponds to the *great saphenous vein* of the lower limb.

Basilic Vein (Figs. 7.4 and 7.5)

The basilic vein (postaxial vein) begins as the continuation of the medial end of the dorsal venous arch of the hand. It runs upwards along the back of the medial border of the forearm, winds round this border near the elbow to reach the anterior aspect of the forearm, where it continues upwards in front of the elbow along the medial side of the biceps brachii up to the middle of the arm, where it pierces deep fascia, unites with the brachial veins and runs along the medial side of the brachial artery to become continuous with the axillary vein at the lower border of the teres major.

N.B.

- Basilic vein is the postaxial vein of the upper limb and corresponds to the *short saphenous vein of the lower limb.*
- About 2.5 cm above the medial epicondyle of humerus, it is joined by the median cubital vein.
- It is accompanied by the *medial cutaneous nerve of the forearm.*

Median Cubital Vein (Fig. 7.5)

It is a communicating venous channel between the cephalic and basilic veins, which shunts blood from the cephalic vein to the basilic vein.

It begins from the cephalic vein, 2.5 cm below the elbow bend, runs obliquely upwards and medially to end in the basilic vein, 2.5 cm above the bend of elbow.

The important features of median cubital vein are as follows:

- It is separated from brachial artery by the bicipital aponeurosis.
- It communicates with the deep veins through a perforator vein, which pierces the bicipital aponeurosis.
- It receives median vein of the forearm.
- It shunts blood from cephalic vein to the basilic vein.

Median Vein of the Forearm

Median vein of the forearm begins from *palmar venous network*, runs upwards in the midline on the anterior aspect of forearm to end in any one of three veins in front of elbow (*viz.* cephalic, basilic, and median cubital veins).

N.B.

Sometimes the upper end of *median vein of the forearm* bifurcates into *median cephalic* and *median basilic veins*, which join the cephalic and basilic veins, respectively. In this situation, the *median cubital vein is absent* (Fig. 7.6B).

COMMON VENOUS PATTERNS IN FRONT OF THE ELBOW (FIG. 7.6)

The veins in front of the elbow commonly form two patterns, *viz.*

1. H-shaped pattern.
2. M-shaped pattern.

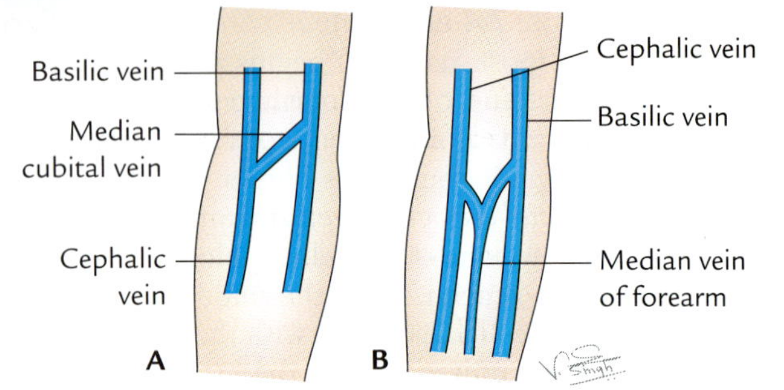

FIG. 7.6 ■ Common venous patterns in front of the elbow: (A) H-shaped pattern and (B) M-shaped pattern.

CLINICAL CORRELATION

- **Venepuncture in the cubital fossa:** The veins in front of the elbow, for example *median cubital vein, cephalic vein*, and *basilic vein* are routinely used for giving intravenous injections and for withdrawing blood from the donors.
  The **median cubital vein** is most preferred for venepuncture due to the following reasons:
  (a) It is the most superficial vein in the body, hence access is easy.
  (b) It is well supported by the underlying bicipital aponeurosis.
  (c) It is well anchored to the deep vein by a perforating vein, hence it does not slip during procedure.
- **Haemodialysis:** The *cephalic vein is preferred for haemodialysis* in the patients with *chronic renal failure* (CRF), to remove waste products from blood.
- **Cardiac catheterization:** The ***basilic vein is preferred for cardiac catheterization*** for the following reasons:
  (a) The diameter of basilic *vein increases as it* ascends from cubital fossa to the axillary vein.
  (b) It is in direct line with the axillary vein. To enter the right atrium the catheter passes in succession as follows:
  Basilic vein→axillary vein→subclavian vein→brachiocephalic vein→superior vena cava→right atrium of the heart
  The ***cephalic vein is not preferred for cardiac catheterization*** due to the following reasons:
  (a) Its diameter does not increase as it ascends.
  (b) It joins the axillary vein at a right angle hence it is difficult to manoeuvre the catheter around sharp cephaloaxillary angle.
  (c) In deltopectoral groove, it frequently divides into small branches. One of these branches ascends over the clavicle and joins the external jugular vein.
- **Cephalojugular communication:** Here cephalic vein communicates with external jugular vein through a small communicating vein which crosses in front of clavicle.
  When a segment of axillary vein is removed during clearance of axillary lymph nodes in breast cancer, this communicating vein enlarges considerably to help the drainage of venous blood from upper limb.
  It is often ruptured in fracture clavicle to cause bleeding.

DEEP VEINS

- The deep veins begin as *venae commitantes* accompanying digital arteries which course proximally along superficial and deep palmar arterial arches as superficial and deep palmar venous arches. Then these veins continue proximally as venae commitantes of larger arteries. Later they unite to form large deep veins lie along the arteries.
- The major deep veins of upper limb comprise:
  (a) venae comitantes, which accompany the large arteries, such as radial, ulnar, arteries;
  (b) venae comitantes of the brachial artery; and
  (c) axillary vein.

Venae comitantes of the radial and ulnar arteries accompany the radial and ulnar arteries, respectively, and join to form the *brachial veins*.

Venae comitantes are small veins, one on each side of the brachial artery. They join axillary vein at the lower border of the teres major muscle. The medial one often joins the basilic vein.

Axillary vein begins as a continuation of basilic vein at the lower border of the teres major muscle and runs through axilla, passes through its apex to continue as *subclavian vein* at the outer border of the first rib (for details see Chapter 4, page 52).

The overview of venous drainage of upper limb is shown in Fig. 7.7.

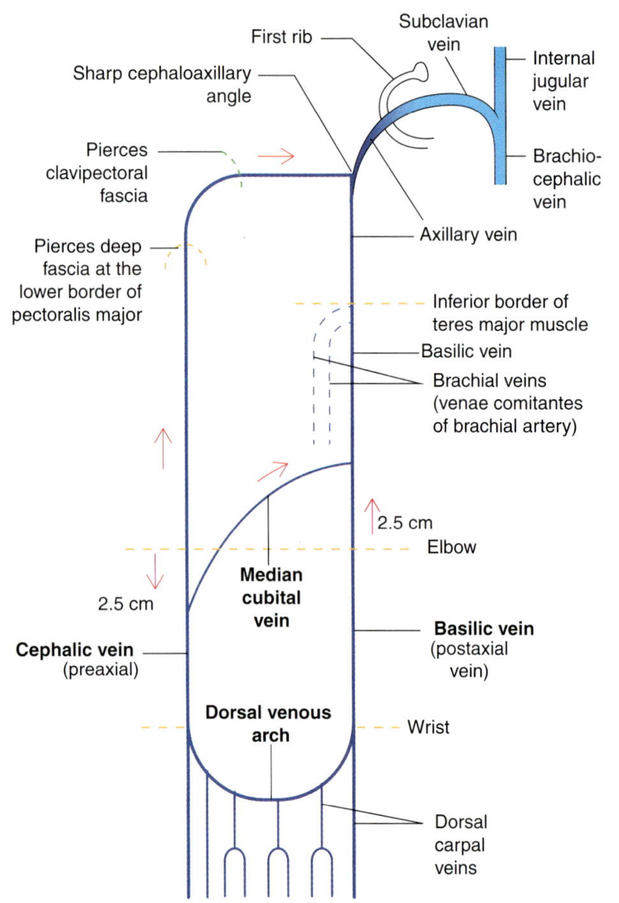

FIG. 7.7 ■ Schematic diagram showing venous drainage of the upper limb.

LYMPHATIC DRAINAGE OF THE UPPER LIMB (FIG. 7.8) AN 13.1

The lymphatic drainage of the upper limb occurs through the unnamed lymph vessels, which originate in the hand and run upwards towards the axilla.

When they reach cubital fossa, the lymph passes through *cubital nodes*. From here lymph vessels run superiorly to drain into the *axillary lymph nodes*.

LYMPH VESSELS

The lymph vessels draining the lymph from the upper limb, as elsewhere in the body, are divided into two groups: superficial and deep.

Generally the **superficial lymph vessels** follow the superficial veins and **deep lymph vessels** follow the deep veins. The lymph collected by both superficial and deep lymph vessels drain into **axillary lymph nodes**. The details are as under:

SUPERFICIAL LYMPH VESSELS

The superficial lymph vessels are located in the subcutaneous tissue. They are much more numerous than the deep lymph vessels. They generally accompany the superficial veins.

The *superficial lymph vessels* drain the lymph from skin and subcutaneous tissue. They course upwards towards the axilla. Most of them end in the axillary lymph nodes.

Those from lateral side of the limb and *lateral two digits* follow the cephalic vein and drain into the *infraclavicular lymph nodes*.

Those from medial side of the limb and *medial three digits* follow the basilic vein and drain into the *lateral group of axillary nodes*.

Some of the medial lymph vessels terminate in the **supratrochlear or epitrochlear nodes**, which are situated just above the medial epicondyle along the basilic vein.

A few lymph vessels drain the thumb end in the *deltopectoral lymph nodes*. The efferents from these nodes pierce the clavipectoral fascia to drain in the apical group of axillary nodes.

N.B.

- Almost all the superficial lymph vessels of the upper limb drain into *lateral group of axillary nodes*.
- Lymph from palm is drained into the lymph plexus on the dorsum of the hand.
- *Vertical area of lymph shed* is in the middle of the back of arm and forearm: The lymph vessels from the back of the arm and forearm curve around the medial and lateral borders of limb to reach the front of the limb, thus forming a vertical area of lymph shed.

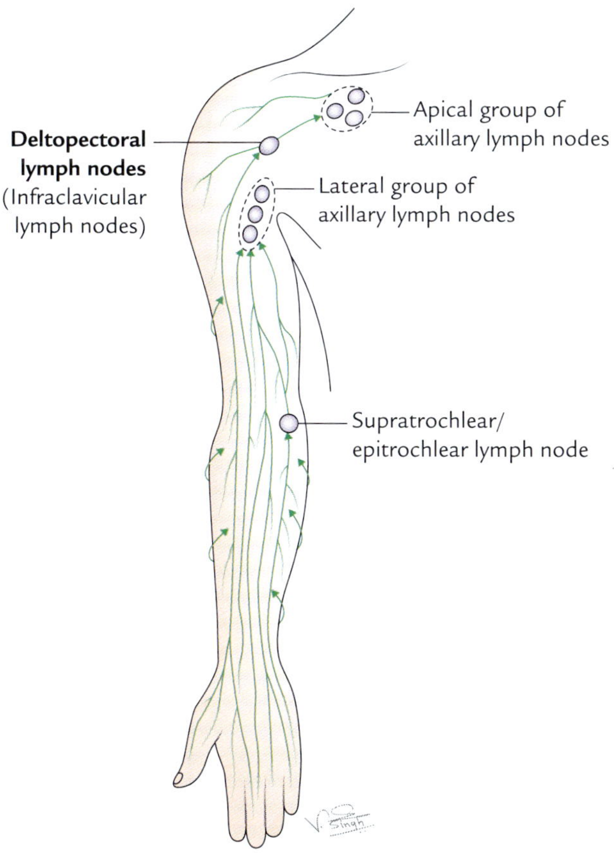

FIG. 7.8 ■ Lymphatic drainage of the upper limb.

DEEP LYMPH VESSELS

The deep lymph vessels are much less numerous than the superficial lymph vessels. They drain structures lying deep to deep fascia, *viz.* muscles. The deep lymph vessels course along the arteries and drain into the *lateral group of the axillary lymph nodes*.

CLINICAL CORRELATION

- **Lymphangitis:** The inflammation of the lymph vessels is termed *lymphangitis*. It usually follows trivial injuries, for examples cuts and pin-pricks, to any part of the upper limb. *In acute lymphangitis*, the lymph vessels may be seen underneath the skin as *red streaks*, which are tender (i.e. painful to touch).
- **Lymphoedema:** The obstruction of lymph vessels may cause oedema (i.e. swelling) in the area of drainage due to accumulation of colloidal tissue fluid. It often occurs due to surgical removal of lymph nodes in cancer surgery.

LYMPH NODES

The lymph nodes draining the upper limb are divided into two groups: (a) superficial and (b) deep.

SUPERFICIAL LYMPH NODES

They lie in the superficial fascia, along the superficial vein. These are as follows:

1. **Deltopectoral nodes/Infraclavicular nodes,** one or two in number, lie in the deltopectoral groove

along the cephalic vein. They drain lymph from thumb including its web and superolateral part of the breast.

2. **Superficial cubital/Supratrochlear nodes** lie 5 cm above the medial epicondyle along the basilic vein. They drain the lymph from the ulnar side of the hand and forearm.

DEEP LYMPH NODES

The deep lymph nodes are as follows:

1. **Axillary lymph nodes** are present in the axilla and are divided into five sets. These are main lymph nodes of the upper limb (for details see Chapter 4, page 53).
2. **A few other deep lymph nodes** lie on the following sites:
   (a) Along the medial side of the brachial artery.
   (b) In the cubital fossa, at the bifurcation of the brachial artery (called *deep cubital node*).
   (c) Occasionally along the arteries of the forearm.

CLINICAL CORRELATION

- The axillary lymph nodes are enlarged (*lymphadenopathy*) and become painful following infection in any part of the upper limb.
- In infection affecting the medial side of the hand and forearm, *supratrochlear lymph node* becomes enlarged and tender.

Golden Facts to Remember

• Most prominent superficial vein in the body • Most commonly used vein for venepuncture	Median cubital vein
• Most preferred vein for cardiac catheterization	Basilic vein
• Commonest pattern of the superficial veins in front of elbow	H-shaped
• Most of the superficial lymph vessels of the upper limb drain into	Lateral group of the axillary lymph nodes
• Most distal superficial lymph node in the upper limb	Supratrochlear/ epitrochlear node
• Commonest cause of lymphoedema of the upper limb	Removal of the axillary lymph nodes during mastectomy
• Longest superficial vein of the upper limb	Cephalic vein
• Area of lymph shed in the arm and forearm	Vertical area in the middle of the back of arm and forearm

CLINICAL CASE STUDY

A 38-year-old female went to the pathologist for routine blood examination. The pathologist asked the technician to collect the blood sample of the lady. While attempting to collect the blood sample from median cubital vein, the technician noticed that the blood in the syringe is bright red. He immediately withdrew the needle.

In second attempt, he inserted the needle slightly medial to the previous puncture. The lady felt sharp pain, which radiated to the lateral three digits. **It was diagnosed as misplaced injection in median cubital vein.**

Questions

1. What is median cubital vein?
2. Name the fascial structure which separates median cubital vein from brachial artery and median nerve.
3. Mention the cause of sharp pain that radiated to the lateral 3½ digits.
4. What does the bright red blood in syringe indicate during collection of the blood sample from the median cubital vein?

Answers

1. It is a communicating vein in front of elbow between the cephalic and basilic veins.
2. Bicipital aponeurosis.
3. Median nerve injury.
4. Puncture of the brachial artery.

Arm

CHAPTER 8

SPECIFIC LEARNING OBJECTIVES

After studying this chapter, the student should be able to:

- Describe and demonstrate muscle groups of arm with emphasis on biceps and triceps brachii. AN 11.1
- Describe the origin, course and relations, branches (or tributaries), and termination of important nerves and vessels in arm. AN 11.2
- Describe the anatomical basis of venepuncture of cubital veins. AN 11.3
- Describe the origin, insertion, nerve supply, and actions of: (a) biceps brachii, (b) brachialis, and (c) triceps brachii.
- Describe anastomoses around elbow joint. AN 11.6
- Write short notes on: (a) musculocutaneous nerve, (b) brachial artery, (c) arterial anastomosis around the elbow, and (d) profunda brachii artery.
- Enumerate: (a) anatomical events/changes occurring at the level of insertion of coracobrachialis, (b) branches given by the radial nerve in the radial/spiral groove, and (c) contents of the cubital fossa.
- Describe the anatomical basis of Saturday night paralysis and wrist drop. AN 11.4
- Describe the boundaries and contents of cubital fossa in brief and discuss its clinical significance. AN 11.5
- Describe the clinical testing of biceps brachii muscle. AN 13.7

The arm (L. brachium = arm) is the part of the upper limb between the shoulder and the elbow. The bone of the arm—the humerus—articulates above with the scapula to form the shoulder joint and below with the radius and ulna to form the elbow joint. The humerus is almost entirely covered by muscles. The **primary neurovascular bundle of the arm** is located on the medial side of the arm, hence protected by the limb, which it serves. It consists of *brachial artery*, with its *venae comitantes*, *basilic vein*, and *median nerve*.

Since the arm is termed brachium in Latin, most of its structures are named accordingly, *viz.* biceps brachii, coracobrachialis, brachialis, triceps brachii, brachial vessels, etc.

SURFACE LANDMARKS

The following bony landmarks and soft tissue structures can be felt in the living individual (Fig. 8.1):

1. **Greater tubercle of the humerus:** It can be felt just below and lateral to the acromion, deep to the deltoid with the arm lying by the side of the trunk. It forms the most lateral bony point of the shoulder region.
2. **Shaft of the humerus:** It can be felt indistinctly in thin individuals.
3. **Medial epicondyle of the humerus:** It is the prominent bony projection felt on the medial side of the elbow. The projection is best seen and felt in the midflexed elbow.
4. **Lateral epicondyle of the humerus:** It can be felt in the upper part of the depression on the posterolateral aspect of the extended elbow.
5. **Medial and lateral supracondylar ridges:** These can be felt in the lower one-fourth of the arm as the upward continuations of the medial and lateral epicondyles, respectively.
6. **Deltoid muscle:** It forms the rounded contour of the shoulder, which becomes prominent on abducting the arm. It covers the upper half of the humerus anteriorly, laterally, and posteriorly, and its apex (i.e. tendon) is attached to the lateral side of the middle of the humerus on deltoid tuberosity.
7. **Biceps muscle:** It forms a conspicuous bulge on the front of the arm, which becomes prominent on flexing the elbow. Its tendon can be felt on the front of the elbow.
8. **Brachial artery pulsations:** These can be felt in front of the elbow just medial to the tendon of the biceps muscle.
9. **Ulnar nerve:** It can be rolled by the middle finger in the groove behind the medial epicondyle of the humerus.
10. **Superficial veins in front of the elbow** (i.e. cephalic, basilic, and median cubital veins): These become visible when they are distended by applying tight pressure around the arm, and then flexing and extending the elbow a few times with clenched fist.
11. **Head of radius:** This can be felt in the depression on the posterolateral aspect of the elbow just distal

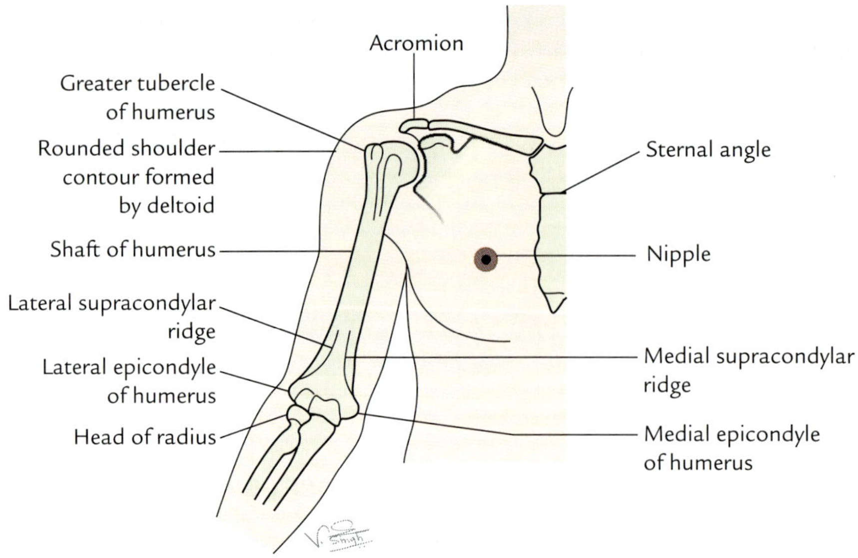

FIG. 8.1 ■ Surface landmarks on the front of the arm.

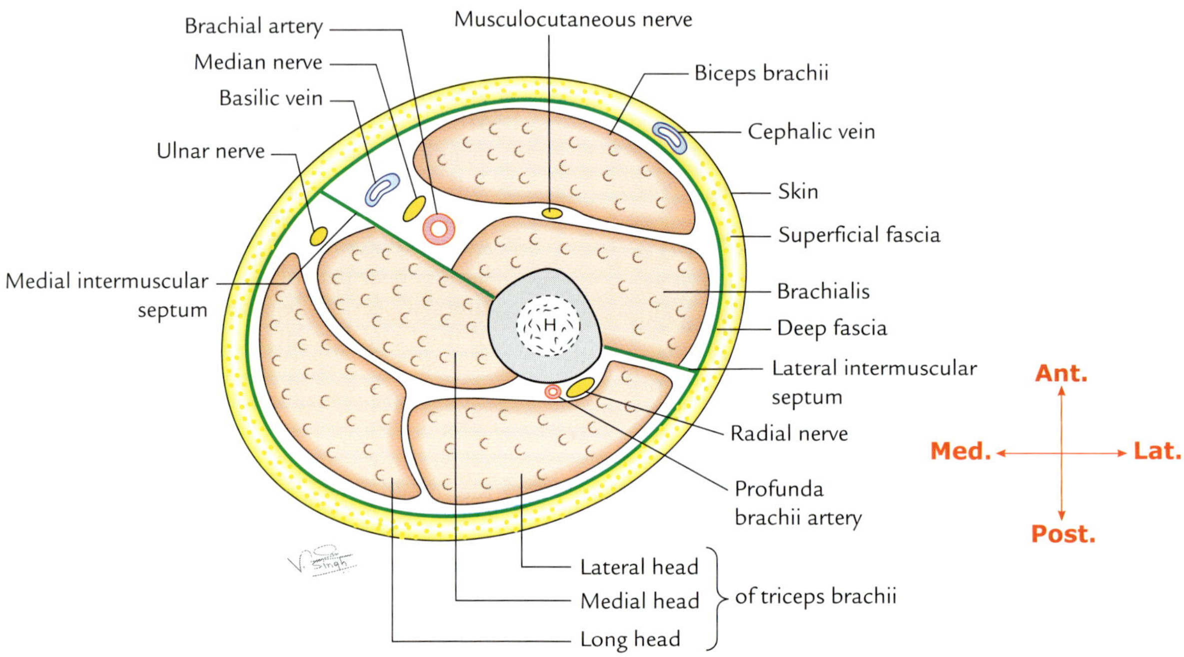

FIG. 8.2 ■ Transverse section of the arm just below the level of insertion of the deltoid muscle (H = humerus).

to the lateral epicondyle. The rotation of the head of radius can be felt by supinating and pronating the forearm.

12. **Olecranon process of ulna (proximal part of ulna):** It is readily palpable on the back elbow between the medial and the lateral epicondyles.

COMPARTMENTS OF THE ARM AN 11.1

The deep fascia encloses the arm like a sleeve. The two intermuscular fascial septa, one on the medial side and one on the lateral side, extend inward from the fascial sleeve and get attached to the medial and lateral supracondylar ridges of the humerus, respectively. These septa and fascial sleeve divide the arm into the anterior and posterior compartments (Fig. 8.2). Each compartment has its own muscles, nerve, and artery.

N.B.

Some structures, however, pierce the intermuscular septa to shift from one compartment to the other, *namely*:

- The ulnar nerve and superior ulnar collateral artery pierce the medial intermuscular septum to enter the posterior compartment.
- The radial nerve and the radial collateral artery pierce the lateral intermuscular septum to enter the anterior compartment.

ANTERIOR COMPARTMENT OF ARM

The contents of the anterior compartment of the arm are:
- **Muscles:** **B**iceps brachii, **B**rachialis, and **C**oracobrachialis.
  Mnemonic: **BBC**.
- **Nerve:** musculocutaneous nerve.
- **Artery:** brachial artery.
- **Vein:** basilic vein.

In addition to the above structures, the following large nerves also pass through the anterior compartment of the arm:
- Median nerve
- Ulnar nerve
- Radial nerve

MUSCLES OF FRONT OF ARM

Biceps brachii

Origin

The biceps brachii muscle arises from scapula by two heads: long and short (Fig. 8.3).

1. **Long head** arises from the **supraglenoid tubercle** within the capsule of the shoulder joint. Its tendon runs above the head of the humerus and emerges from the joint through the intertubercular sulcus. The long head is intracapsular but extra synovial.
2. **Short head** arises along with coracobrachialis from the tip of the coracoid process.

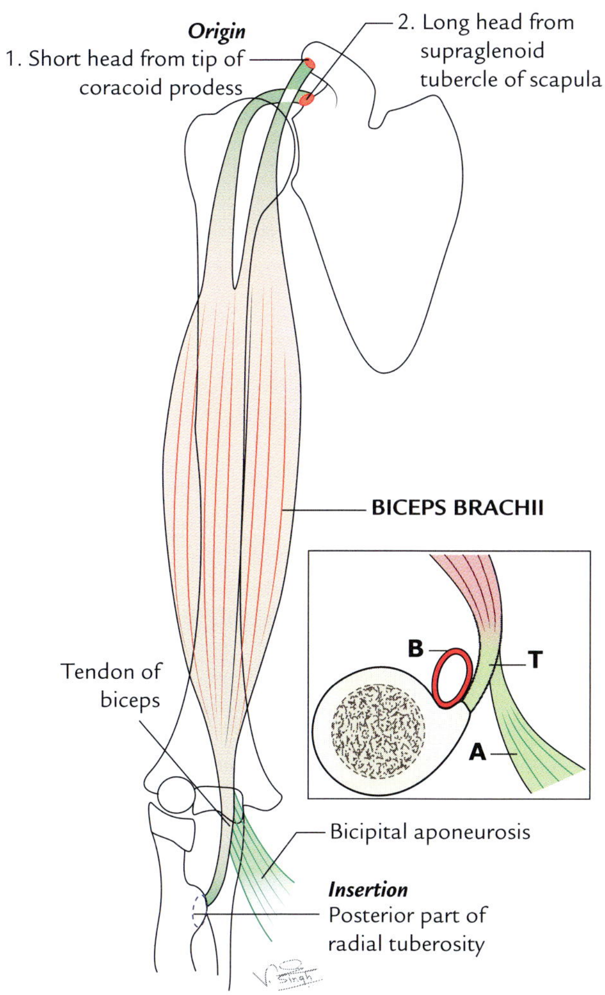

FIG. 8.3 Origin and insertion of the biceps brachii muscle. Figure in the inset shows details at the site of insertion of biceps tendon (A = bicipital aponeurosis; B = synovial bursa; T = biceps tendon).

The two heads join together in the distal third of the arm to form a belly that ends in a tendon, which gives off the ***bicipital aponeurosis*** from its medial aspect, opposite to the bend of the elbow.

It separates the overlying median cubital vein from underlying median nerve and brachial artery from injury. Hence protect artery and nerve during venepuncture. Hence, also called as '**grâce à Dieu fascia**' (which means praise to God) or by grace of God.

The origin of biceps brachii is easily remembered by a following mnemonic.

Mnemonic: **L**ovely **s**ights are **s**een **c**uriously, that is **l**ong head arises from **s**upraglenoid tubercle and **s**hort head from **c**oracoid process.

Insertion

The biceps muscle is inserted into:
(a) The posterior part of the radial tuberosity by its tendon. A bursa intervenes between the tendon and the anterior part of the tuberosity and
(b) The deep fascia on the medial aspect of the forearm by its aponeurosis (bicipital aponeurosis). The aponeurosis protects the underlying brachial artery and the median nerve.

Relations

- **Proximal part** is overlapped by pectoralis major and deltoid muscles.
- Long head passes in intracapsularly through shoulder joint.
- Distal part lies in front brachialis and musculocutaneous nerve.
- Medial border overlaps the neurovascular bundle of arm made up of brachial vessels and median nerve.

Nerve supply

By the musculocutaneous nerve (C5–C7).

Actions

1. It is a strong supinator of the forearm, when the elbow is flexed. This action is used in screwing movements, such as tightening the screw with a screw driver.
2. It is a powerful flexor of the forearm, when the elbow is extended.
3. It is also a weak flexor of the shoulder joint.

Clinical testing

The biceps brachii is tested by asking the patient to flex the elbow against resistance when the forearm is supinated. In this act, the muscle forms a prominent bulge on the front of the arm.

CLINICAL CORRELATION

- **Biceps reflex:** It is tested during physical examination by tapping the tendon of biceps brachii by the reflex hammer with the forearm pronated and partially extended at the elbow. The normal reflex is *brief jerk*-like flexion of the elbow. The normal reflex confirms the integrity of the musculocutaneous nerve and the C5 and C6 spinal segments.
- **Popeye's deformity:** When long head of biceps brachii ruptures due to attrition, the belly of muscle bunch up to form a large ball-shaped painful swelling in front of arm that resembles to the arm of a famous cartoon character Mr Popeye of 1930s. Hence, it is termed Popeye's deformity (Fig. 8.4).

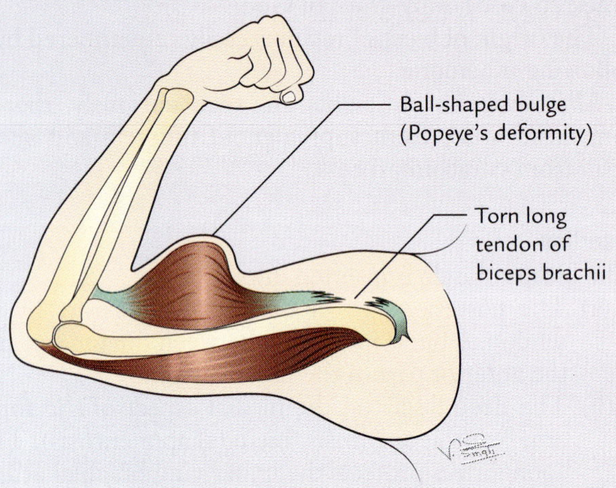

FIG. 8.4 ■ Popeye's deformity.

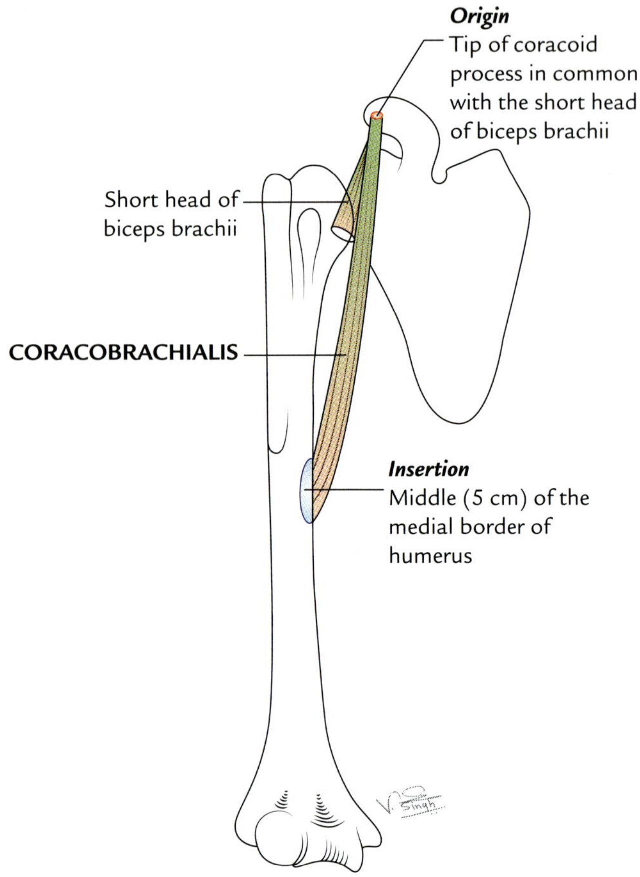

FIG. 8.5 ■ Origin and insertion of the coracobrachialis muscle.

Coracobrachialis (Fig. 8.5)

Origin

Coracobrachialis originates from the tip of the coracoid process of the scapula along with the short head of the biceps brachii.

Insertion

Into the middle of the medial border of the shaft of the humerus.

Nerve supply

By the musculocutaneous nerve.

Actions

It is a weak flexor and adductor of the arm.

N.B.

- **Morphology of the coracobrachialis:** It represents the muscle of the medial compartment of the forelimb of quadrupeds, which is not well developed in human beings. In some animals, this muscle consists of three heads (i.e. tricipital muscle). In human beings, the upper two heads are fused and the musculocutaneous nerve passes between the two fused heads. The lower third head has disappeared in humans. But occasionally the lower third head persists as a fibrous band (**ligament of Struthers**), which extends between the **supratrochlear/trochlear spur** and the medial epicondyle of the humerus (Fig. 2.11). The median nerve and the brachial artery then pass deep to the ligament and may be compressed.
- **Anatomical events occurring at the insertion of the coracobrachialis:** It is an important landmark as many anatomical events occur at this level (Fig. 8.6):
  1. Circular shaft of the humerus becomes triangular below this level.
  2. Brachial artery passes from the medial side of the arm to its anterior aspect.
  3. Basilic vein pierces the deep fascia.
  4. Median nerve crosses in front of the brachial artery from the lateral to the medial side.
  5. Radial nerve pierces the lateral intermuscular septum to pass from the posterior compartment to the anterior compartment.
  6. Ulnar nerve pierces the medial intermuscular septum to go into the posterior compartment.
  7. Medial cutaneous nerve of the arm and the forearm pierces the deep fascia.
  8. Nutrient artery pierces the humerus.

Brachialis

Origin

Brachialis originates from the anterior surface of the lower half of the shaft of the humerus. Superiorly the origin of the brachialis embraces the insertion of the deltoid (Fig. 8.7).

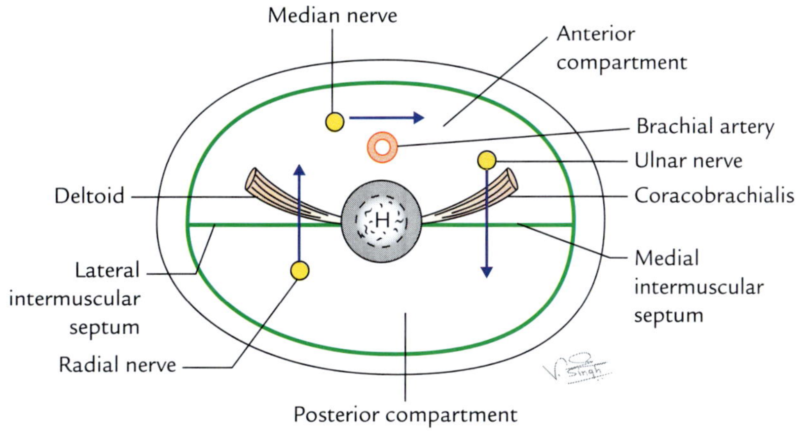

FIG. 8.6 ■ Important anatomical events occurring at the level of insertion of the coracobrachialis.

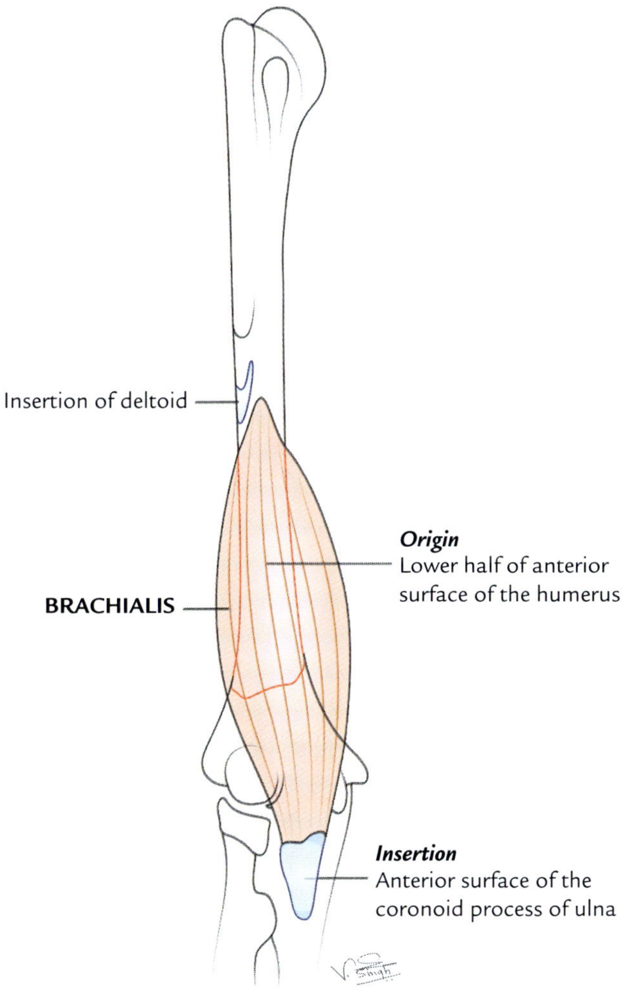

FIG. 8.7 ■ Origin and insertion of the brachialis.

Insertion

Into the anterior surface of the coronoid process of the ulna, including the tuberosity of the ulna.

Nerve supply

It has dual innervation:

1. Medial two-thirds by the *musculocutaneous nerve.*
2. Lateral one-third by the *radial nerve.*

Actions

It is the untiring strong flexor of the elbow joint; hence, it is often called '**work-horse of the elbow joint**'.

Table 8.1 summarizes the origin, insertion, nerve supply, and actions of the muscles of the anterior compartment of the arm.

Musculocutaneous Nerve (VR of C5–C7)

Origin and Course

The musculocutaneous nerve is the **nerve of the front of the arm** (Figs. 8.8 and 13.2). It arises from the lateral cord of the brachial plexus in the lower part of axilla at the lower border of pectoralis minor. It runs downward and laterally, pierces the coracobrachialis, which it supplies, and then passes downwards and laterally between the biceps and brachialis muscles which it supplies. It appears at the lateral margin of the biceps tendon, pierces the deep fascia about 2 cm above the elbow, and descends over the lateral aspect of the forearm as the *lateral cutaneous nerve of the forearm to provide sensory innervation to its lateral aspect.*

Branches and Distribution

1. **Muscular branches** to the biceps brachii, coracobrachialis, and brachialis.
2. **Cutaneous branch** (the *lateral cutaneous nerve of the forearm*) supplies the skin on the front and lateral aspect of the forearm up to wrist.
3. **Articular branch** to the elbow joint through its branch to the brachialis muscle.

CLINICAL CORRELATION

Injury of the musculocutaneous nerve: Although it is rare, if occurs, it leads to the following signs and symptoms:

- Loss of strong flexion and supination.
- Loss of biceps tendon reflex.
- Loss of sensation along the lateral aspect of the forearm.

Brachial Artery **AN 11.2**

Origin and Course

The brachial artery is the **main artery of the arm** (Fig. 8.9). It begins at the lower border of the teres major

TABLE 8.1 Origin, insertion, nerve supply, and main actions of the muscles of the anterior compartment of the arm (i.e. front of the arm)

Muscle	Origin	Insertion	Nerve supply	Actions
Biceps brachii	• *Short head* from the tip of the coracoid process of the scapula • *Long head* from the supraglenoid tubercle of the scapula	Posterior rough part of the radial tuberosity	Musculocutaneous nerve	• Supination of the forearm when the elbow is flexed • Flexion of the forearm when the elbow is extended
Coracobrachialis	Tip of the coracoid process of the scapula along with the short head of biceps	Middle one-third of the medial border of the humerus	Musculocutaneous nerve	Helps in flexion and adduction of the arm
Brachialis	Lower half of the anterior surface of the humerus	On the anterior surface of the coronoid process of the ulna, including ulnar tuberosity	• Musculocutaneous nerve (mainly) • Radial nerve	Flexion of the forearm in all positions

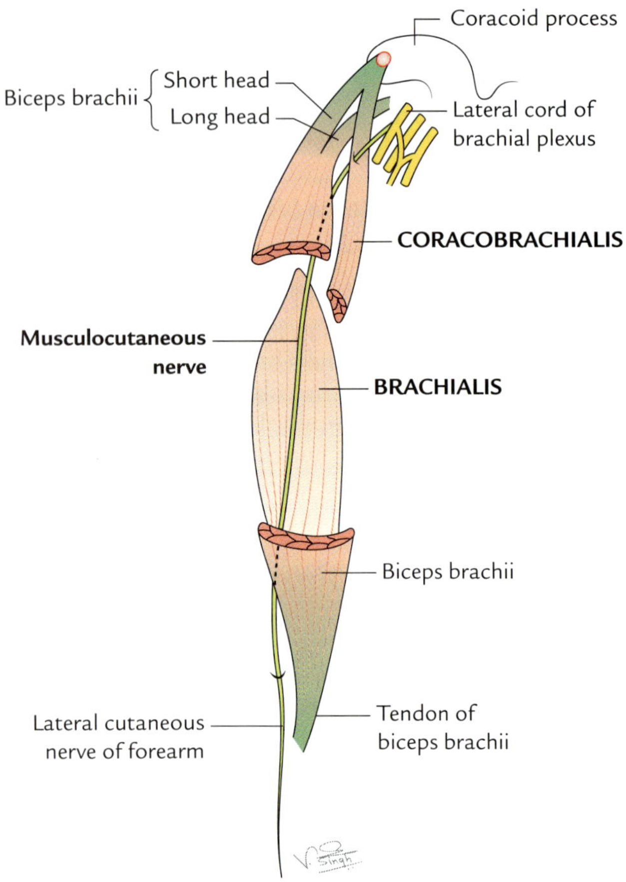

FIG. 8.8 Course and distribution of the musculocutaneous nerve.

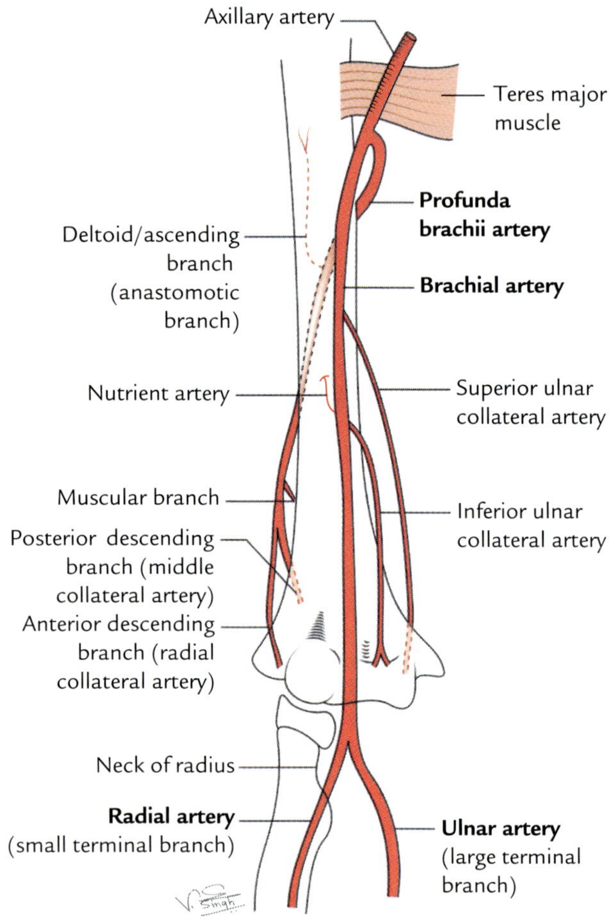

FIG. 8.9 Brachial artery.

muscle as a continuation of the axillary artery. It runs downwards and laterally in front of arm and enters the cubital fossa, to lie medial to tendon of biceps muscle. It terminates in front of the elbow at the level of the neck of radius by dividing into the radial and ulnar arteries (Fig. 8.9).

N.B.

Brachial artery lies near to skin hence susceptible for traumatic injuries.

Relations

Anteriorly
- *In the upper part*, it is related to the medial cutaneous nerve of the forearm, which lies in front of it.
- *In the middle part*, it is crossed by the median nerve from the lateral to the medial side.
- *In the lower part*, in the cubital fossa, it is crossed by the bicipital aponeurosis.

Posteriorly From above downward, the brachial artery lies successively on the long head of the triceps, medial head of the triceps, coracobrachialis, and brachialis muscles.

Medially The ulnar nerve and the basilic vein in the upper part of the arm, and median nerve in the lower part of the arm.

Laterally The median nerve, coracobrachialis, and biceps in the upper part of the arm and the tendon of the biceps in the lower part.

N.B.

The brachial artery is superficial throughout its course, being covered only by the skin and fascia, hence easily accessible.

Branches

1. **Muscular branches** to the muscles of the anterior compartment of the arm.
2. **Profunda brachii artery** (largest and first branch): It arises from the posteromedial aspect of the brachial artery just below the lower border of the teres major. It accompanies the radial nerve with which it immediately leaves the *lower triangular intermuscular space* to enter the *spiral groove* on the posterior surface of the humerus.
3. **Nutrient artery to the humerus** enters the nutrient foramen of the humerus located near the insertion of the coracobrachialis.
4. **Superior ulnar collateral artery** arises near the middle of the arm and accompanies the ulnar nerve.
5. **Inferior ulnar collateral (or supratrochlear) artery** arises near the lower end of the humerus and divides into the anterior and posterior branches, which take part in the formation of arterial anastomosis around the elbow.
6. Radial and ulnar arteries (terminal branches).

CLINICAL CORRELATION AN 11.2

- **Brachial pulse:** The brachial pulse is commonly felt in the cubital fossa medial to the tendon of biceps and its pulsations are auscultated for *recording the* **blood pressure**. The biceps tendon is easily palpable on flexing the elbow. Method of taking blood pressure is taught in physiological practical classes.
- **Compression of brachial artery:** The brachial artery can be effectively compressed against the shaft of the humerus at the level of insertion of the coracobrachialis to stop the haemorrhages in the upper limb occurring from any artery distal to the compression of the brachial artery, for example bleeding wounds of the palmar arterial arches (Fig. 8.10).
- **Volkmann's ischaemic contracture (ischaemic compartment syndrome):** The sudden complete occlusion of brachial artery due to tight plaster cast or its laceration due to supracondylar fracture of the humerus (Fig. 8.11) can cause fibrosis of muscles of the forearm due to their ischaemia and necrosis within a few hours. The muscles can tolerate ischaemia up to 6 hours only. Thereafter they undergo necrosis, and the fibrous tissue replaces the necrotic tissue. As a result, of fibrosis muscles shorten permanently, producing a flexor deformity akin to claw hand characterized by the flexion of the wrist, extension of the MP joints, and flexion of the IP joints, which lead to the loss of hand power.

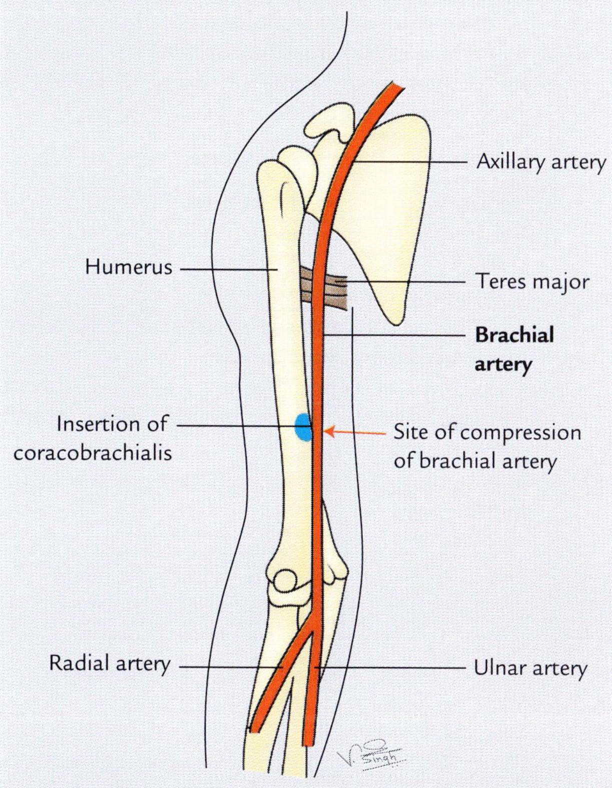

FIG. 8.10 ■ Compression of the brachial artery against the humerus.

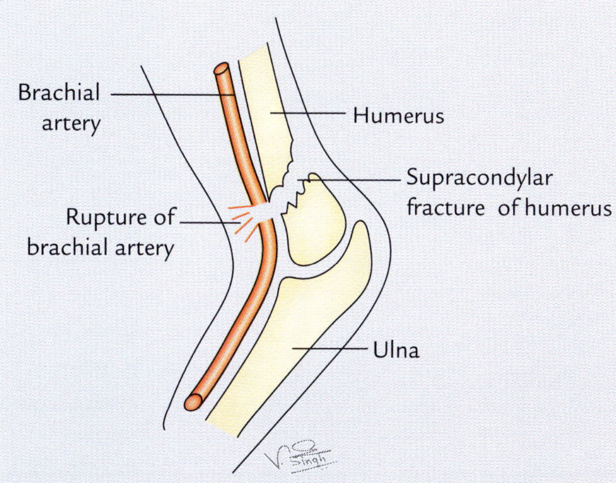

FIG. 8.11 ■ Rupture of the brachial artery in the supracondylar fracture of the humerus.

Arterial Anastomosis Around the Elbow AN 11.6

The arterial anastomosis around the elbow takes place *between the branches of the brachial artery and those from the upper ends of the radial and ulnar arteries* (Fig. 8.12).

For easy remembering, the anastomosis is divided into the following parts:

- **In front of the medial epicondyle:**
  (a) **I**nferior ulnar collateral artery (a branch of the brachial artery), anastomose with
  (b) **A**nterior ulnar recurrent artery (branch of the ulnar artery)
- **Behind the medial epicondyle:**
  (a) **S**uperior ulnar collateral artery (a branch of the brachial artery), anastomose with
  (b) **P**osterior ulnar recurrent artery (a branch of the ulnar artery)

  Mnemonic: **I A**m **P**retty **S**mart.
- **In front of the lateral epicondyle:**
  (a) **A**nterior descending artery (radial collateral artery, a branch of the profunda brachii artery), anastomose with
  (b) **R**adial recurrent artery (a branch of the radial artery)
- **Behind the lateral epicondyle:**
  (a) **P**osterior descending artery (middle collateral artery, a branch of the profunda brachii artery), anastomose with
  (b) **I**nterosseous recurrent artery (a branch of the posterior interosseous artery); which is a branch of common interosseous artery (a branch of the ulnar artery)

  Mnemonic: **A**merican **R**esidents **P**refer **I**ndia.

  Significance of anastomosis:

  1. Provides blood supply to elbow joint
  2. Provides collateral circulation

NERVES OTHER THAN MUSCULOCUTANEOUS NERVE PASSING THROUGH THE ARM AN 11.2

These are **median, ulnar**, and **radial nerves** (Fig. 8.13).

Median Nerve (Root Value: C5–T1)

Origin, course, and termination

The median nerve arises from the lateral and medial cords of the brachial plexus in axilla and descends down on the front of arm. It is closely related to the brachial artery throughout its course in the arm. Initially it lies lateral to the brachial artery, but crosses over it medially in the midarm. As a result in the cubital fossa it lies medial to brachial artery. It is superficially located, except at the elbow where it is crossed by the bicipital aponeurosis.

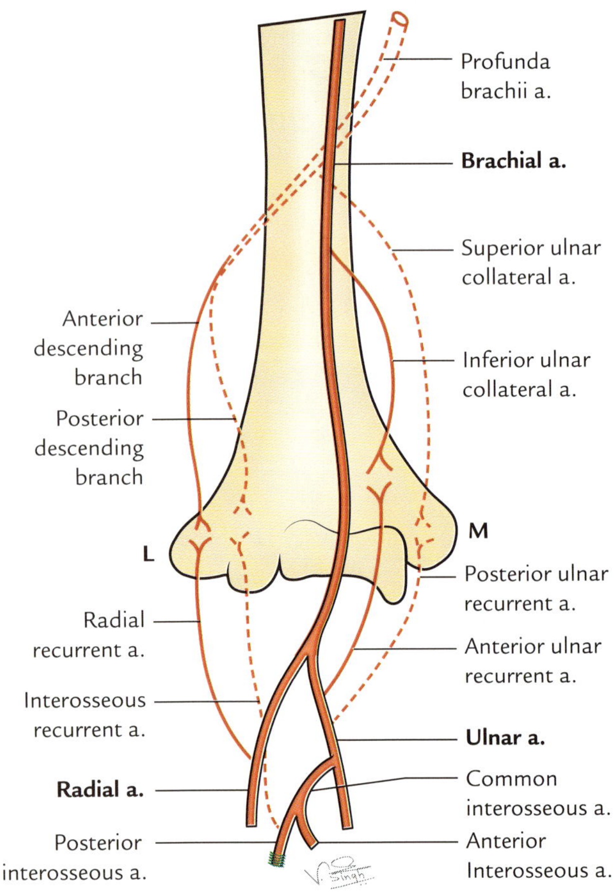

FIG. 8.12 ■ Arterial anastomosis around the elbow joint (L = lateral epicondyle, M = medial epicondyle).

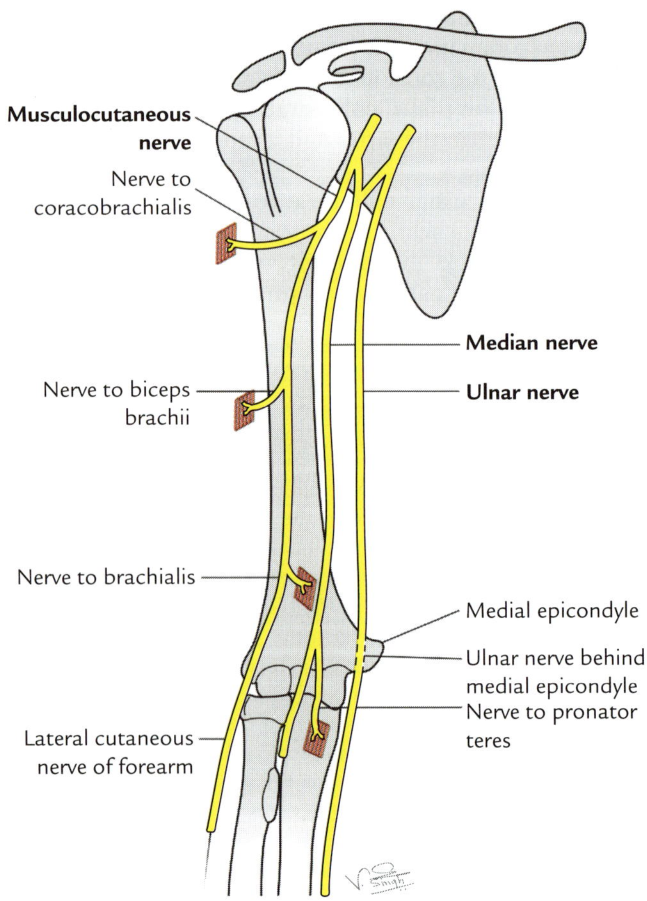

FIG. 8.13 ■ Large nerves passing through the front of the arm. Note, nerve of the front of arm is musculocutaneous nerve.

N.B.

The relationship of median nerve with the brachial artery in the arm is as follows (Fig. 8.14):

1. **In the upper part**, it is lateral to the artery.
2. **In the middle part**, it crosses in front of the artery from the lateral to the medial side.
3. **In the lower part**, it is medial to the artery up to the elbow.

Branches

In the arm, the median nerve gives rise to the following branches:

1. **Nerve to pronator** teres just above the elbow
2. **Vasomotor nerve** to the brachial artery
3. **Articular branch** to the elbow joint at or just below the elbow

Ulnar Nerve (Root Value: C8 and T1)

Origin, course, and termination (Fig. 8.14)

The ulnar nerve arises from the medial cord of the brachial plexus in the axilla. It then runs downward on the medial side of the arm medial to the brachial artery up to the insertion of the coracobrachialis. Here it pierces the medial intermuscular septum along with the superior ulnar collateral artery to enter the posterior compartment of the arm. At the elbow, the ulnar nerve passes behind the medial epicondyle of the humerus where it can be easily palpated (Fig. 8.15). *The ulnar nerve does not give any branch in the arm.*

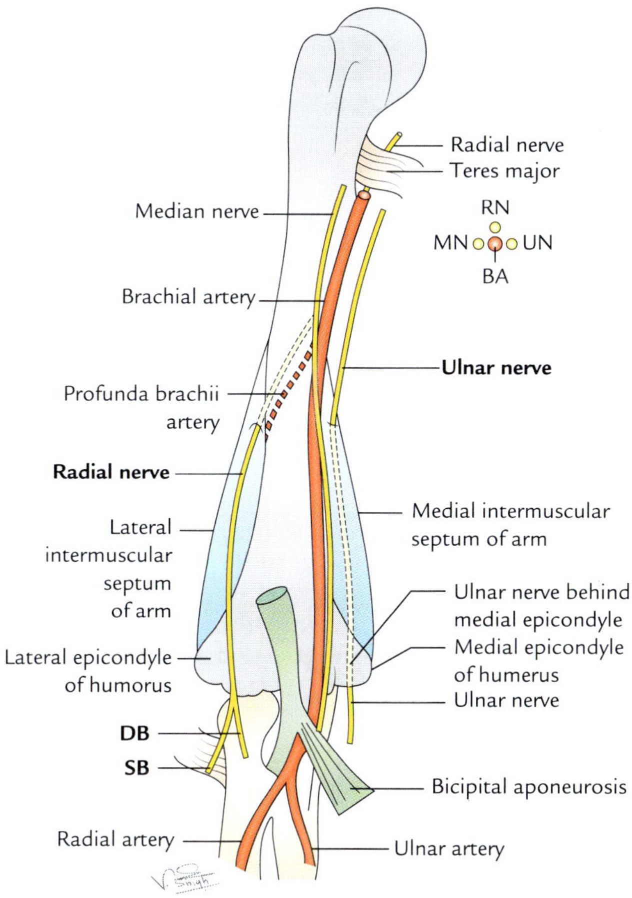

FIG. 8.14 ■ Relations of the median nerve with the brachial artery in the arm. The course of the radial and ulnar nerves in the arm is also shown (SB = superficial branch of radial nerve, DB = deep branch of radial nerve, BA = brachial artery, MN = median nerve, RN = radial nerve, UN = ulnar nerve).

CLINICAL CORRELATION

Funny bone: It is neither funny nor bone but the name given to part of ulnar nerve behind medial epicondyle of humerus. This is because when medical condyle of humerus is knocked/pumped against a hard object, there is a feeling of tingling and numbness along medial side of forearm and hand.

N.B.

'Funny bone' is a nickname to ulnar nerve behind medial epicondyle of humerus because of funny feeling one gets after medial epicondyle is hit against the hard object.

Radial Nerve in Arm (Root Value: C5-T1)

The radial nerve arises from the posterior cord of the brachial plexus in the axilla (Fig. 8.15A). In the arm, the nerve first lies posterior to the brachial artery. Then it winds around the back of the arm to enter the radial/spiral groove of the humerus between the lateral and medial heads of the triceps where it is accompanied by the profunda brachii artery (Fig. 8.15B). At the lower end of the spiral groove, it pierces the lateral intermuscular septum and enters the anterior compartment of the arm. Here it continues downward in front of the elbow in the cubital fossa, between the brachialis and brachioradialis muscles. Then at a variable point, it divides into two terminal branches: (a) a sensory branch, the *superficial radial nerve* and (b) a motor branch, the *deep radial nerve*. The later disappears into the substance of the supinator muscle just below the elbow, passes between superficial and deep layers of supinator to enter the posterior compartment of forearm and now called as *posterior interosseous nerve*. Here it runs downward on the posterior aspect of interosseous membrane up to wrist, where it terminates by forming a **pseudoganglion**.

Branches

1. In the axilla:
   (a) Nerves to the long and medial heads of triceps
   (b) Posterior cutaneous nerve of the arm
2. In the spiral groove:
   (a) Nerves to the lateral and medial heads of triceps
   (b) Nerve to anconeus
   (c) Lower lateral cutaneous nerve of the arm
   (d) Posterior cutaneous nerve of the forearm
3. In the anterior compartment of the arm:
   (a) Nerves to brachialis, brachioradialis, and extensor carpi radialis longus
   (b) Articular branches to the elbow joint
   (c) Deep radial nerve
   (d) Superficial radial nerve

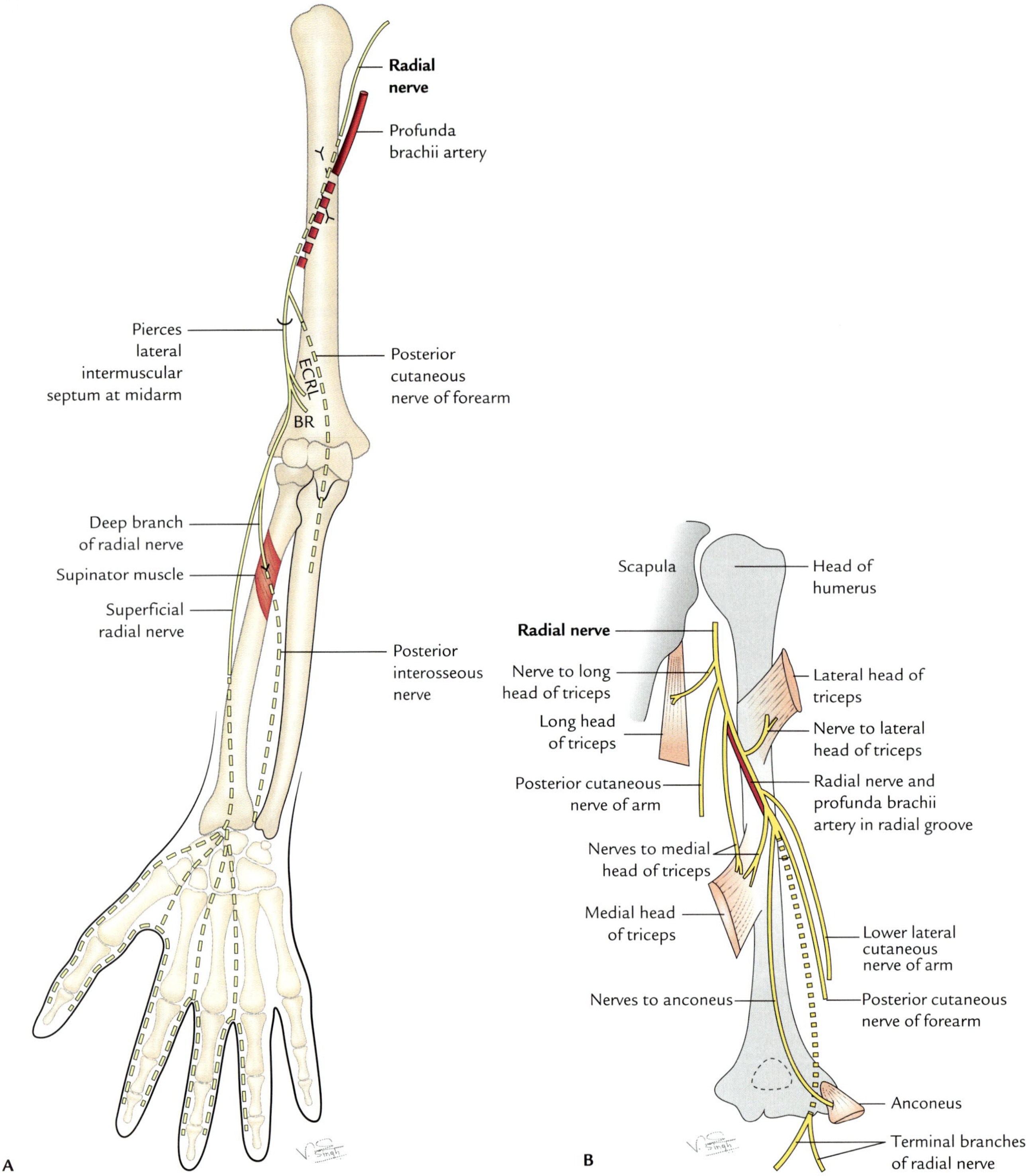

FIG. 8.15 Radial nerve. (**A**) Origin, course, and termination and (**B**) course, relations, and branches of the radial nerve in axilla and the arm (BR = brachioradialis, ECRL = extensor carpi radialis longus).

CLINICAL CORRELATION

The radial nerve is commonly injured in the radial groove due to various reasons, *viz.* fracture shaft of humerus (for detail see Chapter 13, page 174). It leads to: (a) wrist drop, (b) sensory loss over a narrow strip of skin on the back of forearm, (c) tingling and burning sensations on the back of hand involving thumb, index finger, and middle finger.

CUBITAL FOSSA (L. CUBITUS = ELBOW) (FIG. 8.16)

AN 11.5

The cubital fossa is a triangular hollow in front of the elbow. Its base is horizontal and directed upward, whereas its apex is directed downward. It corresponds (i.e. homologous) to the lower half of the popliteal fossa of the lower limb.

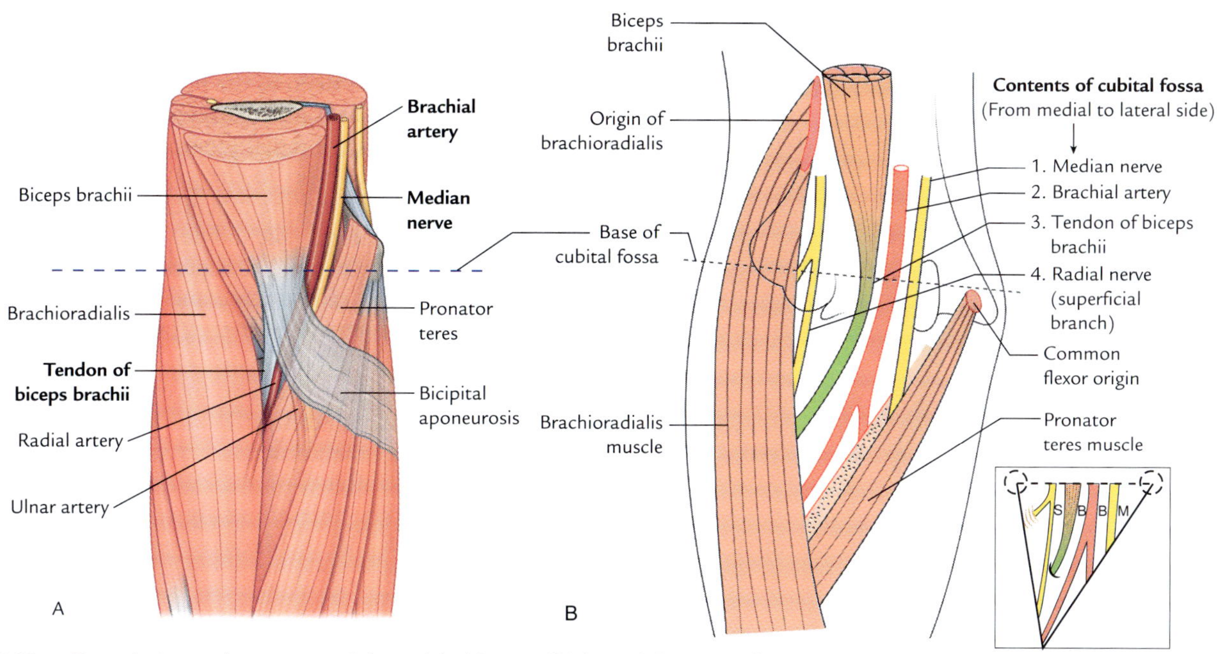

FIG. 8.16 Boundaries and contents of the cubital fossa. (**A**) Actual diagram of cubital fossa and (**B**) schematic diagram showing contents. Diagram in the inset on right side is highly schematic to show the relations of structures. (*Source: Gray's Basic Anatomy, Third Edition:* A. Wayne Vogl, Adam W. M. Mitchell, Richard L. Drake, Fig. 7.61B, Elsevier Inc., 2023.)

Boundaries

Lateral: Medial border of the brachioradialis muscle

Medial: Lateral border of the pronator teres muscle

Base: An imaginary horizontal line, joining the front of two epicondyles of the humerus

Apex: Meeting point of the lateral and medial boundaries. Here the brachioradialis overlaps the pronator teres.

Floor: It is formed by two muscles, *brachialis* in the upper part and *supinator* in the lower part (Fig. 8.17).

Roof: It is formed from the deep fascia of the forearm reinforced on the medial side by the *bicipital aponeurosis.*

N.B.

Superficial to deep fascia lies:
(a) Superficial fascia
(b) Skin

Note: The *superficial fascia* contains (i) median cubital vein connecting the cephalic and basilic veins and (ii) medial and lateral cutaneous nerves of the forearm. The lateral cutaneous nerve lies along the medial side of the cephalic vein and the medial cutaneous nerve along the lateral side of the basilic vein (Fig. 8.18).

Contents

The cubital fossa is actually a narrow space, and, therefore, its contents are displayed only if the elbow is extended and its margins are pulled apart.

The contents of the cubital fossa from the medial to the lateral side are as follows (Fig. 8.16):

1. **Median nerve:** It leaves the fossa by passing between the two heads of pronator teres.
2. **Brachial artery:** It terminates in the fossa at the level of the neck of radius by dividing into the radial

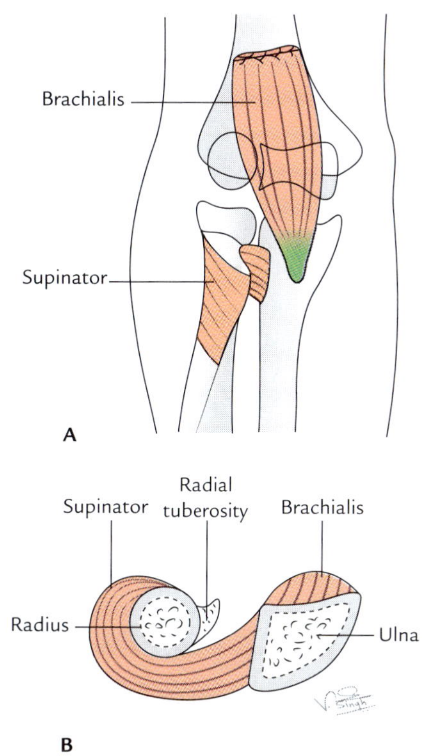

FIG. 8.17 Muscles forming the floor of the cubital fossa. (**A**) Anterior view and (**B**) cross-sectional view.

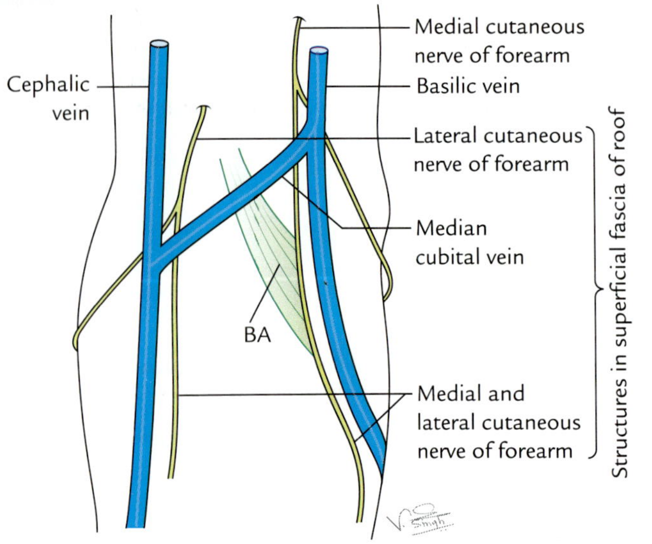

FIG. 8.18 Structures in the roof of the cubital fossa. BA, bicipital aponeurosis.

and ulnar arteries. The radial artery is superficial and leaves the fossa at the apex. The ulnar artery is deep and passes deep to the pronator teres.

3. **Biceps tendon:** It passes backward and laterally to be attached on the radial tuberosity.
4. **Radial nerve:** It lies in the gap between the brachialis medially and the brachioradialis laterally. At the level of lateral epicondyle, it divides into two terminal branches: (a) a superficial branch called the superficial radial nerve and (b) a deep branch called the deep radial nerve/posterior interosseous nerve. The latter disappears in the substance of the supinator muscle. The superficial radial nerve passes downward in front of the forearm under the cover of the brachioradialis.

Mnemonic: The contents of the cubital fossa from the medial to the lateral side are easily remembered by the *mnemonic:* **MBBS** (**M** = **M**edian nerve, **B** = **B**rachial artery, **B** = **B**iceps tendon, **S** = **S**uperficial radial nerve; Fig. 8.16).

CLINICAL CORRELATION

AN 11.3

Clinical significance of cubital fossa: The knowledge of anatomy of the cubital fossa is clinically important for the following reasons:

(a) **Venepuncture of cubital veins:** The venepuncture is a clinical method to pierce vein by a needle for either intravenous injection or removal of blood for doing a laboratory test. The most common site for venepuncture is cubital fossa as it houses three superficial veins: cephalic, median cubital, and basilic.
Out of these median cubital vein is most preferred.
The **median cubital vein** is the vein of choice.

This is because it is:
- Most prominent vein in the body.
- Tends to remain stationary for being connected to deep veins by a perforating vein.
- Does not usually collapse during shock.
- Lies more superficially and not accompanied by a nerve, hence skin over it is less sensitive. Hence, venepuncture is less painful.
- Underlying bicipital aponeurosis acts as a hard platform, when elbow is extended and protects the underlying median nerve and brachial artery from injury (Fig. 8.19).

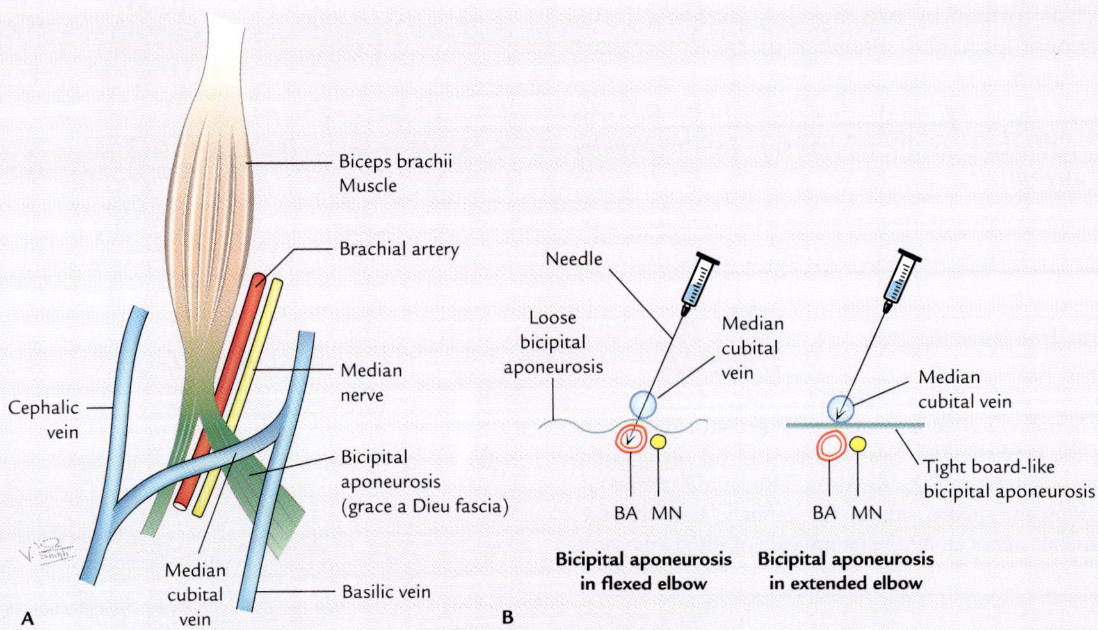

FIG. 8.19 Relations of bicipital aponeurosis with median cubital vein, brachial artery, and median nerve. Note: Bicipital aponeurosis protect the underlying artery and nerve during venepuncture in extended elbow. Note: Bicipital aponeurosis performs two functions: (**A**) Draws posterior border of ulna medially during supination and (**B**) Protects the brachial artery and median nerve during venepuncture. BA = brachial artery, MN = median nerve.

(b) The **brachial artery** in this region is easily located medial to biceps tendon, and auscultated universally for hearing Korokoff sounds while **recording the blood pressure manually**.

(c) To deal with the fractures around elbow, *viz*. supracondylar fracture of the humerus. The contents of cubital fossa especially the brachial artery and median nerve are vulnerable in supracondylar fracture of the humerus.

(d) The contents of cubital fossa particularly median nerve and brachial artery are likely to get injured in supracondylar fracture of humerus.

POSTERIOR COMPARTMENT OF ARM

The contents of the posterior compartment of the arm are as follows (AN 11.1):

- **Muscle:** Triceps brachii
- **Nerve:** Radial nerve
- **Artery:** Profunda brachii artery

In addition to these structures, the following structures also pass through this compartment:

- Ulnar nerve
- Ulnar collateral arteries

Ulnar nerve and ulnar collateral arteries are described on page 99.

MUSCLES OF BACK OF ARM

Triceps Brachii (*Fig. 8.20*)

Triceps brachii is a large muscle, which forms most of the substance on the back of the arm. As its name implies, it has three heads.

Origin (Fig. 8.21)

1. **Long head:** It arises from the infraglenoid tubercle of the scapula.
2. **Lateral head:** It arises from an oblique ridge above the spiral groove on the upper part of the posterior surface of the shaft of humerus.

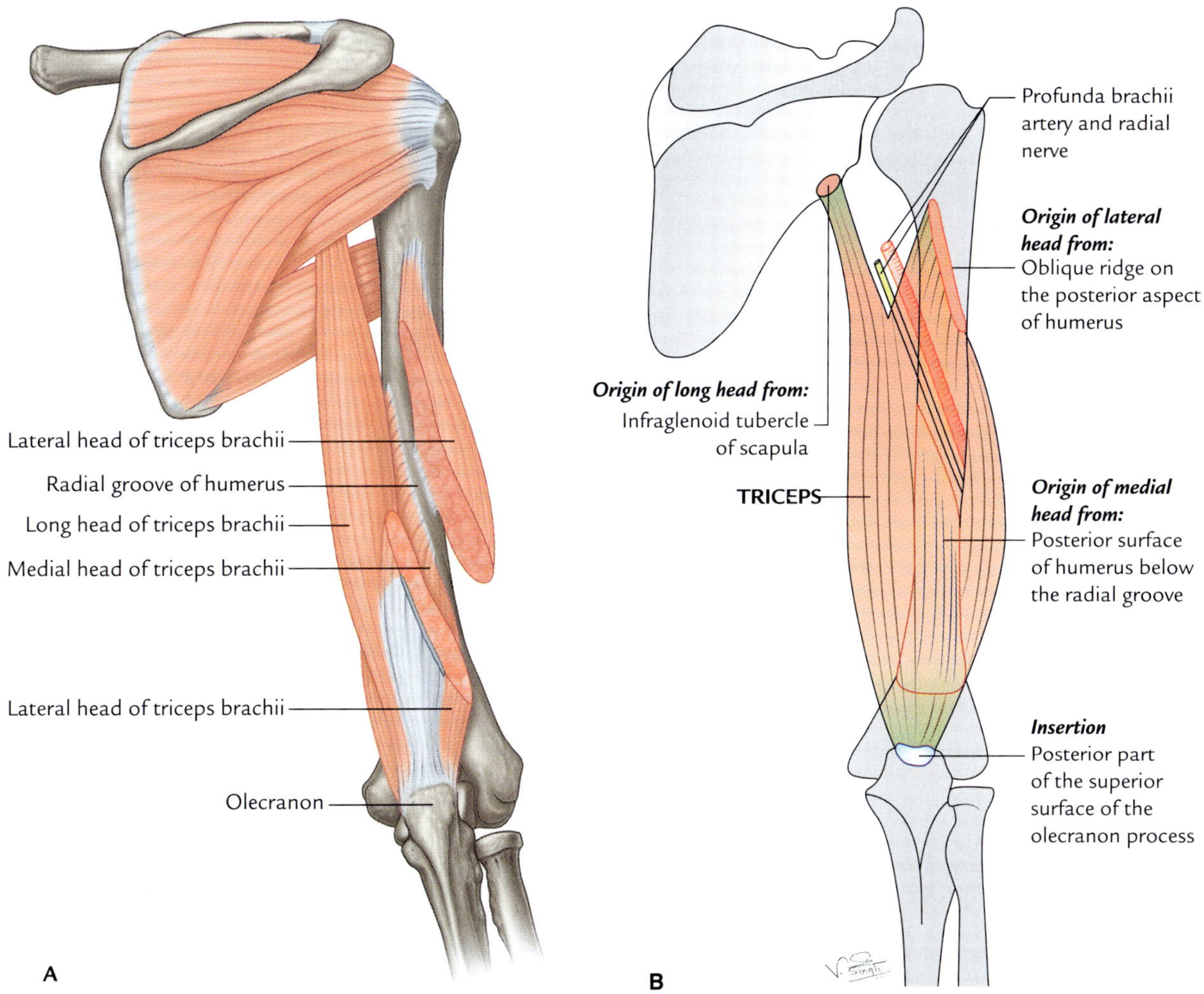

FIG. 8.20 ■ Origin and insertion of the triceps brachii. (**A**) Actual diagram and (**B**) schematic diagram. *Source: Gray's Anatomy for Students, Fourth Edition:* Richard L. Drake, A. Wayne Vogl, Adam W. M. Mitchell, Fig. 2.65, Page 138, Elsevier Inc., 2020.)

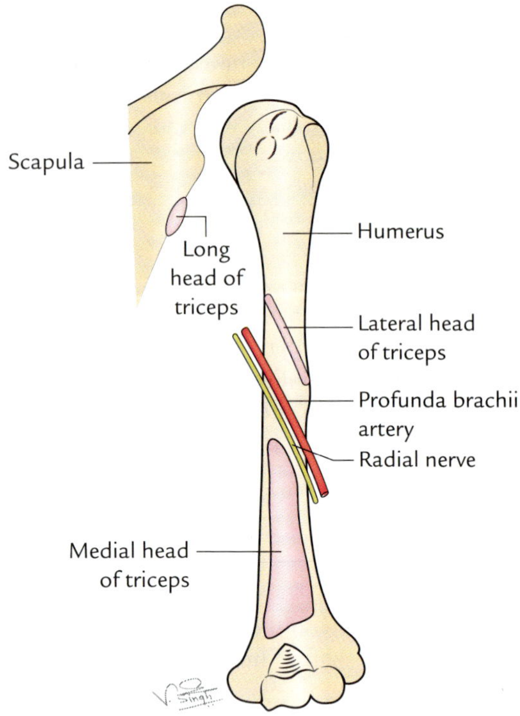

FIG. 8.21 ■ Origin of the triceps brachii.

3. **Medial head:** It arises from the posterior surface of the lower half of the shaft humerus below the spiral groove.

The medial head is actually deep to the other two heads, but it is named medial because at the level of radial groove it lies medial to the lateral head.

Insertion

The common tendon is inserted into the posterior part of the superior surface of the olecranon process of ulna.

N.B.

A few fibres of the medial (deep) head are inserted into the posterior aspect of the capsule of the elbow joint and are referred to as the **articularis cubiti** or **subanconeus muscle**. These fibres prevent the nipping of the capsule during the extension of the arm.

Nerve supply

By the radial nerve (C7 and C8): Each head receives a separate branch from the radial nerve in the following manner:

- *Nerve to long head* arises from the radial nerve in axilla.
- *Nerve to lateral head* arises from the radial nerve in the radial groove.
- *Nerve to medial head* arises from the radial nerve in the radial groove through nerve to anconeus.

N.B.

The long head is sometimes supplied by axillary nerve.

Actions

The triceps brachii is the powerful extensor of the elbow joint. The long head supports the head of the humerus during the hyperabduction of the arm.

Clinical testing: When flexed elbow is extended against resistance, the contracting triceps brachii can be felt on the back of arm.

CLINICAL CORRELATION

Injury of the radial nerve in the radial groove: If the radial nerve is damaged in the radial groove, the *extension of the elbow and triceps reflex is not completely lost* because the nerve to the long head arises from the radial nerve in axilla.

Radial Nerve

AN 11.2

It is described on page 99.

Profunda Brachii Artery (Deep Artery of the Arm)

The profunda brachii artery is the largest branch of the brachial artery (Fig. 8.22). It arises from the posteromedial aspect of the brachial artery just below the teres major. It accompanies the radial nerve through the radial groove and then terminates by dividing into anterior and posterior descending branches, which take part in the arterial anastomosis around the elbow joint.

Branches

1. **Deltoid (ascending) branch:** It ascends between the long and lateral heads of the triceps and anastomoses with the descending branch of the posterior circumflex humeral artery.
2. **Nutrient artery to the humerus:** It enters the shaft of the humerus in the radial groove, just behind the deltoid tuberosity.
3. **Anterior descending (radial collateral) artery:** It is the smaller terminal branch that accompanies the radial nerve and anastomoses with the radial

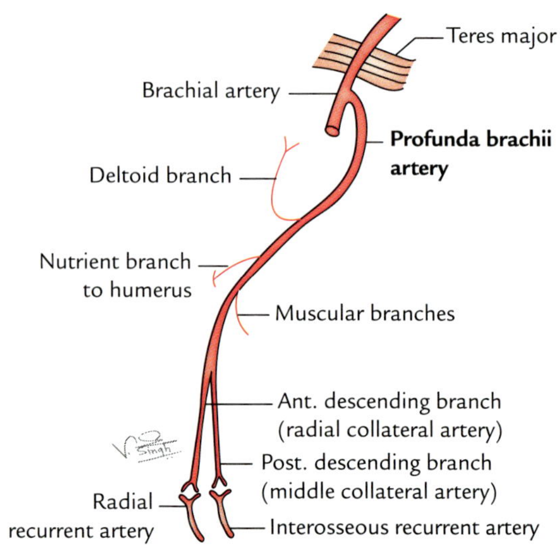

FIG. 8.22 ■ Profunda brachii artery.

recurrent artery in front of the lateral epicondyle of the humerus.

4. **Posterior descending (middle collateral) artery:** It is the larger terminal branch of the profunda brachii artery, which descends behind the shaft of the humerus and anastomoses with the interosseous recurrent artery behind the lateral epicondyle of the humerus.

Golden Facts to Remember

• Most lateral bony point of the shoulder region	Greater tubercle of the humerus
• Work-horse of the forearm flexion	Brachialis muscle
• Most commonly auscultated artery for recording blood pressure	Brachial artery in the cubital fossa
• Best place to compress the brachial artery to stop haemorrhage in the arm and hand	Medial aspect of humerus near the middle of the arm (site of insertion of the coracobrachialis)
• Largest branch of the brachial artery	Profunda brachii artery
• Neurovascular structures jeopardized in midshaft fracture of the humerus	Radial nerve and profunda brachii artery
• Strong supinator elbow	Biceps brachii
• Most preferred vein for venepuncture in the upper limb	Median cubital vein
• Damage of the radial nerve in spiral groove causes only weakness in the extension of the elbow and not the total inability to extend the elbow	Because branches of the radial nerve supplying the long and medial heads of triceps arise in axilla, that is above the radial groove
• Ligament of Struthers (third head of the coracobrachialis)	Fibrous band extending between the supratrochlear spur and medial epicondyle of the humerus
• Work-horse of the forearm extension	Medial head of triceps
• rendre grâce à Dieu (to give praise to God)	Bicipital aponeurosis
• Main source of blood supply to arm and hand	Brachial artery

CLINICAL CASE STUDIES

Case I

A 45-year-old weight lifter while lifting the heavy weight in weight-lifting competition suddenly felt a sudden snap and severe pain in his shoulder region. He dropped the weight and left the platform. He was taken to the hospital for check-up. On examination, the doctor noticed a ball-like bulge near the centre of anterior aspect of the arm. The patient was not able to supinate his arm, and his forearm was pronated and flexed. A diagnosis of the **rupture of the tendon of the long head of biceps** was made.

Questions

1. What are the causes of the rupture of the tendon of the long head of biceps and which age group does it mostly affect?
2. What is the origin of the long and short heads of the biceps brachii?
3. What caused the ball-like bulge in front of the arm and name this deformity?

Answers

1. (a) The rupture of the tendon of the long head of biceps usually occurs from the wear and tear of an inflamed tendon as it moves back and forth in the bicipital groove of the humerus. It may also result from the forceful flexion of the arm against excessive resistance as during weightlifting.
   (b) It usually occurs in individuals of >35 years of age.
2. (a) *Long head* from the supraglenoid tubercle of the scapula.
   (b) *Short head* from the tip of coracoid process of the scapula.
3. (a) Detached belly of the biceps muscle.
   (b) Popeye deformity.

Case II

A young adult man while speeding his motor bike met an unfortunate accident and fractured his upper arm. An X-ray in emergency revealed **fracture midshaft of humerus**.

Questions

1. Which nerve is likely to get injured?
2. What muscles are likely to be affected?
3. Area of sensory loss if any.
4. Obvious effect of an injury.

Answers

1. Radial nerve.
2. All the muscles on the back of arm and forearm except long head of triceps.
3. Sensory loss in the back of forearm and dorsal aspect hand and lateral 3½ digits.
4. Wrist drop.

CHAPTER

9

Forearm

SPECIFIC LEARNING OBJECTIVES

After studying this chapter, the student should be able to:

- Describe the important muscle groups on the anterior aspect of forearm with attachments, nerve supply and actions. AN 12.1
- Describe the origin, insertion, nerve supply, actions, and special features of flexor digitorum profundus (FDP).
- Identify and describe the flexor retinaculum with its attachments. AN 12.3
- Describe the compartments deep to extensor retinaculum. AN 12.14
- Write short notes on: (a) radial artery in the forearm, (b) ulnar artery in the forearm, (c) posterior interosseous nerve and vessels, and (d) radial pulse. AN 12.12
- Enumerate: (a) superficial muscles on the front of the forearm, (b) structures lying in front of the wrist, (c) structures cut in suicidal cut on the radial side of the wrist, and (d) deep muscles on the back of the forearm.
- Identify and describe the origin, course, relations, branches (or tributaries), termination of important nerves and vessels of forearm. AN 12.2
- Describe extensor expansion formation. AN 12.15
- Identify and describe the important muscle groups of dorsal forearm with attachments, nerve supply, and actions. AN 12.11

The forearm extends from the elbow to the wrist and has two bones that are tied together by a thin strong fibrous membrane—the *interosseous membrane* (Fig. 9.1). The head of the radius is at the proximal end of the forearm, whereas the head of the ulna is at the distal end of the forearm. The radius and the ulna at both their ends articulate with each other to form the superior and inferior radioulnar joints. All important movements of the supination and pronation of the forearm occur at these joints. The upper ends of the radius and ulna articulate with the lower end of the humerus to form the elbow joint. The lower end of radius articulates with the carpus to form wrist joint (Fig. 9.1).

The main purpose of the movements of the forearm at the elbow and the radioulnar joints is to place the hand at the desired place to execute the force of shoulder and arm into a desired action. The muscles, nerves, and vessels are present both on the front and back of the forearm.

SURFACE LANDMARKS (FIG. 9.2)

A. On the front of forearm:

1. **Medial and lateral epicondyles of the humerus** can be easily felt at the elbow; the medial epicondyle is more prominent than the lateral epicondyle. The ulnar nerve can be rolled behind the medial epicondyle (see also page 91).
2. **Tendon of the biceps brachii** can be easily palpated in front of the elbow. The pulsations of the brachial artery can be felt just medial to the tendon.
3. Head of radius and olecranon process of the ulna have been described on page 91.
4. **Head of ulna** forms a round elevation on surface, on the medial side of anterior aspect of the wrist.
5. **Pisiform bone** can be felt on the medial side of the base of hypothenar eminence, where the tendon of flexor carpi ulnaris (FCU) muscle ends.

B. On the back of the forearm:

1. **Olecranon process of the ulna** is the most prominent bony elevation on the back of the elbow in the midline. In an extended elbow, the tip of the olecranon process lies on a horizontal line with two epicondyles of the humerus, and in the flexed elbow, the three points when joined form an *equilateral triangle*.
2. **Posterior border of the ulna** is subcutaneous throughout its length. It can be felt in the longitudinal furrow on the back of the forearm with the flexed elbow. It separates the flexor and extensor muscles of the forearm.
3. **Styloid processes of the radius and ulna** can be easily felt on the lateral and medial sides of the wrist, respectively. The styloid process of the radius is located about 1.25 cm more distally. The styloid process of the radius can be felt in the proximal part of the anatomical snuff box. The

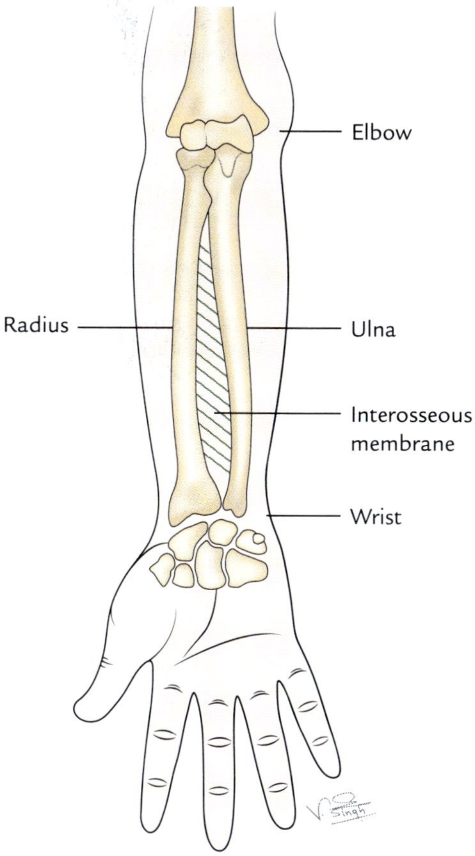

FIG. 9.1 ■ Framework of front of forearm.

styloid process of the ulna can be felt on the posteromedial aspect of the wrist, about 1 cm above the styloid process of the radius.

4. **Dorsal tubercle of the radius (Lister's tubercle)** can be palpated on the posterior aspect of the distal end of the radius in line with the cleft between the index and middle fingers.
5. **Tendons of flexor carpi radialis (FCR), palmaris longus, and FCU** can be felt/identified on the front of the wrist when the fisted hand is flexed against resistance (Fig. 9.2).
6. **Pulsations of brachial, radial, and ulnar arteries** can be felt on the front of the forearm (see Chapter 14, page 189).
7. Transverse creases in front of the wrist:
   a. *Proximal transverse crease* lies at the level of the wrist joint.
   b. *Distal palmar crease* corresponds to the proximal border of the flexor retinaculum.

FASCIAL COMPARTMENTS OF THE FOREARM

The forearm is enclosed in sheath of the deep fascia of the forearm (antebrachial fascia). It is attached to the posterior subcutaneous border of the ulna. From the deep surface of the fascia, septa pass between the muscles, and some of them reach the bone.

This deep fascia, together with the interosseous membrane and fibrous intermuscular septa, divides the forearm into several compartments, each having its own muscles, nerves, and blood supply. Classically, the forearm is divided into two compartments: (a) anterior compartment and (b) posterior compartment (Fig. 9.3)

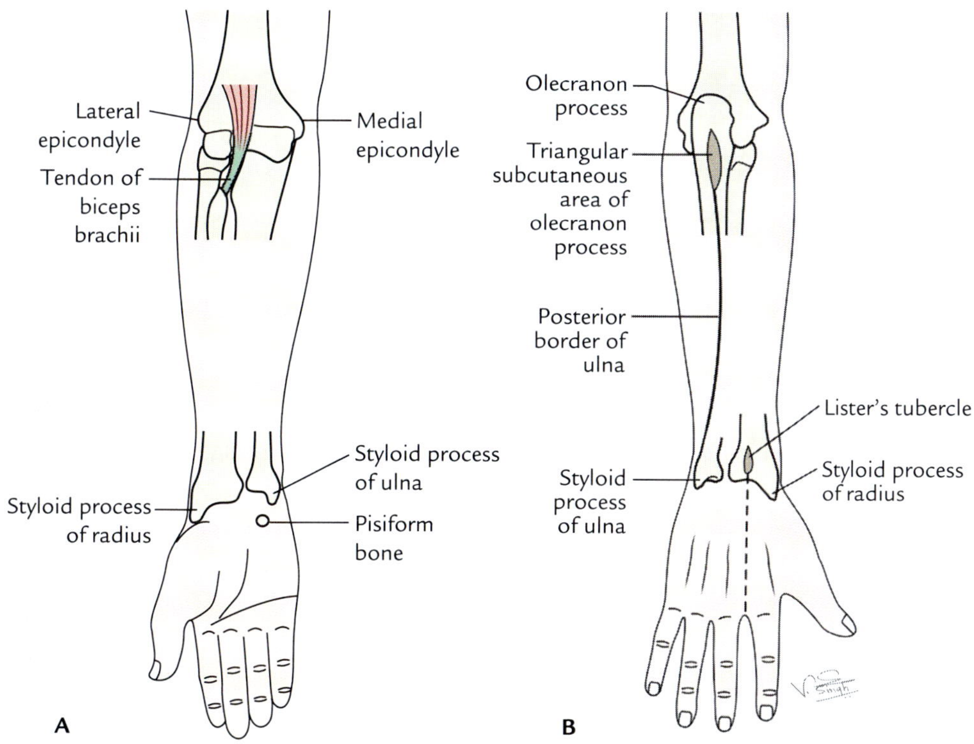

FIG. 9.2 ■ Surface landmarks on the front (**A**) and back (**B**) of forearm.

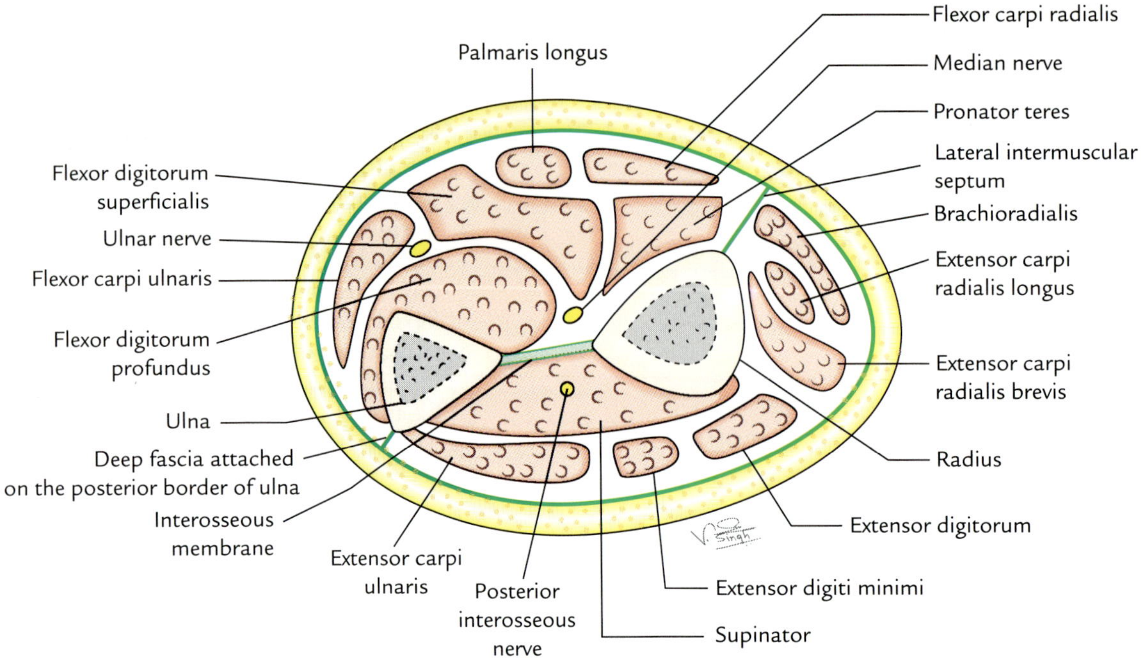

FIG. 9.3 ■ Fascial compartments of the forearm. Cross section through the upper third of the forearm.

by lateral intermuscular septum, interosseous membrane and deep fascia attached on posterior border of ulna.

The anterior compartment contains the structures on the front of the forearm and the posterior compartment contains the structure on the back of the forearm.

Deep fascia over the flexor muscle tendons as they pass in front of the wrist, it is specially thickened to form **flexor retinaculum** (Fig. 11.4). For details see page 140.

Similarly on the back of distal forearm just proximal to hand, it is specially thickened to form **extensor retinaculum** (Fig. 9.22, page 123). Both the flexor and the extensor retinacula, retain the long digital tendons in position during hand movements and prevent them from bowstringing.

ANTERIOR COMPARTMENT/FRONT OF FOREARM AN 12.1

The front of forearm contains following muscles, vessels, and nerves:

1. **Muscles:** Eight muscles arranged in two groups.
2. **Arteries:** Two arteries, radial and ulnar.
3. **Nerves:** Three nerves; median, ulnar, and radial.

The muscles of the front of forearm are generally divided into two groups: *superficial and deep*.

SUPERFICIAL MUSCLES OF THE FRONT OF THE FOREARM

This group comprises five muscles (Fig. 9.4). From the lateral to the medial side, these are:

1. **P**ronator teres
2. **F**lexor carpi radialis
3. **P**almaris longus
4. **F**lexor digitorum superficialis (FDS)
5. **F**lexor carpi ulnaris

These muscles can be easily remembered by a *Mnemonic:* **P**radeep **F**ound **P**raveen **F**or **F**ight.

Some authorities keep the FDS in the intermediate group.

N.B.

All these muscles are flexor of the forearm and have a common tendinous origin—from the front of the medial epicondyle of the humerus called the **common flexor origin**.

Pronator Teres

Pronator teres is the smallest and most lateral of the superficial flexors of the forearm (Fig. 9.5). It forms the medial boundary of the cubital fossa.

Origin

It arises by two heads: (a) *superficial (humeral) head* from the medial epicondyle of the humerus and (b) *deep (ulnar) head* from the medial margin of the coronoid process of the ulna.

Insertion

Into the rough impression on the middle one-third of the lateral surface (most convex part) of the radius.

Nerve supply

By the median nerve.

Actions

It is the main pronator of the forearm. It also helps in the flexion of the elbow.

Clinical testing

The pronator teres is tested by asking the patient to pronate the forearm from supine position against resistance with elbow flexed.

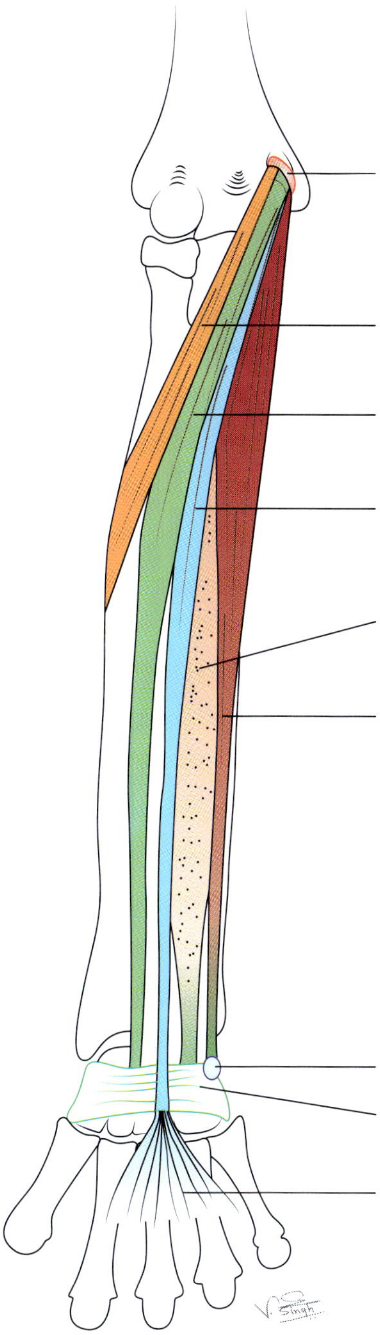

FIG. 9.4 Superficial muscles of the front of the forearm.

N.B.

- *Median nerve* passes between the two heads of the pronator teres.
- *Ulnar artery* passes deep to the deep head of the pronator teres; thus, the ulnar artery is separated from the median nerve by the deep head of the pronator teres in the region of the cubital fossa.

Flexor Carpi Radialis

Origin

FCR originates from the medial epicondyle of the humerus by a common flexor origin (Fig. 9.6).

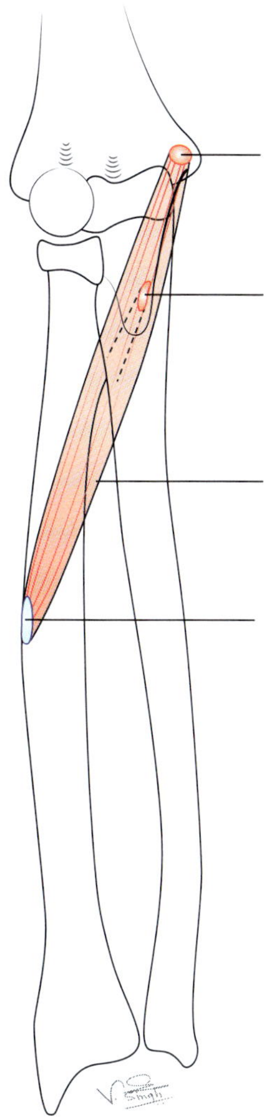

FIG. 9.5 Origin and insertion of the pronator teres.

Insertion

On to the anterior aspects of the bases of the second and third metacarpals.

Nerve supply

By the median nerve.

Actions

1. It flexes the wrist.
2. It abducts the wrist.

N.B.

The tendon of FCR is a good guide to the radial artery that lies just lateral to it at the wrist.

Palmaris Longus

Origin

Palmaris longus originates from the medial epicondyle of the humerus by a common flexor origin.

Insertion

Its long cord-like tendon crosses superficial to the flexor retinaculum and attaches to its distal part, and joins the apex of the palmar aponeurosis.

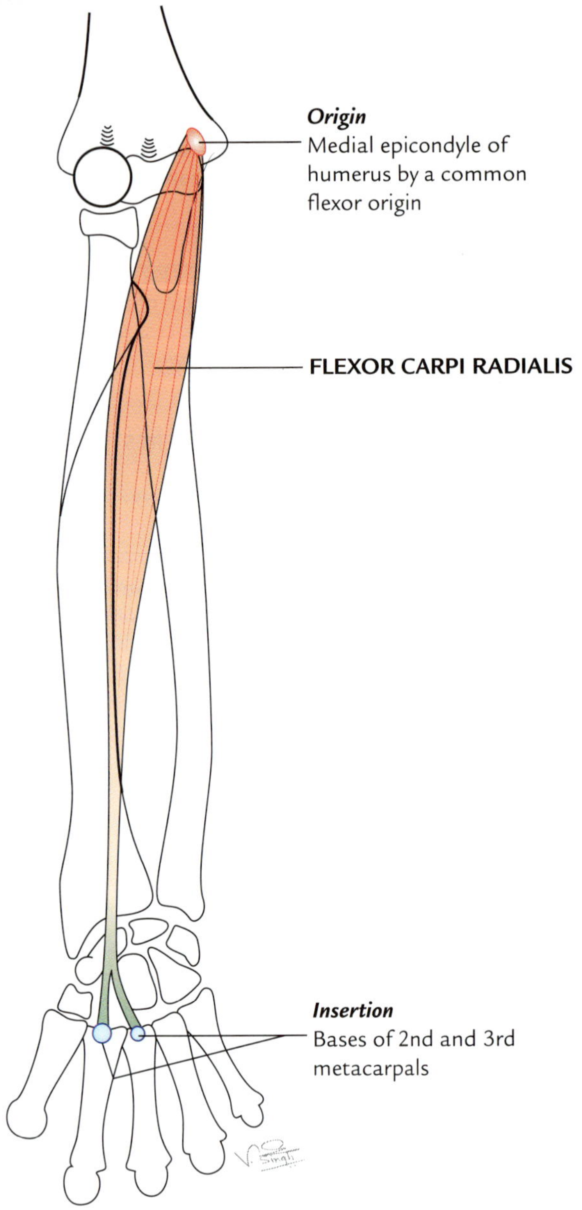

FIG. 9.6 ■ Origin and insertion of the flexor carpi radialis.

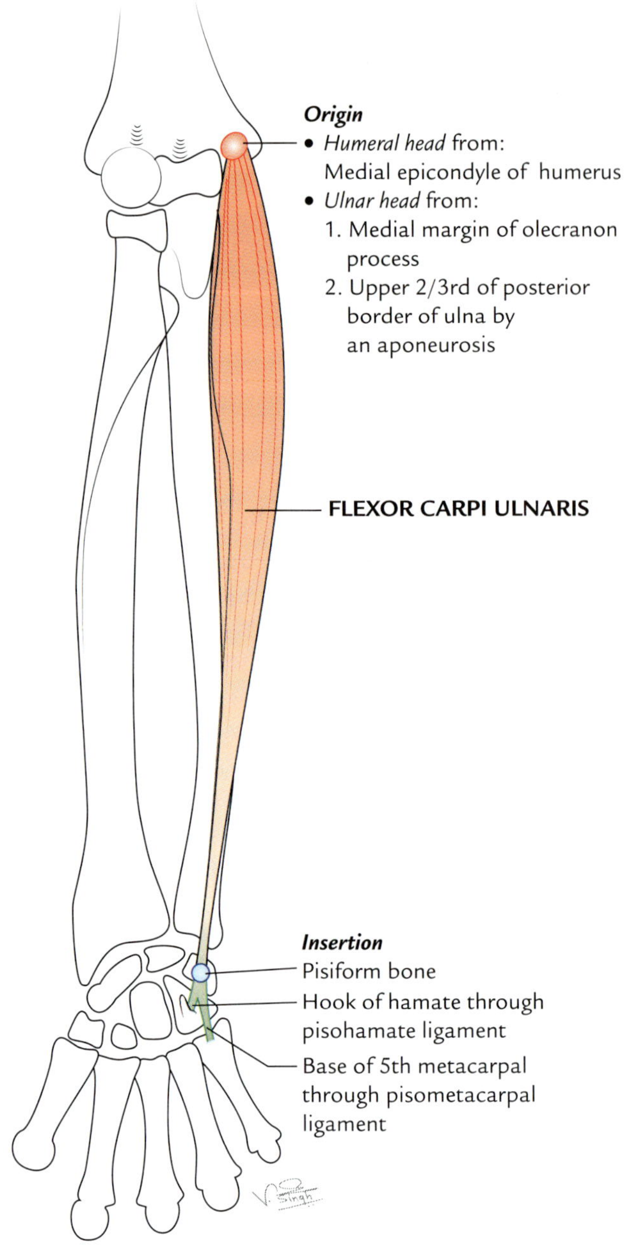

FIG. 9.7 ■ Origin and insertion of the flexor carpi ulnaris.

Nerve supply

By the median nerve.

Actions

It flexes the wrist and makes the palmar aponeurosis tense.

N.B.

- Morphologically, the *palmaris longus* is a degenerating muscle with a small short belly and a long tendon. The *palmar aponeurosis* represents the degenerated tendon of the palmaris longus. The palmaris longus corresponds to the *plantaris* muscle on the back of the leg.
- It is absent on one or both sides (usually on the left) in approximately 10%–15% of people, but its actions are not missed. Hence, its tendon is often used by the surgeons for *tendon grafting*.

Flexor Carpi Ulnaris

The FCU is the most medial of the superficial flexors of the forearm (Fig. 9.7).

Origin

It arises from two heads: a small humeral head and a large ulnar head.

(a) *Humeral head* from the medial epicondyle of the humerus by a common flexor origin.
(b) *Ulnar head* from the medial margin of the olecranon process and by an aponeurosis from the upper two-thirds of the posterior border of the ulna.

Insertion

Into (a) pisiform bone and (b) hook of the hamate and the base of the fifth metacarpal bone (through *pisohamate* and *pisometacarpal ligaments*, respectively). The latter is the true insertion because a sesamoid bone (pisiform) develops in its tendon.

Nerve supply

By the ulnar nerve.

Actions

1. Acting with the extensor carpi ulnaris (ECU), it adducts the wrist joint.
2. Acting with FCR, it flexes the wrist joint.

N.B.

- The *ulnar nerve* enters the forearm by passing between the two heads of FCU, which are connected to each other by a tendinous arch.
- The tendon of FCU is a good guide to the ulnar nerve and ulnar artery that lie on its lateral side at the wrist.

Flexor Digitorum Superficialis (Sublimis; Fig. 9.7)

The FDS is the largest muscle of the superficial group of muscles on the front of the forearm (Fig. 9.8). Actually speaking, it forms the intermediate muscle layer between the superficial and deep groups of the forearm muscles.

Origin

It arises from two heads:

(a) *Humeroulnar head*, from the medial epicondyle of the humerus, sublime tubercle on the medial margin of the coronoid process of the ulna and medial (ulnar) collateral ligament of the elbow joint.

(b) *Radial head*, from the anterior oblique line of the radius, extending from the radial tuberosity to the insertion of the pronator teres (upper half of the anterior border of the radius).

Insertion

Middle phalanges of the medial four digits. The mode of insertion is as follows. The muscles splits into two layers: superficial and deep. The superficial layer forms two tendons that are inserted into middle phalanges of the middle and ring fingers. The deep layer also forms two tendons that are inserted into middle phalanges of the index and little fingers. Before insertion, each of the four tendons splits, opposite to the proximal phalanx, into medial and lateral slips that are inserted into the corresponding sides of the middle phalanx.

Nerve supply

By the median nerve.

Actions

FDS flexes the proximal interphalangeal (PIP) joints of the medial four digits. Acting more strongly, it also helps in the flexion of the metacarpophalangeal and wrist joints.

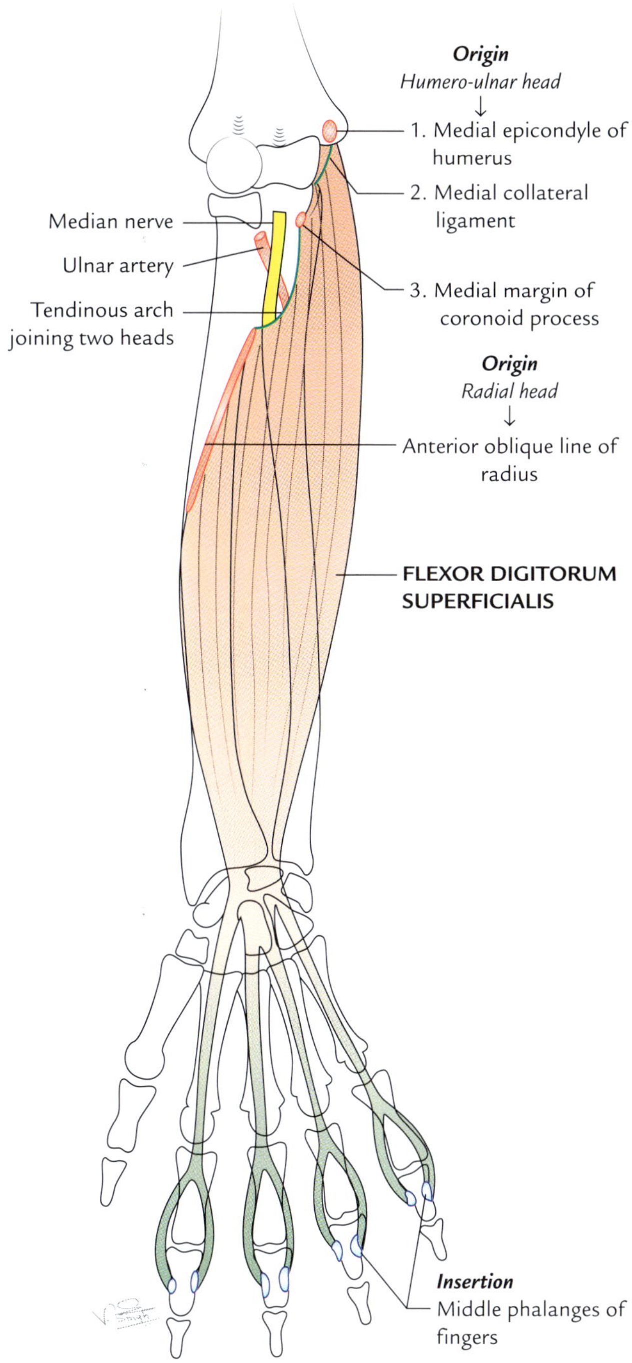

FIG. 9.8 ■ Origin and insertion of the flexor digitorum superficialis.

N.B.

- The **median nerve and the ulnar artery** pass between two heads of FDS, i.e. they pass downward deep to the fibrous arch/tendinous arch connecting the humeroulnar and radial heads of FDS.
- The four tendons of FDS pass deep to the flexor retinaculum enclosed within a common synovial sheath, the *ulnar bursa*.

The brief account of origin, insertion, nerve supply, and actions of muscles of superficial group is given in Table 9.1.

TABLE 9.1 Origin, insertion, nerve supply, and actions of superficial muscles of forearm

Muscle	Origin	Insertion	Nerve supply	Action
1. Pronator teres	• *Humeral head from common flexor origin* • *Ulnar head* from coronoid process of ulna	Lateral aspect of radius in middle	Median nerve	Pronation of forearm
2. Flexor carpi radialis	*Common flexor origin*	Base of second and third metacarpals	Median nerve	Flexion and abduction at the wrist
3. Palmaris longus (absent in 10–15% cases)	*Common flexor origin*	Flexor retinaculum	Median nerve	Flexion of the wrist
4. Flexor carpi ulnaris	• *Humeral head* from common flexor origin • *Ulnar head* from olecranon process and posterior border of ulna	Pisiform bone	Ulnar nerve	Flexion and adduction at the wrist
5. Flexor digitorum superficialis	• *Humeroulnar head* from common flexor origin and coronoid process of ulna • *Radial head* from shaft of radius (oblique line)	Middle phalanges of all fingers	Median nerve	Flexion of PIP joints of all fingers

DEEP MUSCLES OF THE FRONT OF THE FOREARM

There are three deep muscles on the front of the forearm, *namely* (Fig. 9.9A):

1. Flexor pollicis longus (FPL; placed laterally)
2. Flexor digitorum profundus (FDP; placed medially)
3. Pronator quadratus (placed distally)

Flexor Digitorum Profundus

FDP is the most bulky and powerful muscle on the front of the forearm and provides main gripping power to the hand (Fig. 9.9B).

Origin

1. From upper three-fourths of the anterior and medial surfaces of the shaft of the ulna and adjacent medial half of the interosseous membrane.
2. By an aponeurosis from upper three-fourths of the posterior border of the ulna along with the flexor and ECU muscles.
3. From the medial side of the olecranon and coronoid process of the ulna.

Insertion

On to the palmar aspect of the bases of distal phalanges of the medial four digits. The actual mode of insertion is as follows. The muscle forms four tendons that enter the palm by passing deep to the flexor retinaculum. Opposite to the proximal phalanx of the corresponding digit, the tendon perforates the tendon of FDS and passes forward to be inserted in the palmar surface of the distal phalanx.

Nerve supply

1. Medial half by the ulnar nerve.
2. Lateral half by the anterior interosseous nerve—a branch of the median nerve.

Actions

FDP flexes the distal interphalangeal (DIP) joints and helps to flex the PIP and MP joints of the medial four digits. It also helps to flex the wrist joint.

N.B.

FDP:

(a) is the most powerful and bulky muscle of the forearm,
(b) has dual innervation by the median and ulnar nerves,
(c) provides most of the gripping power to the hand,
(d) forms four tendons that enter the hand by passing deep to the flexor retinaculum, posterior to the tendons of FDS in a common synovial sheath—ulnar bursa,
(e) forms most of the surface elevation medial to the palpable posterior border of the ulna, and
(f) provides origin to the lumbrical muscles in the palm.

Clinical testing

The FDP is tested by asking the patient to flex the DIP joint while holding the PIP joint in extension.

The integrity of the median nerve in the forearm is tested in this way by using the index finger and that of the ulnar nerve by using the little finger.

Flexor Pollicis Longus

The FPL lies lateral to the FDP and clothes the anterior aspect of the radius distal to the attachment of the supinator muscle.

Origin

From the upper two-thirds of the anterior surface of the radius below the anterior oblique line and adjoining part of the interosseous membrane.

Insertion

Into the anterior surface of the base of the distal phalanx of the thumb.

Nerve supply

By median nerve.

Actions

Primarily it flexes the distal phalanx of the thumb, and secondarily it flexes the proximal phalanx and first metacarpal

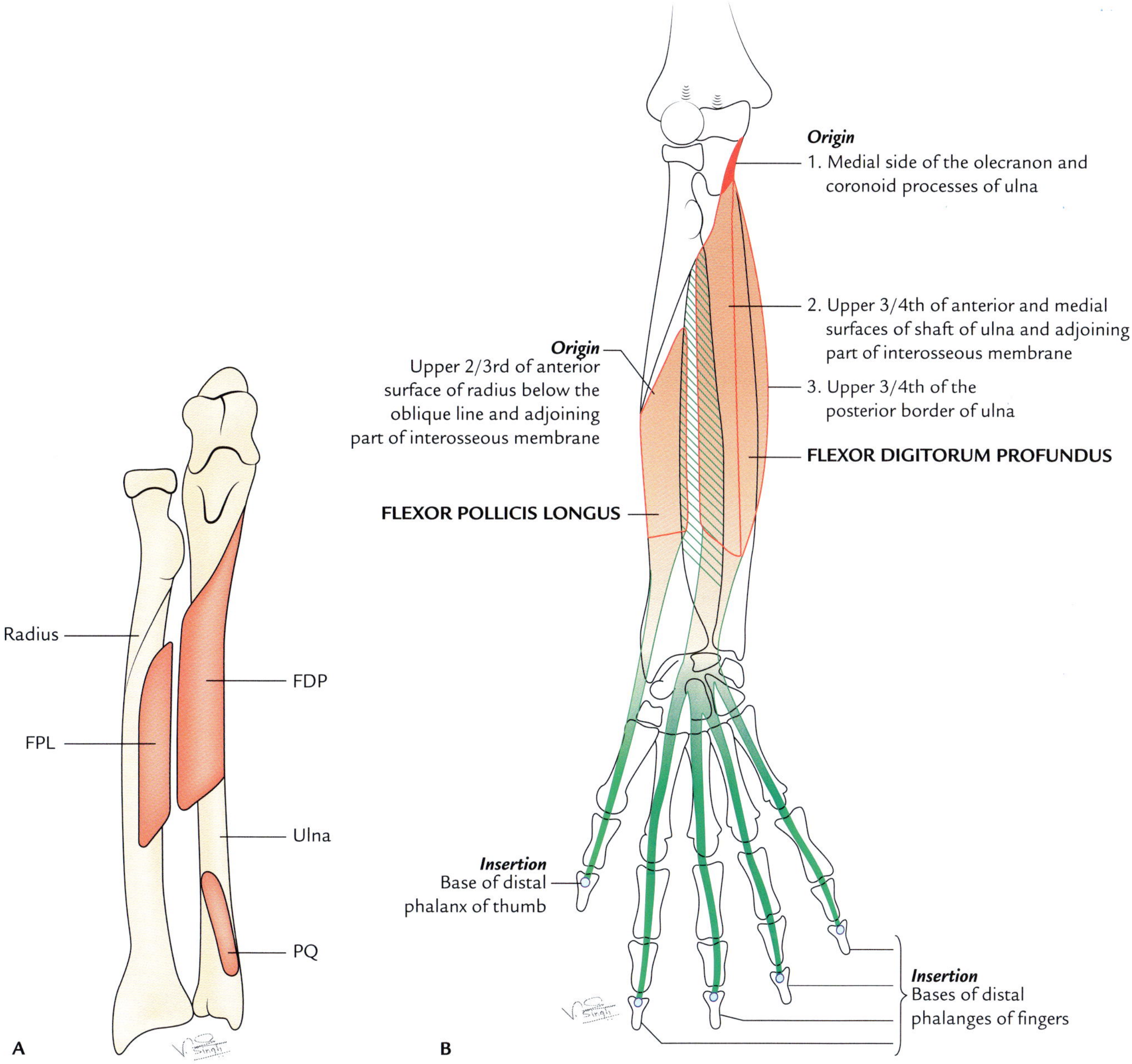

FIG. 9.9 (**A**) Origin of deep muscles of front of forearm on the anterior aspects of radius and ulna. (**B**) Origin and insertion of the flexor digitorum profundus and flexor pollicis longus (FDP = flexor digitorum profundus, FPL = flexor pollicis longus, PQ = pronator quadratus).

at the metacarpophalangeal (MP) and carpometacarpal (CM) joints, respectively.

N.B.

- The *anterior interosseous nerve* and vessels descend on the interosseous membrane between FPL and FDP.
- The FPL is the only muscle which flexes the interphalangeal joint of the thumb.

Clinical testing

The FPL is tested by asking the patient to flex the interphalangeal joint of the thumb, while the proximal phalanx of the thumb is held extended.

Pronator Quadratus

It is a flat quadrilateral muscle that extends across the front of the distal parts of the radius and the ulna (Fig. 9.10).

Origin

From an oblique ridge on the lower one-fourth of the anterior surface of the shaft of the ulna and the medial part of this surface.

Insertion

1. The *superficial fibres* into the distal one-fourth of the anterior border and the anterior surface of the shaft of the radius.
2. The deeper fibres into the triangular area above the ulnar notch of the radius.

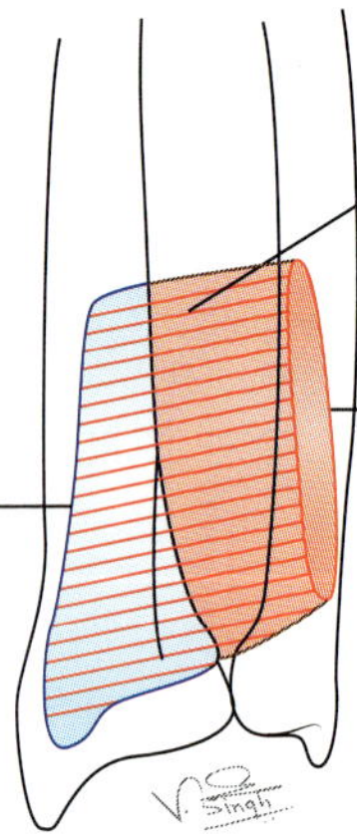

FIG. 9.10 ■ Origin and insertion of the pronator quadratus.

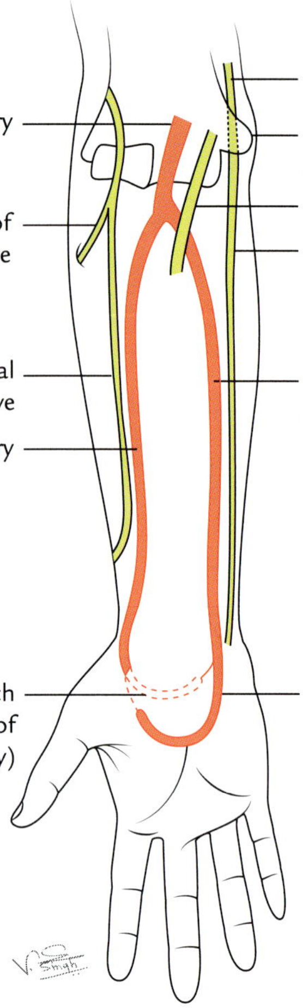

FIG. 9.11 ■ Arteries of the front of the forearm.

Nerve supply

By the anterior interosseous nerve.

Actions

Pronator quadratus is the chief pronator of the forearm and is assisted by the pronator teres only in rapid and forceful pronation.

The brief account of origin, insertion, nerve supply, and actions of deep muscles on the front of forearm is given in Table 9.2.

ARTERIES OF THE FRONT OF THE FOREARM

AN 12.2

The arteries of the front of the forearm are the **ulnar and radial arteries** (Fig. 9.11). They mainly supply blood to the hand through superficial and deep palmar arterial arches.

The blood supply to the forearm is mainly derived from the **anterior and posterior interosseous arteries**, the terminal branches of the common interosseous artery, a branch of the ulnar artery.

Ulnar Artery

Origin, Course, and Termination

The ulnar artery is the **larger terminal branch of the brachial artery**. It begins in the cubital fossa at the level of the neck of the radius (or 1 cm distal to the flexion

TABLE 9.2 **Brief account of origin, insertion, nerve supply, and actions of deep muscles on the front of forearm**

Muscle	Origin	Insertion	Nerve supply	Action
1. Flexor digitorum profundus	Front of upper three-fourths of ulnar shaft and adjoining interosseous membrane	Distal phalanges of four fingers	• Median nerve (ant. interosseous n.) • Ulnar nerve	Flexion of wrist, MP, PIP and DIP joints, especially DIP
2. Flexor pollicis longus	Upper two-thirds of the anterior surface of radius and adjoining interosseous membrane	Distal phalanx of thumb	Median nerve (ant. interosseous n.)	Flexion of MP and IP joints of thumb
3. Pronator quadratus (lies deep to tendons of FDP and FPL)	Lower 1/4th of anterior surface of ulna	Lower 1/4th of anterior surface of radius	Median nerve (ant. interosseous n.)	Pronator of forearm

N.B.

MP = metacarpophalangeal joint
PIP = proximal interphalangeal joint
DIP = distal interphalangeal joint
IP = interphalangeal joint

crease of the elbow). It runs downward and reaches the medial side of the forearm midway between the elbow and the wrist. In the upper one-third of the forearm, the course is oblique (i.e. downward and medially), but in the lower two-thirds, it is vertical.

About 2.5 cm distal to the elbow it is crossed by median nerve from medial to lateral side.

The ulnar nerve lies medial to the distal two-thirds of the artery.

At wrist, it enters the palm by passing in front of the flexor retinaculum lateral to the ulnar nerve and the pisiform bone. It **terminates in the hand** by dividing into large superficial and small deep branches. The superficial branch—the continuation of the artery forms the *superficial palmar arch*, which anastomoses with superficial palmar branch of the radial artery.

Relations

In the upper part of its course, it lies deep to superficial flexor muscles. In the lower part of its course, it becomes superficial and lies between the tendons of the FCU and FDS. The details are as follows.

Anterior: The upper part of the ulnar artery is covered by five superficial muscles of the forearm, namely:

(a) Pronator teres
(b) FCR
(c) Palmaris longus
(d) FDS
(e) FCU

The lower part of the ulnar artery is covered only by the skin and superficial and deep fasciae.

Posterior: Only the origin of the ulnar artery lies on brachialis, while in the remaining whole part of its course, it lies on FDP.

Medial (Fig. 9.14)

(a) Ulnar nerve.
(b) FCU.

Lateral: FDS (tendon).

Branches

1. **Muscular branches** to neighbouring muscles.
2. **Anterior and posterior ulnar recurrent arteries** that take part in the arterial anastomosis around the elbow joint.
3. **Common interosseous artery** that arises from the upper part of the ulnar artery and after a very short course at the upper border of interosseous membrane, it divides into the *anterior* and *posterior interosseous arteries*.
4. **Palmar and dorsal ulnar carpal branches** that take part in the formation of the **palmar and dorsal carpal arches**.
5. Terminal branches are two; the larger superficial branch continues as the *superficial palmar arch*, while the smaller deep branch joins the *deep palmar arch*.

> **CLINICAL CORRELATION**
>
> **Aberrant ulnar artery:** In about 3% of individuals, the brachial artery divides into terminal branches high up in the arm. Therefore the ulnar artery may arise high in the arm and passes superficial to the flexor muscles of the forearm and is termed the *superficial ulnar artery*. This variation should always be kept in mind while withdrawing blood samples or giving intravenous injections, because if the superficial ulnar artery is mistaken for a vein, it may be damaged and produce bleeding. Further, if an irritating drug is injected into the aberrant artery, the result could be fatal.

Anterior Interosseous Artery (Figs. 9.25 and 10.13)

It is a branch of common interosseous artery. It along with *posterior interosseous* artery is the main source of blood supply to the forearm. It is also the *deepest artery on the front of the forearm*.

The *anterior interosseous artery* (Fig. 9.25) descends on the front of the interosseous membrane in company with the anterior interosseous nerve (a branch of the median nerve). It pierces the membrane at the upper border of the pronator quadratus to enter the posterior compartment of the forearm (cf. *peroneal artery of the leg*), where it anastomoses with the posterior interosseous artery and travels underneath the extensor retinaculum to reach the dorsal aspect of the wrist to join the dorsal carpal arch.

Radial Artery

Origin, Course, and Termination

The radial artery is the *smaller terminal branch of the brachial artery*. It begins in the cubital fossa at the level of the neck of the radius. It passes downward to the wrist with lateral convexity. In the upper part, it lies beneath the brachioradialis on the deep muscles of the forearm. Then between the tendons of brachioradialis and flexor carpi radialis in the lower forearm. At wrist, it lies on the anterior surface of the radius lateral to the tendon of flexor carpi radialis and is covered only by the skin and fascia. The superficial radial nerve lies lateral to the middle one-third of the radial artery.

The radial artery leaves the forearm by winding around the lateral aspect of the wrist to reach the anatomical snuff box on the posterior surface of the hand. Its further course in hand is described in the hand later on page 157.

Relations

Anterior: The upper part of the radial artery is overlapped by the brachioradialis, while its lower part is covered only by the skin, and superficial and deep fasciae.

Posterior: The radial artery from above to downward lies on the following structures:

(a) Biceps tendon.
(b) Supinator.
(c) Pronator teres.
(d) FDS.

These structures together form the bed of the radial artery.

N.B.

The radial artery is quite superficial throughout its whole course as compared to the ulnar artery.

Branches in the Forearm

1. **Muscular branches** to the lateral muscles of the forearm.
2. **Radial recurrent artery** arises in the cubital fossa and takes part in the formation of the arterial anastomose around the elbow joint.
3. **Palmar carpal branch** arises near the wrist and anastomoses with the palmar carpal branch of the ulnar artery.
4. **Superficial palmar branch** arises just above the wrist and enters the palm of the hand by passing in front of the flexor retinaculum. It joins the terminal part of the ulnar artery to complete the *superficial palmar arch*.

CLINICAL CORRELATION

- Radial artery is normally used to take pulse and increasingly being used as a main portal for **interventional radiology** (e.g. cardiac angiography/angioplasty).
- **Examination of the radial pulse:** It is felt on the radial side of the front of the wrist where the radial artery lies on the flat anterior surface of the distal end of the radius, and covered only by the skin and fascia. At this site, the radial artery lies between the tendon of FCR medially and the tendon of brachioradialis laterally. While examining the radial pulse, the thumb should not be used because it has its own pulse, which may be mistaken for the patient's pulse. The radial pulse is commonly used for examining the pulse rate.

NERVES OF THE FRONT OF THE FOREARM

AN 12.2

The nerves of the front of the forearm are median, radial, and ulnar (Fig. 9.12).

The radial and ulnar nerves as their names indicate run along the radial and ulnar margins of the forearm outside the radial and ulnar arteries. The median nerve, according its name, runs in the median region of the forearm.

Median Nerve in Forearm

The median nerve is the **principal nerve of the front of the forearm** and supplies all the muscles of the front of the forearm except medial half of the FDP and FCU, which are supplied by the ulnar nerve.

The median nerve leaves the cubital fossa by passing between the two heads of the pronator teres. Here it crosses the ulnar artery (from the medial to the lateral side) from which it is separated by the deep head of the pronator teres. Then along with the ulnar artery, it passes beneath

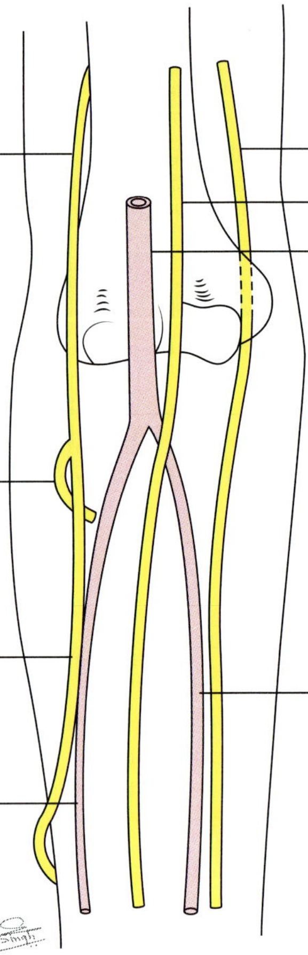

FIG. 9.12 ■ Nerves and arteries on the front of the forearm.

(i.e. deep to) the fibrous arch joining two heads of FDS and runs deep to this muscle on the surface of FDP.

At the wrist, about 5 cm proximal to flexor retinaculum, the median nerve emerges from behind the lateral border of the FDS and lies behind the tendon of the palmaris longus. Note that in front of the wrist, the median nerve becomes superficial lying between the tendons of FDS medially and FCR laterally, and is covered only partly by the tendon of the palmaris longus (Fig. 9.14).

The median nerve enters the palm of the hand by passing deep to the flexor retinaculum through the **carpal tunnel**.

Branches

1. **Muscular branches** in the cubital fossa to the pronator teres, FCR, palmaris longus, and FDS (Fig. 9.13).
2. **Articular branches** to the elbow and the proximal radioulnar joint.
3. **Anterior interosseous** nerve arises in the upper part of the forearm and passes downward on the anterior surface of the interosseous membrane between FPL and FDP. It passes deep to the pronator quadratus and ends on the anterior surface of the carpus. It supplies FPL, lateral half of the FDP, and pronator quadratus. It also provides articular twigs to the distal radioulnar and wrist joints.

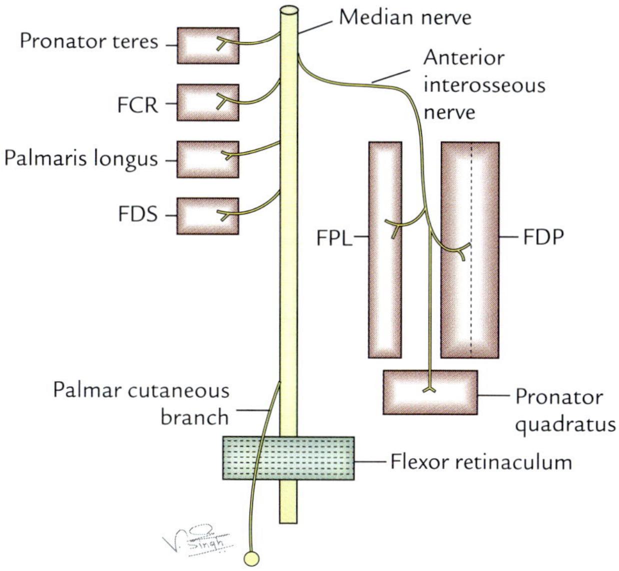

FIG. 9.13 ■ Branches of the median nerve in the forearm.

4. **Palmar cutaneous branch** arises about 5 cm above the wrist and passes forward in front of the flexor retinaculum to supply the skin over thenar eminence and central part of the palm.

For details, see Chapter 13, page 175.

Ulnar Nerve in Forearm

The ulnar enters the front of the forearm by passing through the gap between the two heads of the FCU (*cubital tunnel*). It then runs downward on the medial side of the forearm between the FCU and FDP. It enters the palm of the hand by passing in front of the flexor retinaculum lateral to the pisiform bone.

In the distal two-thirds of the forearm, the ulnar artery is lateral to the ulnar nerve.

Branches

1. **Muscular branches** to the FCU and medial half of the FDP.
2. **Articular branch** to the elbow joint.
3. **Palmar cutaneous branch** arises in the middle of the forearm and supplies the skin over the hypothenar eminence. It sometimes supplies palmaris brevis.
4. **Dorsal cutaneous branch** arises in distal third of the forearm. It passes medially between the tendon of FCU and ulna to reach the dorsum of the hand.

For details, see Chapter 13, page 178.

Radial Nerve in Forearm

The **radial nerve** enters the cubital fossa by descending between the brachioradialis and brachialis muscles. In front of the lateral epicondyle, it divides into two terminal branches—deep and superficial.

The **deep branch of the radial nerve** winds around the neck of the radius between the two heads of the supinator and enters the posterior compartment of the forearm as the *posterior interosseous nerve*.

The superficial branch of the radial nerve (**superficial radial nerve**) is the main continuation of the radial nerve. It runs downward under the cover of brachioradialis on the lateral side of the radial artery. About 7.5 cm above the wrist, the nerve leaves the artery, passes underneath the tendon of the brachioradialis to reach the posterior aspect of the wrist and divides into terminal branches (four or five nerves), which supply the skin of the lateral two-thirds of the posterior aspect of the hand and the posterior surface of the proximal phalanges of the lateral 31/2 digits. The area of skin supplied by the radial nerve on the dorsum of the hand is variable.

For details, see Chapter 13, page 172.

N.B.

The relationship of main nerves and arteries in front of mid-forearm about 7.5 cm above wrist can be remembered by a *Mnemonic:*

From lateral to medial side these are (Fig. 9.12):

Nice: nerve (radial **n**erve)
Aunty: artery (radial **a**rtery)
Never: nerve (median **n**erve)
Allowed: artery (ulnar **a**rtery)
Nuisance: nerve (ulnar **n**erve)

CLINICAL CORRELATION

Surgical safe side of the forearm: The lateral side of the anterior aspect of the forearm is considered to be the 'safe side' by the surgeons because the branches of the median nerve, the main nerve of the front of the forearm, are mostly directed medially to supply the muscles of the front of the forearm. The major nerve on the lateral side is the superficial radial nerve. It is only a sensory branch of the radial nerve and runs deep to the brachioradialis muscle in the proximal forearm.

RELATIONSHIP OF STRUCTURES ON THE FRONT OF THE WRIST

The structures lying in front of the conventional wrist from the *lateral to the medial side* are as follows (Fig. 9.14):

1. Radial **A**rtery
2. **T**endon of FCR
3. Median **N**erve
4. **T**endon of palmaris longus
5. **T**endon of FDS (in a deeper plane)
6. Ulnar **A**rtery
7. Ulnar **N**erve
8. **T**endon of FCU

Mnemonic: **A** **T**rained **N**urse **T**eaches **T**o **A**void **N**ew **T**echniques, i.e. **a**rtery, **t**endon, **n**erve, **t**endon, **t**endon, **a**rtery, **n**erve and **t**endon.

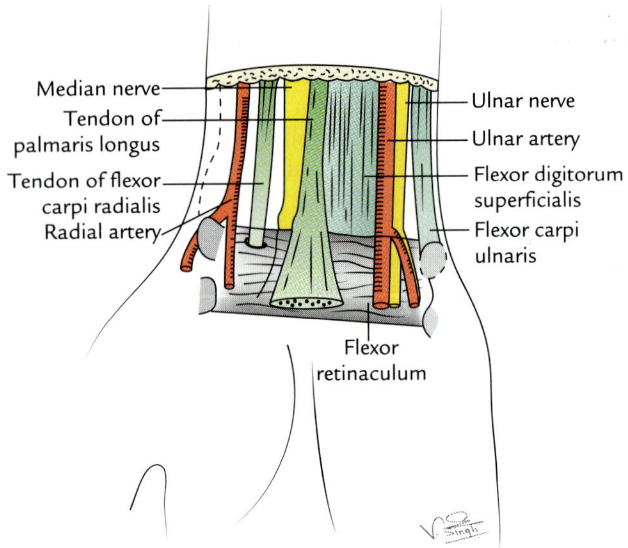

FIG. 9.14 ■ Structures lying in front of the wrist.

N.B.

Median nerve is very superficial in front of the wrist and lies along the lateral edge of the tendon of the palmaris longus.

Median nerve lies deep to the tendon of the palmaris longus.

CLINICAL CORRELATION

Suicidal cuts of the wrist:

- A *deep laceration on the radial side of the wrist* as in a suicide attempt may cut the following structures, from the lateral to the medial side:
  - Radial artery
  - Tendon of FCR
  - Median nerve
  - Tendons of palmaris longus
  - Tendon of FDS
- A *deep laceration on the ulnar side of the wrist* as in suicide attempt may cut the following structures, from the medial to the lateral side:
  - Tendon of FCU
  - Ulnar nerve
  - Ulnar artery

BACK OF THE FOREARM AN 12.11

The following structures are to be studied on the back of the forearm:

1. Muscles of the back of the forearm
2. Posterior interosseous nerve
3. Posterior and anterior interosseous arteries

MUSCLES OF THE BACK OF THE FOREARM

The muscles of the back of the forearm are divided into two groups: (a) superficial and (b) deep.

Superficial Muscles of the Back of the Forearm

The superficial muscles of the back of the forearm are seven in number. From the lateral to the medial side, these are as follows:

Lateral group:
1. Brachioradialis
2. Extensor carpi radialis longus (ECRL)
3. Extensor carpi radialis brevis (ECRB)

Posterior group:
4. Extensor digitorum (ED)
5. Extensor digiti minimi (EDM)
6. Extensor carpi ulnaris (ECU)
7. Anconeus

Of these first three muscles form the lateral group while last four forms the posterior group.

The arrangement of superficial muscles on the back of the forearm is shown in Fig. 9.15.

N.B.

All the superficial muscles arise from lateral epicondyle of humerus except brachioradialis and ECRL which arise separately from lateral supracondylar ridge of humerus.

- Four of the superficial muscles (ECRB, ED, EDM, and ECU) arise by a common tendon from anteriolateral surface of lateral epicondyle of the humerus called the *common extensor origin.*
- All are supplied by posterior interosseous nerve except brachioradialis and ECRL, which are supplied by main trunk of radial nerve.
- All the seven muscles cross the elbow joint.

The origin, insertion, nerve supply, and actions of the superficial muscles of the back of the forearm are presented in Table 9.3.

The origin and insertion of superficial extensors of the forearm is shown in Figs. 9.16–9.19.

Deep Muscles of the Back of the Forearm

There are five deep muscles of the back of the forearm, from above downward these are as follows (Fig. 9.20):

1. Supinator
2. Abductor pollicis longus (APL)
3. Extensor pollicis brevis (EPB)
4. Extensor pollicis longus (EPL)
5. Extensor indicis

The three deep extensors of the forearm, which act on thumb (*APL*, *EPB*, and *EPL*) lie deep to the superficial extensors and in order to gain insertion on the three short long bones of thumb 'crop out' (emerge) from the furrow in the lateral part of the forearm between the lateral and posterior groups of the superficial extensor. These three muscles are therefore termed **outcropping muscles.**

The origin, insertion, nerve supply, and actions of deep muscles of the back of the forearm are presented in Table 9.4.

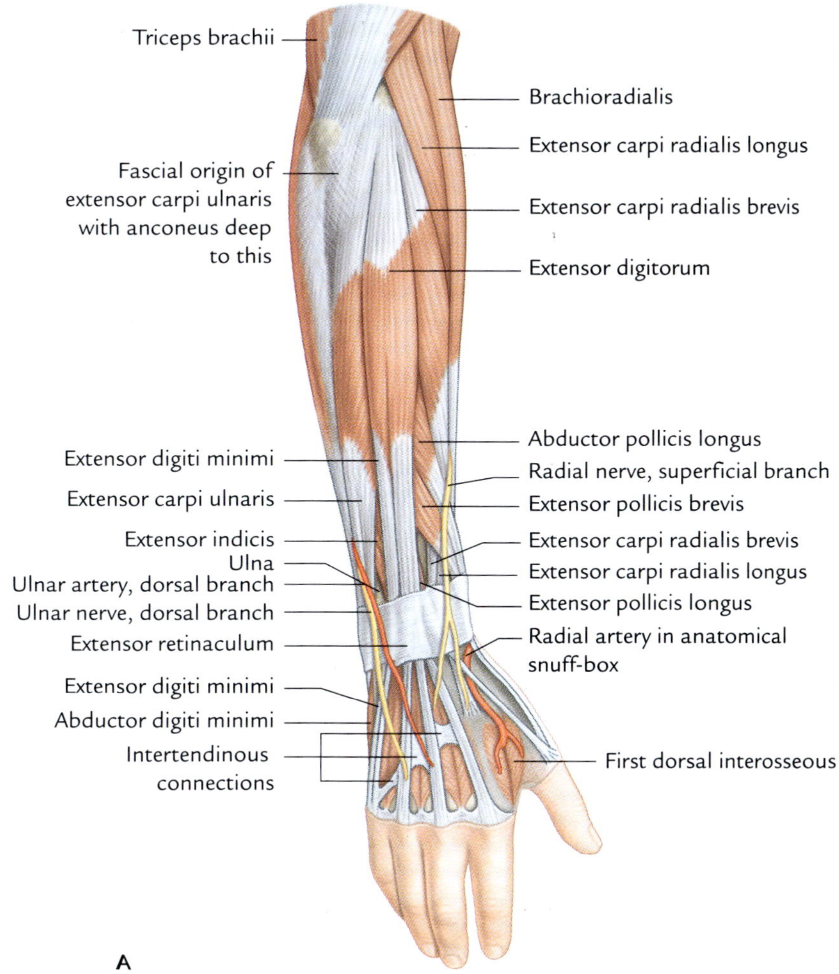

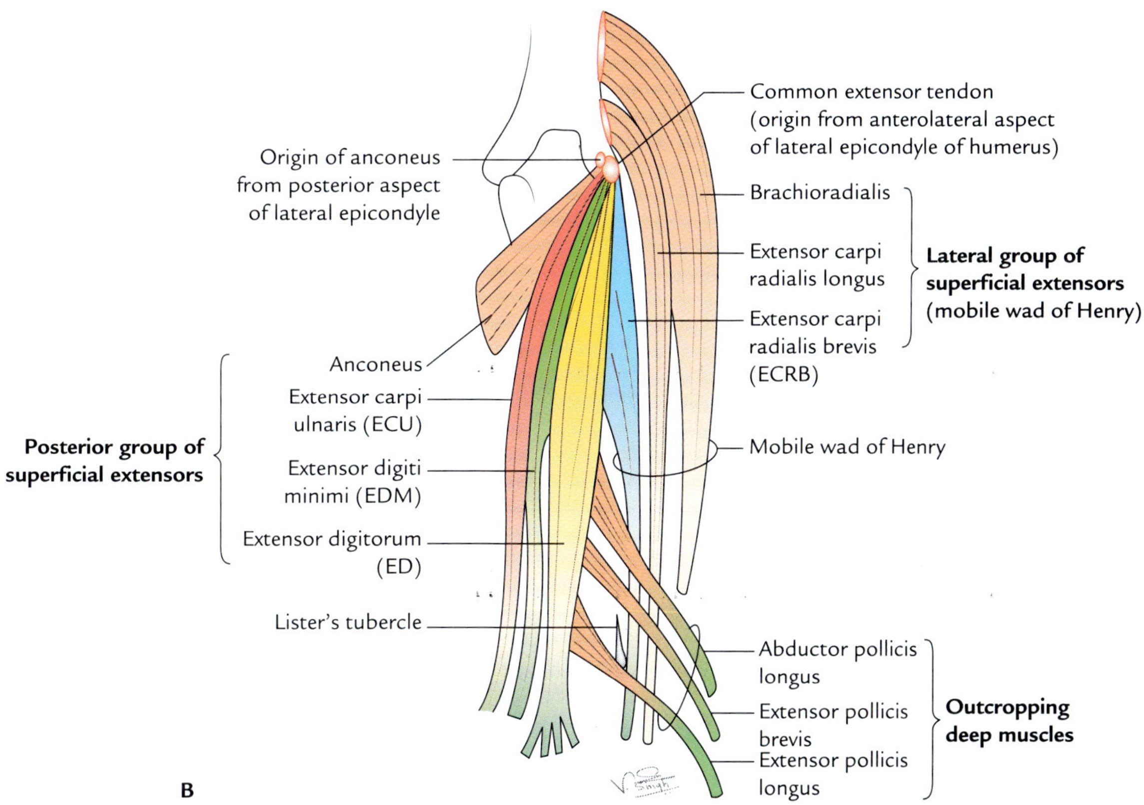

FIG. 9.15 ■ Superficial muscles on the back of the forearm. (**A**) Actual arrangement (*Source: Gray's Anatomy: The Anatomical Basis of Clinical Practice, 41st ed.: Editor-in-Chief Susan* Standring, Fig. 49.23, page 853, Elsevier Limited, 2016.) and (**B**) schematic arrangement.

TABLE 9.3 Origin, insertion, nerve supply, and actions of the superficial muscles of the back of the forearm (superficial extensors)

Muscle	Origin	Insertion	Nerve supply	Actions
Lateral group				
Brachioradialis (Fig. 9.16) (earlier called supinator longus)	Upper two-thirds of the lateral supracondylar ridge of the humerus	Lateral surface of the distal end of the radius just above the styloid process	Radial nerve	• Flexes the elbow joint • Pronates the supinated forearm to midprone position • Supinates the pronated forearm to midprone position
Extensor carpi radialis longus (ECRL)	Lower one-third of the lateral supracondylar ridge of the humerus	Lateral side of the dorsal surface of the base of second metacarpal bone	Radial nerve	• Acting with extensor carpi ulnaris extends the wrist • Acting with flexor carpi radialis abducts the wrist
Extensor carpi radialis brevis (ECRB)	By a common tendon from the lateral epicondyle of the humerus and lateral ligament of the elbow joint	Lateral side of the dorsal surface of the base of third metacarpal bone	Posterior interosseous nerve before piercing the supinator	-Do-
Posterior group				
Extensor digitorum	By a common tendon from the lateral epicondyle	• Gives rise to four tendons for medial four digits • By the extensor expansion, it is inserted into the dorsum of middle and terminal phalanges	Posterior interosseous nerve	Extends the medial four digits. Can also extend the wrist
Extensor digiti minimi	By the common tendon from the lateral epicondyle	• Lies medial to the ED tendon for the little finger • Through the extensor expansion, it is inserted into the dorsum of the middle and terminal phalanges of the little finger	Posterior interosseous nerve	• Extends the little finger • Helps in the extension of the wrist
Extensor carpi ulnaris (ECU)	By the common tendon from the lateral epicondyle and by an aponeurosis from the upper two-thirds of the posterior border of the ulna along with the flexor carpi ulnaris and the flexor digitorum profundus	Into a tubercle on the medial side of the dorsal surface of the base of the fifth metacarpal	Posterior interosseous nerve	• Acting with extensor carpi radialis, it extends the wrist • Acting with flexor carpi ulnaris, it adducts the wrist
Anconeus	From the back of the lateral epicondyle by a separate tendon proximal to that of common extensor tendon	Lateral side of the olecranon process and upper one-fourth of the posterior surface of the ulna	Nerve to anconeus, which arises from the radial nerve in the spiral groove and descends through the medial head of the triceps brachii	Weak extensor of the elbow joint

N.B.

Brachioradialis is paradoxical muscle. Its origin and innervation are characteristic of an extensor muscle, but actually it is a flexor muscle of the elbow.

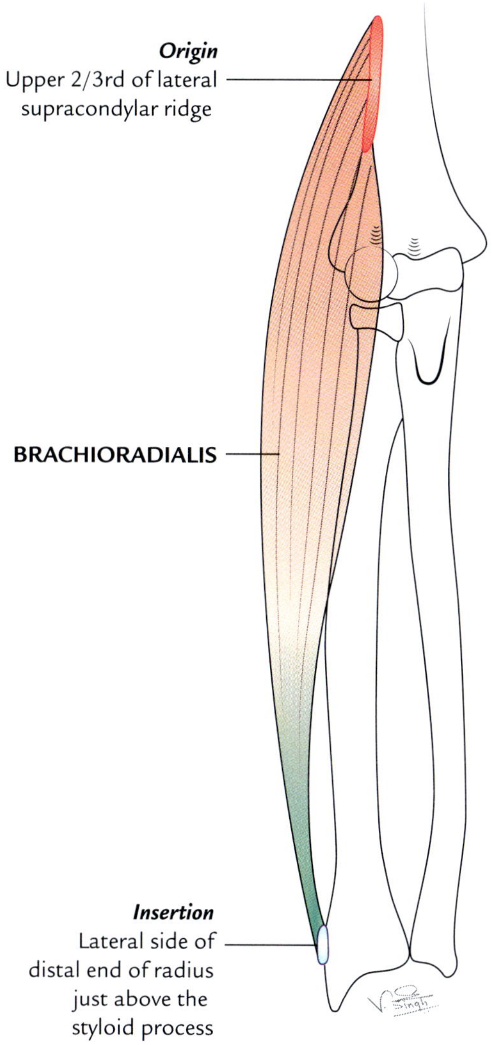

FIG. 9.16 ■ Origin and insertion of the brachioradialis.

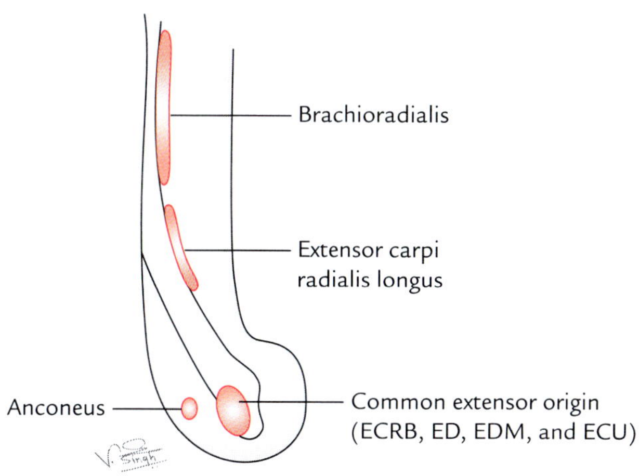

FIG. 9.17 ■ Lateral aspect of the lower end of the humerus showing the origin of seven superficial muscles of the back of the forearm (ECRB = extensor carpi radialis brevis, ED = extensor digitorum, EDM = extensor digiti minimi, ECU = extensor carpi ulnaris).

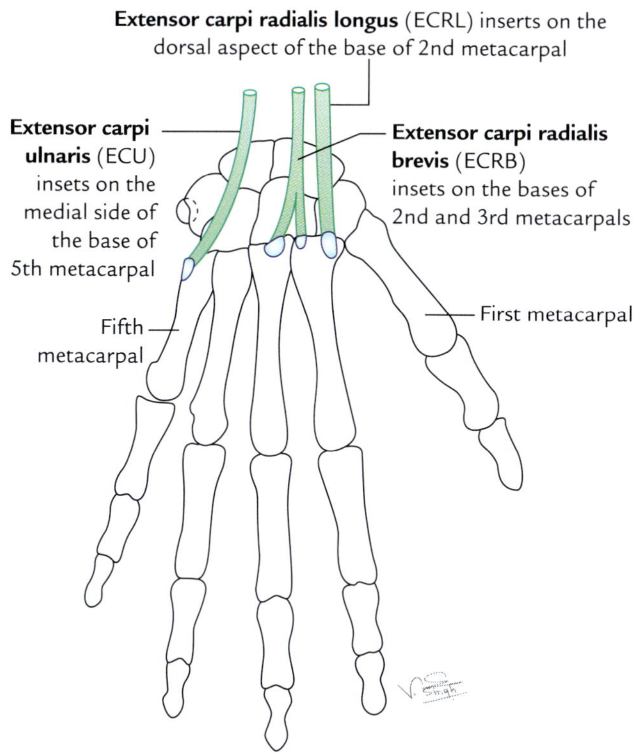

FIG. 9.18 ■ Insertion of the extensor carpi ulnaris, extensor carpi radialis longus, and ECRB.

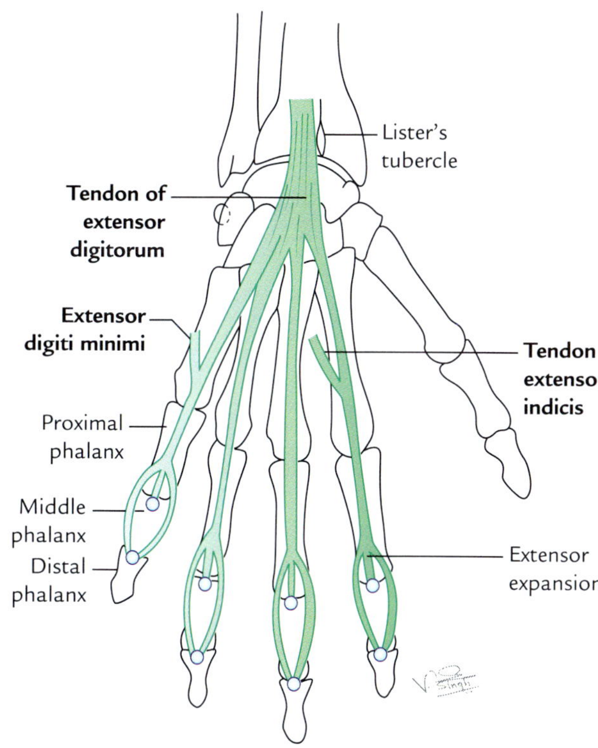

FIG. 9.19 ■ Insertion of the extensor digitorum, extensor carpi ulnaris, and extensor indicis.

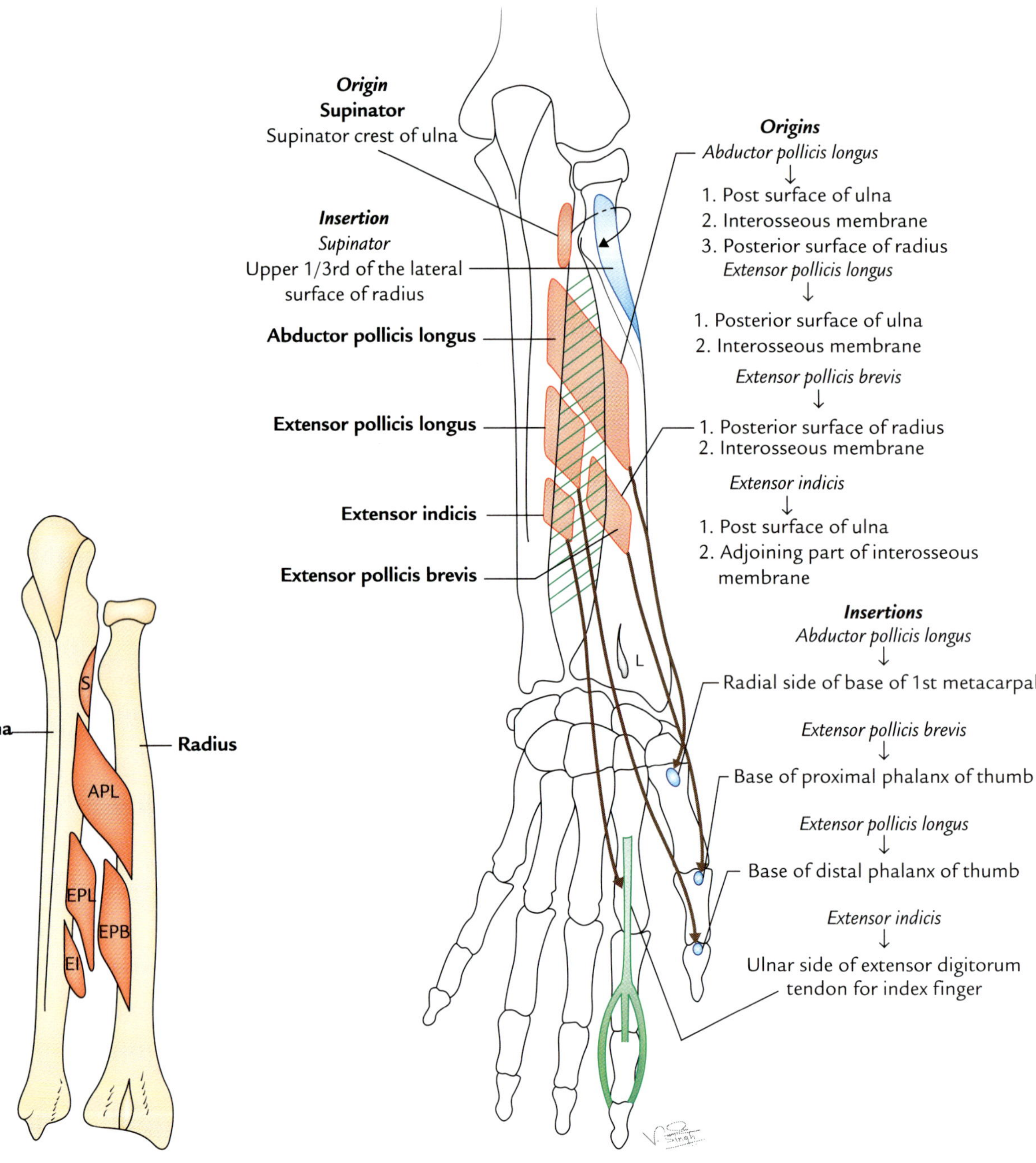

FIG. 9.20 ■ (**A**) Origin of five deep muscles of the back of forearm from the posterior aspects of radius and ulna (S = supinator, APL = abductor pollicis longus, EPL = extensor pollicis longus, EPB = extensor pollicis brevis, EI = extensor indicis). (**B**) Origin and insertion of the deep muscles on the back of the forearm (L = Lister's tubercle).

N.B.

- None of the deep muscles of the back of the forearm cross the elbow joint.
- All of them arise from the radius, ulna, and interosseous membrane.
- All of them are supplied by the *posterior interosseous nerve* (deep branch of the radial nerve).

EXTENSOR RETINACULUM

AN 12.14

The deep fascia on the back of the wrist is thickened to form an oblique fibrous band called the **extensor retinaculum** (Fig. 9.22). It is directed downward and medially, and about 2 cm broad vertically.

Attachments

The *medial end* of the extensor retinaculum is attached to the styloid process of the ulna, triquetral, and pisiform bones (Fig. 9.22).

TABLE 9.4 Origin, insertion, nerve supply, and actions of the deep muscles of the back of the forearm (deep extensors of the forearm)

Muscle	Origin	Insertion	Nerve supply	Action
Supinator (Fig. 9.21)	• Lateral epicondyle • Lateral ligament of the elbow joint • Annular ligament • Supinator crest of the ulna and from the triangular area in front of it	Upper one-third of the posterior, lateral, and anterior surfaces of the radius	Posterior interosseous nerve before piercing the supinator	Supination of the forearm
Abductor pollicis longus (APL)	• Lateral part of the posterior surface of the ulna below the anconeus • Middle one-third of the posterior surface of the radius (below the posterior oblique line) and intervening posterior surface of the interosseous membrane	Lateral side of the base of the first metacarpal	Posterior interosseous nerve	Abducts the thumb
Extensor pollicis brevis (EPB)	From a small area on the posterior surface of radius below the origin of abductor pollicis longus and from adjoining interosseous membrane	Dorsal surface of the base of the proximal phalanx of the thumb	Posterior interosseous nerve	Extends the thumb at metacarpophalangeal joint and extends the carpometacarpal joint
Extensor pollicis longus (EPL)	From lateral part of middle one-third of the posterior surface of ulna and adjoining interosseous membrane	Dorsal surface of the base of the distal phalanx of the thumb	Posterior interosseous nerve	• Extends the joints of thumb • Helps in the extension of the wrist
Extensor indicis	From the posterior surface of ulna below the origin of extensor pollicis longus and also from the adjoining interosseous membrane	• The tendon lies medial to the ED tendon for the index finger • Through the extensor expansion, it is inserted into the dorsum of the middle and distal phalanges of the index finger	Posterior interosseous nerve	• Extends the index finger • Helps in the extension of the wrist

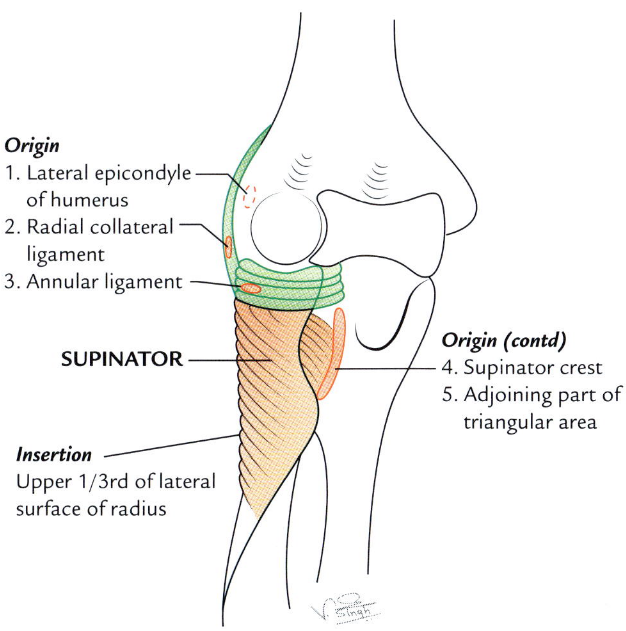

FIG. 9.21 Origin and insertion of the supinator muscle.

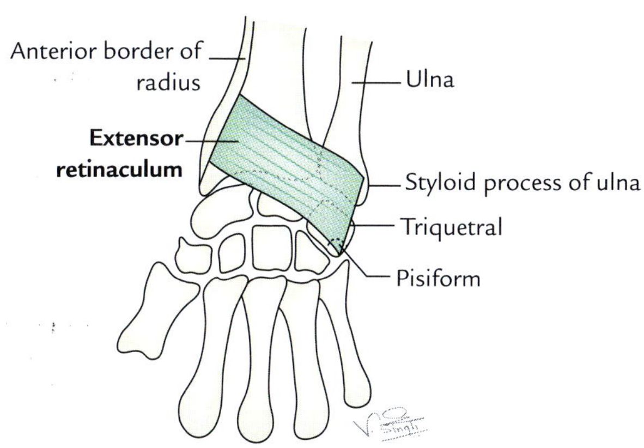

FIG. 9.22 Extensor retinaculum of wrist.

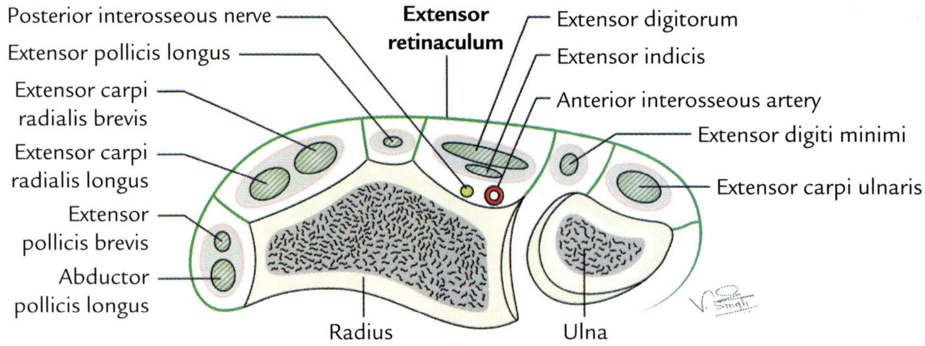

FIG. 9.23 ■ Transverse section of the forearm just above the wrist showing structures passing through various compartments, deep to the extensor retinaculum of the wrist.

Its *lateral end* is attached to the lower part of the anterior border of the radius.

Compartments

The space deep to the extensor retinaculum is divided into six compartments by five septa extending from the retinaculum to the dorsal aspects of the lower ends of the radius and ulna (Fig. 9.23). The compartments are numbered I to VI from the lateral to medial side.

The structures passing through these compartments are listed in Table 9.5.

N.B.

As the tendons pass across the dorsum of the wrist, they are enclosed within synovial sheaths called *synovial tendon sheaths* that reduce the friction of extensor tendons as they pass through the osseofibrous tunnels—the compartments under the extensor retinaculum.

Functions

It holds the extensor tendon in place at the back of the wrist and prevents their bowstringing when the hand is extended at the wrist joint.

TABLE 9.5 **Structures passing through various compartments beneath the extensor retinaculum of the wrist**

Compartment	Structure/structures, passing through
I	• Abductor pollicis longus (APL) • Extensor pollicis brevis (APB)
II	• Extensor carpi radialis longus (ECRL) • Extensor carpi radialis brevis (ECRB)
III	Extensor pollicis longus (EPL)
IV	• Extensor digitorum (ED) • Extensor indicis (EI) • Posterior interosseous nerve • Anterior interosseous artery
V	Extensor digiti minimi (EDM)
VI	Extensor carpi ulnaris (EUC)

POSTERIOR INTEROSSEOUS NERVE (FIG. 9.24) AN 12.12

Origin and Course

The *posterior interosseous nerve* is the deep terminal branch of the radial nerve (Fig. 9.24A). It is the **motor** and **chief nerve of the back of the forearm.** It begins in the cubital fossa as one of the two terminal branches of the radial nerve at the level of lateral epicondyle of the humerus. It leaves the cubital fossa by winding around the lateral side of the neck of the radius in the substance of the supinator. After emerging from the supinator, it runs in the fascial plane between superficial and deep extensor muscles. At the lower border of EPB, it passes deep to the EPL to lie on the posterior surface of the interosseous membrane, on which it runs downward up to the wrist where it ends into a **pseudoganglion** (Fig. 9.24B).

Branches (Fig. 9.24C)

1. Muscular branches:
   (a) *Before piercing the supinator*, it gives branches to the ECRB and supinator.
   (b) *While passing through the supinator*, it gives another branch to the supinator.
   (c) *After emerging from the supinator*, it gives branches to three superficial extensors (ED, EDM, and ECU) and all deep extensors.
2. **Articular branches** to the wrist joint, distal radioulnar joint, and carpal joints.

N.B.

All the muscles on the back of the forearm are supplied by the posterior interosseous nerve except the brachioradialis, ECRL, and anconeus, which are supplied by the radial nerve directly.

CLINICAL CORRELATION

- **Posterior interosseous nerve syndrome:** It occurs when posterior interosseous nerve is entrapped in the **arcade of Frohse,** which is a fibrous band between two heads of supinator muscle. The posterior interosseous nerve passes deep to the arcade into *radial tunnel* between two heads

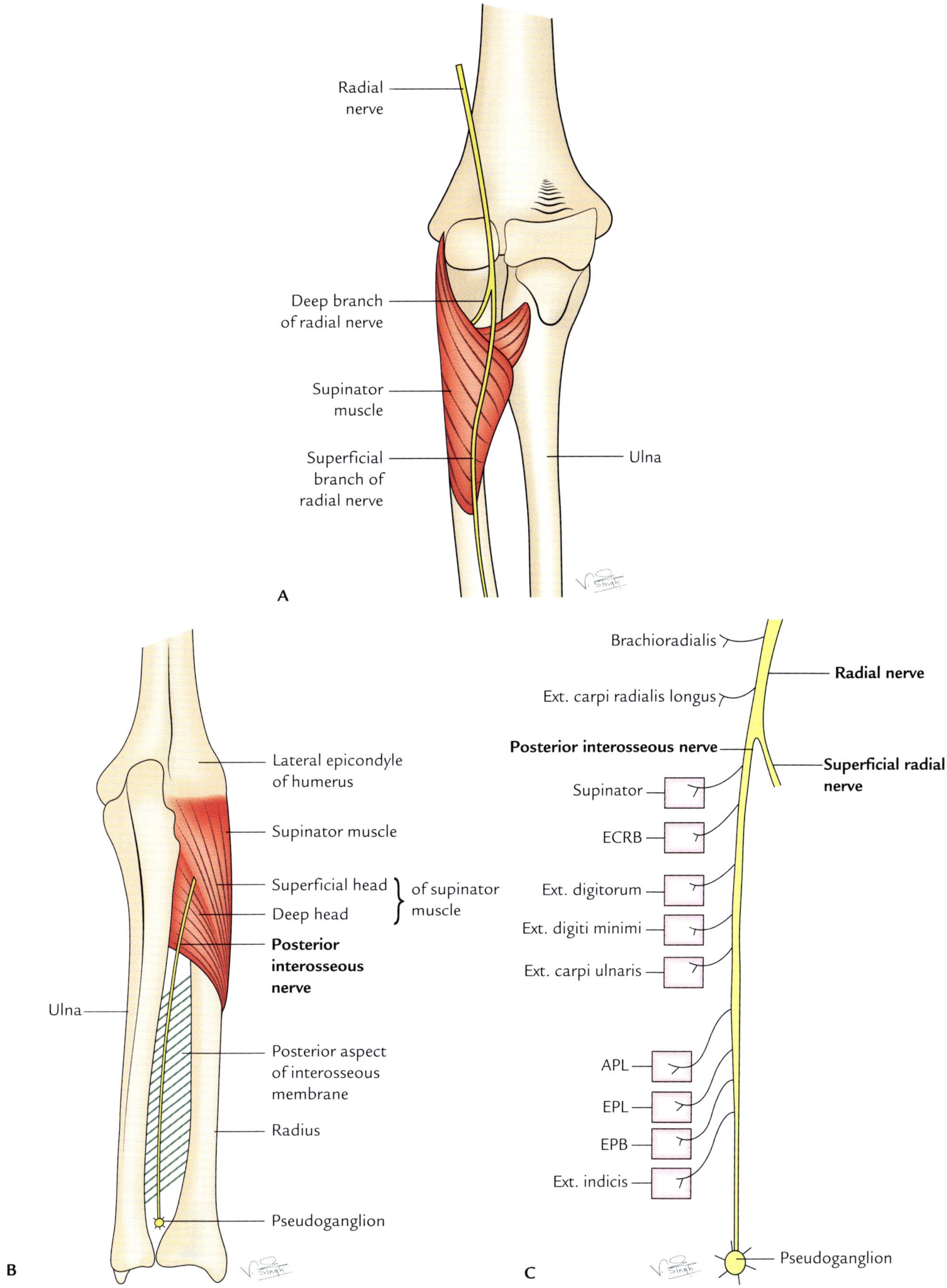

FIG. 9.24 ■ (**A**) Origin of posterior interosseous nerve. (**B**) Course of posterior interosseous nerve on the back of forearm. (**C**) Branches of the posterior interosseous nerve.

(superficial and deep) of supinator muscle. **Clinically** it presents as pain and weakness in forearm causing difficulty in pulling, pushing, and grabbing.

The **posterior interosseous nerve** (i.e. deep terminal branch of the radial nerve) may be damaged during the surgical exposure of the head of the radius, in the fracture proximal end of the radius. Since the ECRL is a spared **wrist drop does not occur**.

Note: Some authorities think that deep terminal branch of radial nerve is termed as posterior interosseous nerve only after energing from supinator muscle.

POSTERIOR INTEROSSEOUS ARTERY (FIG. 9.25A)

The *posterior interosseous artery* (Fig. 9.25) is a smaller terminal branch of the common interosseous artery from the ulnar artery. It begins in the cubital fossa, enters the back of the forearm by passing through the gap between the oblique cord and upper margin of the interosseous membrane. From here, it passes between the supinator and abductor pollicis longus to run on the posterior interosseous nerve. In the lower part of the forearm, it becomes markedly reduced and ends by anastomosing with the anterior interosseous artery. In the lower part of the forearm, the anterior interosseous artery enters the back of the forearm by piercing the interosseous membrane just above the pronator quadratus and supplies a lower one-fourth of the back of the forearm. The posterior interosseous artery in the cubital fossa gives the **interosseous recurrent artery**, which takes part in the formation of anastomosis around the elbow joint.

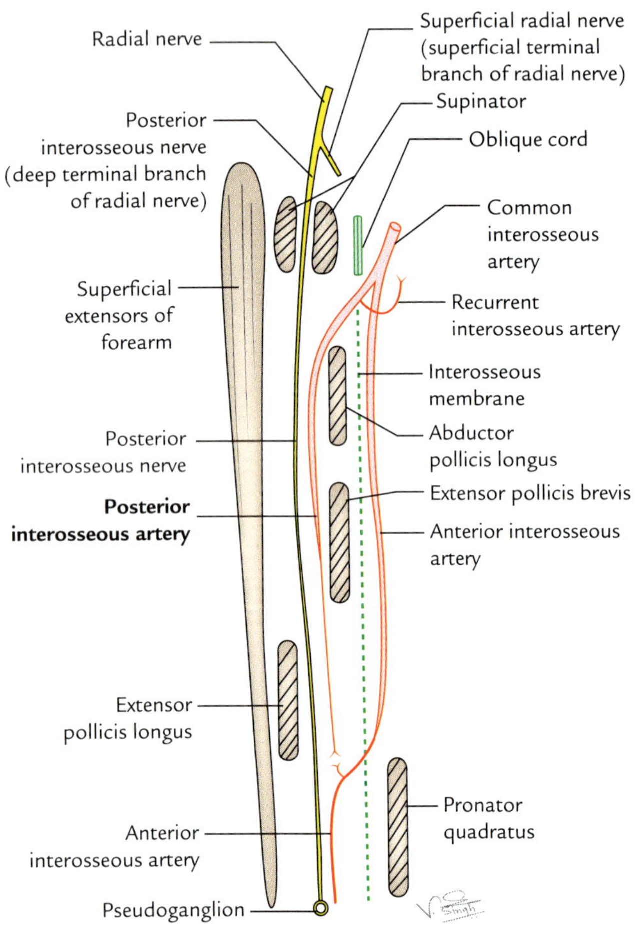

FIG. 9.25 ■ Course and relations of the posterior interosseous artery.

Golden Facts to Remember

• All the flexor muscles of the forearm at elbow lie on the front of forearm except	Brachioradialis, which lies on the back of the forearm
• All the superficial flexors of the forearm are supplied by median nerve except	FCU, which is supplied by the ulnar nerve
• Most powerful and most bulky muscle on the front of the forearm	FDP
• Deepest muscle on the front of the forearm	Pronator quadratus
• Deepest artery on the front of the forearm	Anterior interosseous artery
• Principal nerve of the front of the forearm	Median nerve
• 'Safe side' on the anterior aspect of the forearm for surgeons	Lateral side of the front of the forearm
• Most superficial muscle along the radial side of the forearm	Brachioradialis
• Lister's tubercle	Dorsal tubercle of radius
• Chief nerve of the back of the forearm	Posterior interosseous nerve
• All the muscles on the back of the forearm are extensors except	Brachioradialis, which is a flexor of the forearm
• Commonest site of palpation of arterial pulse	Radial artery at wrist
• Chief source of blood supply to the forearm	Ulnar artery

CLINICAL CASE STUDY

A 25-year-old girl, who was studying in the final MBBS, tried to commit suicide by slashing the front of her wrist with a sharp knife. She was bleeding profusely and was immediately taken to the hospital, where the doctors, on examination, found a lacerated wound on the radial side of her wrist. Surgical procedure was performed and her life was saved. She was diagnosed as a case **suicidal cut in front of her wrist on lateral side**.

Questions

1. Name the structures lying in front of the wrist.
2. Name the structures that are likely to be cut by deep lacerated wound on the radial side of wrist.
3. Injury of which structure leads to profuse bleeding?
4. Name the artery that lies in front of the distal end of the radius between the tendon of FCR and brachioradialis and mention its clinical importance.

Answers

1. From the lateral to the medial side these are: (a) radial artery, (b) tendon of FCR, median nerve (c) tendon of palmaris longus, (d) tendons of FDS, (e) ulnar artery, (f) ulnar nerve, and (g) tendon of FCU (Fig. 9.14).
2. Radial artery, tendon of FCR, tendon of palmaris longus, and median nerve.
3. Radial artery.
4. Radial artery. The ***'radial pulse'*** is felt at the wrist on this site.

CHAPTER 10

Elbow and Radioulnar Joints

SPECIFIC LEARNING OBJECTIVES

After studying this chapter, the student should be able to:

- Describe the elbow joint and superior and inferior radioulnar joints under the following headings: (a) type of joint, (b) articular surfaces, (c) capsule, (d) synovial membrane, (e) ligaments, (f) blood supply, (g) nerve supply, and (h) movements and muscles producing them. AN 13.3
- Write short notes on: (a) carrying angle, (b) ulnar collateral ligament, (c) equilateral or isosceles triangle at the elbow, (d) radioulnar joints, and (e) supination and pronation.
- Enumerate: (a) articulations at the elbow joint and (b) articulations involved in the movements of supination and pronation.
- Give the anatomical basis of: (a) pulled elbow, (b) student's elbow, (c) tennis elbow, and (d) Golfer's elbow.

ELBOW JOINT AN 13.3, AN 13.5

The elbow joint is a joint between the lower end of the humerus and upper ends of the radius and ulna. It actually includes two articulations: (a) **humeroulnar articulation,** between the trochlea of the humerus and the trochlear notch of the ulna and (b) **humeroradial articulation,** between the capitulum of the humerus and the head of the radius. On the surface, the joint line of the elbow is situated 2 cm below the line joining the two epicondyles of the humerus.

The complexity of the elbow joint is further increased by its continuity with the superior radioulnar joint. Thus, there are three articulations in the elbow region, namely (a) humeroulnar, (b) humeroradial, and (c) superior (proximal) radioulnar. These are called **cubital articulations** (Fig. 10.1).

TYPE

It is a hinge type of synovial joint.

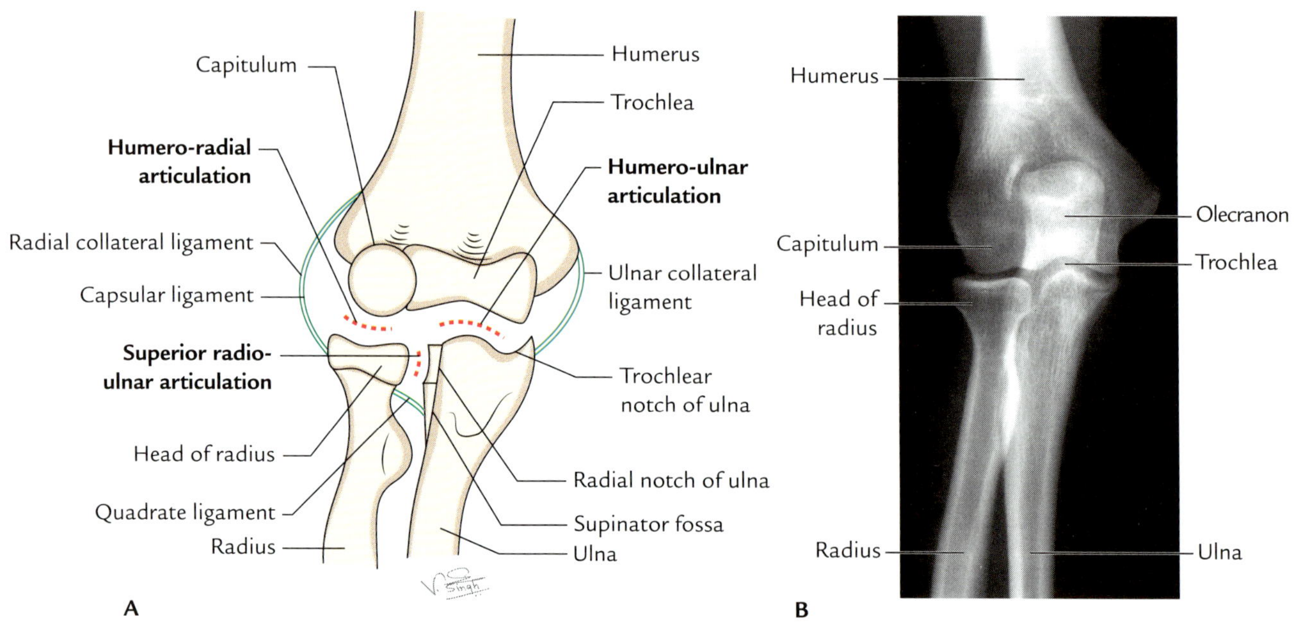

FIG. 10.1 ■ Components of the elbow joint. (**A**) Schematic diagram, (**B**) radiograph of the normal elbow joint (anteroposterior view). (*Source*: *Gray's Anatomy for students:*. Richard L Drake, Wayne Vogl, Adam WM Mitchell, Fig. 7.70D, *Page 681, Elsevier Inc., 2005.*)

ARTICULAR SURFACES

The *upper articular surface* is formed by the **capitulum and the trochlea of the lower end of the humerus.**

The *lower articular surface* is formed by the upper surface of **the head of the radius and the trochlear notch of the ulna**.

The **capitulum** is a rounded hemispherical eminence that possesses a smooth articular surface only on its anterior and inferior aspects.

The **trochlea** is medial to capitulum and resembles a pulley. The medial flange of the trochlea projects to a lower level than its lateral flange.

The **trochlear notch** of the ulna is formed by the upper surface of the coronoid process and the anterior surface of the olecranon process.

The **upper end of the radius** is circular in outline and slightly depressed in the centre.

N.B.

The distal end of the humerus has *three nonarticular fossae:* (a) *olecranon fossa*, a deep hollow above the posterior part of the trochlea, which lodges the tip of the olecranon process of the ulna during the extension of the elbow; (b) *coronoid fossa*, a small hollow above the anterior surface of the trochlea, which lodges the anterior margin of the coronoid process of the ulna during the flexion of the elbow; and (c) *radial fossa*, another small hollow lateral to the coronoid fossa, just above the capitulum, which lodges the anterior margin of the head of the radius during the flexion of the elbow.

JOINT CAPSULE (CAPSULAR LIGAMENT)

It is a fibrous sac enclosing the joint cavity (Fig. 10.2). The inner surface of the capsule is lined by the synovial membrane.

Attachment

Above, it is attached to the medial epicondyle, upper margins of radial, coronoid, and olecranon fossae, and the lateral epicondyle of the humerus, that is it encloses all the nonarticular fossae at the lower end of the humerus.

Below, it is attached to the anterior and medial margins of the coronoid process of the ulna, upper margin of the annular ligament, and upper and medial margins of the olecranon process. Note that it is not attached to the radius.

To facilitate the movements of flexion and extension, the anterior and posterior aspects of the capsule are thinner than the sides.

Synovial Membrane

The inner surface of the joint capsule and nonarticular bony parts inside the capsule are lined by the **synovial membrane** (Fig. 10.3). The synovial membrane forms a crescentic fold between humeroradial and humeroulnar parts, which contains an *extra synovial fat.* Between the synovial membrane and joint capsule, there are *three other fat pads*, occupying olecranon, coronoid, and radial fossae. The synovial membrane of the elbow joint is continuous inferiorly with the synovial membrane of the superior radioulnar joint.

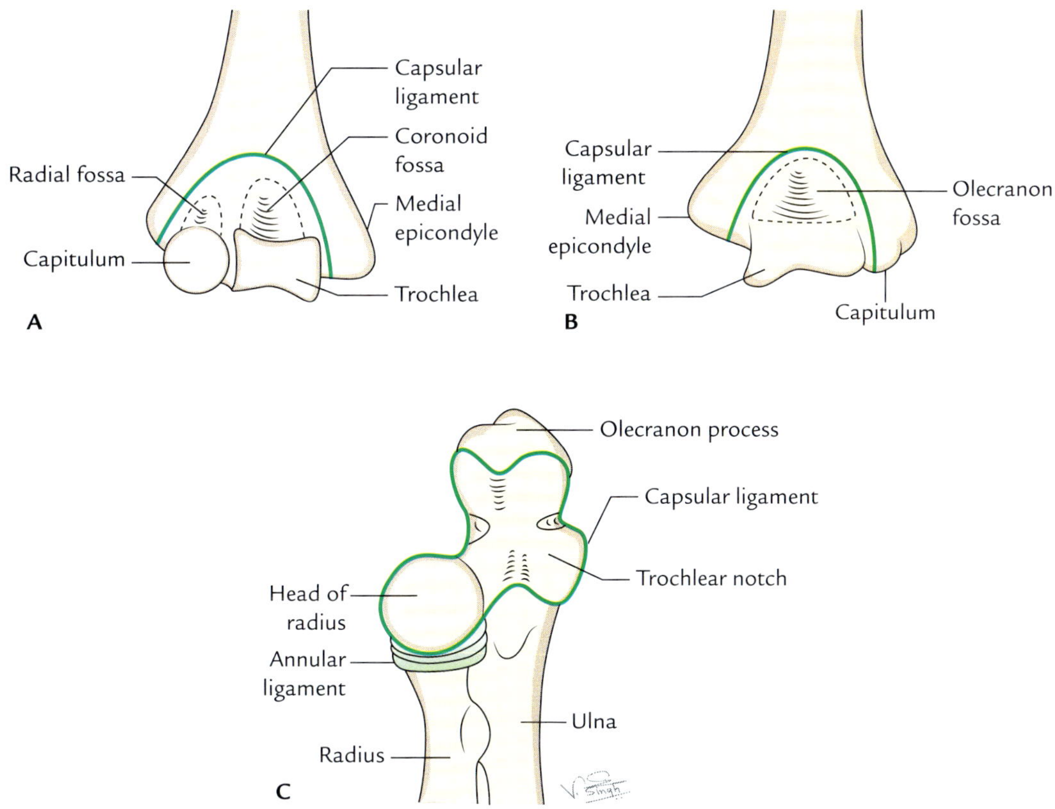

FIG. 10.2 ■ Attachment of the capsular ligament of the elbow joint. (**A**) Anterior aspect, (**B**) posterior aspect, and (**C**) anterosuperior aspect.

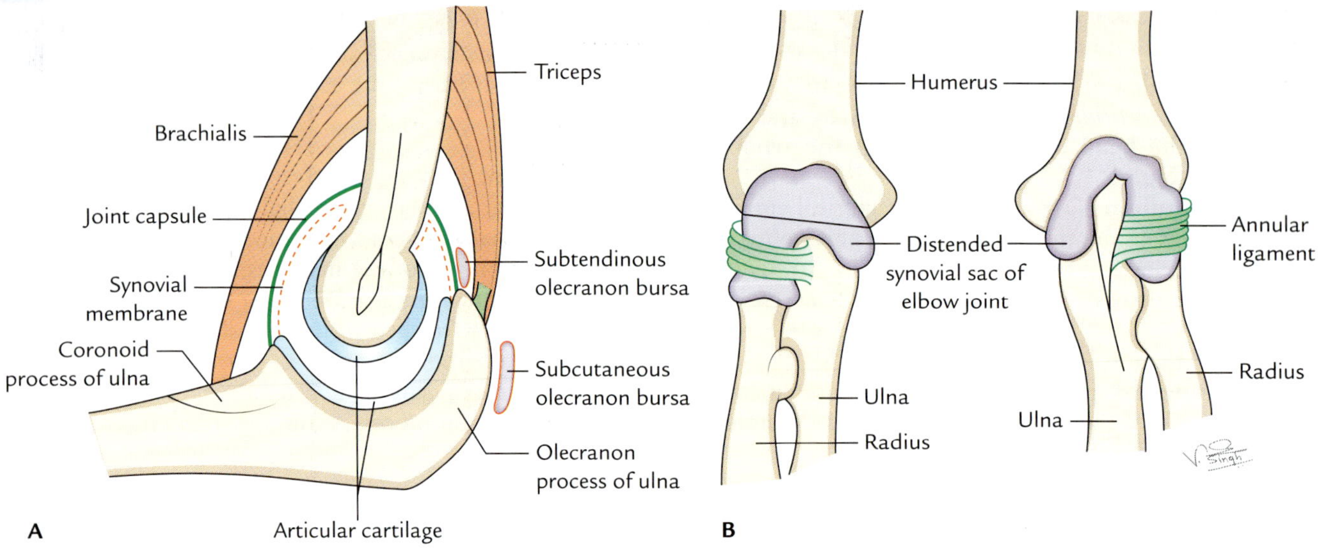

FIG. 10.3 ■ Elbow joint. (**A**) Schematic sagittal section and (**B**) synovial sac (distended).

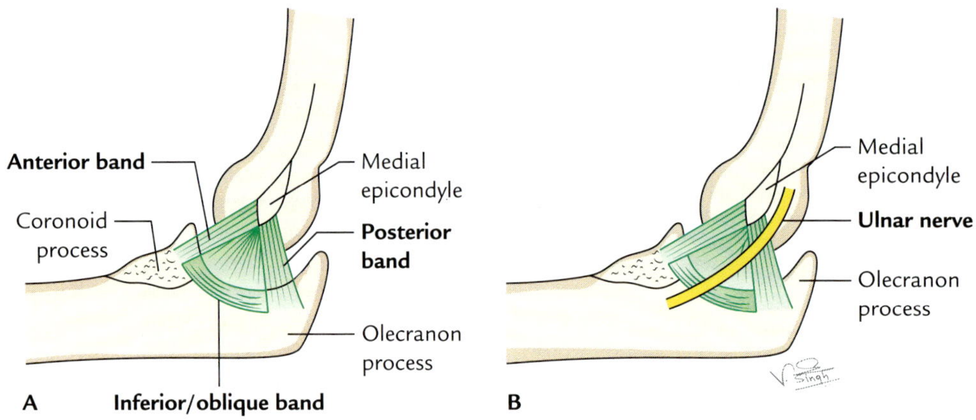

FIG. 10.4 ■ Attachments of the ulnar collateral ligament of the elbow joint. (**A**) Three bands of the ulnar collateral ligament and (**B**) relation of the ulnar nerve with the ulnar collateral ligament.

LIGAMENTS

Medial Ligament (Ulnar Collateral Ligament)

It is triangular in shape, with its apex attached to the medial epicondyle of the humerus and base to the coronoid and olecranon processes of the ulna (Fig. 10.4). It is divided into three parts (or bands): anterior, posterior, and inferior—united by a thin region.

1. The strongest and stiffest *anterior part* extends from front of the medial epicondyle to a tubercle on the medial margin of the coronoid process.
2. The *posterior part* extends from the back of the medial epicondyle of the humerus to the medial margin of the olecranon process.
3. The *inferior part* or the oblique band extends between the olecranon and the coronoid process.

Between the anterior and posterior bands, intermediate fibres descend from the medial epicondyle to the oblique band.

N.B.

The medial collateral ligament is related to the ulnar nerve.

Lateral Ligament (Radial Collateral Ligament)

It extends from the lateral epicondyle of the humerus to the annular ligament with which it blends (Fig. 10.5).

RELATIONS

These are as follows (Fig. 10.6):

Anterior: (a) Brachialis muscle, (b) median nerve, (c) brachial artery, and (d) tendon of biceps brachii. The last three structures are separated from the joint capsule by brachialis.

Posterior: (a) Tendon of triceps and (b) anconeus.

Medially: (a) Flexor carpi ulnaris, (b) ulnar nerve (posteromedially), and (c) common flexor origin of the muscles of the forearm (anteromedially).

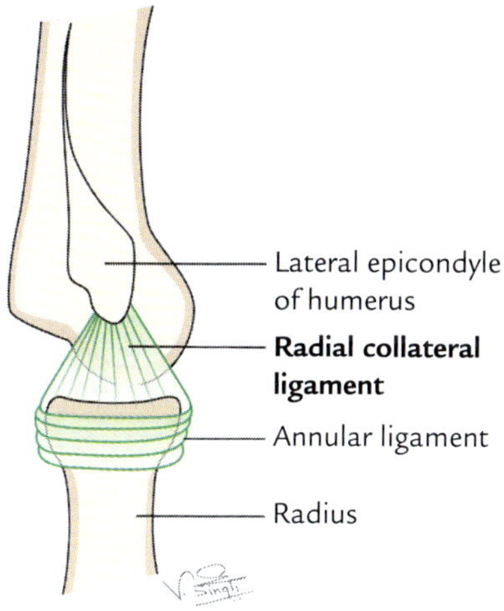

FIG. 10.5 ■ Radial collateral ligament.

Laterally (posterolateral): (a) supinator, (b) common extensor origin of muscles of forearm, and (c) extensor carpi radialis brevis.

BURSAE RELATED TO THE ELBOW JOINT

Four important bursae are related to the elbow joints: (a) two in relation to the triceps insertion and (b) two in relation to the biceps insertion:

1. **Subtendinous olecranon bursa:** A small bursa between the triceps tendon and the upper surface of the olecranon process.
2. **Subcutaneous olecranon bursa:** A large bursa between skin and the subcutaneous triangular area on the posterior surface of the olecranon.
3. **Bicipitoradial bursa:** A small bursa separating the biceps tendon from the smooth anterior part of the radial tuberosity.
4. A small bursa separating the biceps tendon from the oblique cord.

STABILITY OF THE ELBOW JOINT

In adults, the elbow joint is quite stable due to the following two factors:

1. Pulley-shaped trochlea of the humerus fits properly into the jaw-like trochlear notch of the ulna.
2. Strong ulnar and radial collateral ligaments.

BLOOD SUPPLY

The blood supply of elbow joints is by arterial anastomosis around the elbow formed by the branches of brachial, radial, and ulnar arteries.

NERVE SUPPLY

Nerve supply of the elbow joint is by articular branches from:

(a) radial nerve (through its branch to anconeus),
(b) musculocutaneous nerve (through its branch to brachialis),
(c) ulnar nerve, and
(d) median nerve.

MOVEMENTS

Being a uniaxial joint, the elbow joint allows only flexion and extension. The range of flexion is about 140°. These movements and muscles producing them are presented in Table 10.1.

CARRYING ANGLE

The transverse axis of the elbow joint is not transverse but oblique being directed downward and medially. This is because the medial flange of the trochlea lies about 6 mm below to that of the lateral flange. Consequently,

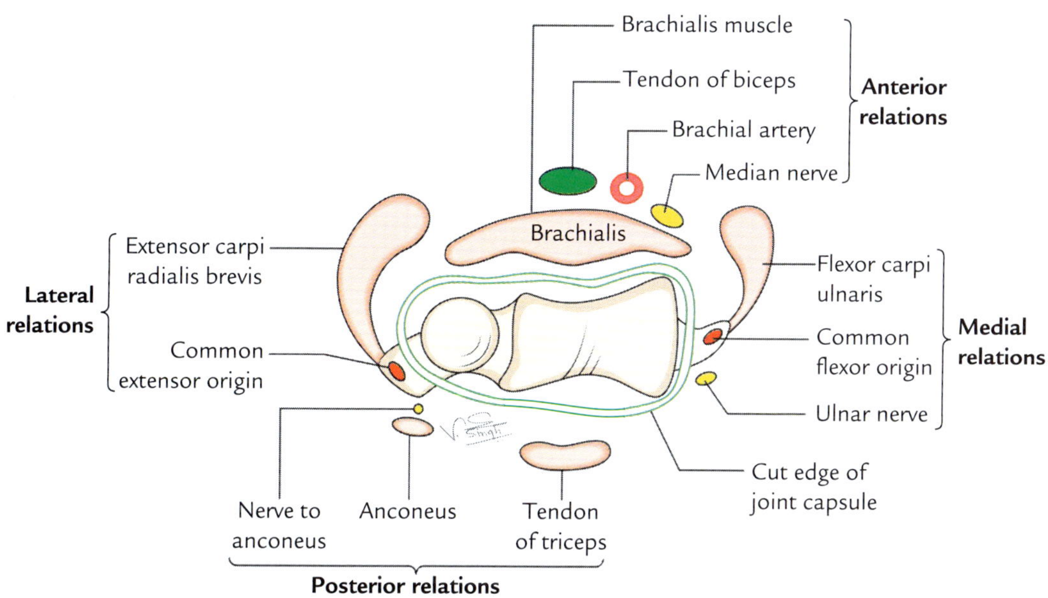

FIG. 10.6 ■ Relations of the elbow joint.

TABLE 10.1 Movements of the elbow joint

Movements	Muscles producing movements
Flexion	• Brachialis • Biceps brachii • Brachioradialis[a]
Extension	• Triceps • Anconeus

[a]The brachioradialis acts most effectively in midprone position as when medical interns walk by putting their aprons over their shoulders.

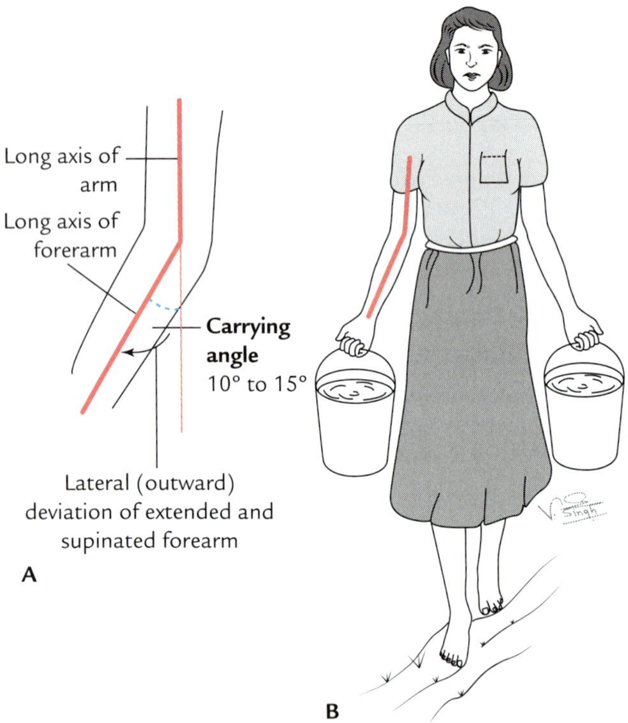

FIG. 10.7 Carrying angle.

when the elbow is extended, the arm and the forearm do not lie in a straight line; rather the forearm is deviated slightly laterally. This angle of deviation of the long axis of the forearm from the long axis of the arm is termed the **carrying angle** (Fig. 10.7).

The carrying angle disappears during pronation and full flexion of the forearm, because the forearm comes into line with the arm in the midprone position—the position in which the hand is mostly used.

The carrying angle varies from 5° to 15° and is more pronounced in females. The wider carrying angle in females avoids rubbing of forearms with the wider female pelvis while carrying loads, for example buckets filled with water from one place to another.

N.B.

The carrying angle is 10°–15° in males and >15° in females.

CLINICAL CORRELATION

- **Aspiration of elbow effusion:** The distension of elbow joint due to effusion within its cavity occurs posteriorly because capsule of the joint is thin posteriorly and covering fascia is also thin. When elbow is distended with effusion, the capsule bulges to either side of triceps tendon. The joint is aspirated by inserting a needle on the posterolateral side, just above the head of radius in a forward (anterior) direction with elbow at the right angle (Fig. 10.8).
- **Dislocation of elbow:** Posterior dislocations of elbow are more common and are often associated with fracture of the olecranon process. The dislocation invariably occurs by falling on an outstretched hand. The triangular relationship between the olecranon and the epicondyles of humerus is lost. Note, in normal flexed elbow the tip of olecranon process and two epicondyles of humerus form an 'equilateral triangle' (Fig. 10.9).

  The reduction, if done early, is achieved fairly easily by first giving traction to overcome spasm and then flexing the forearm to lever joint back into the place.
- **Nursemaid's elbow/pulled elbow (subluxation of head of radius;** Fig. 10.10): It occurs in preschool children, 1–3 years old because in them radial head is still cylindrical and annular ligament is lax. It usually happens when the forearm is suddenly pulled in pronation. The head of radius comes out of annular ligament and the elbow is kept slightly flexed and pronated.

  For example, when nursemaid brings the child home from school by holding his thumb. In the way, she suddenly pulls the forearm in jerk to save the child from speeding car.

  An attempt to supinate the forearm causes severe pain.

  The reduction is easily achieved by supinating and extending the elbow and simultaneously applying direct pressure posteriorly on the head of radius.
- **Tennis elbow (lateral epicondylitis;** Fig. 10.11): It is a clinical condition characterized by pain and tenderness

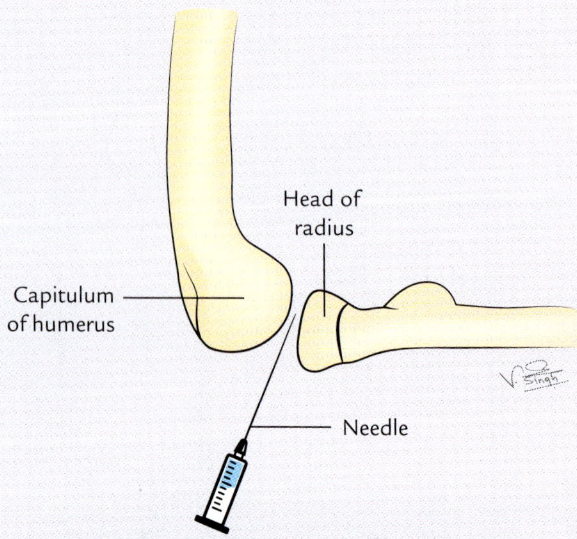

FIG. 10.8 Aspiration of elbow joint.

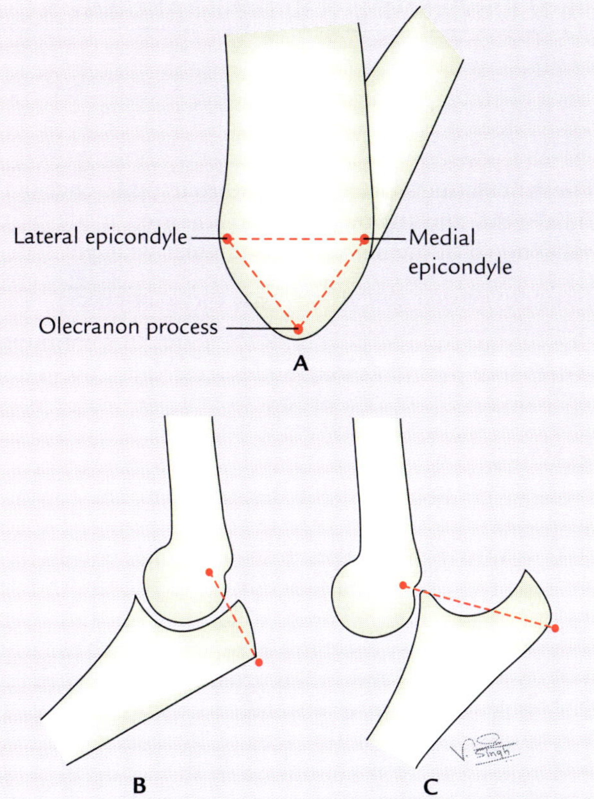

FIG. 10.9 ■ (**A**) Formation of the equilateral triangle by three bony points behind the flexed elbow, (**B**) elbow joint with a normal relationship of three bony points of the elbow, and (**C**) posterior dislocation of the elbow joint causing disturbance in the relationship of three bony points of the elbow due to the backward and upward displacements of the olecranon process. (*Source: Clinical and Surgical Anatomy,* 2ed.: Vishram Singh, Fig. 2.2A (B) and Fig. 2.2B (A and B), Page 52, Elsevier, 2007.)

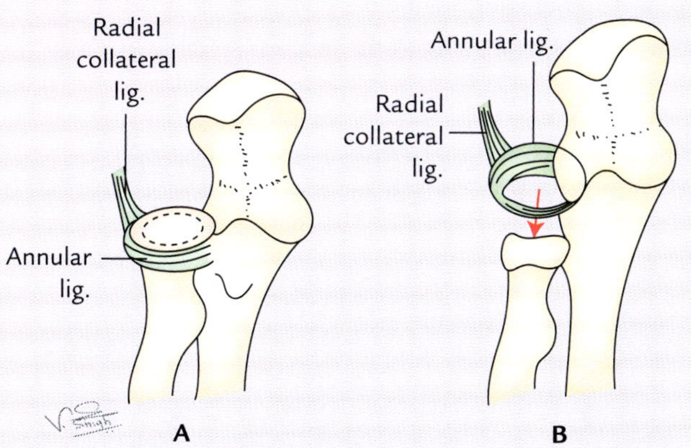

FIG. 10.10 ■ Pulled elbow. (**A**) Head of the radius within the cup-shaped annular ligament and (**B**) head of the radius displaced down from the annular ligament.

over the lateral epicondyle of the humerus during abrupt pronation and extension of wrist. It occurs due to:

(a) sprain of lateral collateral ligament of elbow joint, or (b) a tear of the fibres of extensor carpi radialis brevis, or (c) an inflammation of bursa underneath the extensor carpi radialis brevis, or (d) strain or tear of common extensor origin.

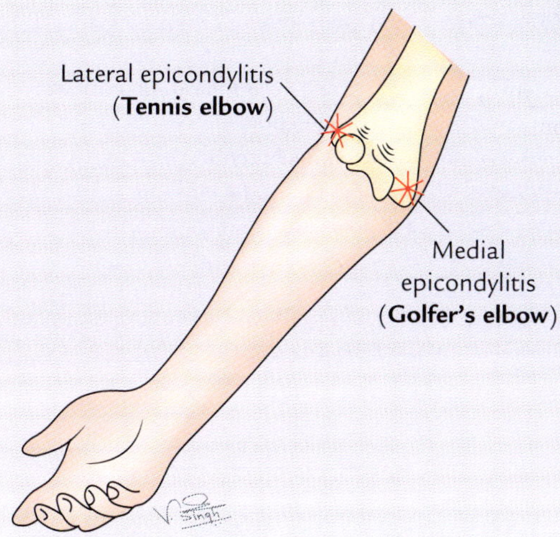

FIG. 10.11 ■ Lateral and medial epicondylitis.

- **Golfer's elbow (medial epicondylitis;** Fig. 10.11): It is a clinical condition characterized by pain and tenderness over the medial epicondyle of the humerus. It occurs due to strain or tear of common flexor origin with subsequent inflammation of medial epicondyle, following repetitive use of superficial flexors of forearm as during playing golf.
- **Student's elbow (Miner's elbow;** Fig. 10.12) is characterized by a round fluctuating painful swelling over the tip of elbow. It occurs due to inflammation of *subcutaneous olecranon bursa* lying over subcutaneous triangular area on the posterior aspect of the olecranon process.
- **Nerve entrapment (compressions) syndromes around elbow:** The nerve entrapments syndromes around elbow are fairly common and cause pain, muscle atrophy, and weakness in the area supplied by the entrapped nerve. The examples are:
  (a) ***Median nerve entrapment***: The median nerve may be compressed: (a) by hypertrophied pronator teres muscles where it passes between the two heads of pronator teres or (b) by abnormally dense aponeurotic edge where it passes deep to fibrous arch between humeroulnar and radial heads of flexor digitorum superficialis.
  (b) ***Ulnar nerve entrapment***: The ulnar nerve may be compressed (a) where it passes posterior to the medial epicondyle of the humerus (commonest site) or (b) where it passes through cubital tunnel formed by tendinous arch joining the humeral and ulnar heads of flexor carpi ulnaris leading to **'cubital tunnel syndrome'**.
  (c) ***Posterior interosseous nerve entrapment***: The posterior interosseous nerve may be compressed (a) where it passes deep to the **arcade of Frohse**, a musculoaponeurotic structure at the proximal edge of supinator muscle or (b) where it passes through the substance of supinator muscle.

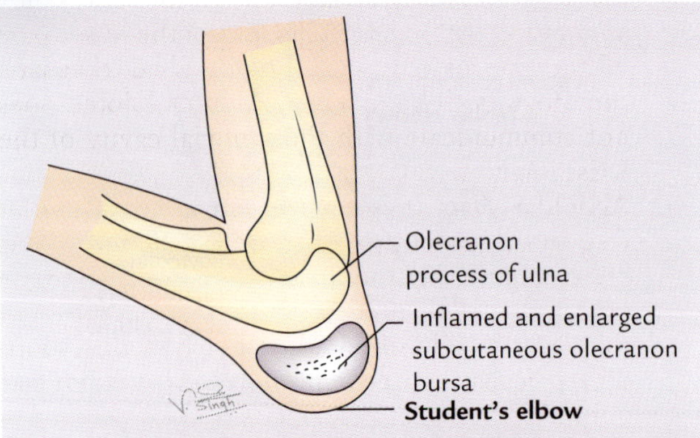

FIG. 10.12 ■ Student's (Miner's) elbow.

RADIOULNAR JOINTS AN 13.3

The radius and the ulna form two joints between them: one at their upper ends and another at their lower ends. They are called the **superior** and **inferior radioulnar joints** (Fig. 10.13). Both these joints are the **synovial joints of pivot variety**. They are **uniaxial** joints permitting only rotation. The shafts of the radius and the ulna are also connected to each other by the **interosseous membrane**. This union between the radius and the ulna is sometimes termed the **middle radioulnar joint**.

SUPERIOR (PROXIMAL) RADIOULNAR JOINT

TYPE

It is a pivot type of the synovial joint.

ARTICULAR SURFACES

The articulating surfaces are: (a) the circumference of the radial head and (b) the fibro-osseous ring made by the radial notch of the ulna and the annular ligament.

JOINT CAPSULE (CAPSULAR LIGAMENT)

The fibrous capsule surrounds the joint. It is continuous with that of the elbow joint and is attached to the annular ligament.

LIGAMENTS

Proximal radioulnar joint has annular and quadrate ligaments.

1. **Annular ligament:** It is a strong fibrous band that encircles the head of the radius and holds it against the radial notch of the ulna. It forms about four-fifths of the fibro-osseous ring within which the head of the radius rotates. Medially, the annular ligament is attached to the margins of the radial notch of the ulna. The upper margin of the ligament is continuous with the capsule of the

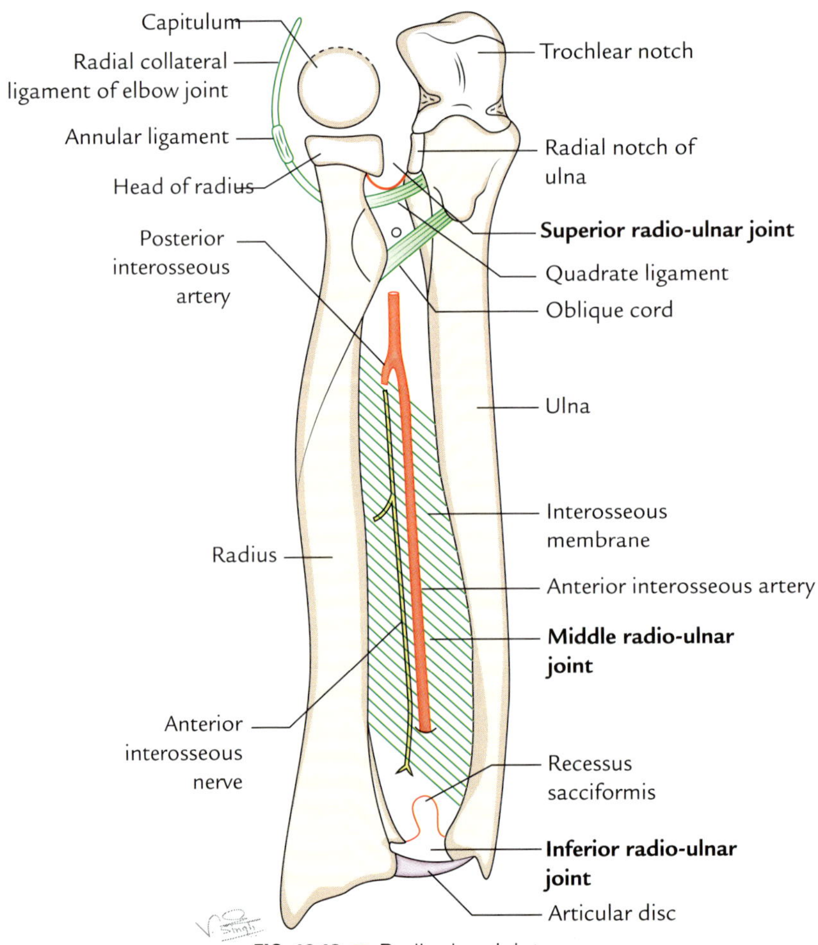

FIG. 10.13 ■ Radioulnar joints.

elbow joint and its lower part becomes narrow and embraces the neck of the radius. The inner surface of the annular ligament is covered by a thin layer of cartilage. Laterally, it blends with the radial collateral ligament.

2. **Quadrate ligament:** It is a thin, fibrous ligament that extends from the neck of the radius to the upper part of the supinator fossa of the ulna just below the radial notch.

SYNOVIAL MEMBRANE

It lines the inner aspect of the joint capsule of the superior radioulnar joint and is continuous with the synovial membrane of the elbow joint. It is prevented from herniation by the quadrate ligament.

RELATIONS

Anteriorly and laterally: Supinator muscle.
Posteriorly: Anconeus muscle.

BLOOD SUPPLY

By articular branches derived from the arterial anastomosis on the lateral side of the elbow joint.

NERVE SUPPLY

By articular branches from the musculocutaneous, median, radial, and ulnar nerves.

MOVEMENTS

Supination and pronation.

INFERIOR (DISTAL) RADIOULNAR JOINT

TYPE

Synovial joint of pivot variety.

ARTICULAR SURFACES

The articulating surfaces are: (a) the convex head of the ulna and (b) the concave ulnar notch of the radius.

LIGAMENTS

1. **Joint capsule (capsular ligament):** It is a fibrous sac that encloses the joint cavity and is attached to the margins of articular surfaces. The inner surface of the joint capsule is lined by the synovial membrane. The synovial lining of the joint sends an upward prolongation in front of the lower part of the interosseous membrane called **recessus sacciformis**. The synovial cavity of joint does not communicate with the synovial cavity of the wrist joint.
2. **Articular disc:** It is a *triangular fibrocartilaginous* disc and is sometimes referred to by clinicians as the **triangular ligament**. Its apex is attached to the base of the styloid process of the ulna and its base to the lower margin of the ulnar notch of the radius. The articular disc separates the inferior radioulnar joint from the wrist joint.

The disc excludes the ulna from the wrist joint and provides a platform for the ulnar head to rotate during supination and pronation.

RELATIONS

Anteriorly: Flexor digitorum profundus.
Posteriorly: Extensor digiti minimi.

BLOOD SUPPLY

By anterior and posterior interosseous arteries.

NERVE SUPPLY

By anterior and posterior interosseous nerves.

A brief comparison of the superior and inferior radioulnar joints is presented in Table 10.2.

MOVEMENTS

Supination and pronation.

RADIOULNAR SYNDESMOSIS

The shafts of radius and ulna are connected to each other by two syndesmoses, *viz.* (a) *oblique cord* and (b) *interosseous membrane* (Fig. 10.13).

INTEROSSEOUS MEMBRANE OF THE FOREARM

It is the fibrous sheet that stretches between the interosseous borders of the radius and the ulna (Fig. 10.9). It holds these bones together and does not interfere with the movements, which take place between them. This union between the radius and the ulna is sometimes termed the **middle radioulnar joint**. This is a **syndesmosis type of fibrous joint**.

TABLE 10.2 **Superior and inferior radioulnar joints**

Features	Superior radioulnar joint	Inferior radioulnar joint
Type	Pivot type of synovial joint	Pivot type of the synovial joint
Articular surfaces	• Circumference of the head of the radius • Fibro-osseous ring formed by the annular ligament and the radial notch of the ulna	• Head of the ulna • Ulnar notch of the radius
Joint cavity	Communicates with the cavity of the elbow joint	Does not communicate with the cavity of the wrist joint
Prime stabilizing factor	Annular ligament	Articular disc
Movements	Supination and pronation	Supination and pronation

Features of the Interosseous Membrane

1. Proximally, it begins 2.3 cm below the tuberosity of the radius and distally it blends with the capsule of the inferior radioulnar joint.
2. The fibres of the membrane run downward and medially from the radius to the ulna.
3. The posterior interosseous vessels pass backward through a gap between the upper border of the interosseous membrane and the oblique cord to reach the back of the forearm.
4. The anterior interosseous vessels enter the back of the forearm by piercing the interosseous membrane 5 cm above its lower margin.

Relations

Anteriorly: Anterior interosseous artery and interosseous nerve.

Posteriorly: Posterior interosseous artery in the upper two-thirds, anterior interosseous artery in the lower one-third and posterior interosseous nerve.

Functions

1. Holds the radius and the ulna together.
2. Transmits compression forces (applied to the radius from hand) to the ulna. Such forces are then transferred to the humerus through the ulna. This mode of transmission is necessary as the radius is the main bone taking part in the formation of wrist joint, while the ulna is the main bone taking part in the formation of the elbow joint (stable humeroulnar component).
3. Provides attachments to muscles.

OBLIQUE CORD

It is a strong fibrous band that extends from the medial side of the tuberosity of the ulna to the lower part of the tuberosity of the radius. Its fibres are directed downward and laterally, that is opposite to that of the interosseous membrane.

N.B.

Morphologically, the **oblique cord** between the ulnar and the radial tuberosities represents the degenerated (atrophied) part of the *flexor pollicis longus muscle.*

SUPINATION AND PRONATION

The **movements of supination and pronation** of the forearm are rotatory movements around a vertical axis. They play an important role in performing the skilled movements of the hand (Fig. 10.14). When the elbow is semiflexed in midprone position, if the palm is turned **upward** it is called **supination** and if turned **downward** it is called **pronation.** These actions can be easily remembered by a *mnemonic: beggars supinate and kings pronate.* The supination and pronation are the rotatory movements of the forearm, which occur at the superior and inferior radioulnar joints around a vertical axis. This axis is oblique and passes from the centre of the head of the radius above to the base of the styloid process of the ulna below. The axis of movement of supination and pronation is not stationary. It moves forward and medially during supination, and backward and laterally during pronation.

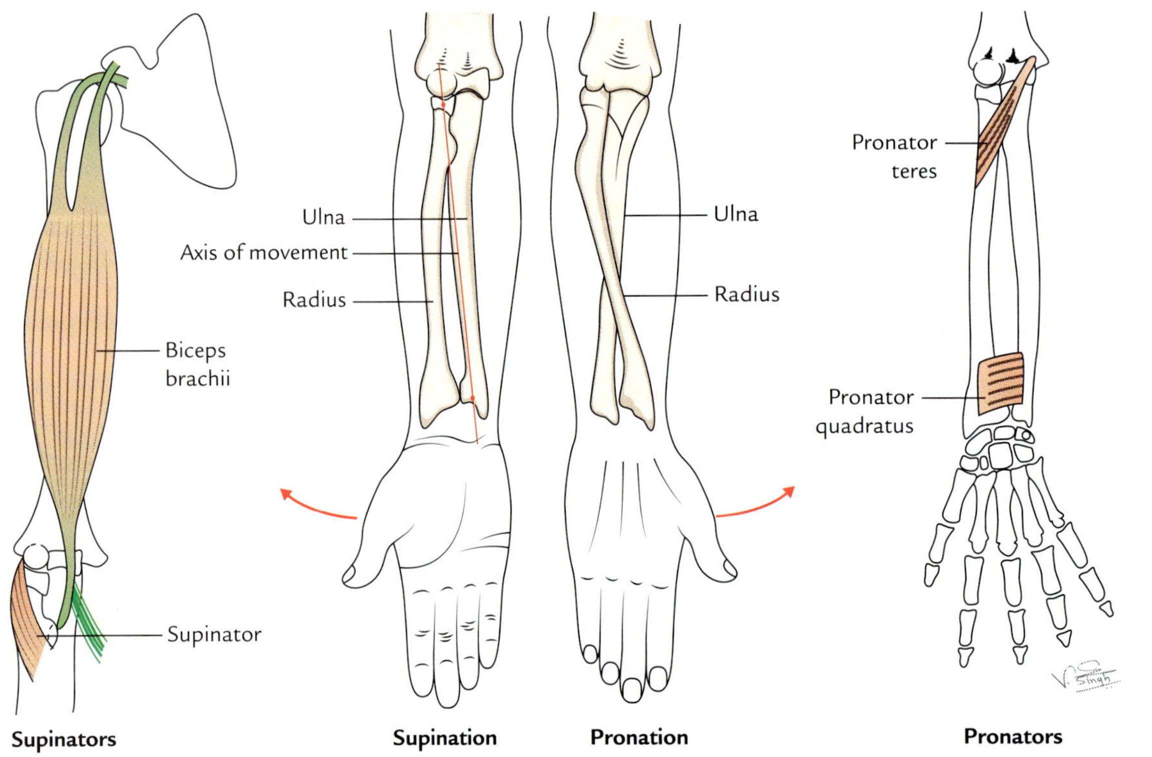

FIG. 10.14 ■ Movements of supination and pronation. Note radius moves around, relatively fixed distal end of ulna.

TABLE 10.3 Movements of supination and pronation

Movements	Muscles producing movements
Supination	• Supinator • Biceps brachii supinates the forearm while the elbow is flexed • Brachioradialis supinates the pronated forearm to midprone position
Pronation[a]	• Pronator quadratus • Pronator teres • Brachioradialis pronates the supinated forearm to midprone position

[a]The flexor carpi radialis, palmaris longus, and gravity also help in pronation.

Morphologically, movements of supination and pronation are evolved for picking up the food and taking it to the mouth. *The food is picked up in pronation and put in mouth in supination*.

In **supination**, the radius and the ulna lie parallel to each other. In **pronation**, there is the rotation of the lower end of the radius along with the articular disc on the head of the ulna. As a result, the lower end of the radius crosses in front of the lower end of the ulna. Simultaneously, the head of the radius rotates within the fibro-osseous ring formed by the annular ligament and the radial notch of the ulna.

The **supination** is chiefly produced by *supinator muscle* and assisted by *biceps brachii muscle* (Fig. 10.14). The **pronation** is produced chiefly by *pronator quadrants* and assisted by *pronator teres* (Fig. 10.14).

During supination the radius and ulna lie parallel to each other. Whereas during pronation radius crosses over ulna.

The movements of the supination and pronation and muscle producing them are given in Table 10.3.

N.B.

The supination is more powerful than pronation simply because: (a) it is antigravity movement and (b) it is performed by powerful muscles, *namely* biceps brachii and supinator. The *pronation is less powerful than supination* because it is performed by less powerful muscles, *namely*, pronator quadratus and pronator teres. Therefore, supination movements are used for tightening the nuts and bolts, whereas pronation movements are used for loosening/opening the nuts and bolts.

Golden Facts to Remember

• Cubital articulations	Humeroradial, humeroulnar, and proximal radioulnar joints
• Student's elbow/Miner's elbow	Subcutaneous olecranon bursitis
• Most important bursa (clinically) around the elbow joint	Subcutaneous olecranon bursa
• Strongest band of the ulnar collateral ligament of the elbow joint	Anterior band
• Chief supinator of forearm	Supinator
• Chief pronator of forearm	Pronator quadrants
• Carrying angle (10°–15° in males and >15° in females)	Angle of deviation of the long axis of the forearm from the long axis of the arm when the elbow is fully extended
• Commonest site of ulnar nerve entrapment (compression)	Behind the medial epicondyle of the humerus
• Most important stabilizing factors of the proximal radioulnar joint	Annular ligament and radial collateral ligament
• Most important stabilizing factor of the distal radioulnar joint	Articular disc (triangular ligament)

CLINICAL CASE STUDY

A 35-year-old mother was crossing the road along with her 3-year-old son. After seeing a speeding car rushing towards them, she suddenly pulled her son away by holding his left hand to avoid the danger of being crushed by the car. The child cried out and later refused to use his left upper limb. The mother took the child to the doctor. On examination, the doctor noticed that the child held his left forearm in a position with the elbow semiflexed and the forearm pronated. A diagnosis of **'pulled elbow'** was made.

Questions

1. What is the pulled elbow?
2. Why is the pulled elbow common in preschool (1–3 years old) children?
3. How can the pulled elbow be reduced/treated?

Answers

1. In a pulled elbow, the head of the radius comes out of the annular ligament of the superior radioulnar joint (i.e. subluxation of the radial head).
2. Because up to 3 years of age, the annular ligament is tubular and has a large diameter, the head of the radius can be easily pulled out of the ligament by traction.
3. The reduction is easily achieved by pulling the forearm downward and then firmly supinating it. By doing so, the subluxation of radius is reduced spontaneously. Finally, the elbow is flexed and held in that position.

CHAPTER

11 Hand

SPECIFIC LEARNING OBJECTIVES

After studying this chapter, the student should be able to:

- Identify and describe the flexor retinaculum with its attachments. AN 12.3
- Explain anatomical basis of carpal tunnel syndrome. AN 12.4
- Write short notes on: (a) palmar aponeurosis, (b) synovial bursae of palm, (c) anatomical snuff box, (d) ulnar nerve in hand, (e) midpalmar space, and (f) arterial arches of hand.
- Give the anatomical basis of: (a) Whitlow and (b) Dupuytren's contracture.
- Identify and describe fibrous flexor sheaths, ulnar bursa, radial bursa, and digital synovial sheaths. AN 12.9
- Identify and describe the muscles of hand. AN 12.5
- Describe the anatomical basis of claw hand. AN 12.8
- Enumerate: (a) thenar and hypothenar muscles, and (b) lumbrical and interosseous muscles of the hand.
- Identify and describe course and branches of important blood vessels and nerves in *hand.* AN 12.7
- Draw the labelled diagrams to show: (a) sensory innervations on the palmar and dorsal surfaces of the hand, (b) cross section of the hand showing the palmar spaces, and (c) pulp spaces of digits.

The **hand** (L. *Manus*) is the distal part/segment of the upper limb. It is a complex and highly evolved anatomic structure that provides primary touch input to the brain and enables humans to perform complex fine motor tasks by way of its free movements, power grip, precision grip, handling, and pinching. The hand is man's great physical asset. It has enabled him to use various tools that his brain has invented. Therefore, a better understanding of its structure and functions is essential. Everything that the doctors do to the hand should be aimed at restoring or maintaining its function. The movements of the hand occur primarily at the wrist joint or radiocarpal joint formed by the articulation of the radius and the first row of the carpal bones (e.g. scaphoid, lunate, and triquetral).

The hand consists of four functional units, namely:

1. Carpus
2. Thumb
3. Index finger
4. A unit comprising the middle, ring, and little fingers

The carpus (first unit) provides a stabilizing platform for the three mobile units (2, 3, and 4).

The hand contains carpal bones, metacarpal bones, and phalanges.

N.B.

Anatomically, the term *wrist* refers to carpus (carpal region) consisting of eight carpal bones and lies between the forearm and the hand, but in general usage, the *wrist* refers to the distal end of the forearm just proximal to the distal ends of the radius and the ulna, around which the wrist watch is worn.

PALMAR ASPECT OF THE HAND

SURFACE LANDMARKS (FIG. 11.1)

1. **Tubercle of scaphoid**: It can be felt at the base of thenar eminence, just lateral to the tendon of the

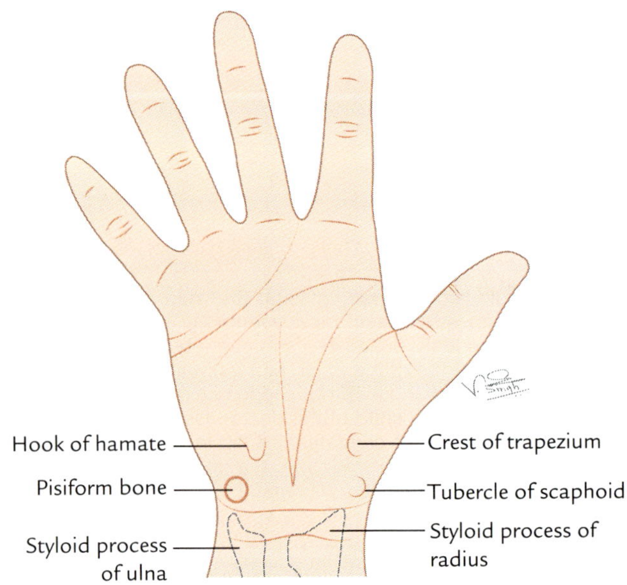

FIG. 11.1 ■ Surface landmarks on the front of the wrist and palm.

flexor carpi radialis (FCR). It is located deep to the lateral part of the distal transverse crease of the wrist.

2. **Tubercle/crest of trapezium**: It can be felt on deep palpation, distolateral to the tubercle of scaphoid.
3. **Pisiform bone**: It can be felt at the base of hypothenar eminence medially. It lies deep to the medial end of the distal transverse crease of the wrist.
4. **Hook of hamate**: It can be felt at one finger's breadth distal to the pisiform bone.

SKIN OF THE PALM

The skin of the palm presents the following characteristic features:

1. It is thick to withstand wear and tear during work.
2. It is richly supplied by the sweat glands but contains no hair or sebaceous glands.
3. It is immobile as it is firmly attached to the underlying palmar aponeurosis.
4. It presents several longitudinal and transverse creases where the skin is firmly bound to the deep fascia.

N.B.

To improve the grip, the skin of the palm is ridged and furrowed and devoid of greasy sebaceous glands.

Flexion Creases of the Wrist, Palm, and Fingers (Fig. 11.2)

1. **Flexion creases of the wrist (wrist creases):** The palmar aspect of the wrist presents two transverse flexion creases, namely:
   (a) Proximal transverse wrist crease.
   (b) Distal transverse wrist crease.
   They are produced as a result of folding of the skin due to the repeated flexion of the wrist. The **distal transverse wrist crease** corresponds to the proximal border of the flexor retinaculum. The **proximal transverse wrist crease** lies at the level of the wrist joint.

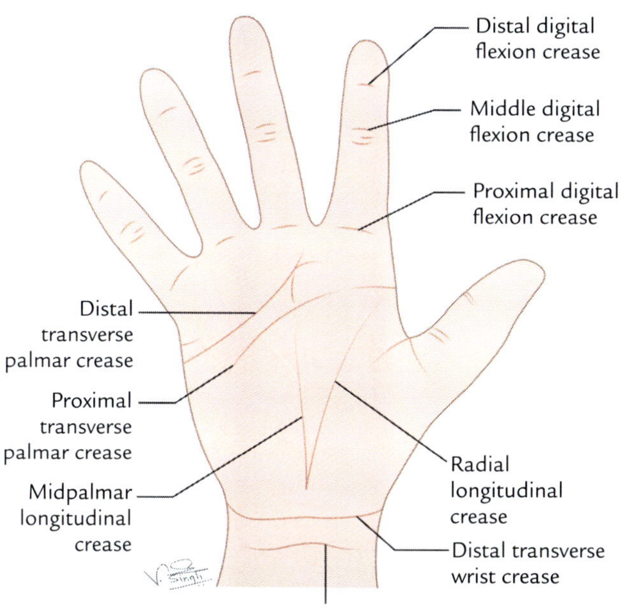

FIG. 11.2 ■ Flexor creases on the palmar aspect of the wrist, palm, and digits.

2. **Palmar flexion creases:** Usually, there are four major palmar creases—two horizontal and two longitudinal that together roughly form an M-shaped pattern:
   (a) Longitudinal palmar creases:
      (i) **Radial longitudinal crease (lifeline of the palmistry):** It partly encircles the thenar eminence (ball of the thumb) and is formed due to the action of the short muscles of the thumb.
      (ii) **Midpalmar longitudinal crease (line of fate in palmistry):** It indicates the lateral limit of the hypothenar eminence (ball of the little finger). It is formed due to the action of the short muscles of the little finger.
   (b) Transverse palmar creases:
      (i) **Distal transverse palmar crease:** It begins at or near the interdigital cleft between the index and middle finger and runs to the ulnar side of palm (with slight distal concavity). Deep to this shafts of the third, fourth, and fifth metacarpals can be palpated.
      (ii) **Proximal transverse palmar crease:** It commences at the lateral border of the palm in common with the radial longitudinal crease, superficial to the head of the second metacarpal. It extends medially and slight proximally across the palm, superficial to the shafts of the third, fourth, and fifth metacarpals.
3. **Digital flexion creases:** Each of the medial four digits have three transverse flexion creases, while the thumb has two transverse creases:
   (a) *Proximal flexion crease:* It lies at the root of the finger about 2 cm distal to the metacarpophalangeal (MP) joint.
   (b) *Middle flexion crease:* It lies over the proximal interphalangeal (PIP) joint.
   (c) *Distal flexion crease:* It lies on or just proximal to the distal interphalangeal (DIP) joint.

The digital flexion creases become deeper when the digits are flexed.

Friction Ridges

The friction ridges are raised ridges with intervening furrows on the surface of skin. They are present in the palms of hands and soles of feet. The friction ridges prevent the slippage when grasping the objects.

The friction ridges present on the tip of fingers/finger pads are used for **fingerprints**. These have basic similarities but are not identical in any two individuals, including identical twins. The four basic types of fingerprints are: (a) arch, (b) whorl, (c) loop, and (d) composite (combination of first three) (Fig. 11.3). The science of classification and identification of fingerprints is called **dermatoglyphics**.

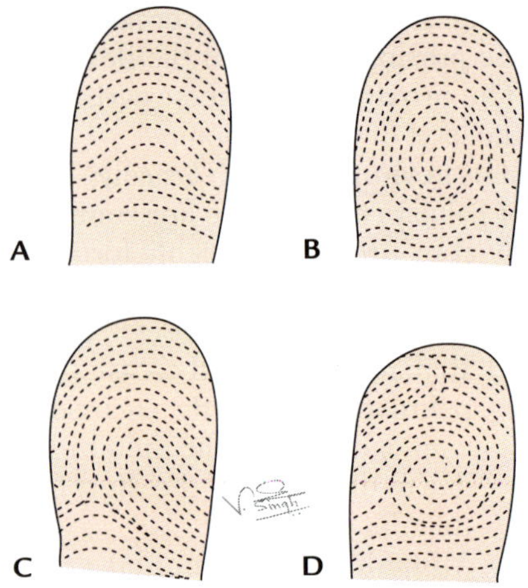

FIG. 11.3 ■ Types of finger prints: (**A**) arch, (**B**) whorl, (**C**) loop, and (**D**) composite.

> **CLINICAL CORRELATION**
>
> - The person with down syndrome (trisomy-21) usually has only one transverse palmar crease called the *simian crease*.
> - Since the fingerprints are not identical in any two individuals including identical twins, they are used in criminal investigations to identify criminals.

SUPERFICIAL FASCIA OF THE PALM

The superficial fascia of the palm is made up of dense fibrous bands that anchor the skin to the deep fascia of the palm. The superficial fascia of the palm presents two important features:

1. It contains a subcutaneous muscle, the **palmaris brevis** on the ulnar side of the palm, which probably helps to improve the grip.
2. It thickens to form a **superficial transverse metacarpal ligament** that stretches across the roots of fingers over the digital nerve and vessels.

Palmaris Brevis Muscle (Fig. 11.7, page 141)

It is the subcutaneous muscle in the superficial fascia of the medial part of the palm. Morphologically, it represents the panniculus carnosus.

Origin

From the flexor retinaculum and palmar aponeurosis.

Insertion

Into the skin along the medial border of the hand.

Nerve Supply

Superficial branch of the ulnar nerve.

Actions

When an object is grasped tightly in the hand, it causes the wrinkling of the medial palmar skin and helps to prevent the ulnar displacement of the hypothenar eminence.

DEEP FASCIA OF THE PALM

The deep fascia on the palmar aspect of the hand is specialized to form three structures:

1. Flexor retinaculum.
2. Palmar aponeurosis.
3. Fibrous flexor sheaths of digits.

Flexor Retinaculum (Transverse Carpal Ligament) AN 12.3

It is a strong fibrous band formed by the thickening of deep fascia in front of carpus (anatomical wrist; Fig. 11.4). It bridges the anterior concavity of carpus (also called carpal arch) and converts it into an *osseofibrous tunnel* called the **carpal tunnel** for the passage of flexor tendons of the digits.

It is rectangular in shape roughly of the size of postage stamp. It has two surfaces and four borders.

Attachments (Fig. 11.5)

Medially: It is attached to the pisiform and the hook of the hamate.

Laterally: It is attached to the tubercle of the scaphoid and the crest of the trapezium.

> N.B.
>
> On either side, the flexor retinaculum gives a slip (Fig. 11.5):
>
> - A superficial slip on the medial side (called the **volar carpal ligament**) is attached to the pisiform bone. The ulnar nerve and vessels pass deep to this slip (Fig. 11.6).
> - A deep slip on the lateral side is attached to the medial lip of the groove of trapezium, converting it into an osseofibrous tunnel for the passage of the tendon of the FCR (Fig. 11.6).

Relations

Structures passing superficial to the flexor retinaculum:

From the medial to the lateral side, these are (Fig. 11.6):

1. Ulnar nerve.
2. Ulnar artery.
3. Palmar cutaneous branch of the ulnar nerve.
4. Tendon of the palmaris longus.
5. Palmar cutaneous branch of the median nerve.
6. Superficial palmar branch of the radial artery.

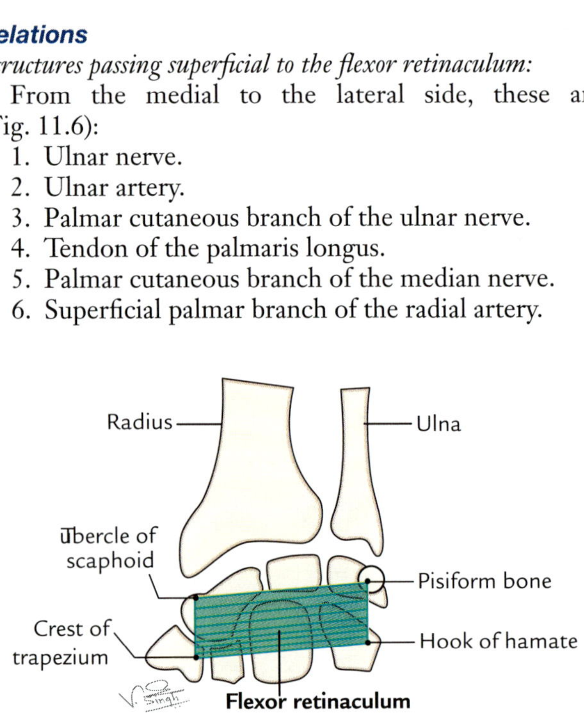

FIG. 11.4 ■ Flexor retinaculum of wrist.

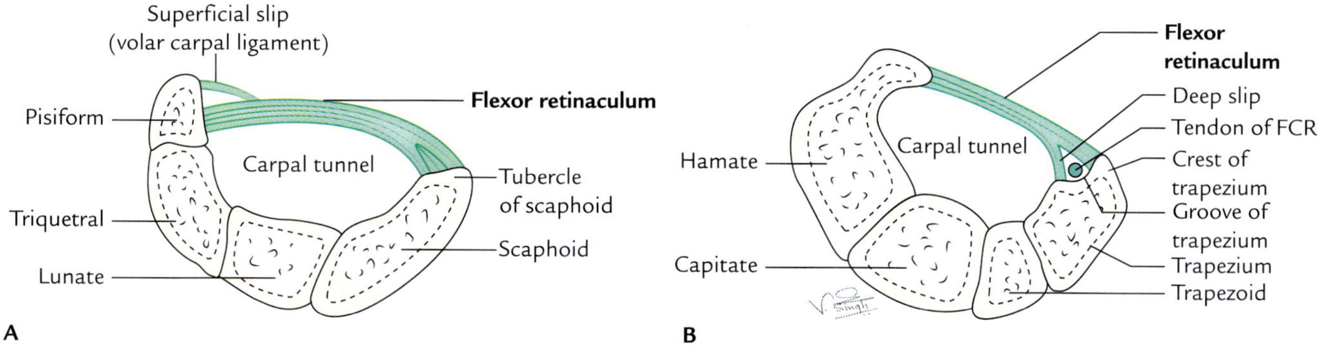

FIG. 11.5 ■ Attachment of the additional medial and lateral slips of the flexor retinaculum. (**A**) At the level of the proximal row of carpal bones and (**B**) at the level of the distal row of carpal bones.

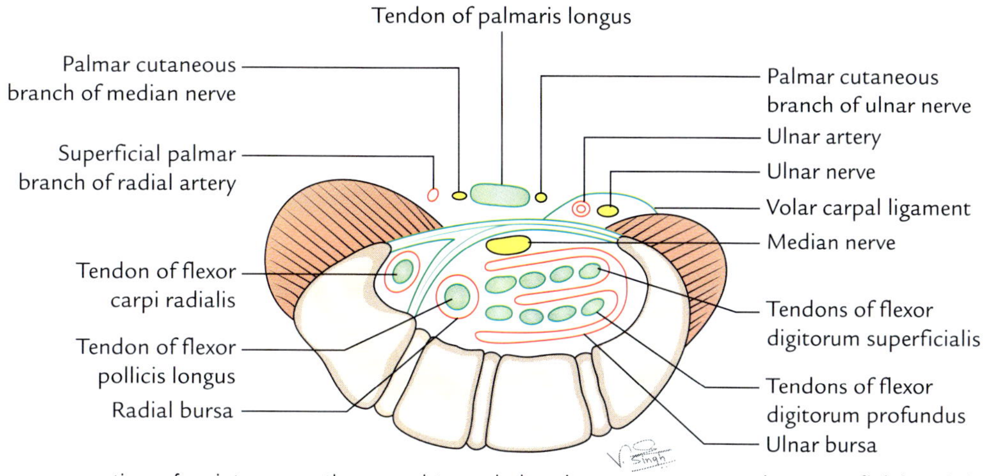

FIG. 11.6 ■ Transverse section of wrist across the carpal tunnel showing structures passing superficial and deep to the flexor retinaculum.

Structures passing deep to the flexor retinaculum (i.e. through the carpal tunnel):

These are as follows (Fig. 11.6):

1. Tendons of flexor digitorum superficialis (FDS).
2. Tendons of flexor digitorum profundus (FDP).
3. Tendon of flexor pollicis longus (FPL).
4. Median nerve.

N.B.

The compression of median nerve in carpal tunnel is called as **carpal tunnel syndrome**. For details see page 178. AN 12.4

- The flexor tendons of fingers (i.e. tendons of FDS and FDP) are enclosed in a synovial sheath called the **ulnar bursa**.
- The tendon of FPL is on the radial side and enclosed in a separate synovial sheath called the **radial bursa**.
- The tendon of the FCR pass through a separate canal in the lateral part of the flexor retinaculum.

Palmar Aponeurosis (Fig. 11.7)

The deep fascia of the palm is thin over the thenar and hypothenar eminences and thick in the central part of the palm where it forms the *palmar aponeurosis.*

The palmar aponeurosis (Fig. 11.7) is a strong well-defined central part of the deep fascia of the palm that covers

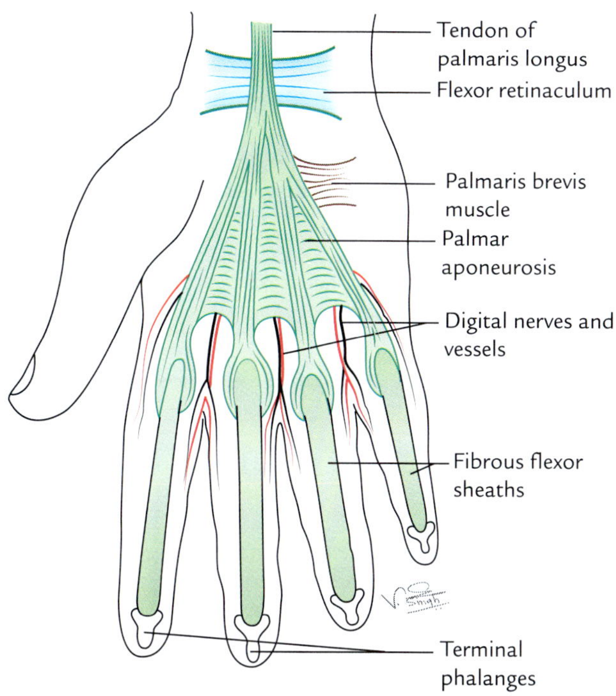

FIG. 11.7 ■ Palmar aponeurosis.

the long flexor tendons and superficial palmar arch. It is **triangular in shape** and made up mainly of longitudinal fibres and few transverse fibres intersecting the former.

Its apex is directed proximally towards the wrist and its base is directed distally towards the roots of the fingers.

Features

The palmar aponeurosis presents the following features:

1. Apex
2. Base
3. Medial border
4. Lateral border

Apex: It is the narrow proximal end of the palmar aponeurosis which blends with the flexor retinaculum. Its superficial fibres are continuous with the tendon palmaris longus.

Base: It is the broad distal end of the palmar aponeurosis. Just proximal to the heads of the metacarpals, the base divides into four longitudinal slips, one each for medial four digits. Each slip further divides into two slips that blend with the fibrous flexor sheaths of the corresponding digits.

The digital nerve and vessels and tendons of the lumbrical emerge through the intervals between the four longitudinal slips.

Medial border: The medial edge of the aponeurosis is continuous with the deep fascia covering the hypothenar muscles and gives origin to the palmaris brevis.

The *medial palmar septum* extends inward from this edge to the fifth metacarpal.

Lateral border: The lateral edge of the aponeurosis is continuous with the deep fascia covering the thenar muscles. The *lateral palmar septum* extends inward from this edge to the first metacarpal.

The *intermediate palmar septum* extends inward from near this edge obliquely to the third metacarpal (Fig. 11.20).

Functions

1. Helps to improve the grip of the hand by fixing the skin.
2. Protects the underlying tendons, nerves, and vessels.

N.B.

Morphologically, palmar aponeurosis represents the degenerated tendons of the *palmaris longus muscle*.

CLINICAL CORRELATION

Dupuytren's contracture (Fig. 11.8): It is a progressive fibrosis (interstitial increase in the fibrous tissue) in the medial part of the palmar aponeurosis. Consequently, the **medial part of the aponeurosis may undergo** progressive thickening to form **permanent contracture**, resulting in the flexion deformity of the little and ring fingers. The ring finger is most commonly affected. The proximal and middle phalanges are acutely flexed but distal phalanges remain unaffected. A surgical fasciectomy is required if the hand function is grossly impaired.

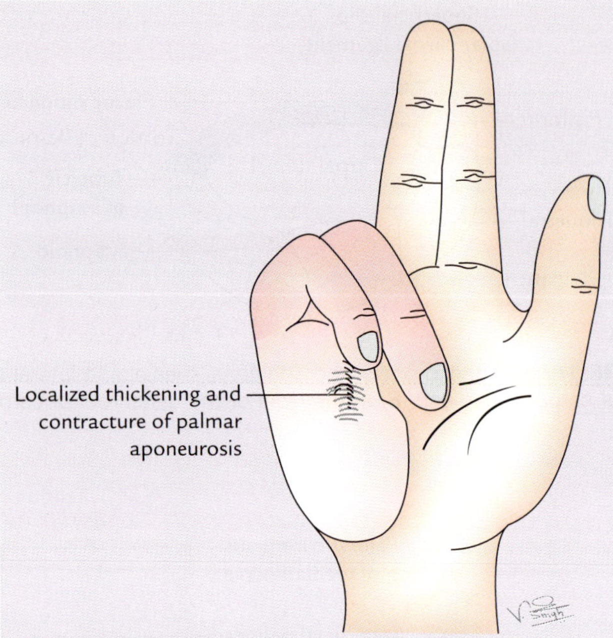

FIG. 11.8 Dupuytren's contracture.

FIBROUS FLEXOR SHEATHS OF THE FINGERS

AN 12.9

The deep fascia on the anterior surface of each digit thickens and arches over the long flexor tendons to form the *fibrous flexor sheath of the finger*, which extends from the head of the metacarpal to the base of the distal phalanx (Fig. 11.9).

Attachments

The arched fibrous sheath is attached to the margins of the phalanges and palmar ligaments of interphalangeal joints. The proximal end of the sheath is open. Here its margins are continuous with the distal slips of the palmar aponeurosis. The distal end of the sheath is attached to the palmar surface of the distal phalanx just distal to the insertion of FDP. Thus, the sheath along with the anterior surfaces of the phalanges and palmar ligaments of interphalangeal joints form a *blind osseofibrous tunnel* through which passes long flexor tendons enclosed in the *digital synovial sheath*.

The osseofibrous tunnel of each finger contains a pair of tendons (tendon of FDS and that of FDP).

The osseofibrous tunnel of the thumb contains the tendon of FPL.

The fibrous sheath is thick over the phalanges, and thin and lax over the interphalangeal joints to permit flexion.

The *annular* and *cruciform parts* (referred to as *pulleys by the clinicians*) are thickened reinforcements of the fibrous flexor sheaths.

Function

The fibrous flexor sheaths hold the tendons in position during the flexion of digits.

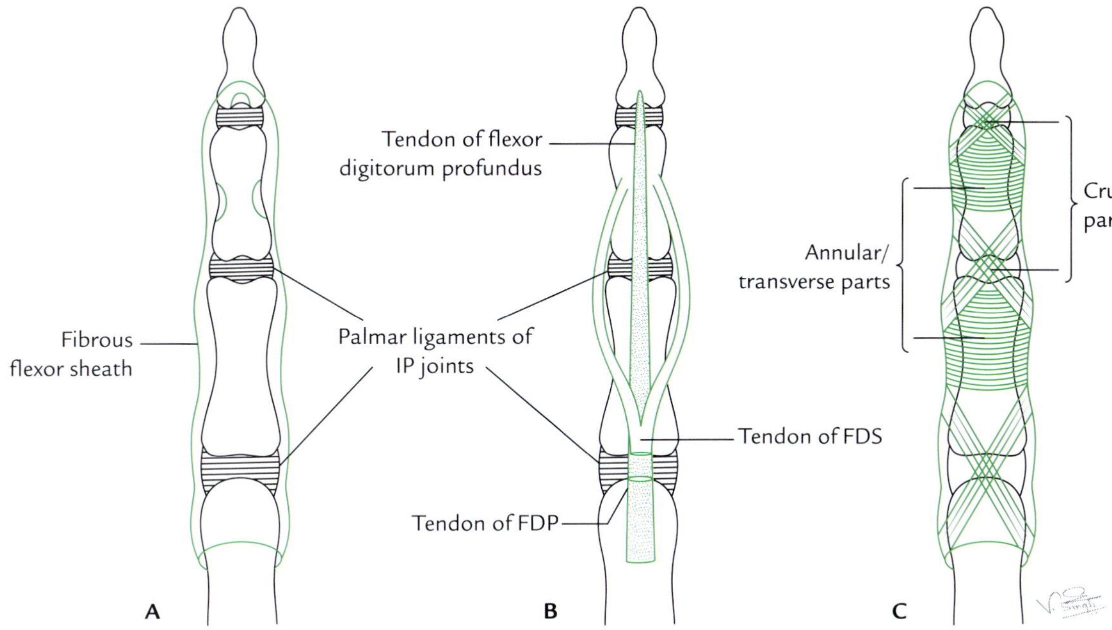

FIG. 11.9 Fibrous flexor sheaths of the fingers. (**A**) Attachment of the sheath, (**B**) tendons passing through the sheath, and (**C**) arrangement of fibres within the sheath—cruciate fibres in front of the joints and transverse fibres in front of bones (FDS = flexor digitorum superficialis, FDP = flexor digitorum profundus, IP = interphalangeal).

CLINICAL CORRELATION

Trigger finger: It is a clinical condition in which a finger gets locked in full flexion and can be extended only after excessive voluntary effort or with the help of the other hand. When extension begins it occurs suddenly and with a click, hence the name the—*trigger finger*. This condition is caused by the presence of a localized thickening of fibrous flexor sheath or a long flexor tendon, preventing the movement of the tendon within the fibrous flexor sheath of the digit. When the tendon tries to move, its thickened part is caught in the osseofibrous tunnel momentarily. This condition can be relieved surgically by incising the fibrous flexor sheath.

SYNOVIAL SHEATHS OF LONG FLEXOR TENDONS **AN 12.9**

The synovial sheaths around the long flexor tendons serve as lubricating devices to prevent their friction, while moving within the osseofibrous tunnels.

The synovial sheath around each tendon is double layered, consisting of an outer and inner layers with lubricating synovial fluid between the two layers.

Every digital synovial sheath has a mesotendon of the synovial membrane that conveys vessels to the tendon (*cf.* mesenteries of the gut; Fig. 11.10 inset).

Ulnar Bursa

The long flexor tendons of the fingers (four of FDS and four of FDP) while passing through the osseofibrous carpal tunnel are enclosed in a common synovial sheath called the *ulnar bursa* (Figs. 11.10 and 11.11). The tendon invaginates the sheath from the lateral side.

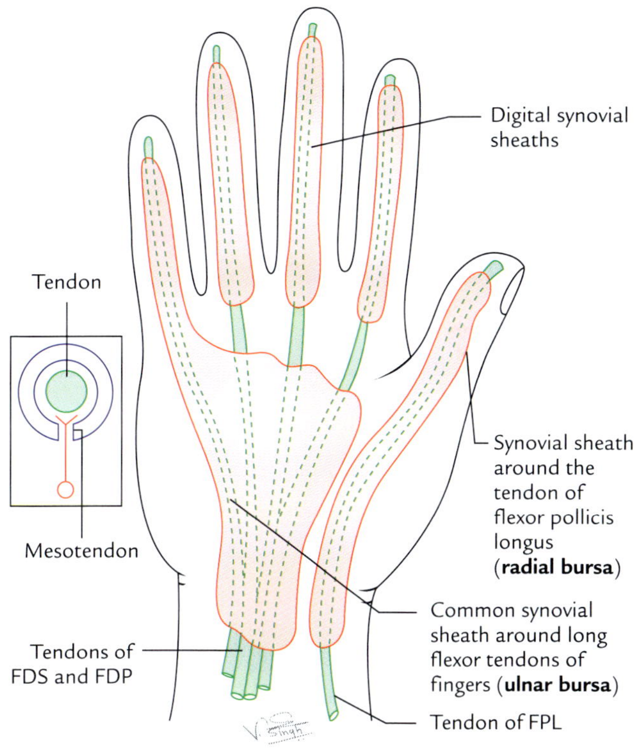

FIG. 11.10 Synovial sheaths around the long flexor tendons. The figure in the inset shows two layers of synovial sheath and mesotendon (FDS = flexor digitorum superficialis, FDP = flexor digitorum profundus, FPL = flexor pollicis longus).

The *ulnar bursa* extends proximally into the forearm about a finger breadth (2.5 cm) proximal to the flexor retinaculum. Distally, it extends in the palm up to the middle of the shafts of the metacarpal bones.

The distal medial end of the ulnar bursa is continuous with the digital synovial sheath of the little finger.

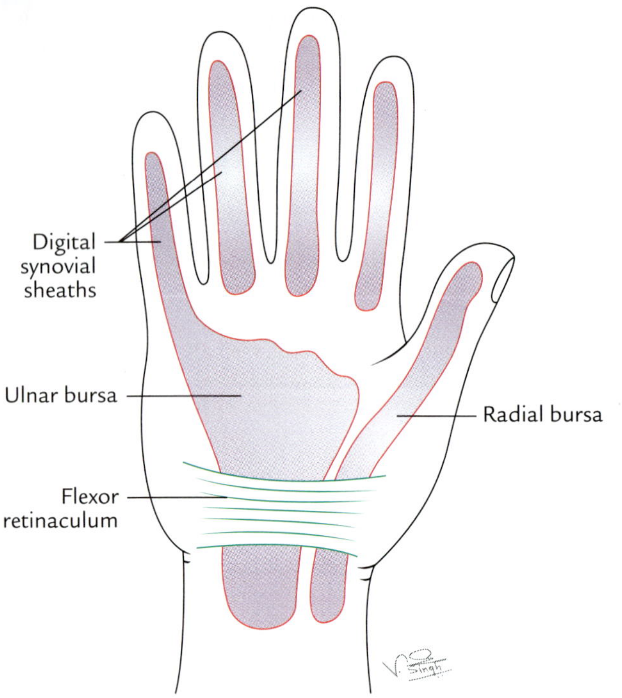

FIG. 11.11 ■ Ulnar bursa, radial bursa, and digital synovial sheaths.

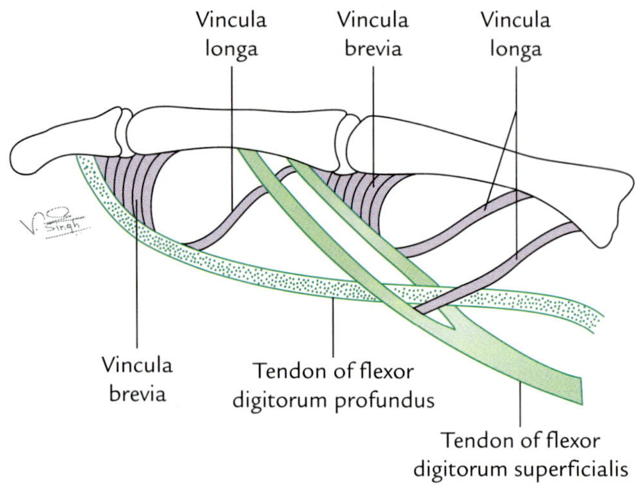

FIG. 11.12 ■ The long flexor tendons of the fingers showing the vincula longa and vincula brevia.

Radial Bursa

The tendon of FPL while passing through the osseofibrous carpal tunnel is enclosed in a synovial sheath called the **radial bursa** (Figs. 11.10 and 11.11). Proximally, it extends into the forearm about a finger breadth proximal to the flexor retinaculum. Distally, it is continuous with the digital synovial sheath of the thumb.

N.B.

The *radial bursa* is usually separate from the ulnar bursa, but it may communicate with the *ulnar bursa* deep to the flexor retinaculum.

Digital Synovial Sheaths

The long flexor tendons of digits connect the muscles of forearm to the bones of digits. These are two to each finger and one of thumb. While passing beneath the tunnels of fibrous flexor sheaths of digits are enclosed in the synovial sheath (Figs. 11.10 and 11.11). The digital synovial sheath extends from the head of the metacarpals to the distal phalanges of the digits.

N.B.

- The digital synovial sheath of the little finger is continuous with the *ulnar bursa*.
- The digital synovial sheath of the thumb is continuous with the *radial bursa*.
- Parts of long flexor tendons of the index, middle, and ring fingers between the ulnar bursa and digital synovial sheaths are devoid of synovial sheaths.

Functions

The function of the ulnar bursa, radial bursa, and digital synovial sheaths is to allow the long tendons of digits to move freely/smoothly with minimum friction beneath the flexor retinaculum and fibrous flexor sheaths.

Vincula Longa and Vincula Brevia

As the tendons lie within the fibrous flexor sheaths, they are connected to the phalanges by the thin bands of the connective tissue, called the **vincula.** *In each digital sheath, there are five vincula—two short and three long.* The short ones are called the vincula brevia and the long ones are called the **vincula longa** (Fig. 11.12). The vincula brevia are small triangular bands attached to the palmar aspect of the IP joints and the distal part of adjoining phalanx. The vincula longa are long, narrow bands that extend from the dorsal aspect of the tendon to the proximal part of the palmar surface of adjoining phalanx. The blood vessels reach the tendons through these vincula.

CLINICAL CORRELATION

- **Tenosynovitis of the synovial sheaths of the flexor tendons:** It is the infection and inflammation of the synovial sheaths of long flexor tendons, which mostly result from small penetrating wounds caused by pin prick or insertion of thorn. The infection of digital synovial sheaths results in the distension of the sheath with pus. The digit gets swollen and becomes very painful due to the stretching of the sheath by pus. The infection may extend from digital synovial sheaths to the palmar spaces.
- **Space of Parona's infection:** In the case of the infection of digital synovial sheaths of the little finger and thumb, the infection may quickly reach out to the ulnar and radial bursae due to their continuity, if these bursae are involved and neglected. The proximal ends of these bursae may burst and pus may enter into the fascial space of the forearm (space of Parona) between FDP anteriorly and the interosseous membrane and the pronator quadratus posteriorly.

INTRINSIC (SMALL) MUSCLES OF HAND AN 12.5

These are short muscles whose origin and insertion are confined within the territory of the hand. They are responsible for the skilled movements of the hand and also help the hand in adjusting for proper gripping. There are 20 intrinsic muscles in the hand. They have small motor units; hence, they can act with precision to carry out skilled movements.

The intrinsic muscles of the hand are arranged into the following five groups:

1. Thenar muscles
2. Adductor of thumb
3. Hypothenar muscles
4. Lumbricals
5. Interossei

Thenar Muscles (Fig. 11.13)

They are three in number, namely:

1. Abductor pollicis brevis
2. Flexor pollicis brevis
3. Opponens pollicis

Relationship

1. Abductor pollicis brevis lies laterally.
2. Flexor pollicis brevis lies medially.
3. Opponens pollicis lies deep between the above two muscles.

Features

1. They form the thenar eminence of the palm of the hand (a muscular bulge) on the radial side of the palm at the base of the first digit (thumb).
2. They are chiefly responsible for the opposition of the thumb.
3. All of them are supplied by the recurrent branch of the median nerve (C8 and TI).

N.B.

The actions of the thenar muscles are indicated by their names to some extent; however, they all are involved in opposition providing a pincer-like grip between the thumb and the index finger.

Hypothenar Muscles (Fig. 11.13)

They are also three in number, namely:

1. Abductor digiti minimi
2. Flexor digiti minimi
3. Opponens digiti minimi

Some authorities also consider palmaris brevis as one of the hypothenar muscles.

Relationship

1. Abductor digiti minimi lies medially.
2. Flexor digiti minimi lies laterally.
3. Opponens digiti minimi lies deep to the above two muscles.

Features

1. They form the hypothenar eminence of the palm of the hand, a muscular bulge on the ulnar side of the palm at the base of the first digit (little finger).
2. All of them are supplied by the deep branch of the ulnar nerve. The origin, insertion, and actions of the thenar and hypothenar muscles are presented in Table 11.1.

N.B.

- The *flexor pollicis* brevis has dual nerve supply: superficial head by the median nerve and deep head by the deep branch of the ulnar nerve.
- Tendons of insertion of the flexor digiti minimi along with the abductor digiti minimi on the medial side of the base of the first phalanx contain a sesamoid bone.

Adductor Pollicis Muscle (Fig. 11.14)

This fan-shaped muscle is located deep in the palm in contact with the metacarpal and interossei. It consists of two heads: (a) oblique and (b) transverse.

Origin

1. *Oblique head* arises from the anterior aspects of the capitate bone and bases of the second and third metacarpal bones—forming a crescentic shape (Fig. 11.13A).
2. *Transverse head* arises from ridge on distal two-thirds of the anterior surface of the shaft of the third metacarpal.

Insertion

Into the medial side of the base of the proximal phalanx of the thumb.

Nerve Supply

Deep branch of the ulnar nerve (C8 and TI).

Actions

Adduction of the thumb to provide power to the grip.

N.B.

- The tendons of insertion of the adductor pollicis on the medial side of the base of the proximal phalanx of the thumb contain a *sesamoid bone*.
- The *deep palmar arch* and deep branch of *ulnar nerve* pass between the two heads of the adductor pollicis.

Clinical Testing (Froment's Sign)

Give the patient a thin book and ask him to grasp it firmly between the thumbs and the index fingers of both hands. If the adductor pollicis muscles are healthy and acting normally, the thumbs will be straight and able to hold the book. But if the muscle is paralyzed and not acting, the thumbs are flexed at IP joints (Fig. 13.17). This occurs because when adductor pollicis longus are not acting, the actions of flexor pollicis longus compensates for it to maintain the grip.

Lumbrical Muscles

There are four lumbrical muscles and they are numbered first, second, third, and fourth from the lateral to medial

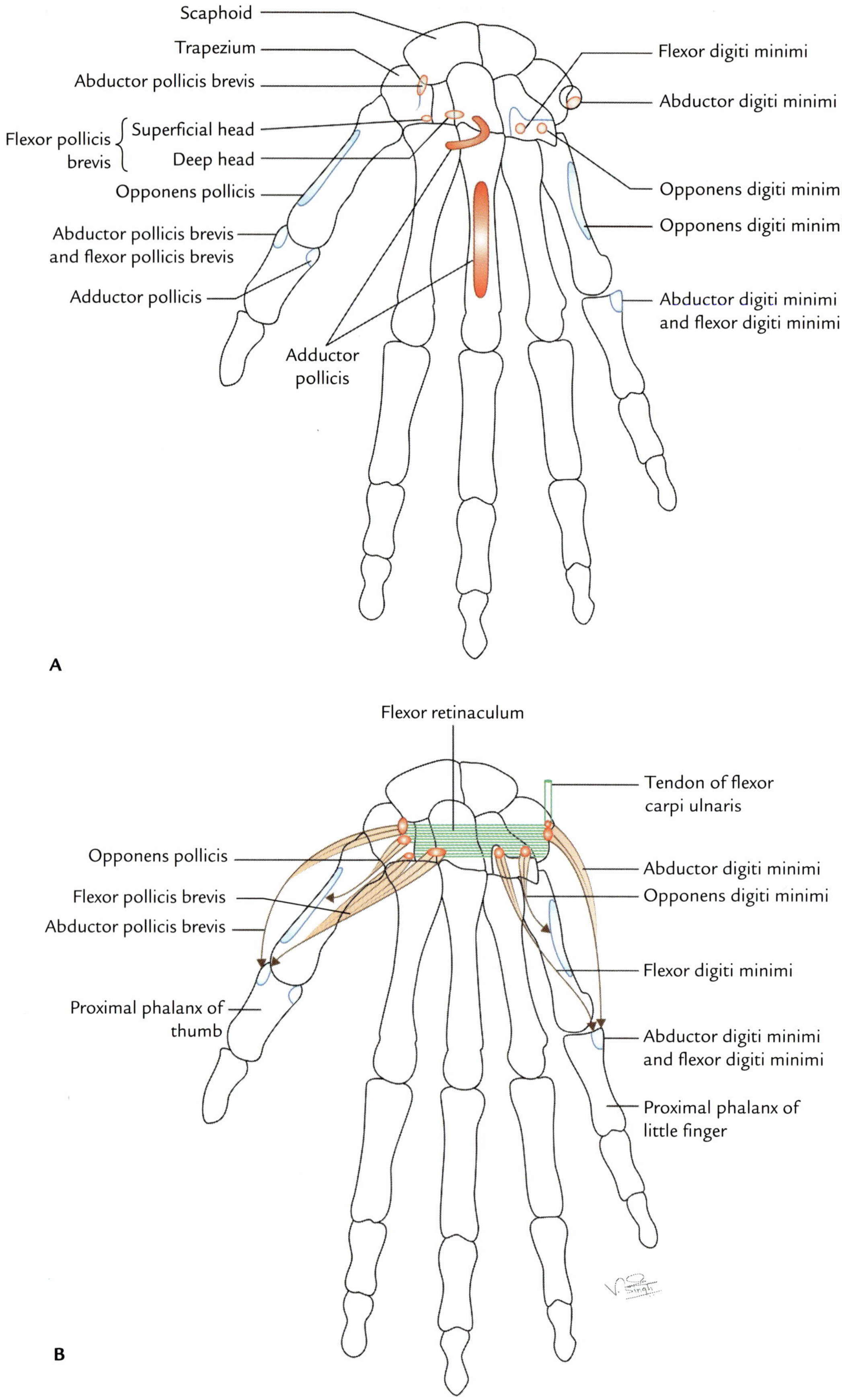

FIG. 11.13 ■ Thenar and hypothenar muscles. (**A**) Bony attachment and (**B**) origin and insertion (FPB = flexor pollicis brevis). Origins and insertions of these muscles are marked red and blue respectively on palmar aspect hand skeleton

TABLE 11.1 Origin, insertion, and actions of the thenar and hypothenar muscles

Muscles	Origin	Insertion	Action
Thenar Muscles			
Abductor pollicis brevis	• Tubercle of the scaphoid • Crest of the trapezium • Flexor retinaculum	Lateral side of the base of the proximal phalanx of the thumb	Abduction of the thumb
Flexor pollicis brevis	• Superficial head from the distal border of the flexor retinaculum • Deep head from the trapezoid and capitate bones	Lateral side of the base of the proximal phalanx of the thumb	Flexion of the thumb
Opponens pollicis	• Flexor retinaculum • Crest of the trapezium	Lateral border and adjoining lateral half of the palmar surface of the first metacarpal bone	• Opposition of the thumb • Deepens the hollow of the palm
Hypothenar Muscles			
Abductor digiti minimi	• Pisiform bone • Tendon of the flexor carpi ulnaris	Ulnar side of the base of the proximal phalanx of the little finger	Abduction of the little finger
Flexor digiti minimi	• Flexor retinaculum • Hook of hamate	Ulnar side of the base of the proximal phalanx of the little finger along with the tendon of the abductor digiti minimi	Flexion of the little finger
Opponens digiti minimi	• Flexor retinaculum • Hook of the hamate	Medial surface of the shaft of the fifth metacarpal bone	• Opposition of the tip of the little finger with the tip of the thumb • Deepens the hollow of the palm

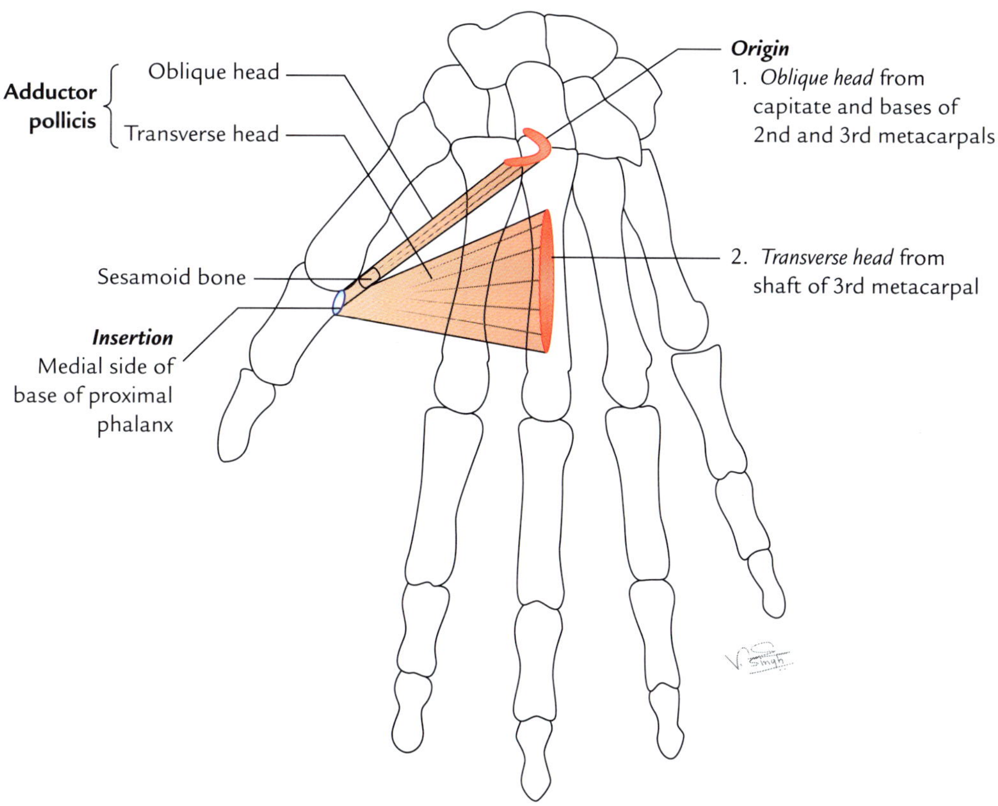

FIG. 11.14 Origin and insertion of the adductor pollicis muscle.

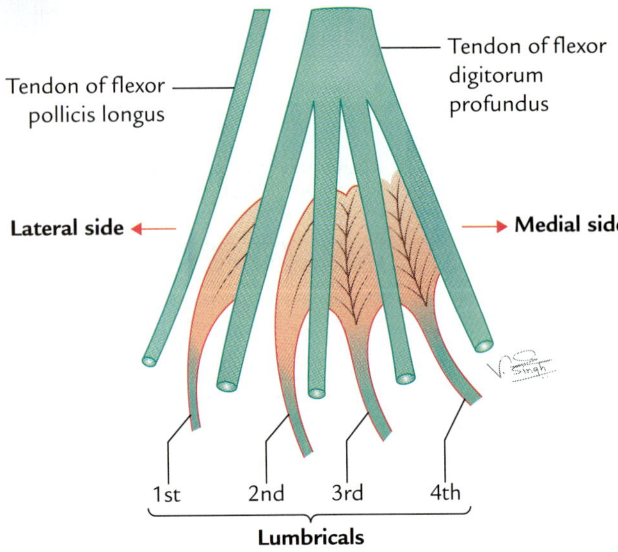

FIG. 11.15 ■ Lumbrical muscles.

side. They are small slender muscles one for each finger. They are named the *lumbricals* because of their elongated worm-like shape (L. lumbrical = earthworms; Fig. 11.15).

Origin

1. **Lumbricals 1 and 2** (unipennate): From the lateral side of the lateral two tendons of the FDP.
2. **Lumbricals 3 and 4** (bipennate): From adjacent sides of the medial three tendons of the FDP.

Insertion

The tendons cross the radial side of the MP joints to be inserted into the lateral side of the dorsal digital expansion of the corresponding digit from second to fifth.

Nerve Supply

- First and second lumbricals by the median nerve (C8 and T1).
- Third and fourth lumbricals by the deep branch of the ulnar nerve (C8 and T1).

Actions

Lumbricals flex the MP joints and extend the proximal and distal interphalangeal (PIP and DIP) joints.

Interossei

The eight small interosseous muscles, as their name indicates, are located between the metacarpal bones. They are arranged into two groups: palmar and dorsal (Fig. 11.16).

Palmar Interossei (Fig. 11.16A)

Palmar interossei are four small muscles located between the palmar surfaces of the metacarpals. They are numbered 1–4 from the lateral to medial side.

Dorsal Interossei (Fig. 11.16B)

Dorsal interossei are four small muscles located between the shafts of the metacarpals and numbered from 1 to 4 from the lateral to medial side.

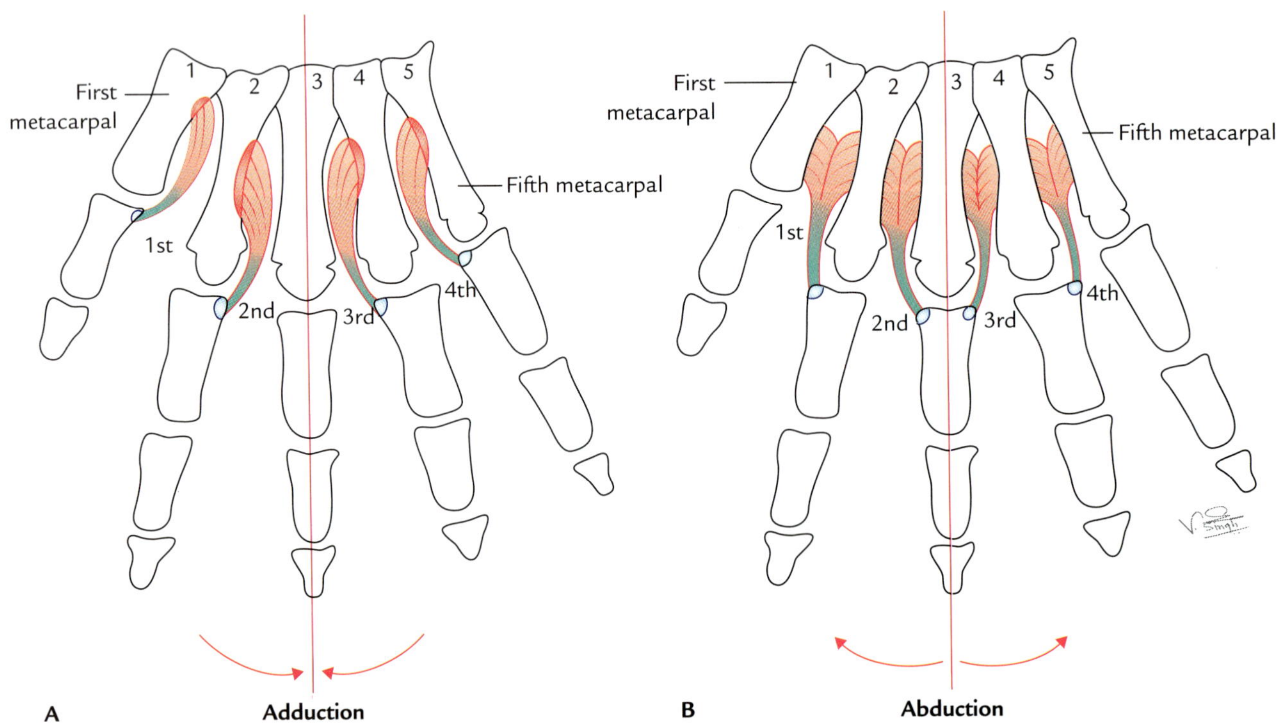

FIG. 11.16 ■ Interosseous muscles. (**A**) Palmar interossei and (**B**) dorsal interossei.

TABLE 11.2 **Origin and insertion of the palmar and dorsal interossei**

Muscles	Origin	Insertion
Palmar Interossei		
• First palmar interosseous	Medial side of the base of the first metacarpal	Each palmar interosseous muscle is inserted into the dorsal digital expansion and base of proximal phalanx of the corresponding digit – First and second into medial sides of the thumb and index fingers, respectively – Third and fourth into lateral sides of the fourth and fifth digits, respectively
• Second palmar interosseous	Medial half of the palmar aspect of the second metacarpal	
• Third and fourth palmar interossei	Lateral parts of the palmar aspects of the shafts of the fourth and fifth metacarpals	
Dorsal Interossei		
• First dorsal interosseous	Adjacent sides of the shafts of first and second metacarpals	Each dorsal muscle is inserted into the dorsal digital expansion and base of the proximal phalanx of the digit – First and second on the lateral sides of the index and middle fingers, respectively – Third and fourth on the medial sides of the middle and ring fingers, respectively
• Second dorsal interosseous	Adjacent sides of the shafts of second and third metacarpals	
• Third dorsal interosseous	Adjacent sides of the shafts of third and fourth metacarpals	
• Fourth dorsal interosseous	Adjacent sides of the shafts of fourth and fifth metacarpals	

N.B.

- There is one palmar interossei muscle for the first, second, fourth, and fifth digits but not for the third digit.
- Dorsal interossei are attached only on second, third, and fourth digits.

The origin and insertion of the palmar and dorsal interossei are presented in Table 11.2.

The insertion of the lumbricals and interossei in dorsal digital expansion is shown in Fig. 11.25 on page 156.

Nerve supply

All the palmar and dorsal interossei are supplied by the deep branch of the ulnar nerve.

Actions

Palmar interossei adduct the digits, whereas the dorsal interossei abduct the digits. The axis of adduction and abduction passes vertically through the centre of the middle finger.

A *mnemonic* to remember the action of interossei is: palmar adduct (PAD) and dorsal abduct (DAB).

N.B.

Acting together, the palmar and dorsal interossei and the lumbricals produce flexion of MP joints and the extension of proximal and distal interphalangeal (PIP and DIP) joints, this action is termed *Z-movement*.

Clinical testing

The palmar interossei are tested by asking the patient to grasp the paper between two adjacent fingers. If muscles are healthy and acting properly, the paper will be firmly held and some resistance is offered when the clinician tries to withdraw it.

The differences between the palmar interossei and dorsal interossei are listed in Table 11.3.

TABLE 11.3 **Differences between the palmar and dorsal interossei**

Features	Palmar interossei	Dorsal interossei
Location	On the palmar surface between the metacarpals	Between the metacarpals
Type	Unipennate	Bipennate
Origin	From palmar aspects of the metacarpals	From the side of metacarpals
Action	Adduction of digits	Abduction of digits

CLINICAL CORRELATION

Claw-hand: It is a deformity of hand in which fingers are bent in such a position that hand looks like a claw (see Fig. 13.18, page 181).

Clinical features

- Hyperextension of metacarpophalangeal (MP) joints
- Flexion of proximal and distal interphalangeal (PIP and DIP) joints
- Loss of abduction and adduction of fingers
- Flattening of arches of hand
- Sensory loss along the distribution of ulnar and median nerves

Cause: Lesions of median and ulnar nerves leading to paralysis of flexors of wrist, MP, PIP and DIP joints.

ARTERIES OF THE PALM OF HAND AN 12.7

The hand is richly supplied with the blood. There are two major arteries of the hand, namely terminal parts of the ulnar and radial arteries. On entering the palm, the branches of these arteries unite to form **superficial** and **deep palmar arterial arches**, respectively.

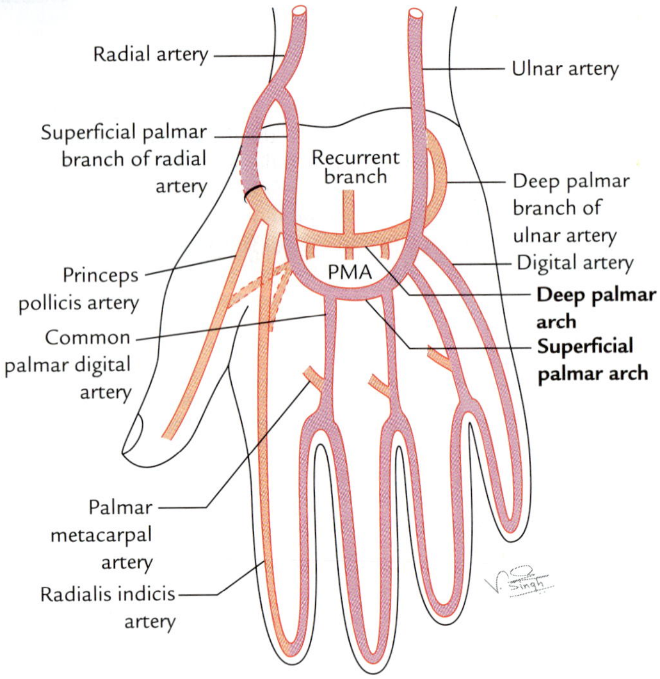

FIG. 11.17 ■ Superficial and deep palmar arterial arches (PMA = palmar metacarpal arteries).

Superficial Palmar Arterial Arch

Formation

The superficial palmar arterial arch is the direct continuation of the ulnar artery (i.e. superficial palmar branch of the ulnar artery) beyond the flexor retinaculum (Fig. 11.17). On entering the palm, the artery curves laterally deep to palmar aponeurosis and in front of long flexor tendons. The convexity of the arch is directed towards the digits.

The arch is completed laterally by anastomosing with the superficial palmar branch of the radial artery.

N.B.

The *ulnar artery* enters the palm by passing in front of flexor retinaculum just lateral to ulnar nerve and pisiform bone.

After entering the palm, it gives rise to deep palmar branch which passes deep between abductor and flexor digiti minimi to anastomose with radial artery, then continues laterally as **superficial palmar arch**.

Relations

Superficial: Palmar aponeurosis.

Deep:

1. Long flexor tendons of FDS and FDP
2. Lumbricals
3. Digital branches of the median and ulnar nerves

Branches

1. *Three common palmar digital arteries* go to the interdigital clefts between the fingers and each divides into two proper digital arteries, which supply their adjacent sides. In the interdigital clefts, they are joined by the palmar metacarpal arteries.
2. *One proper digital artery* runs along the medial side of the little finger which it supplies.
3. *Cutaneous branches to the palm* which supply the skin and superficial fascia of the palm.

Surface Anatomy

The superficial palmar arch lies across the centre of the palm at the level of the distal border of the fully extended thumb.

Deep Palmar Arch

Formation

The deep palmar arch is the direct continuation of the radial artery (Fig. 11.17). The arch is completed medially (at the base of the fifth metacarpal) by anastomosing with the deep palmar branch of the ulnar artery.

The radial artery enters the palm from the dorsal aspect of the hand by passing between the two heads of the first dorsal interosseous muscle. Immediately after entering the palm, the radial artery gives off two branches: *arteria princeps pollicis and arteria radialis indicis.*

In the palm, it passes between the two heads of adductor pollicis to continue as a deep palmar arch.

N.B.

The *radial artery* enters the dorsum of hand by passing backwards deep to tendons of abductor pollicis longus and extensor pollicis brevis to enter anatomical snuff box. Then to enters proximal end of first interosseous space to reach palm.

Relations

Deep:

(a) Proximal parts of shafts of the metacarpals.
(b) Interosseous muscles.

Superficial:

(a) Long flexor tendons of the fingers.
(b) Lumbricals.

N.B.

The deep branch of the ulnar nerve lies in the concavity of the deep palmar arch.

Branches

1. **Three palmar metacarpal arteries** that join the common palmar digital arteries, the branches of the superficial palmar arch.
2. **Three perforating arteries** that pass through the second, third, and fourth interosseous spaces to anastomose with dorsal metacarpal arteries (not seen in the figure).
3. **Recurrent branch/branches** run proximally in front of the carpus to end in the *palmar carpal arch*.

Surface Anatomy

The deep palmar arch lies about 1.2 cm proximal to the superficial palmar arch (for details see Chapter 14).

The differences between the superficial and deep palmar (arterial) arches are given in Table 11.4.

TABLE 11.4 Differences between the superficial and deep palmar arches

	Superficial palmar arch	Deep palmar arch
Formation	By anastomosis between the direct continuation of the ulnar artery (i.e. superficial palmar branch) with the small superficial branch of the radial artery	By anastomosis between the direct continuation of the radial artery with the small deep palmar branch of the ulnar artery
Location	Superficial to long flexor tendons	Deep to long flexor tendons
Branches	• Three common palmar digital arteries • One proper digital artery • Cutaneous branches	• Three palmar metacarpal arteries • Three perforating arteries • Recurrent branches

CLINICAL CORRELATION

Laceration of palmar arterial arches: The lacerated wounds of palmar arterial arches usually cause profuse and uncontrollable bleeding. The compression of the brachial artery against the humerus on medial side of midarm is the most effective method to control the bleeding.

The ligation or clamping of the radial artery or ulnar artery or both proximal to the wrist fails to control the bleeding because of connections of these arches with the palmar and dorsal carpal arches.

NERVES IN THE PALM OF THE HAND **AN 12.7**

There are two nerves in the palm of the hand, namely:

1. Ulnar nerve.
2. Median nerve.

N.B.

The *ulnar nerve* is the main motor nerve of the hand, whereas the *median nerve* is the main sensory nerve of the hand.

Ulnar Nerve

The ulnar nerve enters the palm by passing superficial to the flexor retinaculum between the pisiform bone and the ulnar artery (Figs. 11.18 and 11.19). At the distal border of the flexor retinaculum, it divides into the superficial and deep terminal branches.

Superficial Branch

It enters the palm deep to the *palmaris brevis*, which it supplies and then divides into digital branches. The digital nerves supply the skin of the medial 1½ fingers. The digital nerves cross over the tips of digits and supply the skin on the dorsum of distal phalanges. The superficial branch of the ulnar nerve is accompanied by the superficial branch of the ulnar artery.

Deep Branch

It dips in the interval between abductor digiti minimi and flexor digiti minimi muscles, and then pierces opponens digiti minimi to reach the deep part of the palm. It turns laterally within the concavity of the deep palmar arch to end by supplying the adductor pollicis.

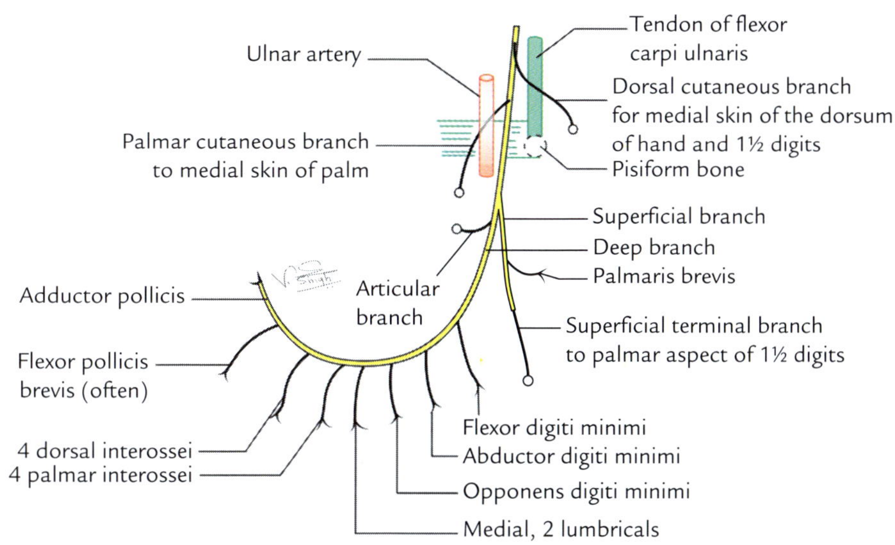

FIG. 11.18 ■ Course and distribution of the ulnar nerve in hand.

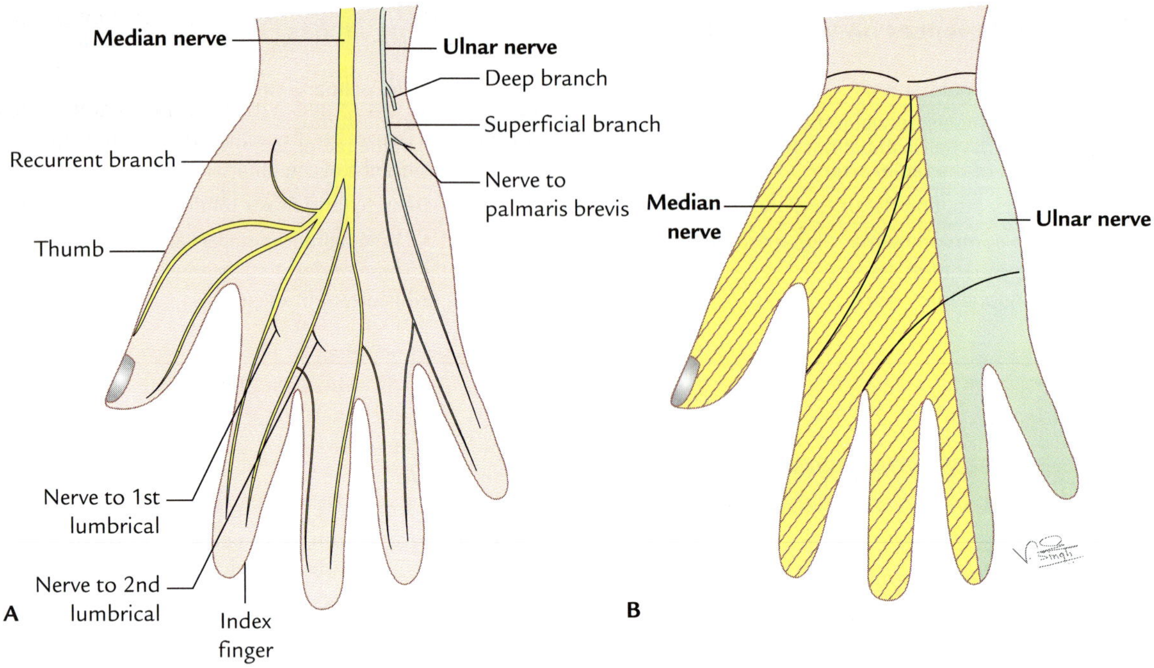

FIG. 11.19 ■ Sensory innervation of the palm of the hand. (**A**) Branches of median and ulnar nerves (**B**) areas of sensory innervation on the palmar aspect of the hand by median and ulnar nerves.

The deep branch supplies:

- *Articular branches* to intercarpal, carpometacarpal, and intermetacarpal joints.
- *Muscular branches* to
  - three hypothenar muscles,
  - adductor pollicis,
  - four dorsal interosseous muscles,
  - four palmar interosseous muscles, and
  - medial two lumbricals.

The distribution of ulnar nerve in the palm of the hand is summarized in Table 11.5.

N.B.

The ulnar nerve supplies all the intrinsic muscles of the hand (except thenar muscles and lateral two lumbricals), which are concerned with the fine movements of the hand as performed by musicians. Hence, the ulnar nerve is also termed the **musician's nerve**.

CLINICAL CORRELATION

Ulnar canal syndrome/Guyon's tunnel syndrome: It is a clinical condition which occurs due to the compression of the ulnar nerve in Guyon's canal[a] at the wrist. Clinically, it presents as:
(a) hypoaesthesia in medial 1½ fingers and
(b) weakness of intrinsic muscles of the hand.

[a]**Ulnar tunnel/Guyon's canal** is an osseofibrous tunnel formed by the pisohamate ligament, bridging the concavity between the pisiform bone and the hook of the hamate.

Median Nerve (Fig. 11.19)

The median nerve enters the hand by passing through the carpal tunnel (i.e. deep to flexor retinaculum) along with nine tendons (four each of FDS and FDP and one of FPL; Fig. 11.6). Just after emerging from the carpal tunnel, it divides into the lateral and medial divisions (Fig. 11.19).

TABLE 11.5 Distribution of the ulnar nerve in the palm of the hand (Figs. 11.18 and 11.19)

Branches	Distribution
Palmar cutaneous branch[a]	Skin on the medial 1/3rd of the palm
Dorsal cutaneous branch[b]	Skin on the medial half of the dorsum of the hand and dorsal aspect of medial 1½ fingers
Superficial terminal branch	• Skin of the palmar aspect of medial 1/3rd of palm • Palmaris brevis muscle
Deep terminal branch	• All the intrinsic muscles of the hand except lateral two lumbricals/and thenar muscles • Intercarpal, carpometacarpal, and intermetacarpal joints

[a]Palmar cutaneous branch of the ulnar nerve arises just proximal to the wrist.
[b]Dorsal cutaneous branch of the ulnar nerve arises 5 cm proximal to the wrist.

TABLE 11.6 Distribution of the median nerve in the hand

Median nerve	
Sensory distribution	• Skin on the lateral half of the palm • Palmar surface of lateral 3½ digits including dorsal surfaces of their distal phalanges
Motor distribution	• Muscles of thenar eminence • Lateral two (first and second) lumbricals

Lateral division gives off:

(a) *Recurrent branch*, which curls upward to supply thenar muscles (e.g. abductor pollicis brevis, flexor pollicis brevis, and opponens pollicis) and

(b) *Three proper palmar digital branches*, which provides sensory innervation to the thumb and lateral side of the index finger. The digital branch to the index finger sends a twig to the first lumbrical.

Medial division gives off:

Two common digital nerves that provide sensory innervation to the medial side of the index finger, middle finger, and lateral side of the ring finger. The lateral common digital nerve sends a twig to second lumbrical.

The distribution of the median nerve in the palm of the hand is summarized in Table 11.6.

FASCIAL SPACES OF THE HAND (FIG. 11.20)

By virtue of the arrangement of various fascia and fascial septa, many fascial spaces are formed in the region of the hand. Normally, they are potential spaces filled with the loose connective tissue, but they become obvious only when fluid or pus collects in them. These spaces are of great surgical importance because they may get infected and distended with pus. The knowledge of their boundaries is essential because they may limit the spread of infection in the palm.

The various spaces of the hand are as follows:

A. Palmar spaces
1. Midpalmar space
2. Thenar space
3. Pulp spaces of digits

B. Dorsal spaces
1. Dorsal subcutaneous space
2. Dorsal subaponeurotic space

C. Space of Parona

FASCIAL SPACES OF THE PALM (FIG. 11.20)

Midpalmar Space (Fig. 11.20)

The triangular midpalmar space is located under the medial half of the hollow of the palm (Fig. 11.20).

Boundaries

Anterior: From superficial to deep, it is formed by:
1. Palmar aponeurosis.
2. Superficial palmar arch.
3. Digital nerve and vessels supplying medial 3½ fingers.
4. Ulnar bursa enclosing flexor tendons of the medial three fingers.
5. Medial three (second, third, and fourth) lumbricals.

Posterior: Fascia covering interossei and medial three metacarpals.

Lateral: Intermediate palmar septum extending obliquely from near the lateral edge of the palmar aponeurosis to the third metacarpal bone. This septum separates the midpalmar space from the thenar space.

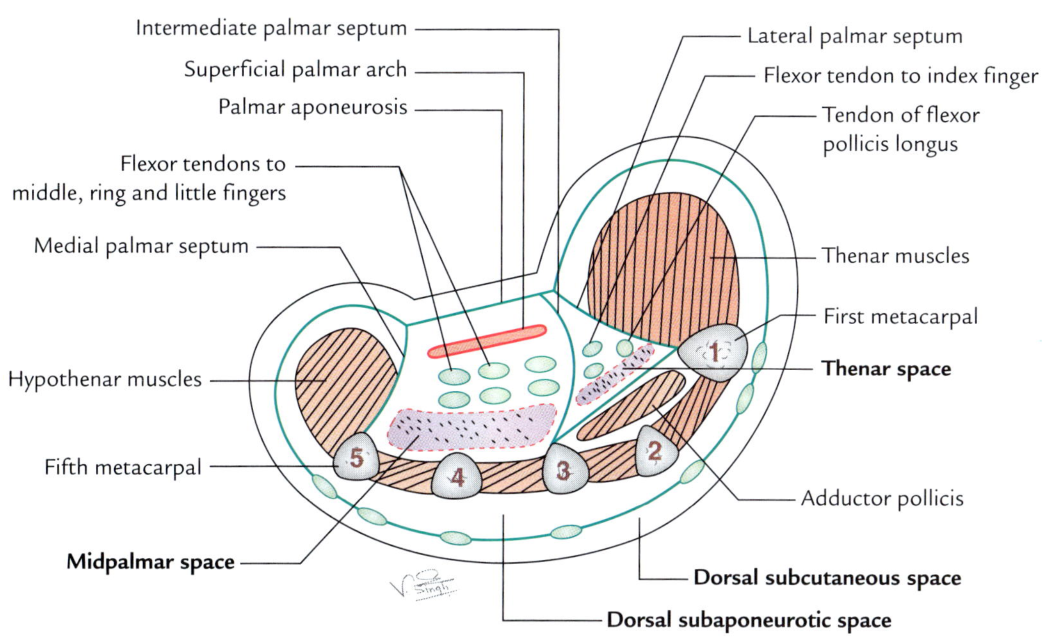

FIG. 11.20 ■ Cross section of the hand showing palmar spaces and spaces on the dorsum of the hand.

Medial: Medial palmar septum extending from the medial edge of the palmar aponeurosis to the fifth metacarpal. This septum separates the midpalmar space from the hypothenar space occupied by the hypothenar muscles.
Proximal: Midpalmar space is continuous with the forearm space of the Parona through carpal tunnel.
Distal: Midpalmar space is continuous with the medial three web spaces through the medial three lumbrical canals.

N.B.

Web spaces: The web space is a subcutaneous space in each interdigital cleft and is filled with loose areolar tissue. It contains the lumbrical tendon, interosseous tendon, digital nerve, and vessels.

The web space extends from the free margin of the web, as far proximally as the level of transverse metacarpal ligaments.

Thenar Space (*Fig. 11.20*)

The triangular thenar space is located under the outer half of the hollow of the palm.

Boundaries

Anterior: From superficial to deep, it is formed by:
1. Palmar aponeurosis (lateral part).
2. Digital nerve and vessels of lateral 1½ digits.
3. Radial bursa enclosing tendon of FPL.
4. Flexor tendons of the index finger.
5. First lumbrical.

Lateral: Lateral palmar septum extending from lateral edge of palmar aponeurosis to the first metacarpal.
Medial: Intermediate palmar septum.
Posterior: Fascia covering the transverse head of adductor pollicis.
Proximal: Forearm space of Parona through carpal tunnel.
Distal: The space communicates with the first web space through the **first lumbrical canal**.

The surface projections of midpalmar and thenar spaces are given in Fig. 11.21.

Pulp Spaces of the Digits (*Fig. 11.22*) AN 12.10

The pulp spaces of the digits are subcutaneous spaces on the palmar side of tips of the fingers and thumb. The pulp space is filled with subcutaneous fatty tissue.

Boundaries

Superficially: Skin and superficial fascia.
Deeply: Distal two-thirds of distal phalanx.

Features

1. The space is traversed by numerous fibrous septa extending from skin to the periosteum of the terminal phalanx, dividing it into many loculi.
2. The deep fascia of pulp of each finger fuses with the periosteum of terminal phalanx distal to the insertion of FDP tendon.
3. The digital artery that supplies the diaphysis of phalanx runs through this space. The epiphysis of distal phalanx receives its blood supply proximal to the pulp space.

CLINICAL CORRELATION

- **Infections of fascial spaces of the palm:**
  - *Infection of midpalmar space* (Figs. 11.20 and 11.21): The ulnar bursa is considered as the inlet for infection and lumbrical canals as the outlets of infection in midpalmar space. The pus from this space is drained by incisions in the medial two web spaces.
  - *Infection of thenar space* (Figs. 11.20 and 11.21): The infection may reach the thenar space from infected radial bursa or synovial sheath of the index finger.

The pus from thenar space is drained by an incision in the first web space (web space of the thumb).

The midpalmar and thenar spaces and their surface projection in the palm are shown in Fig. 11.21.

- **Pulp space infection of digit (Fig. 11.22):** Being the most exposed parts of the digits, the pulp spaces are prone for infection. An abscess in the pulp-space is called

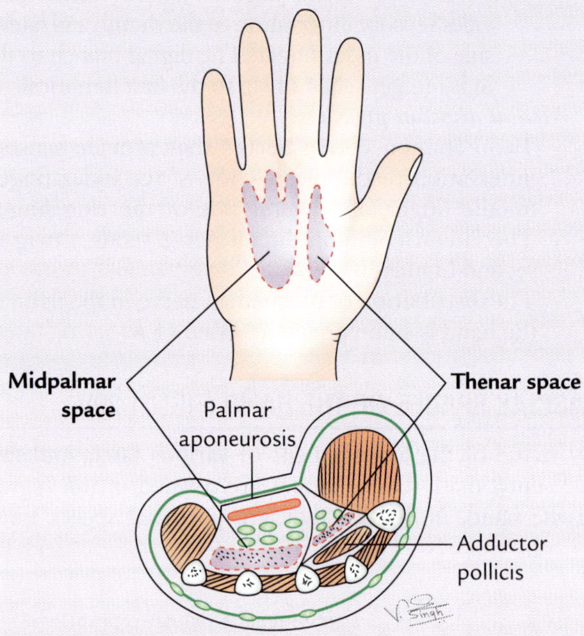

FIG. 11.21 Midpalmar and thenar spaces of the hand and their surface projections in the palm.

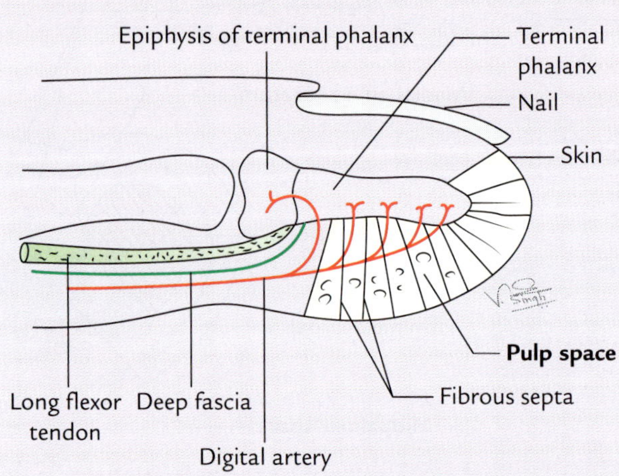

FIG. 11.22 Pulp space of the digit.

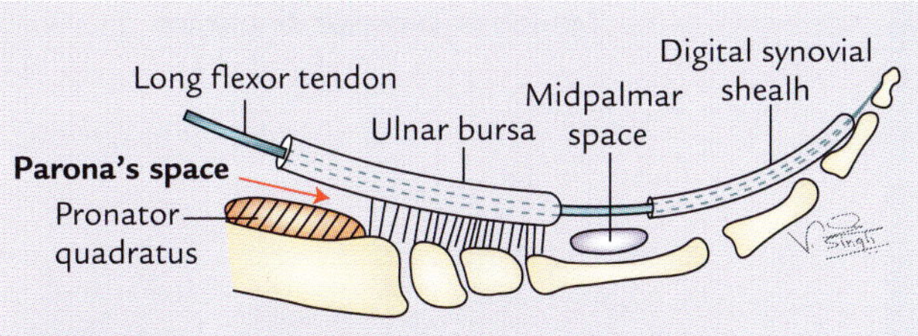

FIG. 11.23 ■ Forearm space (Parona's space) as seen in section along the long axis of the hand. The red arrow lies in Parona's space.

whitlow or **felon**. The rising tension in the pulp space causes severe throbbing pain. The pus from pulp space is drained by a lateral incision, opening all loculi and avoiding tactile skin sensation on the front of the finger.

If neglected, the whitlow may lead to avascular necrosis of distal four-fifths of the terminal phalanx due to occlusion of digital artery as result of pressure. The proximal one-fifth phalanx (i.e. epiphysis) is not affected because the branch of digital artery supplying it does not traverse the pulp space.

Space of Parona (Forearm Space; Fig. 11.23)

It is merely a fascial interval underneath the flexor tendons on the front of distal part of the forearm.

Boundaries

Anterior:

(a) Tendon of FDP and FDS surrounded by a synovial sheath (ulnar bursa).

(b) Tendon of FPL surrounded by a synovial bursa (radial bursa).

Proximal: Proximally, it is continuous with the intermuscular spaces of the forearm.

Distal: Distally it becomes continuous with midplamar and thenar spaces through carpal tunnel.

Lateral: Outer border of the forearm.

Medial: Inner border of the forearm.

CLINICAL CORRELATION

The forearm space (Parona's space) becomes infected from infected ulnar bursa. Pus collects behind the long flexor tendons.

SURGICAL INCISIONS ON THE FRONT OF WRIST AND HAND (FIG. 11.24)

The surgical incisions in the palm should be well planned and given carefully to avoid contractures:

- Incisions should be parallel to major skin creases of the hand as far as possible.
- An incision should not cross the skin crease at a right angle.

Guidelines for some incisions are as follows (Fig. 11.24**):**

- To drain abscess of the *thenar space*, a vertical incision is given in first web space (A).
- To drain abscess from *midpalmar space*, small vertical incision should be given in the medial two web spaces (B).

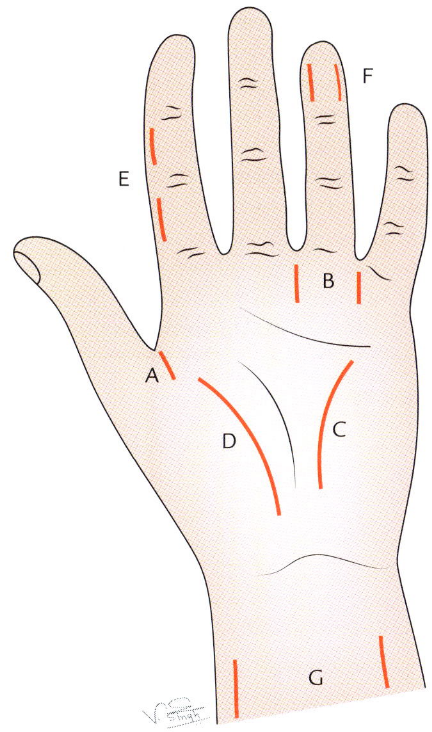

FIG. 11.24 ■ Incisions on the front of wrist and hand for draining abscess from: (**A**) thenar space, (**B**) midpalmar space, (**C**) ulnar bursa, (**D**) radial bursa, (**E**) digital synovial sheath, (**F**) pulp space, (**G**) space of Parona.

- To drain abscess from *ulnar bursa*, incision should be given along the radial margin of hypothenar eminence (C).
- To drain abscess from *radial bursa*, incision should be given along the medial margin of thenar eminence (D).
- To drain pus from *digital synovial sheath*, vertical incisions should be given along the side of proximal and middle phalanges (E).
- To drain pus from pulp space, vertical incision should be given along the sides of pulp (F).
- To drain pus from space of Parona, vertical incisions should be given on the distal part of forearm (G).

DORSUM OF THE HAND

SURFACE LANDMARKS

1. **Knuckles**, the bony prominences at the junction of hand and digits, which become visible prominently when a fist is made. They are produced by the heads of metacarpals.
2. **Anatomical snuff box**, a triangular depression, which appears on the dorsolateral aspect of the hand when the thumb is hyperextended. The pulsations of radial artery can be felt in this box. The beginning of cephalic vein can also be seen at this site. The tendon of extensor pollicis longus forming its posteromedial boundary and tendons of abductor pollicis longus and extensor pollicis brevis forming its anterolateral boundary are clearly visible.

3. **Extensor tendons of fingers** stand out clearly when the wrist is extended and digits are abducted. These tendons are not visible far beyond knuckles because they flatten here to form extensor expansions.
4. **Dorsal venous network** is clearly visible and forms the prominent feature of the dorsum of hand.
5. **Base of first metacarpal (thumb)** can be readily felt in the angle between the tendons of abductor pollicis longus and extensor pollicis longus.
6. Whole of the **radial border** and most of the **dorsal surface of the second (index) metacarpal** can be readily felt. Its base forms the prominence of the back of the hand.

N.B.

The dorsal surfaces of *metacarpals* of the middle, ring, and little fingers are obscured by the extensor tendons.

SKIN ON THE DORSUM OF THE HAND

The skin on the dorsum of the hand is thin and loose when the hand is relaxed. The hairs are present on the dorsum of the hand and on the proximal parts of the digits, especially in males.

Superficial Fascia

The superficial fascia on the dorsum of the hand contains dorsal venous arch, cutaneous branches of the radial nerve, and dorsal cutaneous branch of the ulnar nerve.

The ***dorsal venous arch*** is already described in Chapter 7.

The superficial radial nerve and dorsal cutaneous branch of ulnar nerve are described on page 158.

Deep Fascia

The deep fascia on the back of the wrist is thickened to form thick fibrous band—the extensor retinaculum, which holds the extensor tendons in place (for details see pages 122–124).

EXTENSOR TENDONS OF DIGITS ON THE DORSUM OF THE HAND

These are as follows:

1. **Tendons of the thumb:** They are three in number; one for each bone of the thumb (Figs. 11.28 and 11.29):
   (a) Tendon of *abductor pollicis longus* (APL) is inserted on the base of first metacarpal.
   (b) Tendon of *extensor pollicis brevis* (EPB) is inserted on the base of proximal phalanx.
   (c) Tendon of *extensor pollicis longus* (EPL) is inserted on the base of distal phalanx.
2. **Tendons of extensor digitorum for fingers:** These are four in number which diverge across the dorsum of the hand, where they are usually connected to one another by three oblique fibrous intertendinous bands. The tendons are united in such a way as to form with deep fascia an aponeurotic sheath, which is attached to the borders of the second and fifth metacarpals.

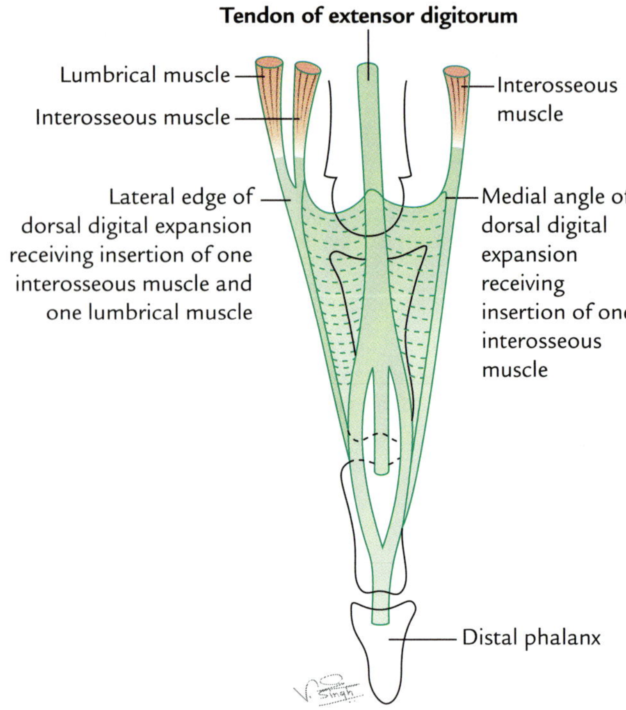

FIG. 11.25 ■ Formation of dorsal digital expansion and insertion of the lumbricals and interossei into it.

FORMATION OF DORSAL DIGITAL EXPANSIONS (FIG. 11.25) AN 12.15

Each tendon of extensor digitorum expands over the MP joint to cover its dorsal aspect and sides like a hood and fuses anteriorly with the fibrous flexor sheath. The tendons of lumbricals and interossei are inserted into this expansion. The expansion narrows as the tendons of lumbricals and interossei converge towards it on the dorsum of the proximal phalanx and splits into three slips. The central slip is inserted into the base of the middle phalanx and the lateral slips to the base of terminal phalanx.

N.B.

- The dorsal digital expansion forms a *functional unit* to coordinate the actions of long extensors, long flexors, lumbricals, and interossei on the digit.
- On the index finger and little finger, the expansion is strengthened by extensor indicis and extensor digiti minimi, respectively, which blends with it.

CLINICAL CORRELATION

- **Mallet finger/baseball finger/cricketer's finger** (Fig. 11.26): The insertion of extensor tendon into the base of the terminal phalanx may be torn by a forceful blow on the tip of the finger, which causes sudden and strong flexion of the phalanx. Occasionally, small flakes of the bone may be avulsed. Consequently, the distal phalanx assumes a flexed position with swan neck deformity and voluntary extension is impossible. This condition commonly occurs in *cricketers* and *baseball players*.

- **Boutonniere (button-hole) deformity** (Fig. 11.27): It is opposite to mallet finger deformity. It is characterized by flexion of PIP joint and hyperextension of distal phalanx. It occurs when the flexed PIP joint pokes through the extensor expansion following rupture of its central portion of dorsal digital expansion due to a direct end on trauma to the finger.

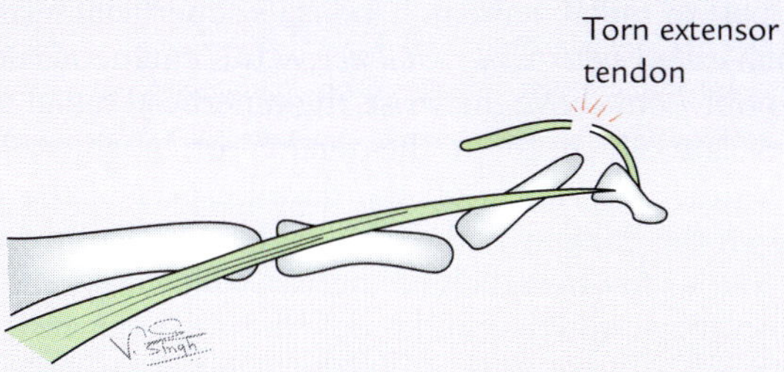

FIG. 11.26 ■ Mallet finger with swan neck deformity.

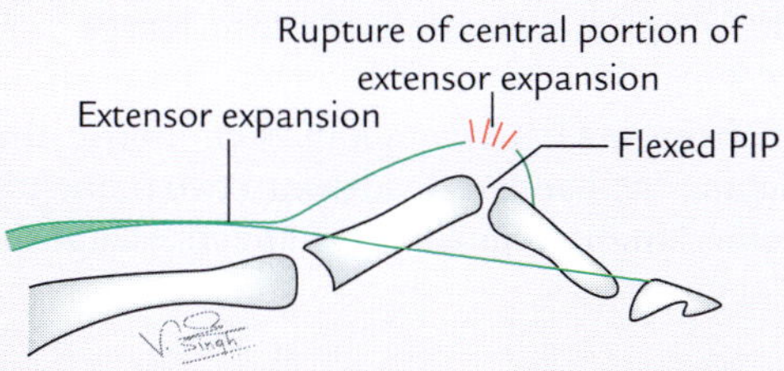

FIG. 11.27 ■ Boutonniere (button-hole) deformity. Note proximal interphalangeal (PIP) joint is poking through the extensor expansion.

ANATOMICAL SNUFF BOX (FIGS. 11.28 AND 11.29)

The anatomical snuff box is an elongated triangular depression seen on the lateral side of the dorsum of hand when the thumb is hyperextended.

Boundaries (Fig. 11.28)

Posterolaterally, it is bounded by:

1. Tendon of abductor pollicis longus.
2. Tendon of extensor pollicis brevis.

Posteromedially: Tendon of extensor pollicis longus.

Floor: It is formed by:

1. Scaphoid and
2. Trapezium.

Roof: It is formed by:

1. Skin and
2. Superficial fascia.

The roof deep to skin is crossed by (Fig. 11.29):

1. Cephalic vein, from medial to lateral side.
2. Terminal branches of the superficial radial nerve, from lateral to medial side.

Contents: Radial artery.

CLINICAL CORRELATION

Clinical significance of anatomical snuff box:

- The pulsations of radial artery can be felt in the anatomical box.
- The tenderness in the anatomical box indicates fracture of scaphoid bone.
- The cephalic vein at this site is often used for giving intravenous fluids.
- The superficial branches of the radial nerve can be rolled over the tendon of extensor pollicis longus.

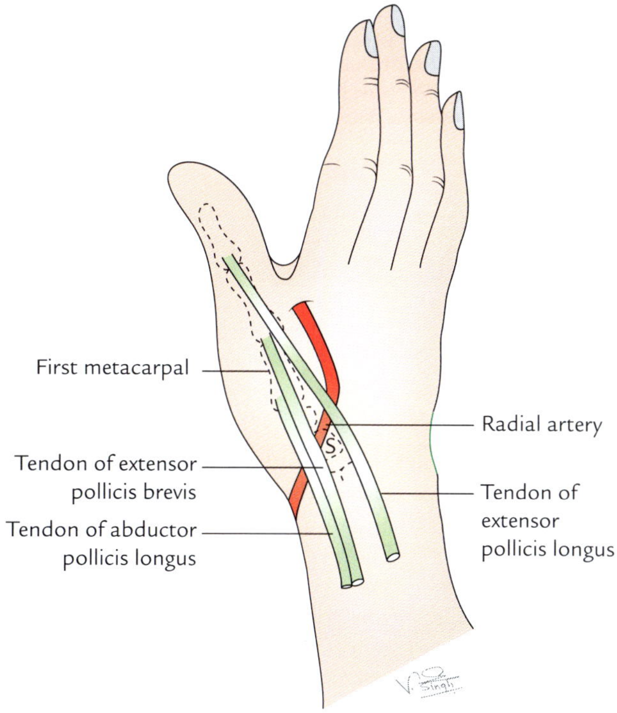

FIG. 11.28 ■ Boundaries and contents of the anatomical snuff box (S = scaphoid).

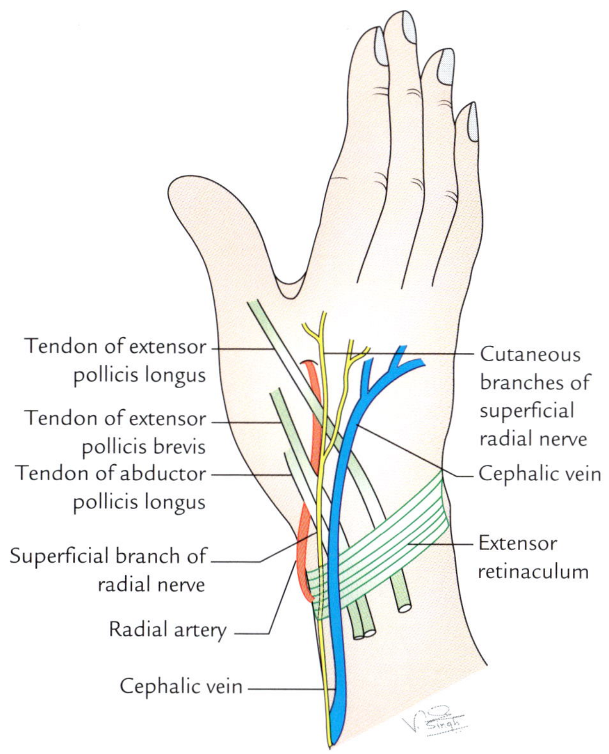

FIG. 11.29 ■ Structures crossing the roof of anatomical snuff box.

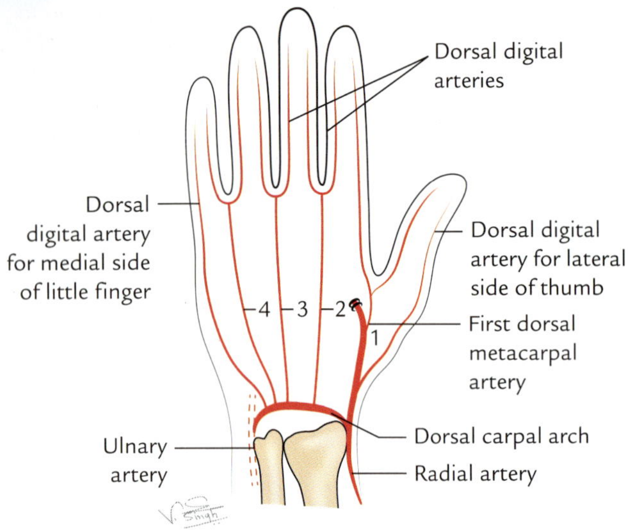

FIG. 11.30 ■ Arterial supply of dorsum of the hand. 1, 2, 3, and 4 = first, second, third, and fourth dorsal metatarsal arteries.

ARTERIES OF THE DORSUM OF THE HAND

The dorsum of hand is supplied directly or indirectly by the branches of radial and ulnar arteries through dorsal metacarpal arteries (Fig. 11.30).

Dorsal carpal arch, formed on the dorsal aspect of carpus by the dorsal carpal branches of radial and ulnar arteries. It gives rise to **second, third and fourth dorsal metacarpal arteries.**

First dorsal metacarpal artery, arising from radial artery before it passes deep into the palm by passing between the two heads of first dorsal interosseous muscle.

NERVES OF THE DORSUM OF THE HAND (FIG. 11.31A)

The nerves of the dorsum of the hand are two, namely:

1. **Superficial radial nerve** (superficial cutaneous branch of the radial nerve).
2. **Dorsal cutaneous branch of the ulnar nerve.**

Superficial Radial Nerve (Fig. 11.31A)

The part of radial nerve in hand is its superficial terminal branch called *superficial radial nerve*. It is cutaneous nerve.

About 7 cm above the wrist, the superficial radial nerve passes laterally deep to the tendon of brachioradialis, pierces the deep fascia on the dorsal aspect of the wrist to reach the dorsum of the hand and immediately divides into four or five dorsal digital nerves, which cross the roof of anatomical snuff box and supply the skin over the lateral two-thirds of the dorsum of hand and dorsal aspects of lateral 3½ digits except the skin over their distal phalanges.

Dorsal Cutaneous Branch of Ulnar Nerve (Fig. 11.31A)

It arises from ulnar nerve about 5 cm above the wrist. On reaching the hand, it divides into two branches which supply the skin of the medial 1½ fingers except their distal phalanges.

Sensory Innervation of the Dorsum of the Hand (Fig. 11.31B)

1. Lateral two-thirds of dorsum of the hand and lateral 3½ digits except distal phalanges by the radial nerve.
2. Medial one-third of dorsum of the hand and medial 1½ digits except their distal phalanges by the ulnar nerve.

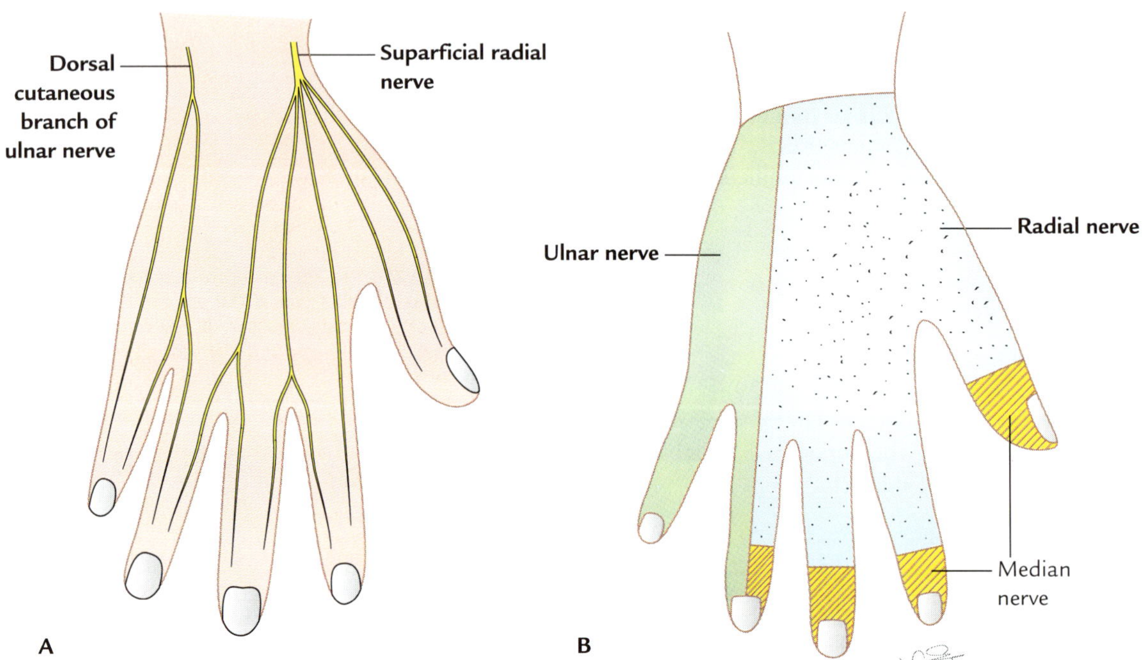

FIG. 11.31 ■ Sensory innervation of dorsum of the hand. (**A**) Branches of dorsal cutaneous branch of ulnar nerve and superficial radial nerve on the dorsum of the hand, (**B**) areas of the sensory innervation of the dorsum of the hand by ulnar and radial nerves.

SPACES ON THE DORSUM OF THE HAND

There are two potential spaces on the dorsum of the hand (Fig. 11.20), namely:

1. Dorsal subcutaneous space.
2. Dorsal subaponeurotic space.

Dorsal subcutaneous space: It lies deep to skin on the dorsum of the hand.

Dorsal subaponeurotic space: The extensor tendons on the dorsum of hand along with deep fascia of the dorsum of hand forms an aponeurotic sheet which is attached to the borders of the second and fifth metacarpals.

The space between dorsal surface of the medial four metacarpals and interosseous muscles anteriorly and aponeurotic sheet (vide supra) posteriorly is called *dorsal subaponeurotic space*.

The dorsal subaponeurotic space is limited proximally at the bases of metacarpals and distally at the MP joints by fibrous partitions.

CLINICAL CORRELATION

- **Infection of subcutaneous space:** The infection of subcutaneous space is uncommon but sometimes it may get infected after injury over the knuckles. Collection of pus in this space produces large swelling due to looseness of the skin. The pus points through skin and can be drained by incision given at the pointing site.
- **Infection of subaponeurotic space:** The septic infection of subaponeurotic space is generally *primary*, following wounds on the dorsum of the hand. It may, however, get involved *secondarily* to the infection of the midpalmar space. The pus collected in the subaponeurotic space is limited proximally at the bases of metacarpal bones and distally at the MP joints. On each side, it is limited opposite the borders of second and fifth metacarpal bones. To drain the pus from this space, incisions are made in the aponeurosis between the tendons distally. Alternatively, two incisions may be made, one on the radial side and one along the ulnar side of extensor tendons.

Golden Facts to Remember

• All intrinsic muscles of the hand are supplied by ulnar nerve *except*	Muscles of thenar eminence and first two lumbricals
• *Life line* of palmistry in the hand	Radial longitudinal palmar crease
• Digit to which maximum number of muscles are attached	Thumb (eight muscles)
• Most fixed digit in hand	Middle finger
• Musician's nerve	Ulnar nerve
• Most prominent feature on the dorsum of hand	Dorsal venous network
• Cricketer's finger/ baseball finger	Flexion deformity of the finger
• Trigger finger	Locking of finger in full flexion
• Eye of the hand/ peripheral eye	Median nerve

CLINICAL CASE STUDY

A 27-year-old dental student while going to the college fell from the motorcycle with an outstretched right hand. He got up and went to the college to attend his classes. In the class, he felt pain in his right wrist. He went to emergency department for check-up. The resident doctor over there, on examination, noticed tenderness in the region of anatomical snuff box of his right hand. The X-ray of hand did not reveal any fracture. The doctor made a diagnosis of sprained wrist. The elastic bandage was applied around the wrist and sent back. Three weeks later the student was still experiencing pain on moving his hand. He went to a senior orthopaedic surgeon, who after careful examination, made a diagnosis of **fracture of the right scaphoid bone**.

Questions

1. Name the carpal bones which form the floor of anatomical snuff box.
2. Why fracture of scaphoid bone was wrongly diagnosed as sprained wrist?
3. The scaphoid bone is prone to avascular necrosis after its fracture. Why?
4. Why scaphoid bone is difficult to immobilize?

Answers

1. Scaphoid and trapezium.
2. In fracture of scaphoid, the X-ray examination often does not reveal fracture immediately after injury because displacement of fractured segments does not occur.
3. The scaphoid bone most commonly fractures through its narrow part called *waist*. The proximal segment undergoes avascular necrosis because it receives its arterial supply through the distal part of the bone, which is severed during fracture.
4. Because of its position and small size.

CHAPTER 12

Wrist Joint, Joints of the Hand, and Movements of the Hand

SPECIFIC LEARNING OBJECTIVES

After studying this chapter, the student should be able to:

- Give brief description of wrist joint and first carpometacarpal joint under following headings: (a) type of joint, (b) articular surfaces (c) ligaments, and (d) movements and muscles producing them. AN 13.3
- Describe the carpometacarpal and metacarpophalangeal joints. AN 13.4
- Give brief account of first carpometacarpal joint.
- Describe and demonstrate the movements of thumb and muscles involved. AN 12.6

The hand is the region of the upper limb distal to the forearm. It consists of three parts: (a) Carpus (wrist), (b) metacarpus, and (c) digits.

The study of wrist joint and joints of hand is essential to understand the various movements of the hand. Of these, radiocarpal (wrist), mid-carpal, and first carpometacarpal joints need to be studied in detail as they execute wide range of movements.

N.B.

The radiocarpal and midcarpal joints together form the **wrist complex**.

WRIST JOINT (RADIOCARPAL JOINT) AN 13.3, AN 13.5

The joint between forearm and hand is called wrist joint.

TYPE

The wrist joint is a **synovial joint of ellipsoid variety** between lower end of radius and carpus (Fig. 12.1).

ARTICULAR SURFACES

1. **Proximal articular surface** is formed by *inferior surface of the lower end of radius* and *inferior surface of the triangular articular* disc of inferior radioulnar joint.
   This articular surface is almost elliptical in shape and concave from side to side.
2. **Distal articular surface** is formed by the proximal surfaces of scaphoid, lunate, and triquetral bones. It is smooth, oval and convex surface.

N.B.

- Although wrist joint is an articulation between forearm and hand, the medial bone of forearm—the ulna is excluded from this articulation by an articular disc.
- In the neutral position of the wrist, only the scaphoid and lunate are in contact with the radius and articular disc; the triquetral comes into contact with the articular disc only in the full adduction of the wrist.

The pisiform bone also does not participate in this articulation because it acts primarily as a sesamoid bone to increase the leverage of the flexor carpi ulnaris and lies in a plane anterior to the other carpal bones.

LIGAMENTS (FIG. 12.2)

1. **Capsular ligament (joint capsule):** It is the fibrous covering of the joint and is attached above to the distal ends of radius and ulna, and below to the proximal row of carpal bones.
2. **Synovial membrane:** It lines the inner surface of the fibrous capsule and extends up to the margins of the articular surfaces.
3. **Radial collateral ligament:** It extends from the tip of styloid process of radius to lateral aspects of the scaphoid and trapezium. It is related to the radial artery.
4. **Ulnar collateral ligament:** It extends from the tip of styloid process of ulna to the medial aspects of the triquetral and pisiform bones.
5. **Palmar radiocarpal ligament:** It extends from anterior margin of the lower end of radius to the anterior surfaces of the scaphoid, lunate, and triquetral bones. It is formed due to thickening of the lateral part of the anterior aspect of the fibrous capsule.
6. **Palmar ulnocarpal ligament:** It extends vertically downwards from the base of styloid process and adjoining part of articular disc to the anterior surface of the lunate and triquetral. It is formed due to thickening of the medial part of the anterior aspect of the fibrous capsule.

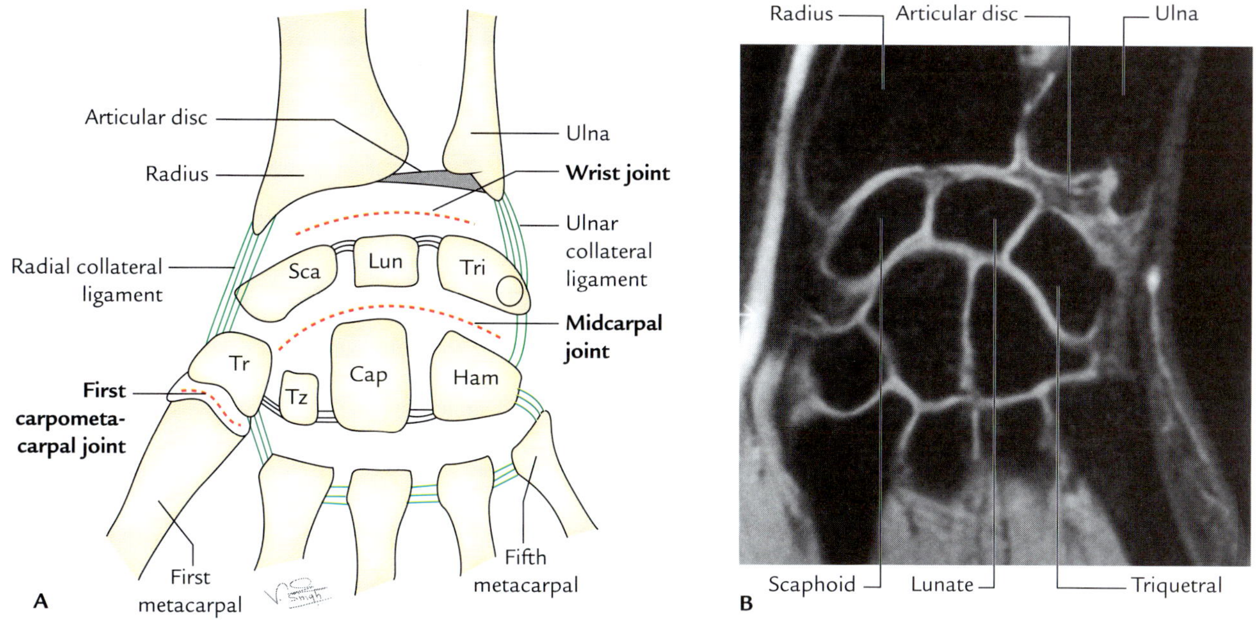

FIG. 12.1 Coronal section through wrist region: (**A**) schematic diagram; (**B**) as seen in magnetic resonance imaging, showing wrist joint, midcarpal joint, intercarpal joints, carpometacarpal joints. (*Source B: Gray's Anatomy for Students:* Richard L Drake, Wayne Vogl, Adam WM Mitchell, Fig. 7.91 C, Page 710, Elsevier Inc. 2005.)

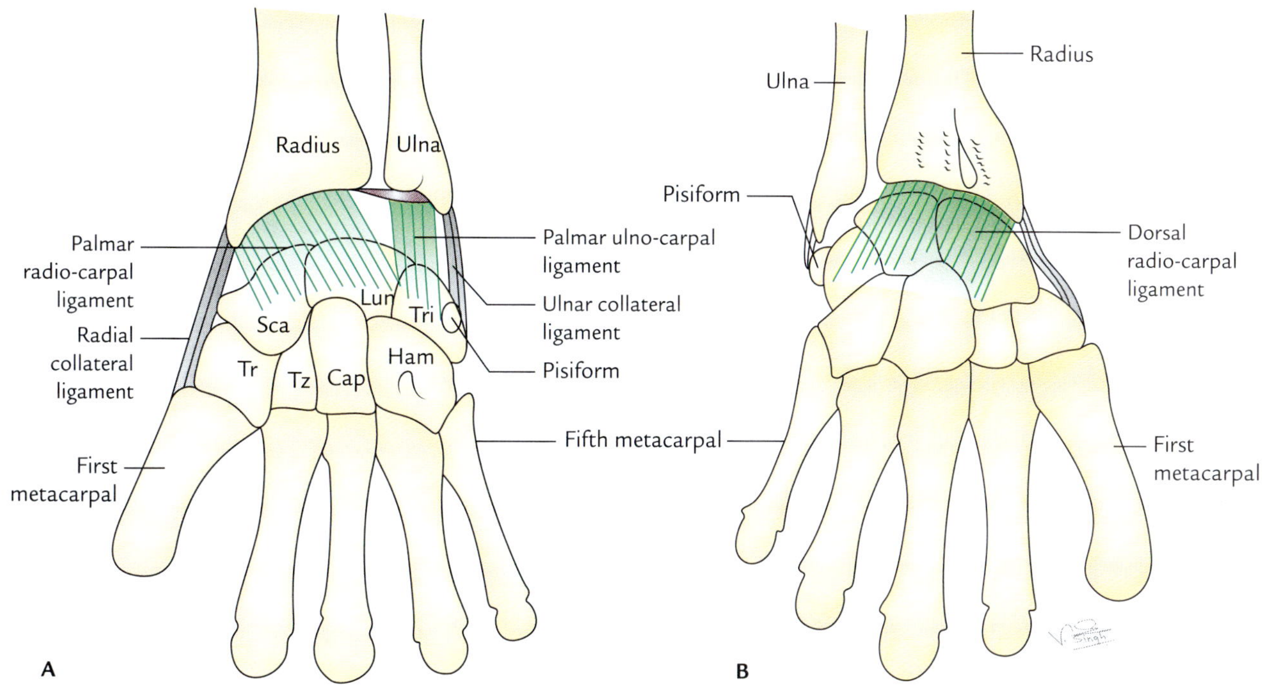

FIG. 12.2 Ligaments of the radiocarpal (wrist) joint: (**A**) palmar radiocarpal and ulnocarpal ligaments, (**B**) dorsal radiocarpal ligaments.

7. **Dorsal radiocarpal ligament:** It extends downwards and medially from the posterior margin of the lower end of radius to the dorsal surface of the scaphoid, lunate, and triquetral bones.

N.B.

The strongest bonds of union of wrist joint are ulnar and radial collateral ligaments.

RELATIONS (FIG. 12.3)

Anterior

1. Tendons of flexor digitorum superficialis (FDS), flexor digitorum profundus (FDP), and associated synovial sheath (ulnar bursa).
2. Tendon of flexor pollicis longus (FPL) and associated synovial sheath (radial bursa).
3. Median nerve.

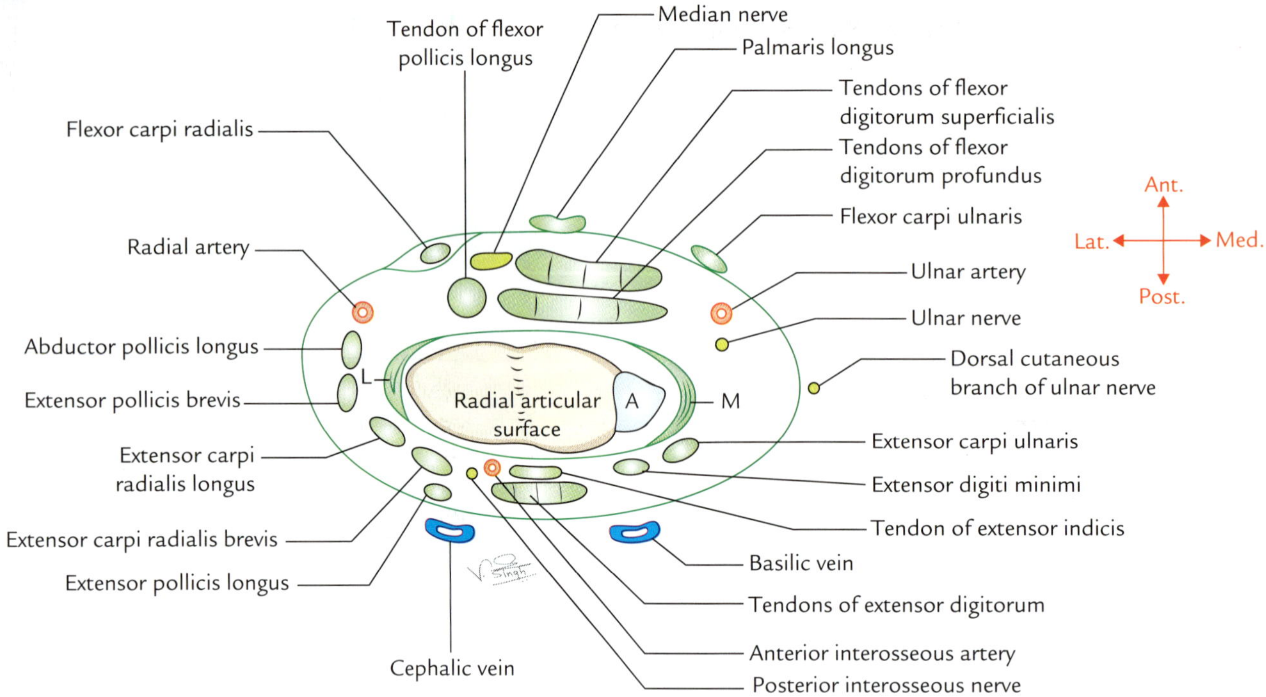

FIG. 12.3 Relations of the right wrist joint [A = articular disc, M = medial (ulnar) collateral ligament, L = lateral (radial) collateral ligament].

4. Tendon of flexor carpi radialis and associated synovial bursa.
5. Ulnar nerve and vessels.

Posterior

1. Extensor tendons of wrist and fingers, and associated synovial sheaths.
2. Anterior interosseous artery.
3. Posterior interosseous nerve.

Lateral

1. Radial artery (across the radial collateral ligament).
2. Tendon of abductor pollicis longus (APL).
3. Tendon of extensor pollicis brevis (EPB).

Medial

Dorsal cutaneous branch of ulnar nerve.

Movements

It is a **biaxial joint** and permits the following movements:

1. Flexion.
2. Extension.
3. Abduction.
4. Adduction.
5. Circumduction.

Flexion and extension occur along the *transverse axis*, and abduction and adduction occur along the *anteroposterior axis*.

N.B.

- The movements at the wrist joint are usually associated with movements at the **midcarpal joint** (joint between the proximal and distal rows of carpal bones). The wrist and midcarpal joints together are considered as *link joint*.
- Rotation is not possible at the wrist joint because the articular surfaces are ellipsoid in shape. The lack of rotation at wrist is compensated by the movements of pronation and supination of the forearm.
- The **wrist complex** consists of radiocarpal joint and midcarpal joint.

The movements at the wrist joint and muscles producing them are listed in Table 12.1 and Flowchart 12.1.

TABLE 12.1 Movements at the wrist joint and muscles producing them

Movement	Muscles
Flexion (upward bending of the wrist)	• Flexor carpi radialis (FCR) • Flexor carpi ulnaris (FCU) • Palmaris longus (PL)
Extension (backward bending of the wrist)	• Extensor carpi radialis longus (ECRL) • Extensor carpi radialis brevis (ECRB) • Extensor carpi ulnaris (ECU)
Abduction (lateral bending of the wrist)	• Flexor carpi radialis (FCR) • Extensor carpi radialis longus (ECRL) • Extensor carpi radialis brevis (ECRB) • Abductor pollicis longus (APL)
Adduction (medial bending of the wrist)	• Flexor carpi ulnaris (FCU) • Extensor carpi ulnaris (ECU)

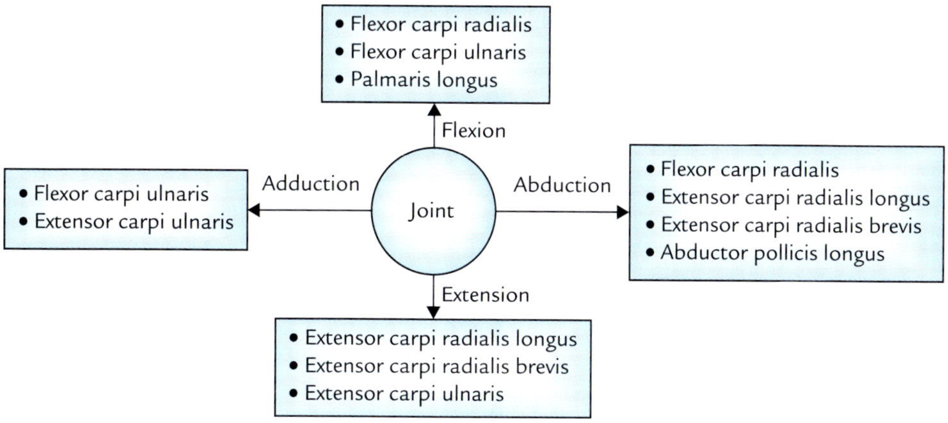

FLOWCHART 12.1 ■ Muscles producing various movements of the wrist.

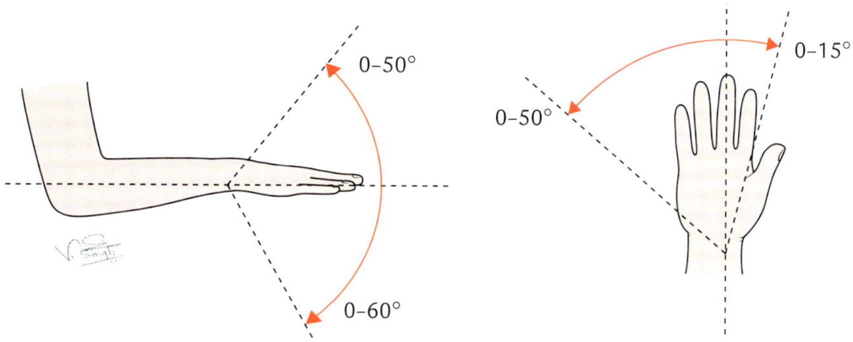

FIG. 12.4 ■ Range of movements of the wrist joint.

N.B.

- Flexion is assisted by long flexor tendons of digits (e.g. FDS, FDP, and FPL). It occurs more at the midcarpal joint than at the wrist joint.
- Extension is assisted by extensors of the digits (e.g. extensor digitorum, extensor digiti minimi, and extensor indicis). It occurs more at wrist than at midcarpal joint.
- Abduction occurs more at midcarpal joint than the wrist joint.
- Adduction mainly occurs at wrist joint.
- Flexion and extension of the hand are actually initiated at the midcarpal joint.

Range of Movements

The range of movements (ROM) of the wrist joint is given in the box below (Fig. 12.4):

Range of movements of the wrist joint

Movement	Range
Flexion	0°–60°
Extension	0°–50°
Abduction	0°–15°
Adduction	0°–50°

CLINICAL CORRELATION

Colles' fracture: It is fracture distal end of radius. For details see page 25, Chapter 2.

- Superficial positions of nerves, vessels, and tendons at wrist make them exceedingly vulnerable to injury.
- **Ganglion** (*Gk* = swelling or knot): It is a nontender cystic swelling which sometimes appears on wrist most commonly on its dorsal aspect (Fig. 12.5). Its size varies from a small grape to a plum. It usually occurs due to mucoid degeneration of synovial sheath around the tendon. The cyst is thin walled and contains clear mucinous fluid. The flexion of wrist makes the cyst to enlarge and it may become painful.
- **Aspiration of the wrist joint:** It is usually done by introducing the needle posteriorly, immediately below the

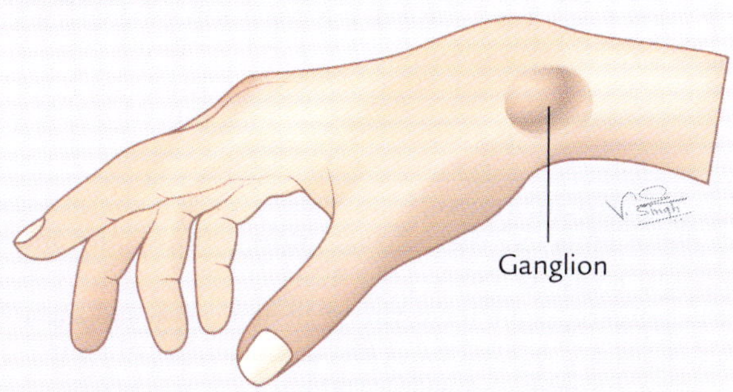

FIG. 12.5 ■ Ganglion on the dorsal aspect of wrist.

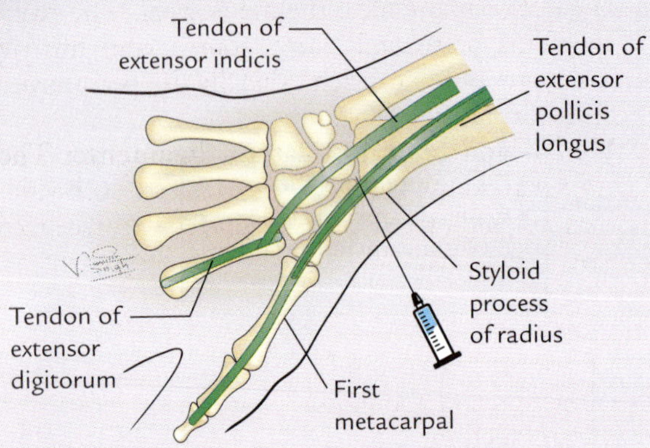

FIG. 12.6 Aspiration of wrist joint.

styloid process of radius between the tendons of extensor pollicis longus and extensor indicis (Fig. 12.6).

- **Immobilization of the wrist joint:** The wrist joint is immobilized in its optimum position of 30° dorsiflexion.
- **Osteoarthritis and rheumatoid arthritis** commonly involves wrist and interphalangeal joints. They are the common cause of pain and swellings in hand.

JOINTS OF THE HAND AN 13.4

The joints of hand are as follows:

1. Intercarpal joints.
2. Midcarpal joint.
3. Carpometacarpal joints.
4. Intermetacarpal joints.

Intercarpal joints: These are plane type of synovial joints which interconnect the carpal bones. They include the following joints:

a. Joints between the carpal bones of the proximal row.
b. Joints between the carpal bones of the distal row.

(*Pisotriquetral joint* formed between pisiform and palmar surface of triquetral bone.)

Midcarpal joint between the proximal and distal rows of the carpal bones.

Carpometacarpal joints: The carpometacarpal joints are plane type of synovial joints except for the carpometacarpal joint of the thumb, which is a saddle joint. The distal surfaces of the carpals of distal row articulate with the bases of metacarpals. Functionally and clinically, first carpometacarpal joint is the most important carpometacarpal joint and hence described in detail later.

Intermetacarpal joints: These are plane type of synovial joints and formed by the articulation of the bases of adjacent metacarpals of the fingers.

N.B.

Joint cavities of intercarpal, carpometacarpal, and intermetacarpal joints: These are the following three joint cavities among the above-mentioned joints (Fig. 12.1):

1. A continuous common cavity of all intercarpal and metacarpal joints, except that of first carpometacarpal joint.
2. Cavity of first carpometacarpal joint.
3. Cavity of pisotriquetral joint.

TABLE 12.2 Movements at the intercarpal, carpometacarpal (except first), metacarpophalangeal, and interphalangeal joints

Joints	Movements
• Intercarpal (IC) joints	Gliding movements
• Carpometacarpal (CM) joints	
– CM joint of thumb	– Freely mobile
– CM joints of second and third fingers	– Almost no moment
– CM joint of fourth finger	– Slightly mobile
– CM joint of fifth finger	– Moderately mobile

Movements of the intercarpal and carpometacarpal joints are listed in Table 12.2.

FIRST CARPOMETACARPAL JOINT (FIG. 12.1) AN 13.3

Type

It is synovial joint of saddle variety.

Articular Surfaces

Proximal: Distal surface of the trapezium.

Distal: Proximal surface of the base of first metacarpal.

Both proximal and distal articular surfaces are reciprocally concavo-convex; hence permit wide range of movements at this joint.

Ligaments

1. **Capsular ligament (joint capsule):** It is thick loose fibrous sac which encloses the joint cavity. It is attached proximally to the margins of articular surface of the trapezium and distally to the circumference of the base of first metacarpal bone. The inner surface of the capsule is lined by the *synovial membrane*.
2. **Lateral ligament:** It is a broad fibrous band stretching from lateral surface of the trapezium to the lateral side of the base of first metacarpal bone.
3. **Anterior (palmar) ligament:** It extends obliquely from palmar surface of trapezium to the ulnar side of the base of first metacarpal.
4. **Posterior (dorsal) ligament:** It also extends obliquely from dorsal surface of trapezium to the ulnar side of the base of first metacarpal.

Relations

The joints are surrounded by various muscles and tendons of the thumb. In addition, it is related to:

(a) Radial artery on its posteromedial sides.
(b) First dorsal interosseous muscle on its medial side.

Blood Supply

By radial artery.

Nerve Supply

By median nerve.

Movements

The various movements which take place at the first carpometacarpal joint are as follows:

1. Flexion and extension.
2. Abduction and adduction.
3. Opposition.
4. Medial and lateral rotation.
5. Circumduction.

The various movements of thumb at first carpometacarpal joint are described in detail on pages 167 to 169.

JOINTS OF THE DIGITS (FIG. 12.7)

The joints of digits are as follows:

1. Metacarpophalangeal joints.
2. Interphalangeal joints.

METACARPOPHALANGEAL (MP) JOINTS (FIG. 12.7A)

Type: They are synovial joints of ellipsoid/condylar variety.

Articular surfaces: They are formed by heads of metacarpals and bases of proximal phalanges.

Ligaments

1. **Palmar ligaments:** The palmar ligament is a fibrocartilaginous plate which is more firmly attached to the phalanx than to the metacarpal. The palmar ligaments of second, third, fourth, and fifth MP joints are joined to each other by **deep transverse metacarpal ligament**.
2. **Medial and lateral collateral ligaments:** These are cord-like fibrous bands present on each side of the joint and extend from head of metacarpal to the base of phalanx.

Movements

- Flexion and extension
- Adduction and abduction
- Circumduction
- Limited rotation

INTERPHALANGEAL (IP) JOINTS (FIG. 12.7B)

Both proximal and distal IP (PIP and DIP) joints are synovial joints of hinge variety. Their structure is similar to that of MP joints.

Movements

Flexion and extension

MOVEMENTS OF THE HAND

To perform the various movements, the hand adopts a specific posture. Hence, students must first understand the positions of hand at rest and during function.

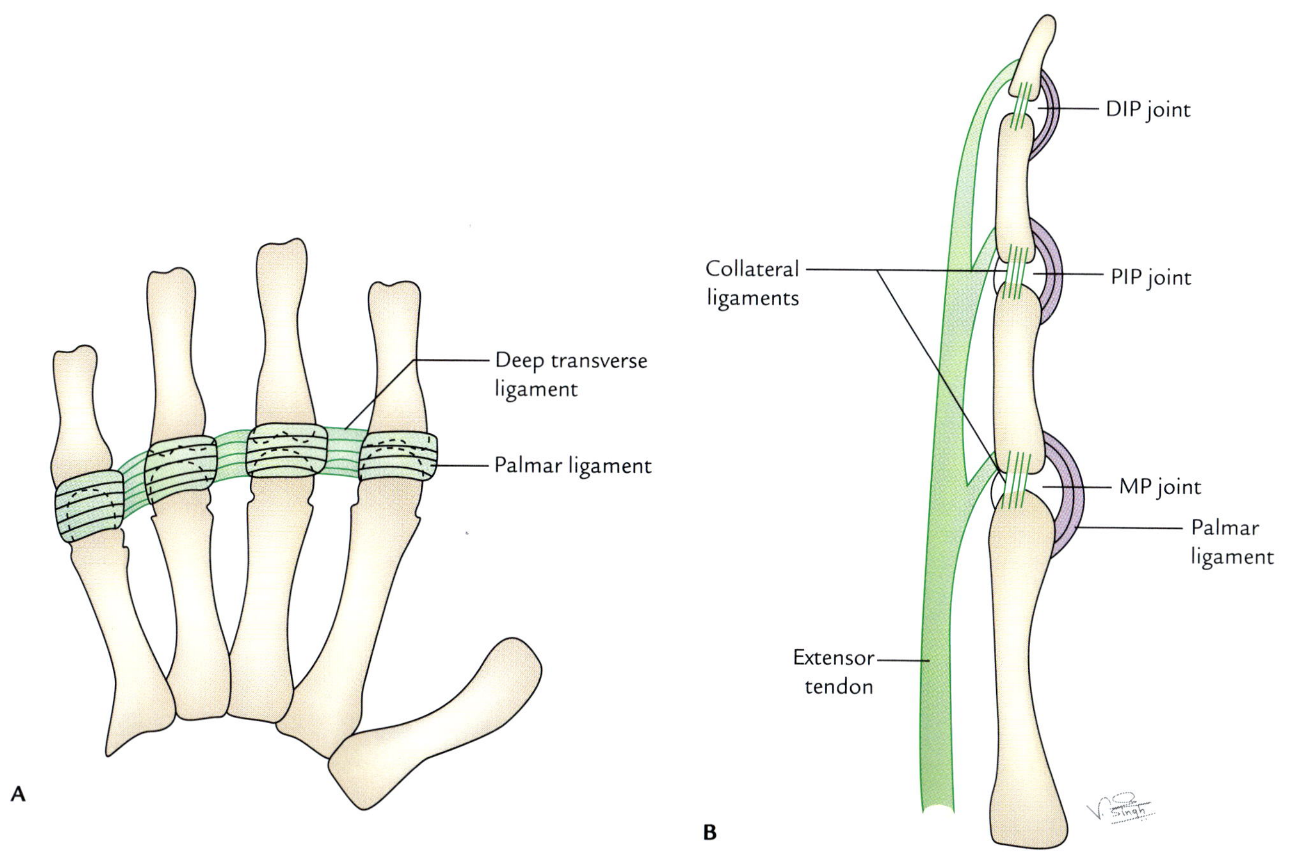

FIG. 12.7 Joints of the fingers: (**A**) MP joints showing palmar and deep transverse ligaments; (**B**) MP, PIP, and DIP joints showing palmar and collateral ligaments (DIP = distal interphalangeal, PIP = proximal interphalangeal, MP = metacarpophalangeal).

POSITION OF THE HAND

Position of the Hand at Rest (Fig. 12.8)

It is the posture adopted by the hand when it is at rest (i.e. not performing any action).

The characteristic features of this position are as follows:

1. Forearm is in semiprone position.
2. Wrist joint is slightly extended.
3. Fingers are partially flexed (index finger is not flexed as much as the other fingers).
4. Plane of thumb nail is at right angle to the plane of finger nails.

Position of Hand During Function (Fig. 12.9)

It is the posture adopted by hand when it is going to grasp an object between the thumb and index finger. The characteristic features of this position are as follows:

1. Forearm is in semiprone position.
2. Wrist joint is slightly extended (more than that in position of rest).
3. All the fingers, including index finger, are partially flexed.
4. Thumb is rotated in such a way that the plane of thumb nail lies parallel with that of index finger and pulps of thumb and index finger are in contact.

N.B.

- Forearm bones are most stable when the forearm is in midprone position.
- When the wrist is partially extended: (a) flexor and extensor tendons of digits work to their best mechanical advantage and (b) flexors and extensors of carpus provide a stable base for movements of the digits.

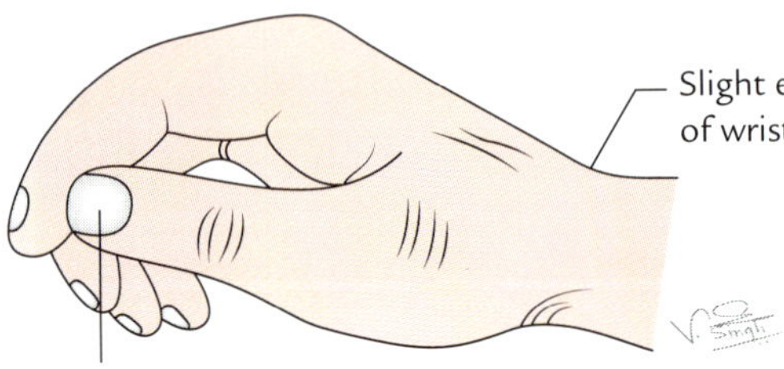

FIG. 12.8 ■ Position of the hand at rest.

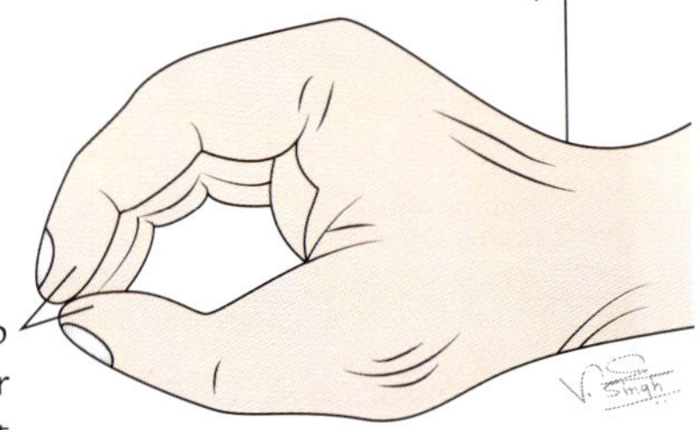

FIG. 12.9 ■ Position of the hand during function.

CLASSIFICATION OF MOVEMENTS OF THE HAND

The movements of hand are classified into the following two types:

1. Nonprehensile.
2. Prehensile.

Nonprehensile movements: These are the movements in which objects are manipulated by pushing, tapping, or lifting and involve movements of individual digits.

Prehensile movements (Fig. 12.10): These are of two types: (a) *precision grip* and (b) *power grip*. A third type called *hook grip* is used to suspend or pull the objects.

These movements are used for transmission of forces and not for skilled manipulation.

To understand the functions of hand, we must know about arches of hand and functional components of hand.

ARCHES OF THE HAND (FIG. 12.11)

Like foot, the hand also has arches. The hand is composed of a series of three flexible bony arches. Their preservation following an injury is of supreme functional importance to the hand.

The arches of the hand are as follows:

1. **Proximal transverse carpal arch:** It is formed by the concavity of the carpus with flexor retinaculum stretching between its pillars.
2. **Distal transverse metacarpal arch:** It is formed by the heads of the metacarpal bones, which are bound together by the deep transverse metacarpal ligaments.
3. **Longitudinal arches:** They formed by the palmar concavity of the metacarpals and associated phalanges of digits. Note slightly flexed posture of the digits. The axis of this arch is centred between second and third metacarpals. These arches are also called *longitudinal rays*.

Factors Maintaining Arches of Hand

These are as follows:

1. Palmar aponeurosis
2. Palmar metacarpal ligaments
3. Muscles of thenar and hypothenar eminences
4. Interossei
5. Long flexor tendons

Function of Arches

The arches of the hand provide room for grasping objects in the hollow of palm.

The more accentuated the arches are, the more secure is the grip. The thenar and hypothenar muscles and palmaris brevis play an important role in providing adjusting power of the arches.

CLINICAL CORRELATION

Abnormalities of arches of the hand: The disturbances of palmar arches result in flat *hand* with impairment of gripping power. The flattening *of carpal arch* seriously affects the gripping power of the thumb. It occurs due to surgical division of flexor retinaculum or injury to the carpus.

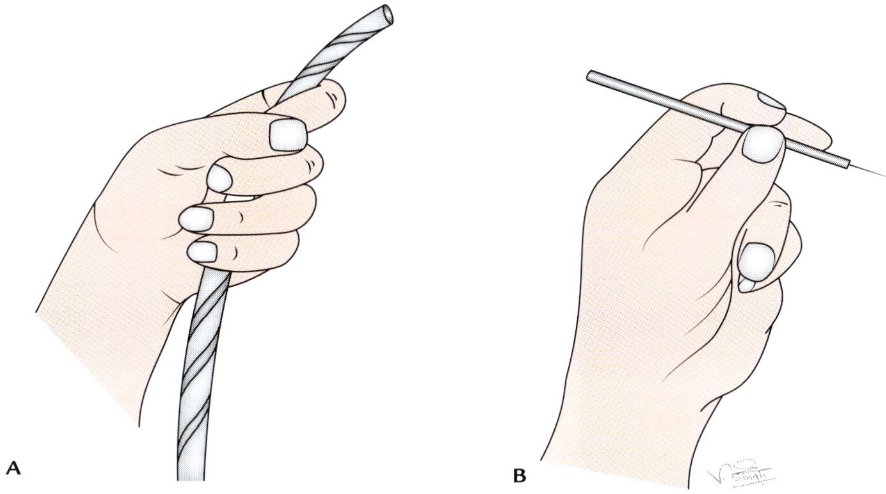

FIG. 12.10 ■ Prehensile movements of the hand: (**A**) power grip, (**B**) precision grip.

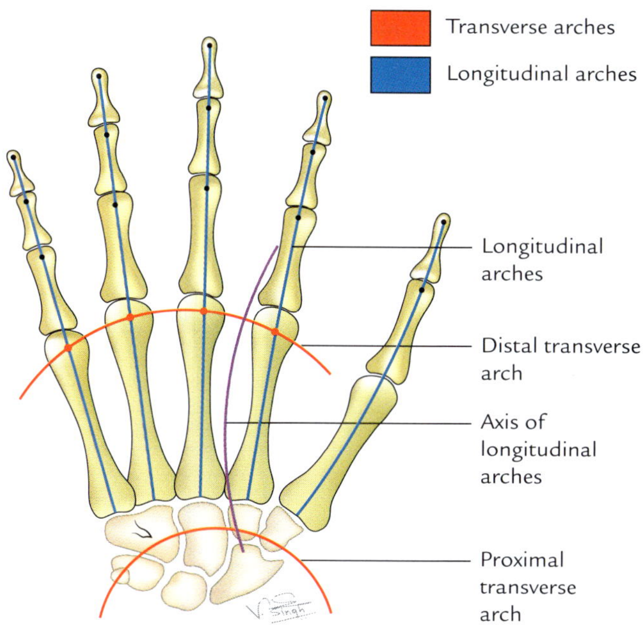

FIG. 12.11 ■ Arches of hand.

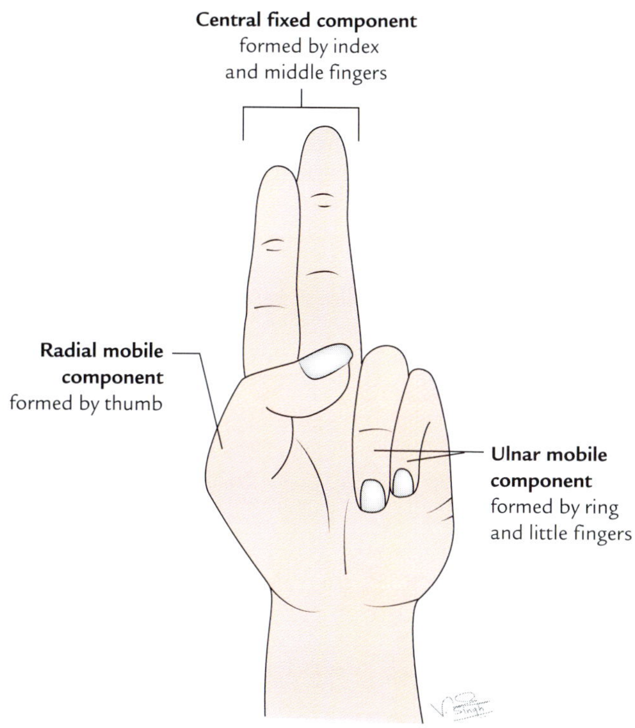

FIG. 12.12 ■ Functional components of the hand.

FUNCTIONAL COMPONENTS OF THE HAND

The hand consists of the following three functional components (Fig. 12.12):

1. Central fixed component.
2. Radial mobile component.
3. Ulnar mobile component.

The **central fixed component** is formed by the metacarpals of index and middle fingers.

The **mobile radial component** is formed by the thumb.

The **mobile ulnar component** is formed by the ring and little fingers.

N.B.

The *mobile radial component* (thumb) comes into play in precision manipulations against the index finger:

- The thumb, index finger, and middle finger together form the so-called *radial digital tripod.*
- The mobile ulnar component is termed *ulnar hook* which provides for stable power grip with palm or in 'hook grip'.
- The little finger is important for power grip whereas thumb is important for both power and precision grip.

MOVEMENTS OF THE THUMB **AN 12.6**

The metacarpal of the thumb (i.e. first metacarpal) does not lie in the same plane as the metacarpals of the fingers, but occupies a more anterior position (Fig. 12.13).

In addition, it is rotated medially through 90°, and as a result its extensor surface is directed laterally and not backwards. For this reason, the movements of the thumb occur in planes at right angles to the planes of the corresponding movements of the fingers. The movements of thumb occur at carpometacarpal, MP, and IP joints.

The movements at the carpometacarpal joint of thumb are much freer than that of any other finger.

The various movements of thumb are (Fig. 12.14):

1. Flexion.
2. Extension.
3. Abduction.
4. Adduction.
5. Opposition.
6. Circumduction.

The movements of thumb, plane of movements, and muscles producing them are enumerated in Table 12.3.

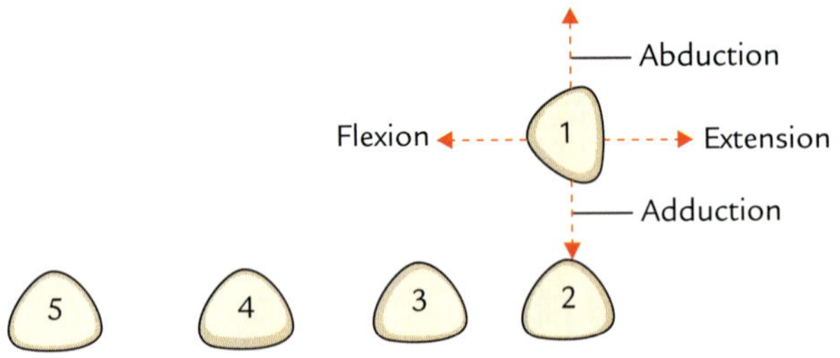

FIG. 12.13 ■ Position of the metacarpals.

N.B.

In addition to movements mentioned in Table 12.3, the following movements of thumb also take place:

- *Circumduction*, a combination of flexion, extension, abduction, and adduction.
- *Medial and lateral rotation* which occurs along the long axis. *Medial rotation* is produced by opponens and flexors and *lateral rotation* by extensors.

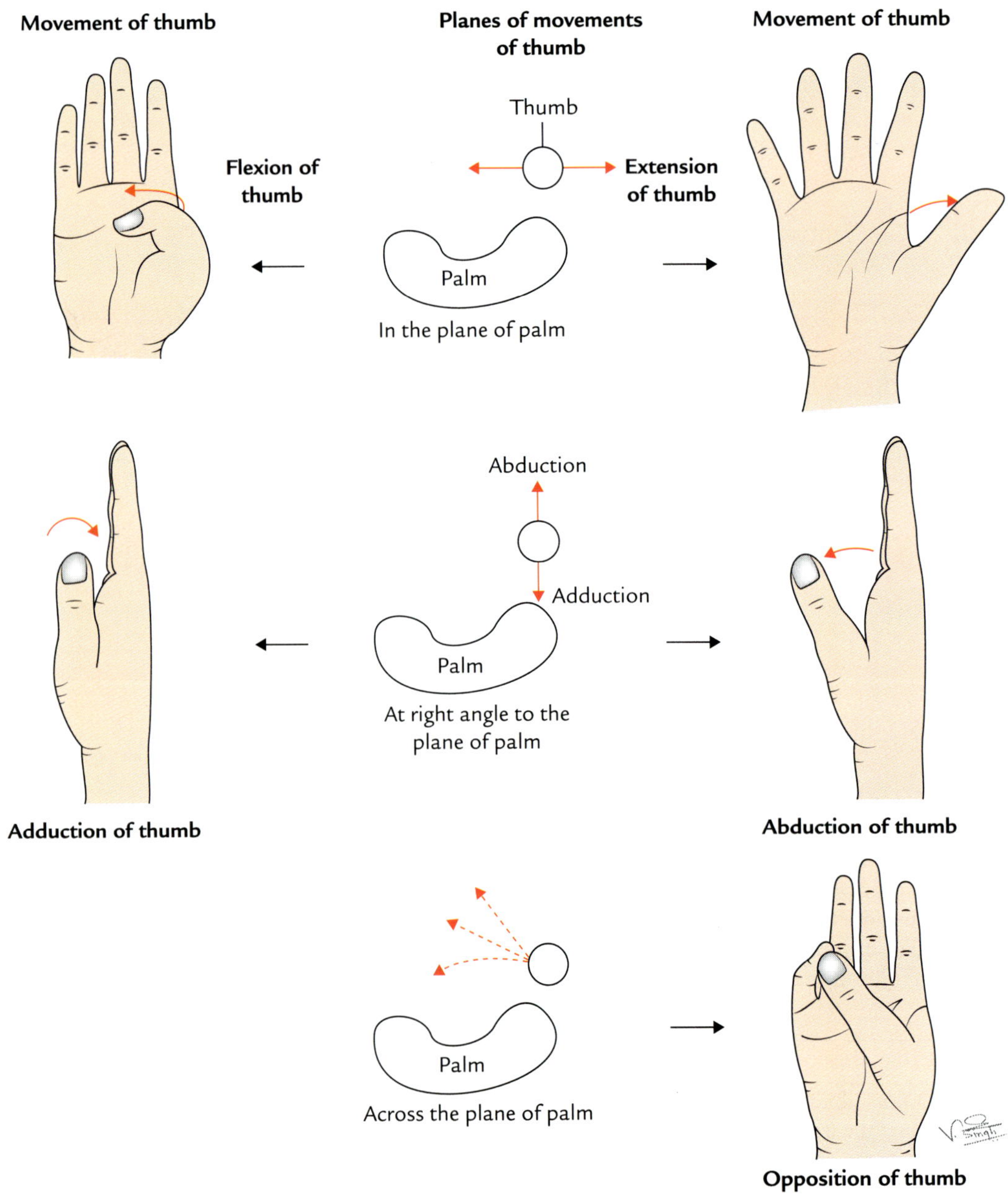

FIG. 12.14 ■ Movements of the thumb.

TABLE 12.3 Movements of the thumb, their plane, and muscles producing them

Movement	Plane of movement	Muscles producing movement
Flexion	Occurs in the plane of palm	• Flexor pollicis longus • Flexor pollicis brevis (FPB) • Opponens pollicis
Extension	Occurs in the plane of palm	• Extensor pollicis longus (EPL) • Extensor pollicis brevis (EPB)
Abduction	Occurs at right angle to the plane of palm (i.e. anteroposterior plane) away from palm	• Abductor pollicis longus (APL) • Abductor pollicis brevis (APB)
Adduction	Occurs at right angle to the plane of palm (i.e., anteroposterior plane) towards the palm	Adductor pollicis
Opposition	Occurs across the palm in such a manner that anterior surface of the tip of the thumb comes into contact with anterior surface of the tip of any other finger	Opponens pollicis

MOVEMENTS OF THE FINGERS

The movements of fingers occur at MP and proximal interphalangeal and distal interphalangeal (PIP and DIP) joints. The movements of fingers are as follows:

1. Flexion and extension.
2. Abduction and adduction.

The movements of finger are given in Table 12.4.

Flexion: It is a forward movement of fingers in the anteroposterior plane and occurs at MP, PIP, and DIP joints.

Extension: It is a backward movement of finger in the anteroposterior plane and occurs at MP, PIP, and DIP joints.

Abduction: It is an away movement of finger from the imaginary midline of the middle finger and occurs at MP joint.

Adduction: It is movement of fingers towards the imaginary midline of the middle finger and occurs at MP joint.

TABLE 12.4 Movements of the fingers and muscles producing them

Movement	Muscles producing them
Flexion	
• Flexion of proximal phalanx (MP joint)	• Lumbricals and interossei
• Flexion of middle phalanx (PIP joint)	• Flexor digitorum superficialis
• Flexion of distal phalanx (DIP joint)	• Flexor digitorum profundus
Extension	
• Extension of proximal phalanx (MP joint)	• Extensor digitorum (in addition by extensor indicis for index finger and extensor digiti minimi for little finger)
• Extension of middle and distal phalanges (PIP and DIP joints)	• Lumbricals and interossei
Abduction	Dorsal interossei (abductor digiti minimi abducts the little finger)
Adduction	• Palmar interossei

N.B.

The movements of abduction and adduction fingers are possible only when fingers are in extended position because in this position the collateral ligaments of MP joints are slack. In flexed position of fingers the collateral ligaments of MP joint are taut.

The movements of fingers and muscles producing them are given in Table 12.4.

CLINICAL CORRELATION

- **Position of immobilization** (Fig. 12.15): The collateral ligaments of the MP and IP joints extend from the side of the head of proximal bone to the side of base of the distal bone. The ligaments of MP joints are on full stretch only when the joint is fully flexed to 90°; on the other hand, ligaments of IP joint are stretched/taut only when the joint is fully extended. This knowledge is of vital importance when immobilizing the hand because contracture of the joints occurs within 2 weeks, if the joints are immobilized when the ligaments are lax/slack. Then the shortening of ligaments will cause irreversible joint contractures. Therefore, the position of immobilization of hand should be such that the MP joints are fully flexed and the IP joints are fully extended.

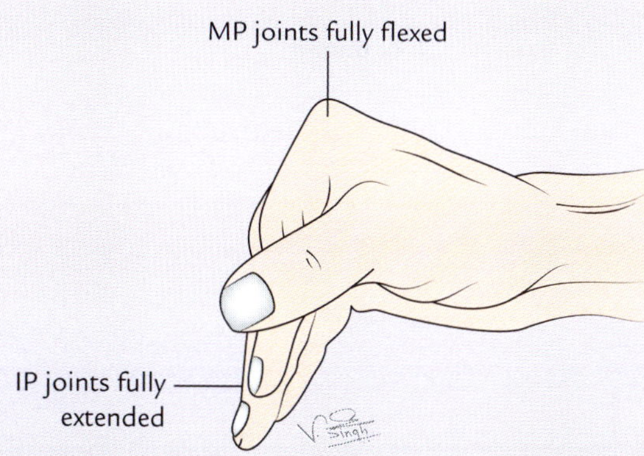

FIG. 12.15 Position of immobilization (MP = metacarpophalangeal joint, IP = interphalangeal joint).

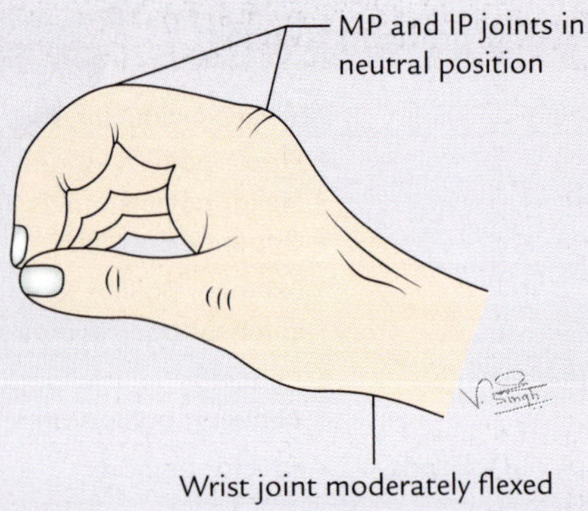

FIG. 12.16 Position of arthrodesis (MP = metacarpophalangeal joint, IP = interphalangeal joint).

- **Position of arthrodesis*** (Fig. 12.16): The position of arthrodesis is one in which wrist joint is moderately dorsiflexed (15°–20°), and the MP and IP joints are set in neutral position.

*__Arthrodesis__ is a surgical procedure consisting of the obliteration of a joint space by doing bony fusion so that no movement can occur at the joint.

Golden Facts to Remember

• Wrist joint complex consists of	Radiocarpal and midcarpal joints
• Most important carpometacarpal joint	First carpometacarpal joint
• Position of forearm in which forearm bones are most stable	Midprone position
• All fingers are abducted by dorsal interossei *except*	Little finger, which is abducted by abductor digiti minimi
• Palmar interossei are attached on all the metacarpals *except*	Third metacarpal (metacarpal of middle finger)
• Axis of movements of adduction and abduction of fingers	Passes through middle finger
• Most important movement of thumb	Opposition

CLINICAL CASE STUDY

An elderly man fell on the road with an outstretched right hand while trying to get into the moving bus. He developed localized pain and swelling on the dorsal aspect of his right wrist. He was taken to the nearby hospital, where on examination, the doctors observed a typical dinner fork deformity in the right hand. The X-ray of the region revealed a fracture of distal end of radius with posterior displacement of the distal fragment. A diagnosis of **Colles' fracture** was made.

Questions

1. What is Colles' fracture and how does it differ from Smith's fracture?
2. Which nerve is likely to be injured in Colles' fracture?
3. What is the position of styloid processes of radius and ulna before and after fracture?

Answers

1. It is the fracture of distal end of radius, about 1 in proximal to the wrist joint with posterior displacement of the distal fragment. If the distal fragment is displaced anteriorly, it is called *Smith's fracture* (Fig. 2.16, p. 26).
2. Median nerve.
3. Before fracture (i.e. in normal state) the tip of styloid process of radius lies about 2 cm distal to that of ulna but after fracture, the tips of styloid processes of radius and ulna come to lie at the same level due to shortening of radius as its distal fragment gets displaced proximally.

CHAPTER 13

Major Nerves of the Upper Limb

SPECIFIC LEARNING OBJECTIVES

After studying this chapter, the student should be able to:

- Describe the origin, course, and distribution of: (a) radial nerve, (b) median nerve, and (c) ulnar nerve. AN 11.2
- Give the anatomical basis of **Saturday night paralysis** and **wrist drop.** AN 11.4, AN 12.13
- Write short notes on: (a) axillary nerve, (b) musculocutaneous nerve, and (c) ulnar nerve in hand.
- Give the anatomical basis of: (a) extension of elbow is possible following lesion of radial nerve in spiral groove, how? (b) carpal tunnel syndrome, and (c) complete claw hand. AN 12.4, AN 12.8

The nerve supply to the upper limb is provided by the **brachial plexus** (described in detail in Chapter 4, page 54).

The five major nerves supplying the upper limb are as follows:

1. Axillary nerve.
2. Musculocutaneous nerve.
3. Radial nerve.
4. Median nerve.
5. Ulnar nerve.

The study of five major nerves of the upper limb should be studied thoroughly and carefully because of their frequent involvement in various injuries and peripheral neuropathies.

AXILLARY NERVE (FIG. 13.1)

The axillary nerve (C5 and C6) arises from posterior cord of brachial plexus. It provides motor innervation to the deltoid and teres minor muscles and sensory innervation to the shoulder joint and to the skin over the lower lateral part of the shoulder (**regimental badge area**). The branches of axillary nerve are shown in Fig. 13.1 (for details see Chapter 5, page 71).

MUSCULOCUTANEOUS NERVE (FIG. 13.2)

The **musculocutaneous nerve** arises from lateral cord of the brachial plexus (C5, C6, and C7). It provides motor innervation to the muscles on the front of the arm and sensory innervation to the skin of the lateral aspect of the forearm. The overview of motor and sensory innervation musculocutaneous nerve is given in the box below (for details see Chapter 8, page 95).

Musculocutaneous nerve (C5, C6, and C7) innervation

Motor innervation:
- Biceps brachii
- Coracobrachialis
- Brachialis

Cutaneous/sensory innervation:
Lateral aspect of forearm.

N.B.

Musculocutaneous innervations in arm is purely motor while in forearm is purely sensory.

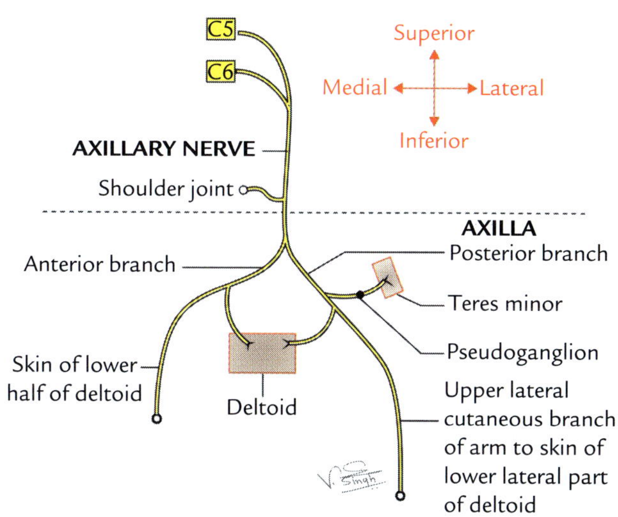

FIG. 13.1 ■ Course and distribution of the axillary nerve.

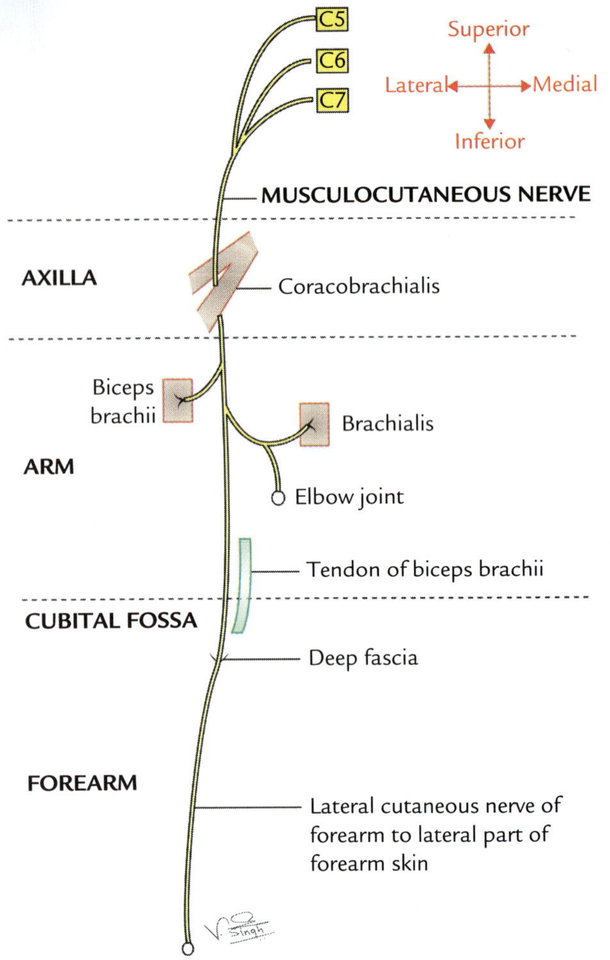

FIG. 13.2 ■ Course and distribution of the musculocutaneous nerve.

RADIAL NERVE (FIG. 13.3)

The radial nerve is the continuation of posterior cord of brachial plexus in the axilla. It is the *largest nerve of the upper limb and largest branch of brachial plexus*. It carries fibres from all the roots (C5, C6, C7, C8, and T1) of brachial plexus (but T1 fibres are not constant).

- **In the axilla**, the radial nerve lies posterior to the third part of the axillary artery and anterior to the muscles forming the posterior wall of the axilla.

In the axilla, it gives off the following three branches:

1. *Posterior cutaneous nerve of arm* (which provides sensory innervation to skin on the back of the arm up to the elbow).
2. *Nerve to the long head of triceps.*
3. *Nerve to the medial head of triceps.*

- **In the arm**, the radial nerve enters the arm at the lower border of the teres major. It passes between the long and medial heads of triceps to enter the lower triangular space, through which it reaches the spiral groove along with profunda brachii artery. The radial nerve in the spiral groove lies in direct contact with the humerus.

N.B.

Boundaries of the spiral groove:

Anteriorly: Middle one-third of the shaft of humerus.
Above: Origin of the lateral head of triceps.
Below: Origin of the medial head of triceps.
Posteriorly: Fibres of lateral and long head of triceps.

- **In the spiral groove**, it gives off the following five branches:
  1. *Lower lateral cutaneous nerve of the arm*, which provides sensory innervation to the skin on the lateral surface of the arm up to the elbow.
  2. *Posterior cutaneous nerve of the forearm*, which provides sensory innervation to the skin down the middle of the back of the forearm up to the wrist.
  3. Nerve to lateral head of triceps.
  4. *Nerve to medial head of triceps.*
  5. *Nerve to anconeus* (it runs through the substance of medial head of triceps to reach the anconeus).

At the lower end of the spiral groove, the radial nerve pierces the lateral intermuscular septum of the arm and enters the anterior compartment of the arm. Here, it first descends between the brachialis and brachioradialis, and then between brachialis and extensor carpi radialis longus before entering the cubital fossa.

- **In the anterior compartment of arm** above the lateral epicondyle, it gives off the following three branches:
  1. Nerve to brachialis (small lateral part).
  2. Nerve to brachioradialis.
  3. Nerve to extensor carpi radialis longus (ECRL).
- **In the forearm:** Radial nerve enters the forearm by passing anterior to lateral epicondyle.

At the level of lateral epicondyle of humerus, it *terminates by dividing into superficial and deep branches* in the lateral part of the cubital fossa.

The **deep branch** is motor. In the cubital fossa it supplies two muscles, namely:

1. Extensor carpi radialis brevis.
2. Supinator.

After supplying these two muscles, it passes through the substance of supinator and enters the posterior compartment of the forearm as **posterior interosseous nerve** and supplies all the other extensor muscles of the forearm. It also gives articular branches to the *distal radioulnar, wrist*, and *carpal joints*.

The **superficial branch** (also called **superficial radial nerve**) is sensory. It runs downwards over the supinator, pronator teres, and flexor digitorum superficialis deep to brachioradialis. About one-third of the way down the forearm (at about 7 cm above wrist), it passes posteriorly, emerging from under the tendon of brachioradialis, proximal to the styloid process of radius and then passes over the tendons of anatomical snuff box, where it terminates as cutaneous branches which provide sensory innervation to skin over the lateral part of the dorsum of hand and dorsal surfaces of lateral 3½ digits proximal to the nail beds.

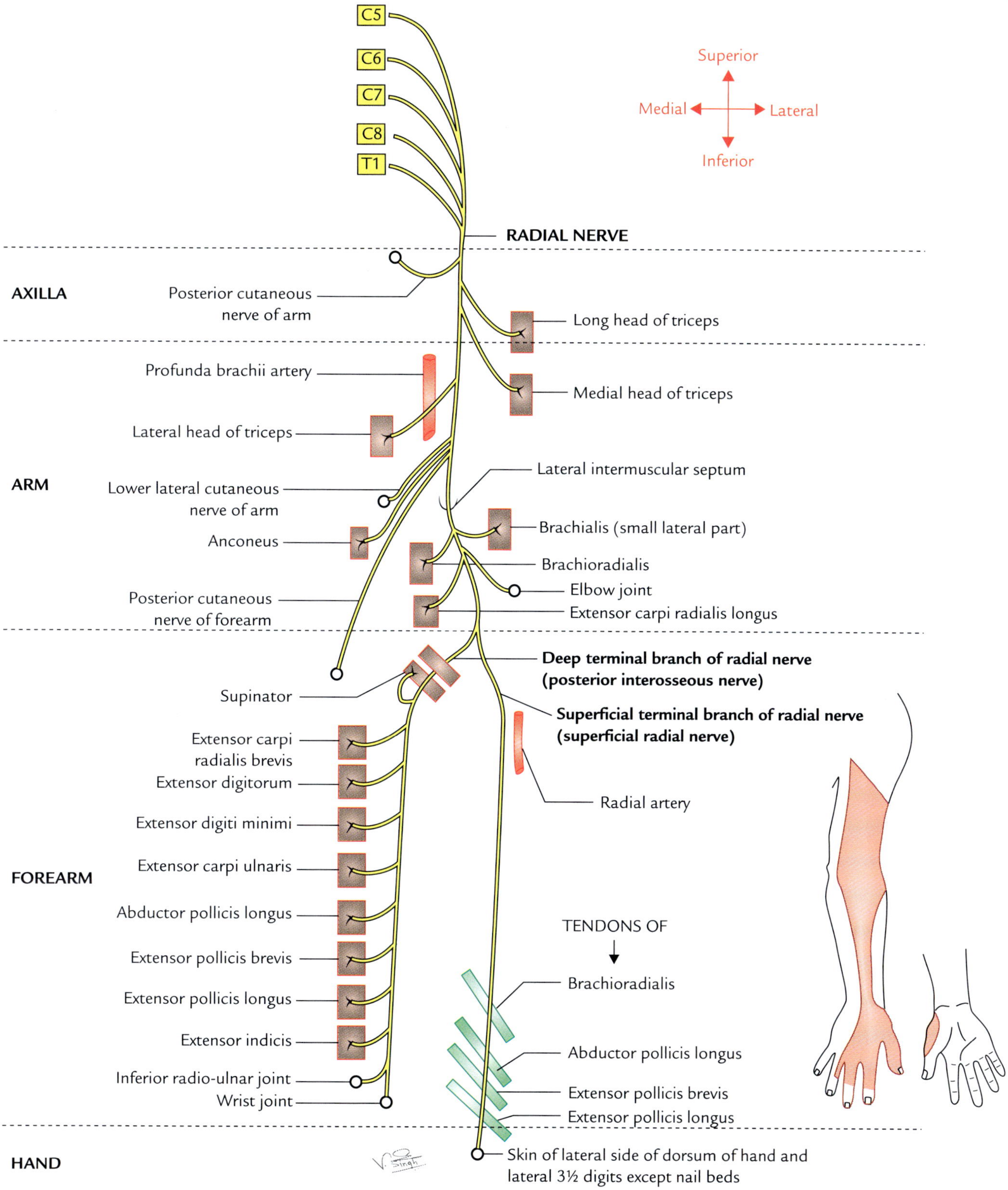

FIG. 13.3 ■ Course, branches, and motor innervations of the radial nerve. Figure on the right lower part shows its sensory (cutaneous) distribution (coloured areas).

The overview of motor and sensory of radial nerve is summarized in the box below.

Radial nerve (C5-T1) innervation

Motor innervation

Triceps brachii
Anconeus
Brachialis (Lat. part)
Brachioradialis
Extensor carpi radialis longus
Extensor carpi radialis brevis
Supinator
Extensor digitorum
Extensor digiti minimi
Extensor indicis
Extensor carpi ulnaris
Abductor pollicis longus
Extensor pollicis longus
Extensor pollicis brevis

} All the muscles on the back of arm and forearm

Cutaneous/sensory innervation

Posterior surface of arm and forearm, lateral two-thirds of dorsum of hand lateral to the axial line of ring finger (Fig. 13.3).

CLINICAL CORRELATION AN 11.4, AN 12.13

Injuries of the radial nerve: The radial nerve may be injured at three sites: (a) in the axilla, (b) in the spiral groove, and (c) at the elbow.

A. **Injury of radial nerve in the axilla:**
In the axilla, the radial nerve may be injured by the pressure of the upper end of crutch (crutch palsy).
Characteristic clinical features in such cases will be as follows:
Motor loss:
- Loss of extension of elbow—due to paralysis of triceps.
- Loss of extension of wrist (wrist drop)—due to paralysis of wrist extensors. This causes **wrist drop** due to unopposed action of flexor muscles of the forearm (Fig. 13.4).
- Loss of extension of digits—due to paralysis of extensor digitorum, extensor indicis, extensor digiti minimi, and extensor pollicis longus.

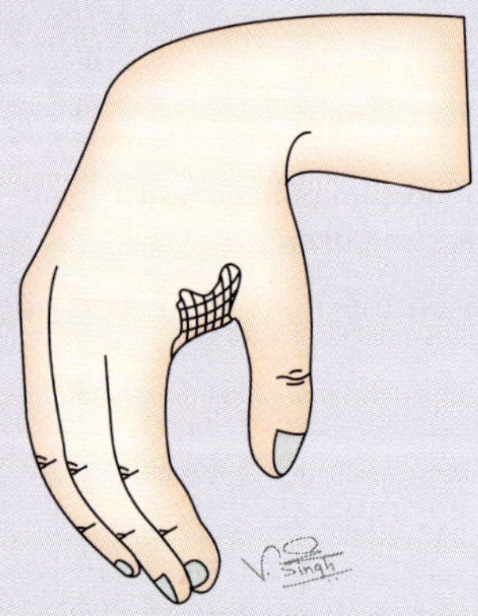

FIG. 13.4 ■ Wrist drop resulting from radial nerve injury.

- Loss of supination in extended elbow because supinator and brachioradialis are paralyzed but supination becomes possible in flexed elbow by the action of biceps brachii.

Sensory loss:
- Sensory loss on small area of skin over the posterior surface of the lower part of the arm.
- Sensory loss along narrow strip on the back of forearm.
- Sensory loss on the lateral part of dorsum of hand at the base of thumb and dorsal surface of lateral 3½ digits except over distal phalanges. More often, there is an isolated sensory loss on the dorsum of hand at the base of the thumb (Fig. 13.5).

B. **Injury of radial nerve in the radial/spiral groove:**
In radial groove, the radial nerve may be injured due to:
(a) Midshaft fracture of humerus,
(b) Inadvertently wrongly placed intramuscular injection, and
(c) Direct pressure on radial nerve by a drunkard falling asleep with his one arm over the back of the chair (**Saturday night paralysis**; Fig. 13.6).

Injury to radial nerve occurs most commonly in the distal part of the groove beyond the origin of nerve to triceps and cutaneous nerves.
Characteristic clinical features in such cases will be as follows:
Motor loss:
- Loss of extension of the wrist and fingers.
- Wrist drop.
- Loss of supination when the arm is extended.

Sensory loss: It is restricted only to a variable small area over the dorsum of hand between the first and second metacarpals.

N.B.

Extension of the elbow is possible in above lesion but may be little weak because nerve to long heads of triceps arises in the axilla, that is before the site of lesion.

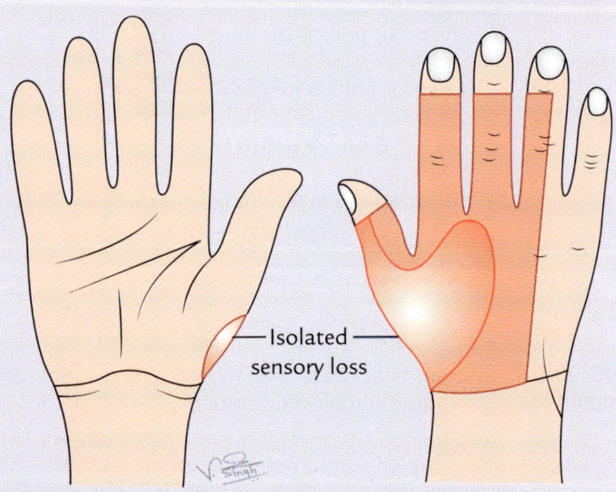

FIG. 13.5 ■ Area of sensory loss in hand following radial nerve injury above the elbow. The light shade shows isolated areas of sensory loss as detected during clinical examination.

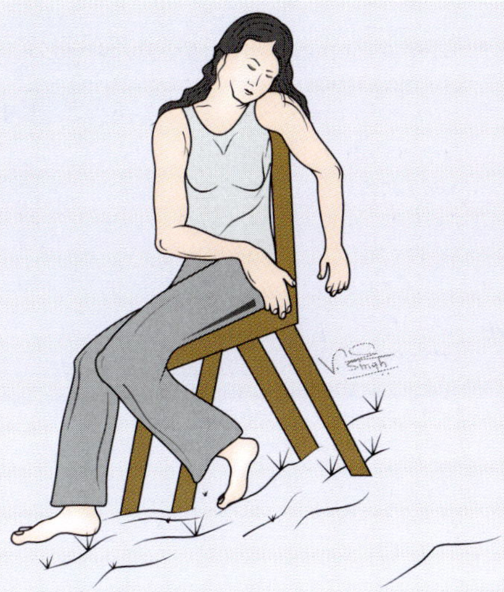

FIG. 13.6 Saturday night paralysis. Note drunk lady falling asleep with arm over the back of chair.

C. **Injury of radial nerve at elbow:**

Radial tunnel syndrome: It is an entrapment neuropathy of the deep branch of radial nerve at elbow. The compression of radial nerve at elbow may be caused by the following four structures:

(a) Fibrous bands, which can tether the radial nerve to the radiohumeral joint.
(b) Sharp tendinous margin of extensor carpi radialis brevis.
(c) Leash of vessels from the radial recurrent artery.
(d) Arcade of Frohse, a fibro-aponeurotic proximal edge of the superficial part of the supinator muscle.

Characteristic clinical features:

- Loss of extension of the wrist and fingers but no wrist drop.
- Pain over the extensor aspect of the forearm.

MEDIAN NERVE (FIG. 13.7)

The **median nerve** arises from brachial plexus in axilla by two roots: (a) lateral and (b) medial. The lateral root (C5, C6, and C7) arises from lateral cord of brachial plexus and medial root (C8 and T1) arises from medial cord of the brachial plexus. The medial root crosses in front of the third part of axillary artery to unite with lateral root in a Y-shaped manner either in front of or on the lateral side of the artery to form the median nerve. So the **root value of median nerve is C5, C6, C7, C8, and T1.**

In the axilla, the median nerve lies on the lateral side of the third part of the axillary artery. It enters the arm at the lower border of teres major.

In the arm, initially, median nerve lies lateral to brachial artery and then crosses in front of the artery from lateral to medial side at the level of midhumerus (i.e. level of insertion of coracobrachialis). After crossing, it runs downwards to enter cubital fossa.

In the cubital fossa, the median nerve lies medial to the brachial artery and tendon of biceps brachii. Here it is covered by bicipital aponeurosis, which separates it from the median cubital vein.

In the cubital fossa, it gives muscular branches from its medial side to supply all the superficial flexors of the forearm-pronator teres, flexor carpi radialis, palmaris longus, and flexor digitorum superficialis except flexor carpi ulnaris.

Median nerve leaves the cubital fossa by passing between the two heads of pronator teres. At this point, it gives off **anterior interosseous nerve.**

The anterior interosseous nerve is purely motor and supplies 2½ deep muscles:

1. Flexor pollicis longus.
2. Lateral half of the flexor digitorum profundus (FDP).
3. Pronator quadratus.

In the forearm, the median nerve passes downwards behind the tendinous arch/bridge between the two heads of flexor digitorum superficialis and runs deep to the flexor digitorum superficialis. About 5 cm proximal to the flexor retinaculum, the median nerve emerges from the lateral side of the FDS and becomes superficial, lying lateral to the tendons of FDS and posterior to the tendon of palmaris longus.

In the midforearm, the median nerve gives muscular branch to the radial head of flexor digitorum superficialis, which gives rise to tendon for index finger.

Before entering the carpal tunnel, it gives off its *palmar cutaneous branch*, which passes superficial to the flexor retinaculum to supply the skin over the thenar eminence and lateral part of the palm.

Median nerve enters the palm by passing through carpal tunnel where it lies deep to flexor retinaculum and superficial to the tendons of FDS, FDP, and FPL and their associated ulnar and radial bursae.

In the palm, the median nerve flattens at the distal border of the flexor retinaculum and divides into lateral and medial divisions. The lateral division gives a **recurrent branch**, which curls upwards to supply thenar muscles except the deep head of flexor pollicis brevis. It then divides into three palmar digital branches. The medial divisions give off two palmar digital nerves.

The five palmar digital nerves supply:

(a) Sensory innervation to the skin of the palmar aspect of the lateral 3½ digits including nail beds and skin on the dorsal aspect of distal phalanges and
(b) First and second lumbricals.

N.B.

- Median nerve is also termed **labourer's nerve** because the coarse movements of the hand required by labourers (e.g. digging the ground, lifting weight, etc.) are performed by long flexors of the forearm which are mostly supplied by the median nerve.
- It is also termed **'eye of the hand'** or **'peripheral eye'** because it provides sensory innervation to the pulp of the thumb and index finger which are used to see the thinness and texture of cloth and are also used for performing fine movements, for example buttoning a coat.

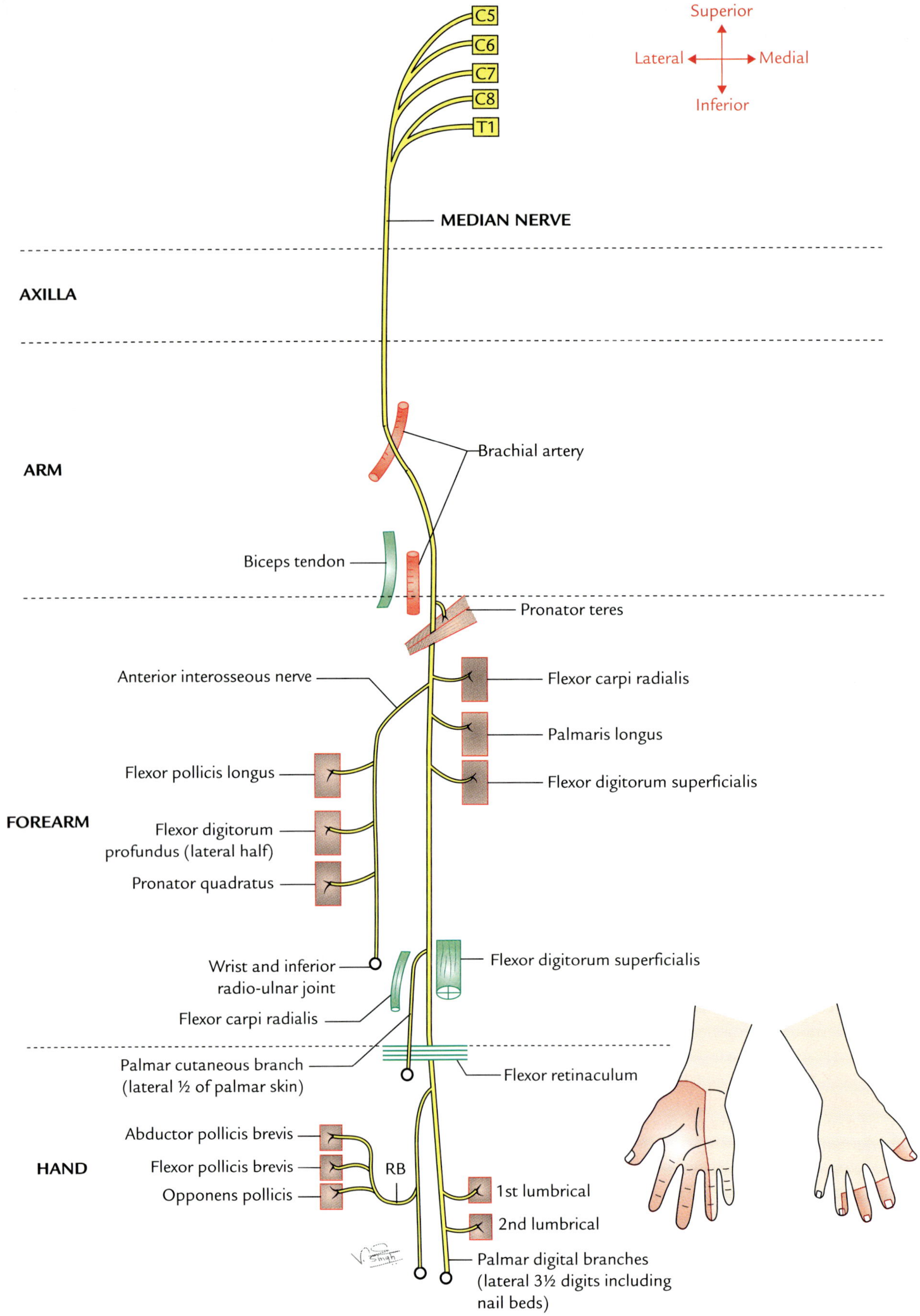

FIG. 13.7 ■ Course, branches, and motor distribution of the median nerve (RB = recurrent branch). Figure on the right lower part shows its sensory (cutaneous) distribution.

The overview of motor and sensory distribution of median nerve is summarized in the box below.

Median nerve (C5-T1) innervation

Motor innervation

Muscles	
Pronator teres Pronator quadratus Flexor carpi radialis Palmaris longus Lateral part of flexor digitorum profundus Flexor digitorum superficialis Flexor pollicis longus	All the muscles on the front of forearm except flexor carpi ulnaris and medial half of flexor digitorum profundus
Abductor pollicis brevis Opponens pollicis Flexor pollicis brevis Two lateral (radial) lumbricals	Thenar muscles and later two lumbricals in hand

Cutaneous innervation

Lateral two-thirds of palm of hand, thumb, index, and middle fingers and the lateral half of ring finger and dorsal tips of the same fingers.

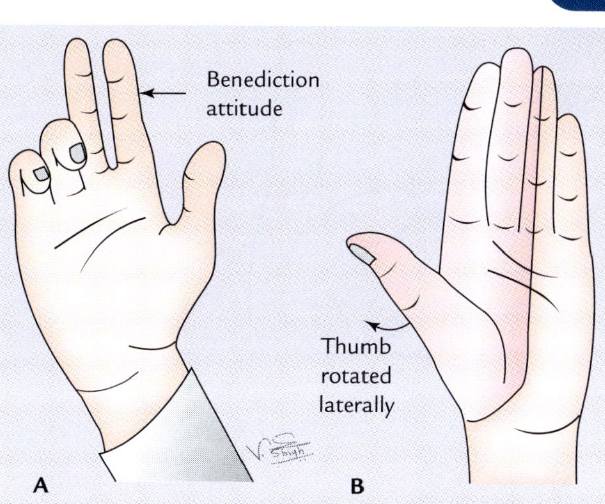

FIG. 13.8 Effects of the median nerve injury: (**A**) benediction deformity of the hand (benediction attitude of hand); (**B**) ape-thumb deformity.

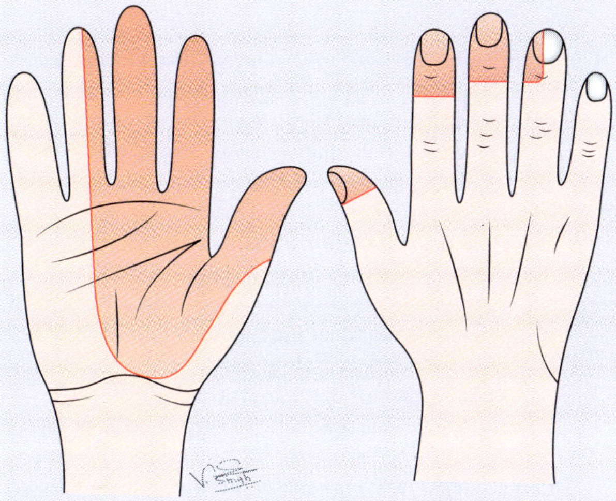

FIG. 13.9 Area of sensory loss in hand following injury of the median nerve.

CLINICAL CORRELATION

Injuries of the median nerve: The lesions of median nerve may occur at the following four sites: (a) at elbow, (b) at midforearm, (c) at wrist (distal forearm), and (d) in the carpal tunnel.

A. **Injury of the median nerve at the elbow:** At elbow the median nerve can be injured due to:
   (a) Supracondylar fracture of humerus,
   (b) Application of tight tourniquet during venepuncture, and
   (c) Entrapment of nerve between two heads of pronator teres or under the fibrous arch connecting the two heads of flexor digitorum superficialis.

   Characteristic clinical features in such cases will be as follows:
   - Forearm kept in supine position (loss of pronation), due to paralysis of pronator teres and pronator quadratus.
   - Wrist flexion is weak—due to paralysis of all the flexors of forearm except medial half of FDP and flexor carpi ulnaris.
   - Adduction of wrist—due to paralysis of FCR and unopposed action of FCU and medial half of FDP.
   - No flexion is possible at the interphalangeal (IP) joints of index and middle fingers.
   - *Benediction type of deformity of the hand* (Fig. 13.8A), that is when patient tries to make fist, the index and middle fingers remain straight, due to paralysis of both superficial and deep flexors (FDS and FDP) of these fingers leading to loss of flexion at PIP and DIP joints. The ring and the little finger can be kept in flexed position due to intact nerve supply of medial half of the FDP.

N.B.

The *Benediction deformity* is clasically an *ulnar claw hand*, where medial 2 digits are extended at MCP joints and flexed at PIP and DIP joints due to paralysis of medial two lumbricals and interossei due to injury of ulnar nerve (ulnar neuropathy). Because it resembles the hand gesture of a Pope (a Christian priest) giving his blessings (a papal benediction). Historically St. Peter had suffered from ulnar claw hand but he continued to give his blessings to his followers by his stretched ulnar claw hand, hence the name *benediction hand* (Flutterman B).

   - Loss of flexion of terminal phalanx of thumb due to paralysis of FPL.
   - ***Ape-thumb deformity*** (Fig. 13.8B), in which thenar eminence is flattened and thumb lies adducted, due to paralysis of muscles of thenar eminence and normal adductor pollicis, respectively.
   - Loss of sensation in lateral half of the palm and lateral 3½ digits and also on the dorsal aspects of same digits (Fig. 13.9).

B. **Injury of the median nerve at the midforearm:** The injury of median nerve at midforearm results in ***pointing index finger*** (Fig. 13.10) due to paralysis of radial head of FDS muscle that continues as tendon of index finger; other signs and symptoms will be same as those which occur in lesion at distal forearm and wrist.

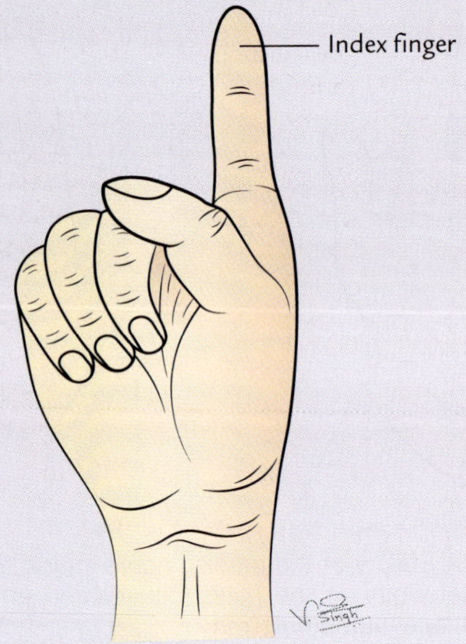

FIG. 13.10 Pointing index finger.

C. **Injury of the median nerve at wrist (distal forearm):** At wrist, median nerve and its palmar cutaneous branch may be injured just proximal to the flexor retinaculum by deep lacerated wounds (cut injury), for example suicidal cuts. *Characteristic clinical features* in such a case will be as follows:
   - ***Ape-thumb deformity***, due to paralysis of muscles of thenar eminence as described in lesion A.
   - Loss of sensation on the lateral part of the palm (including that over the thenar eminence) and lateral 3½ digits including loss of sensation on the dorsal aspect of these digits (Fig. 13.9).

D. **Injury in the carpal tunnel/carpal tunnel syndrome:** The median nerve is injured in the carpal tunnel due to its compression and produces a clinical condition called **carpal tunnel syndrome.** AN 12.4
   The carpal tunnel is formed by anterior concavity of carpus and flexor retinaculum. The tunnel is tightly packed with nine long flexor tendons of fingers and thumb with their surrounding synovial sheaths and median nerve. The median nerve gets compressed in the tunnel due to its narrowing following a number of pathological conditions such as:
   (a) Tenosynovitis of flexor tendons (idiopathic),
   (b) Myxoedema (deficiency of thyroxine),
   (c) Retention of fluid in pregnancy,
   (d) Fracture dislocation of lunate bone, and
   (e) Osteoarthritis of the wrist.
   Characteristic clinical features of the carpal tunnel syndrome are as follows:
   - Feeling of burning pain or *'pins and needles'* along the sensory distribution of median nerve (i.e. lateral 3½ digits) especially at night.
   - There is no sensory loss over the thenar eminence because skin over thenar eminence is supplied by the palmar cutaneous branch of the median nerve, which passes superficial to flexor retinaculum.
   - Weakness of thenar muscles.
   - *'Ape-thumb deformity'* may occur, if left untreated, due to paralysis of the thenar muscles.

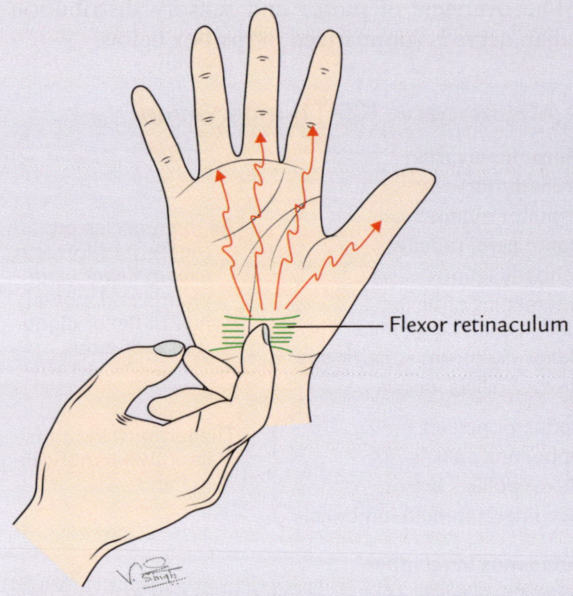

FIG. 13.11 Tinel's sign. Percussion over flexor retinaculum reproduces patient's symptoms.

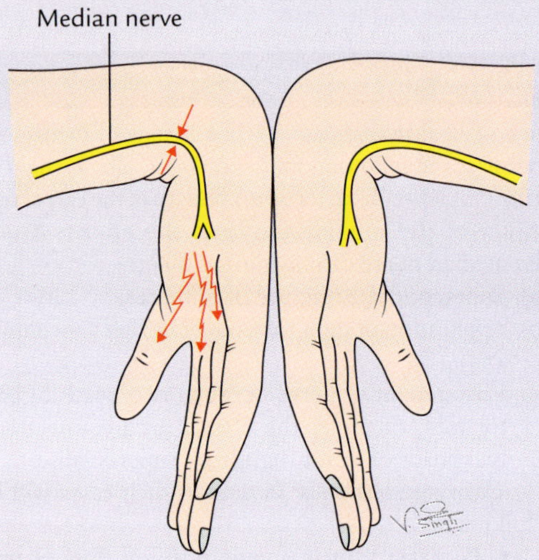

FIG. 13.12 Phalen's test. Flexion of both wrists against each other for 1 minute reproduces patient's symptoms.

   - Positive **Tinel's sign** (Fig. 13.11) and **Phalen's test** (Fig. 13.12).
   - Reduced conduction velocity in the median nerve (<30 m/s) is diagnostic.

N.B.

The signs and symptoms of the carpal tunnel syndrome are dramatically relieved by decompressing the tunnel by giving a longitudinal incision through flexor retinaculum.

ULNAR NERVE (FIG. 13.13)

The ulnar nerve arises in the axilla from the medial cord of brachial plexus (C8 and T1). It receives a contribution from the ventral ramus of C7. The C7 fibres in the ulnar nerve supply flexor carpi ulnaris.

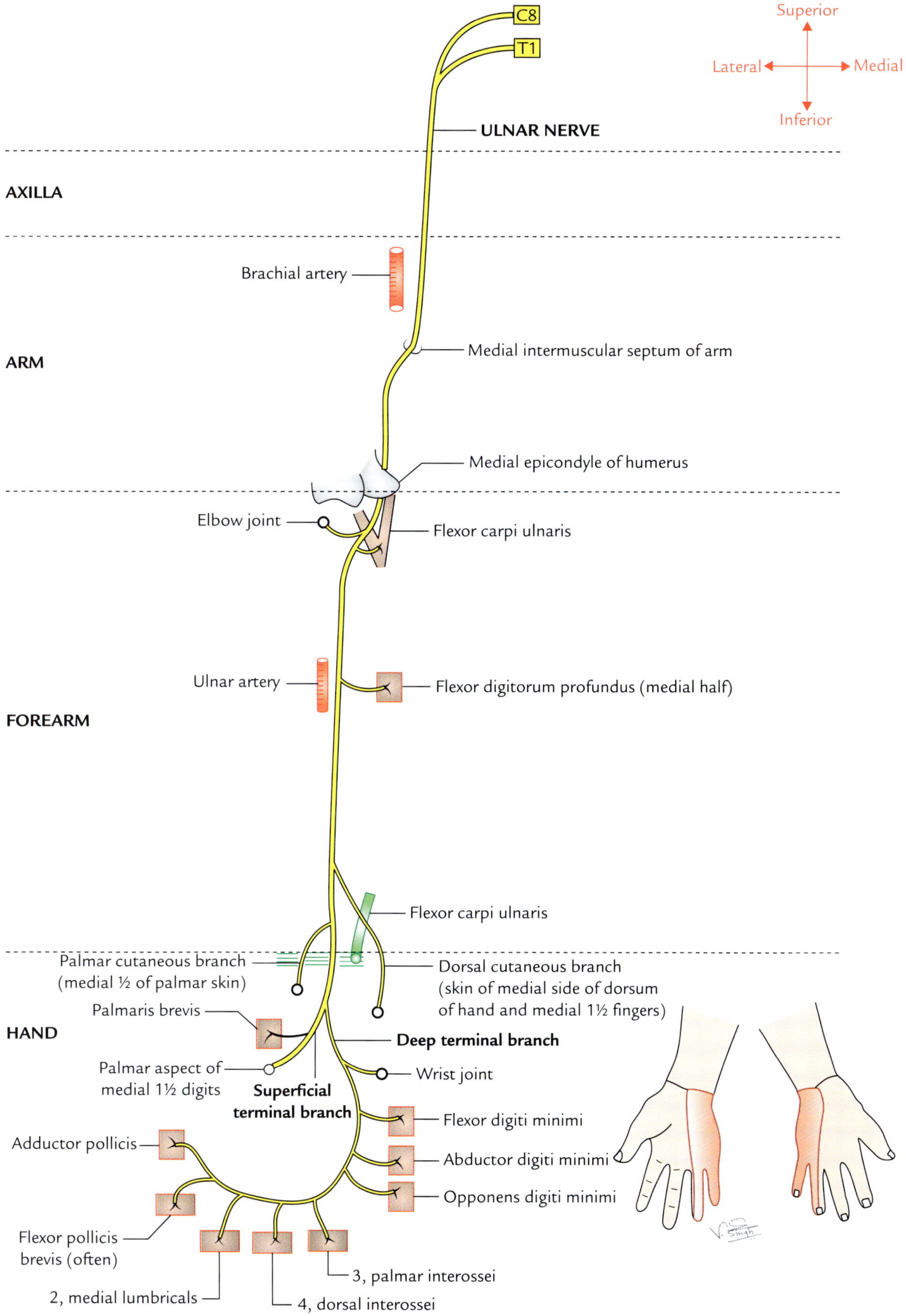

FIG. 13.13 ■ Course, branches, and motor distribution of the ulnar nerve. Figure on the right lower part shows its sensory (cutaneous) distribution.

In the axilla, the nerve lies medial to third part of axillary artery (between axillary artery and vein).

It enters the arm as part of main neurovascular bundle and runs distally along the medial side of the brachial artery up to the midarm (level of insertion of coracobrachialis) where it pierces the medial intermuscular septum to enter the posterior compartment of the arm and runs downwards to the back of the medial epicondyle of humerus. On the back of medial epicondyle, it is lodged in a groove where it can be easily palpated. The groove is converted into a tunnel called **cubital tunnel** by a fibrous band extending between medial epicondyle and olecranon process. The ulnar nerve crosses the ulnar collateral ligament in the floor of the tunnel.

The ulnar nerve does not give any branch in the axilla and in the arm.

The *nerve enters the forearm* by passing between the two heads of flexor carpi ulnaris. In the upper third of forearm, it runs almost vertically downwards under flexor carpi ulnaris. In the lower two-thirds of the forearm, it becomes superficial and lies lateral to the flexor carpi ulnaris. In this part of its course the ulnar nerve and artery descend together, artery being on the lateral side of the nerve.

In the forearm, it gives off the following branches:

1. In the **proximal forearm**, it gives muscular branches to:
   (a) Flexor carpi ulnaris and
   (b) Medial half of flexor digitorum profundus.
2. In the **midforearm**, it gives off *palmar cutaneous branch*, which enters the palm superficial to the flexor retinaculum to provide sensory innervation to the skin over the hypothenar eminence.
3. In the **distal forearm**, about 5 cm proximal to the wrist, it gives off *dorsal cutaneous branch* which provides sensory innervation to the skin over the medial third of the dorsum of the hand and medial 1½ finger.

The ulnar nerve enters the palm by passing superficial to the flexor retinaculum lying just lateral to the pisiform. Here the ulnar nerve is covered by a fascial band (*volar carpal ligament*). The space under this fascial band is termed **ulnar tunnel**. Just distal to pisiform, the ulnar nerve divides into its terminal superficial and deep branches. The *superficial terminal branch* supplies palmaris brevis provides sensory innervation to the skin on the palmar surface of hand and medial 1½ fingers.

The *deep terminal branch* enters *Guyon's canal* (pisohamate tunnel) under cover of pisohamate ligament extending from proximal border of pisiform bone to the hook of hamate turns laterally within concavity of deep palmar arterial arch and ends within substance of adductor pollicis which it supplies. The *deep branch of ulnar nerve is purely motor and supplies all the intrinsic muscles of the hand except the muscles of thenar eminence and first two lumbricals.*

N.B.

The ulnar nerve is often referred to as '*nerve of fine movements*'/ '**musician's nerve**' because it innervates most of the intrinsic muscles of the hand that are involved in the fine intricate hand movements as required by the musicians while playing musical instruments.

The ulnar nerve behind medial epicondyle of humerus is termed 'funny bone' because when the medial part of the elbow hits a hard surface, tingling sensations occur along the ulnar side of the forearm and hand.

The motor and sensory distribution of ulnar nerve is given in the box below.

Ulnar nerve (C8-T1)

Motor innervation

Muscles	
Flexor carpi ulnaris Medial part of the flexor Digitorum profundus	Two muscles on the front of forearm
Adductor pollicis Flexor digiti minimi brevis Abductor digiti minimi Opponens digit minimi Medial two lumbricals Interossei dorsal and palmar	All intrinsic muscles of hand except thenar muscles and two lateral lumbricals

Cutaneous innervation

Medial one-third of hand, little finger and medial one half of ring finger (Fig. 13.15).

CLINICAL CORRELATION AN12.8

Injuries of the ulnar nerve: The ulnar nerve is commonly injured at two sites: (a) at elbow and (b) at wrist.

A. **Injury of the ulnar nerve at elbow:** The injury of ulnar nerve at elbow may occur due to:
   (a) Fracture dislocation of the medial epicondyle,
   (b) Thickening of the fibrous roof of the cubital tunnel (***cubital tunnel syndrome***),
   (c) Compression between the two heads of flexor carpi ulnaris (FCU) muscle, and
   (d) Valgus deformity of elbow (tardy or late ulnar nerve palsy).

   Characteristic clinical features in such cases will be as follows:
   - Atrophy and flattening of hypothenar eminence.
   - ***Ulnar claw-hand deformity (main en griffe)*** affecting ring and little fingers. The first phalanges of these fingers are extended and middle and distal phalanges are flexed (Fig. 13.14A).
   - It is not a true claw hand.
   - Loss of abduction and adduction of fingers.
   - Flattening of hypothenar eminence and depression of interosseous spaces on dorsum of hand due to atrophy of interosseous muscles, respectively (Fig. 13.14B).
   - Loss of adduction of thumb.
   - Loss of sensation over the palmar and dorsal surfaces of the medial third of the hand and medial 1½ fingers (Fig. 13.15A and B).
   - *Card test* and *Froment's sign* are positive (Figs 13.16 and 13.17).

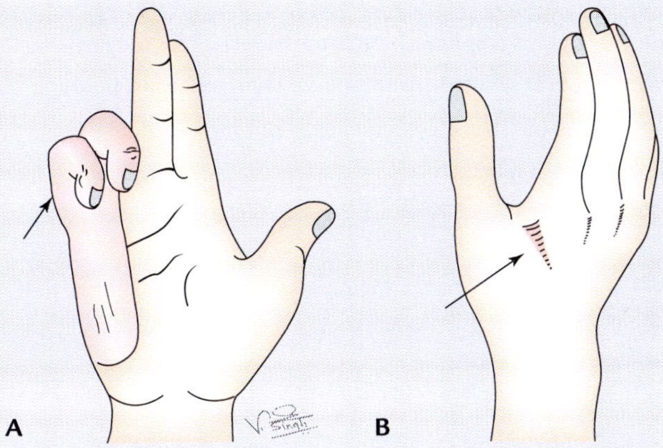

FIG. 13.14 ■ Effects of the ulnar nerve injury: (**A**) ulnar claw hand; (**B**) hollowing of skin in the first web space on dorsal aspect of hand.

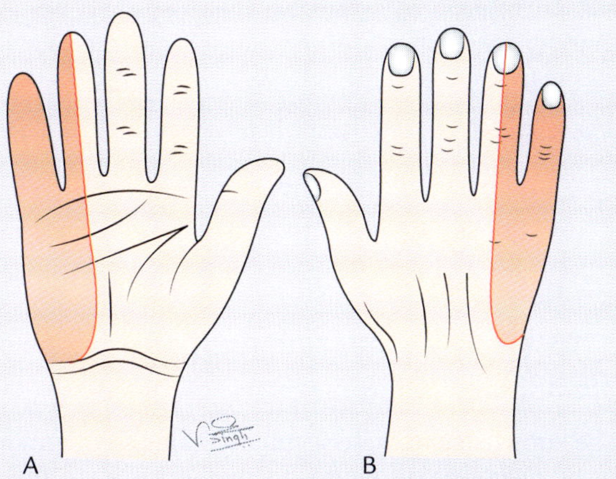

FIG. 13.15 ■ Sensory loss in the hand following ulnar nerve injury: (**A**) palmar aspect; (**B**) dorsal aspect.

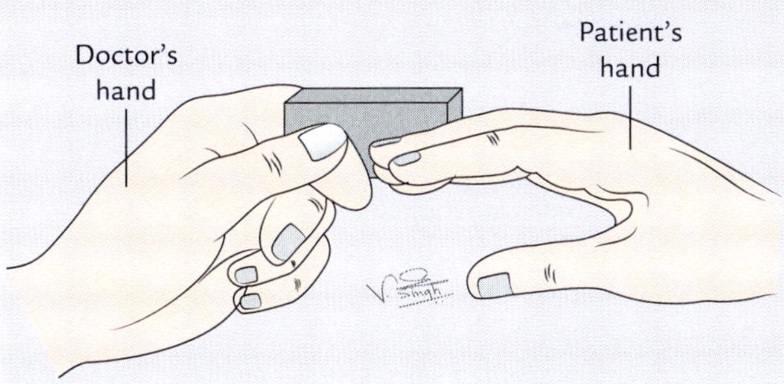

FIG. 13.16 ■ Card or paper test for the integrity of palmar interossei.

B. **Injury of the ulnar nerve at wrist:** The ulnar nerve at wrist is injured due to:
   (a) Superficial position of ulnar nerve at this site makes its vulnerable to cuts and wounds and
   (b) Compression in the Guyon's canal/pisohamate tunnel.
   Characteristic clinical features:
   - Claw-hand deformity affecting ring and little fingers (ulnar claw hand) but it is more pronounced (*ulnar paradox*) because the FDP is not paralyzed; therefore there is a marked flexion of DIP joints.
   - Atrophy and flattening of hypothenar eminence.
   - Loss of abduction and adduction of fingers.
   - Card test and Froment's sign is positive.

N.B.

- **Card test for palmar interossei** (Fig. 13.16)**:** Ask the patient to grasp a piece of paper/card firmly between the sides of adjacent fingers. When the examining doctor pulls the card/paper, if the palmar interossei are acting, this paper will be firmly held in position and some resistance is felt on its withdrawal.
- **Froment's sign/test** (Fig. 13.17)**:** This test is done to assess the *paralysis of adductor pollicis*. Give the patient a thin book and ask him to grasp it between the thumbs and fingers of both hands firmly. If the adductor pollicis are healthy on both sides, the thumbs will be straight, if the adductor pollicis is paralyzed, the last phalanx of thumb will be fully flexed by flexor pollicis longus on that side as it is supplied by median nerve.
- **Complete claw hand** (Fig. 13.18): The *combined lesions of the median and ulnar nerves* at elbow cause a true/complete claw-hand deformity. The *characteristic clinical features of a true claw hand* are as follows:
  – Hyperextension of the wrist and metacarpophalangeal (MP) joints.
  – Flexion of IP joints. Also see page 165.

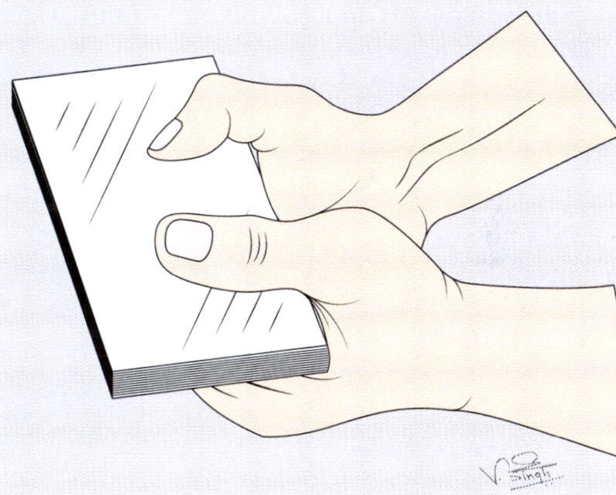

FIG. 13.17 ■ Froment's sign.

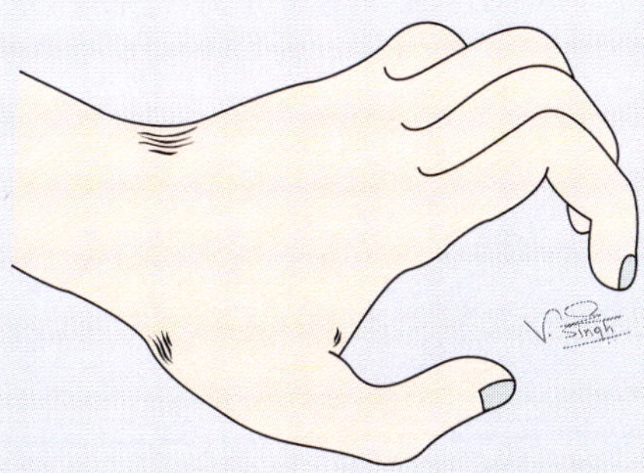

FIG. 13.18 ■ Complete claw hand following combined lesions of the median and ulnar nerves.

TABLE 13.1 Characteristics of radial, median, and ulnar nerves of the upper limb

Nerve	Radial nerve	Median nerve (syn. labourer's nerve)	Ulnar nerve (syn. musician's nerve)
Origin	Posterior cord of brachial plexus	Medial and lateral cords of brachial plexus	Medial cord of brachial plexus
Root value	C5-T1	C5-T1	C8-T1
Motor innervation	Supplies all the muscles on the back of arm and forearm	Supplies: • All the muscles on the front of forearm except flexor carpi ulnaris and medial half of flexor digitorum profundus • Muscle of thenar eminence and first two lumbricals	Supplies: • One-and-half muscles of the forearm (flexor carpi ulnaris and medial half of the flexor digitorum profundus) • All the intrinsic muscles of the hand, except first two lumbricals and muscles of thenar eminence
Sensory innervation	• Posterior surface of the arm and forearm • Dorsal aspect of lateral two-thirds of hand and lateral 3½ digits	Palmar aspect of lateral two-thirds of hand and lateral 3½ digits including their dorsal tips	Palmar and dorsal aspects of medial one-third of hand and medial 1½ fingers
Effects of lesion	• Wrist drop • Absence of extension of MP joints of digits • Loss of sensation to a variable small area over the root of the thumb	• Ape-thumb deformity (Simian's hand) • Wasting of thenar eminence • Absence of abduction of thumb • Pointing index finger • Absence of opposition of thumb • Loss of sensation on the palmar aspect of lateral part of hand and lateral 3½ digits	• Ulnar claw-hand deformity (*main en griffe*) • Wasting of hypothenar eminence • Absence of abduction and adduction of fingers • Loss of sensation on the ulnar side of the hand and medial 1½ digits • Froment's sign and card test are positive

The features of the three principal nerves (radial, median, and ulnar) of upper limb are summarized in Table 13.1.

AUTONOMOUS SENSORY AREAS OF THE HAND

An autonomous sensory area is that part of the dermatome that has no overlap from the adjacent nerves.

The autonomous sensory areas of the hand are used to test the integrity of nerves supplying the hand (e.g. ulnar, median, and radial). The autonomous sensory areas of the radial, median, and ulnar nerves are shown in Fig. 13.19.

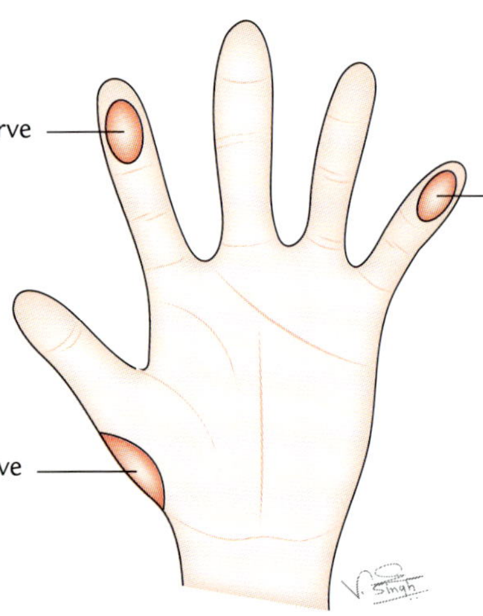

FIG. 13.19 Autonomous sensory areas of the radial, median, and ulnar nerves.

SEGMENTAL INNERVATION OF THE MUSCLES OF THE UPPER LIMB

The knowledge of these segmental values is of importance in the diagnosis of injuries to the nerves or to the spinal cord from which they arise. The segmental innervation of the muscles of the upper limb is given in Table 13.2. These are based on the clinical data observed by Kocher.

TABLE 13.2 Segmental innervation of the muscles of the upper limb

Segment	Muscles innervated
C5	• Deltoid • Supraspinatus, infraspinatus, and teres minor • Rhomboideus major and minor • Coracobrachialis, biceps brachii, and brachialis • Brachioradialis and supinator (*Abductors and lateral rotators of the shoulder; flexors and supinators of the forearm*)
C6	• Pectoralis major and minor • Subscapularis, latissimus dorsi, and teres major • Serratus anterior • Triceps • Pronator teres and pronator quadratus (*Adductors and medial rotators of the shoulder; extensors and pronators of the forearm*)
C7	Extensors and flexors of the wrist
C8	Long flexors and extensors of the fingers
T1	Small muscles of the hand

Golden Facts to Remember

• Largest nerve of the upper limb	Radial nerve
• Most serious disability of the median nerve lesion	Loss of ability to oppose the thumb to other fingers
• Largest nerve/thickest branch of brachial plexus	Radial nerve
• Most common site of the median nerve injury	Carpal tunnel
• Commonest peripheral neuropathy in the upper limb	Carpal tunnel syndrome (compression of median nerve in the carpal tunnel)
• Commonest cause of the carpal tunnel syndrome	Tenosynovitis of flexor tendons
• Commonest site of the ulnar nerve injury	At elbow, where it lies behind the medial epicondyle of the humerus
• Most reliable clinical test for the carpal tunnel syndrome	Cuff compression test (of Gilliatt and Wilson)
• Most common site of the radial nerve injury	Spiral groove
• Labourer's nerve	Median nerve
• Musician's nerve	Ulnar nerve
• Eye of the hand/peripheral eye	Median nerve in hand

CLINICAL CASE STUDY

A 50-year-old female with history of rheumatoid arthritis complained of pain and 'pins and needles sensations' in lateral two-thirds of palm and palmar aspect of lateral 3½ digits of her right hand, which becomes severe at night and compels her to wake up at night. The examination revealed wasting of the thenar eminence, and hypoesthesia to light touch and pinprick over the palmar aspect of lateral 3½ digits. However, skin over the thenar eminence was not affected. The cuff compression test (of Gilliatt and Wilson) was positive.

Questions

1. Name the clinical condition on the basis of signs and symptoms.
2. Name the boundaries of carpal tunnel and enumerate its contents.
3. Compression of which nerve leads to the above condition?
4. Why does pain increase during night which makes the patient to wake up?
5. What is the most reliable clinical diagnostic test for the **carpal tunnel syndrome**? Give its brief account.

Answers

1. **Carpal tunnel syndrome.**
2. The carpal tunnel is bounded posteriorly by carpal bones and anteriorly by inelastic flexor retinaculum (transverse carpal ligament). It contains nine tendons of long flexors (e.g. tendons of FDS, FDP, and FPL) enclosed in synovial sheaths and median nerve.
3. Median nerve.
4. Due to accumulation of tissue fluid in the absence of the pump action of forearm muscles with arm at rest during night.
5. Cuff compression test (of Gilliatt and Wilson), when blood pressure (sphygmomanometer) cuff around the arm is inflated above the point of systolic blood pressure, the pain and paraesthesia are aggravated.

CHAPTER

14

Surface Anatomy of the Upper Limb

SPECIFIC LEARNING OBJECTIVES

After studying this chapter, the student should be able to:

- Palpate important surface landmarks in the upper limb.
- Do the surface marking of the major blood vessels of the upper limb.
- Do the surface marking of the major nerves of the upper limb.
- Enumerate the various sites where arterial pulse can be felt in the upper limb.

The surface marking is the projection of deeper structures on the body surface. It is clinically very important for physicians and surgeons to perform various medical and surgical procedures. This chapter deals with the surface markings of only those structures which are required in day to day practice.

BREAST

The breasts are most prominent superficial structures on the front of chest particularly in females. In adult females, they are hemispherical bulges/bodies one on either side of median region. They are separated from each other by intermammary cleft. Its superior border is not well demarcated from anterior aspect of the chest but its lateral and inferior borders are well defined.

The breast is marked on the surface as follows (Fig. 14.1):

- Mark a point 'a' at the sternal margin at the sternal angle/angle of Louis.
- Mark a point 'b' at the sternal end of sixth costal cartilage.
- Mark a point 'c' on the second rib in the midclavicular line.
- Draw midaxillary line.
- Mark a point 'd' on the lower part of axillary artery under cover of anterior axillary fold.

Now make the outline of the breast on surface by drawing a circular line passing through above four points. Then draw an axillary tail of breast as small tongue-like process from its upper lateral aspect directed upwards and laterally up to midaxillary line (Fig. 14.1). In nulliparous females, the nipple lies in fourth intercostal space about 10 cm from anterior median line.

ARTERIES OF UPPER LIMB AN 13.7

AXILLARY ARTERY (FIG. 14.2)

- Abduct the arm at right angle, that is 90°.
- Mark a point 'a' at midpoint of clavicle.
- Mark a point 'b' on lower end of lateral wall of axilla. Just in front of posterior axillary fold, that is at lower end of lateral wall of axilla.

Now mark the axillary artery on the surface by joining these points by a broad line.

BRACHIAL ARTERY (FIG. 14.3)

- Abduct the arm at right angle, that is 90°.
- Mark a point 'b' in the lateral wall of axilla in front of posterior axillary fold at the lower end of axillary artery.
- Mark a point 'c' in anterior midline of forearm at the level of neck of radius, medial to the tendon of biceps brachii.
- The brachial artery is now marked on the surface by joining these points by a little broad line.

N.B.

Brachial artery is located on medial side of arm in the cleft between biceps and triceps brachii muscles. The axillary artery ends and brachial artery begins at the lower end of the lateral wall of axilla.

RADIAL ARTERY (FIG. 14.4)

- Mark a point 'a' in front of elbow (in the midline of cubital fossa) opposite to the neck of radius on the medial side of biceps tendon.
- Mark a point 'b' on the lateral side, in front of distal forearm at the site of 'radial pulse', between anterior border of radius laterally and tendon of flexor carpi radially medially.
- The radial artery is now marked on the surface by joining these points with gentle convexity to the lateral side.

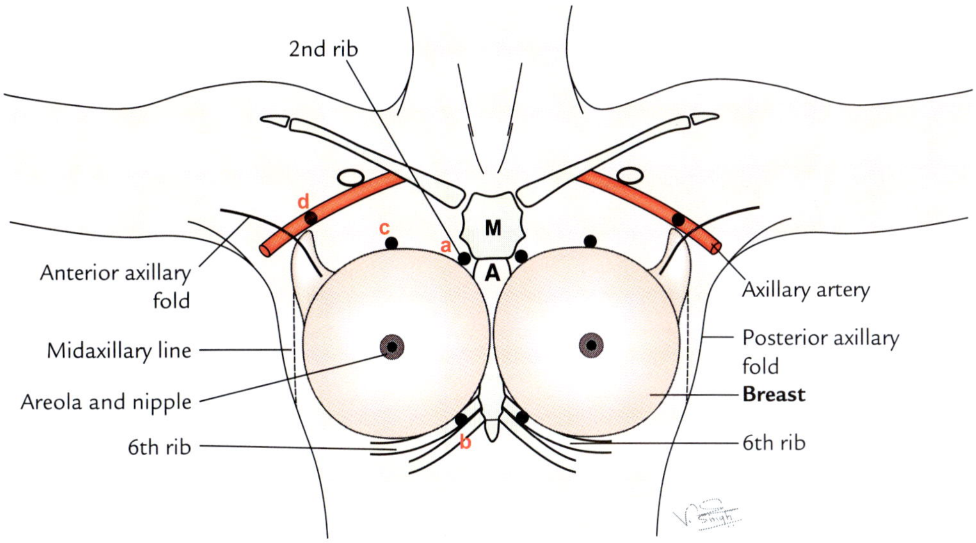

FIG. 14.1 ■ Surface marking of the breast. A = sternal angle, M = manubrium sterni.

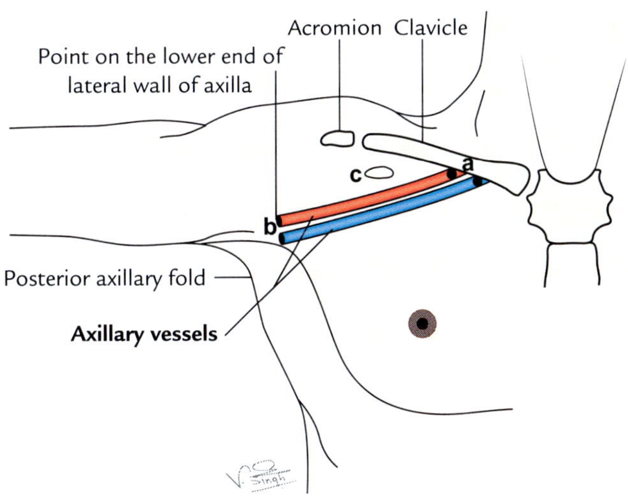

FIG. 14.2 ■ Surface marking of the axillary artery. C = coracoid process.

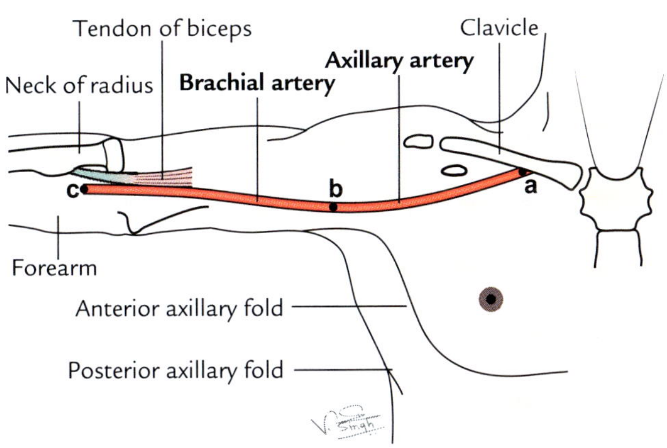

FIG. 14.3 ■ Surface marking of the brachial artery.

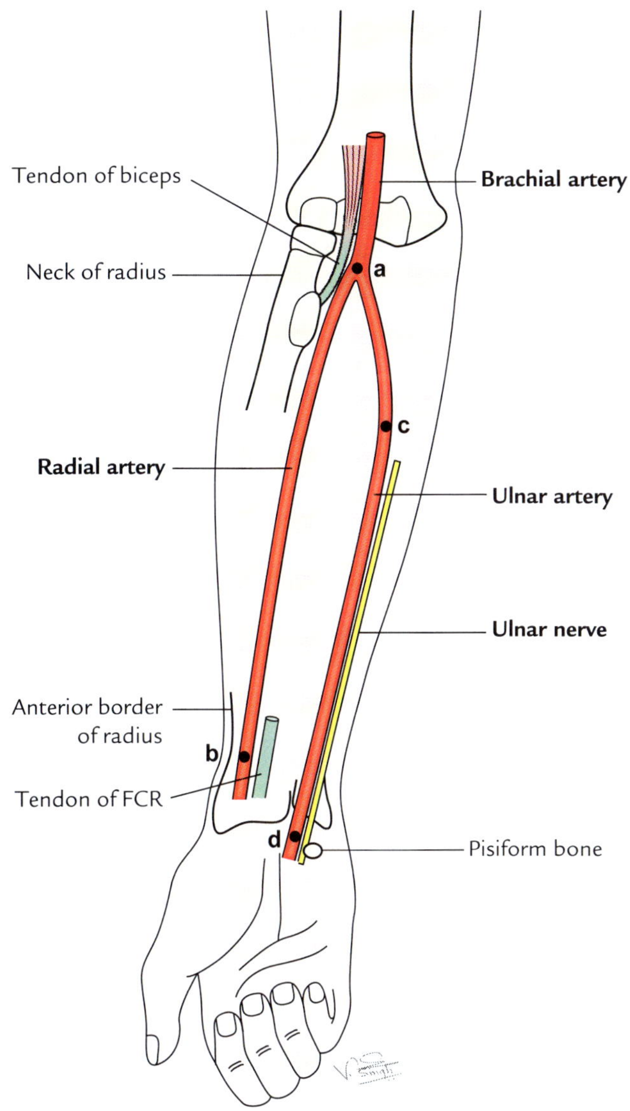

FIG. 14.4 ■ Surface marking of the radial and ulnar arteries.

ULNAR ARTERY (FIG. 14.4)

- Mark a point 'a' on the front of elbow (in the cubital fossa) in the midline on the medial side of biceps tendon.
- Mark a point 'c' near the medial border of forearm at the junction of its upper one-third and lower two-thirds.
- Mark a point 'd' lateral to the pisiform bone.

Now the ulnar artery is marked on the surface by joining these points.

N.B.

- The course of ulnar artery is oblique in its upper one-third and vertical in its lower two-thirds.
- Ulnar nerve lies on medial side of lower two-thirds of ulnar artery.
- Ulnar artery is continuous in the palm as 'superficial palmar arch'.

SUPERFICIAL PALMAR ARCH (FIG. 14.5)

- Mark a point 'a' on the lateral side of pisiform bone.
- Mark a point 'b' medial to the hook of hamate.
- Mark a point 'c' in the centre of palm at the level of distal border of the extended thumb.
- Mark a point 'd' on the distal border of thenar eminence in line with the cleft between index and middle fingers.

Now superficial palmar arch is marked in the palm by joining these points by an arched line with its convexity directed distally towards fingers.

N.B.

Most distal point of superficial palmar arch lies at the level of distal border of fully extended thumb.

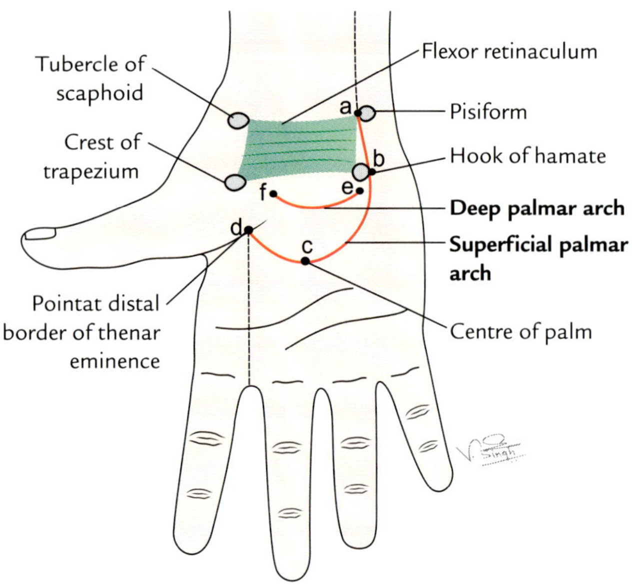

FIG. 14.5 ■ Surface marking of the superficial and deep palmar arterial arches.

DEEP PALMAR ARCH

- Mark a point 'e' just distal to the hook of hamate.
- Mark a point 'f' at the proximal end of first intermetacarpal space.

Now deep palmar arch can be marked in the palm by joining these points by about 4-cm long horizontal line with very slight convexity towards fingers and about 1.2 cm or one finger's breadth proximal the level of superficial palmar arch.

VEINS

AXILLARY VEIN

It is marked on the surface in same way as axillary artery except that the line representing axillary vein is drawn slightly medially (see page 184 and Fig. 14.2).

CEPHALIC VEIN (FIG. 14.6)

The cephalic vein runs upwards on the anterolateral aspect of the arm. It is marked as under:

- Mark a point 'a' in the deltopectoral groove below to the coracoids process.
- Mark a point 'b' in front of elbow in a groove between biceps brachii and brachioradialis muscles.

The cephalic vein is marked on the surface by joining these points by a broad line.

Note: This line passes upwards with slight inclination towards medial side till the coracoids process and then it arches medially towards to join axillary vein.

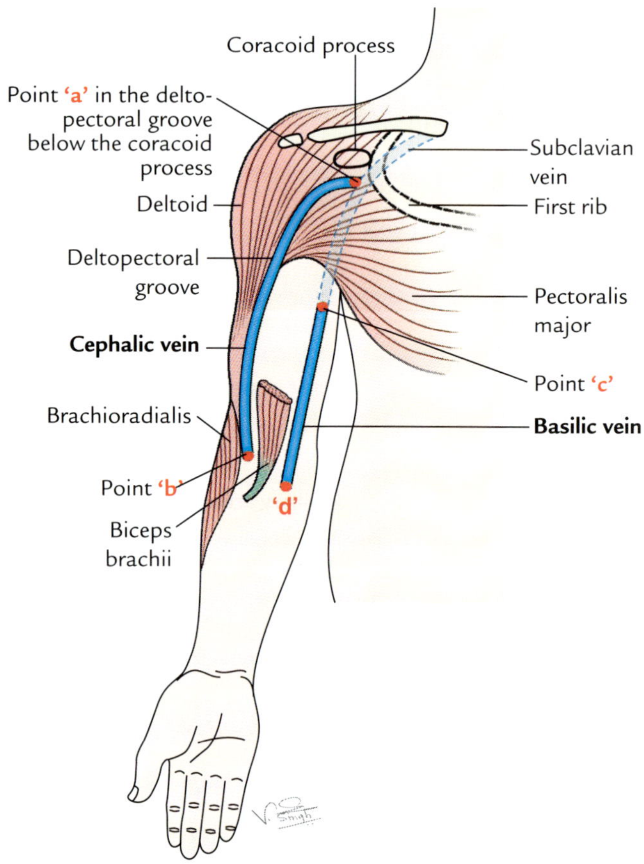

FIG. 14.6 ■ Surface marking of the cephalic and basilic veins.

BASILIC VEIN (FIG. 14.6)

- Mark a point 'c' on the medial side of arm halfway between axilla and medial epicondyle.
- Mark a point 'd' below the elbow on medial side on medial epicondyle.

The basilic vein is now marked on the surface by joining these points by a little wide line.

N.B.

Basilic vein continues above as **axillary vein** which at the outer border of first rib becomes **subclavian vein**.

NERVES

AXILLARY NERVE (FIG. 14.7)

- Mark a point 'a' on the acromion process.
- Mark a point 'b' on the insertion of deltoid muscle.
- Mark a point 'c', 2 cm above the midpoint between the tip of acromion process and deltoid tuberosity.

Now the axillary nerve and its branches are marked on the surface by a curved horizontal line.

N.B.

The idea of surface marking of axillary nerve is important for intramuscular injections.

RADIAL NERVE IN THE ARM (FIG. 14.8)

- Mark a point 'a' on the lateral wall of axilla, at the beginning of axillary artery.
- Mark a point 'b' at the junction of upper one-third and lower two-thirds of a line joining the lateral epicondyle and insertion of deltoid.
- Mark a point 'c' on the front of elbow at the level of lateral epicondyle 1 cm lateral to the tendon of biceps brachii muscle.

Now the radial nerve is marked on the surface by (I) joining first two points by a line crossing the elevation of long and lateral heads of triceps brachii, to represent the oblique course of nerve in radial groove in the posterior compartment of arm and (II) by joining second and third points in front of the arm to show the vertical course of nerve in the anterior compartment of the arm.

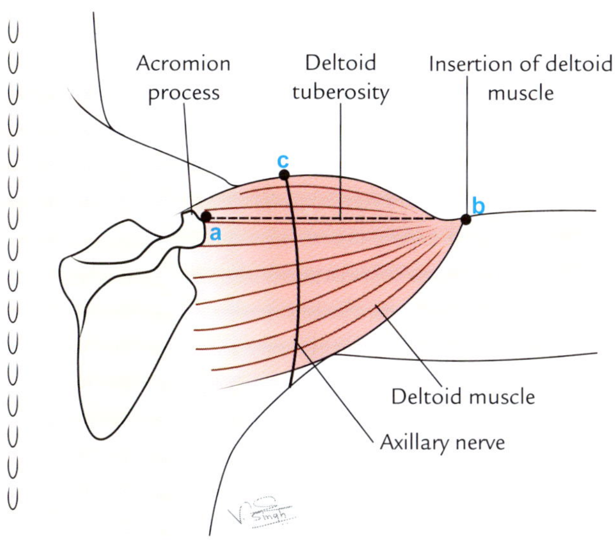

FIG. 14.7 ■ Surface marking of the axillary nerve.

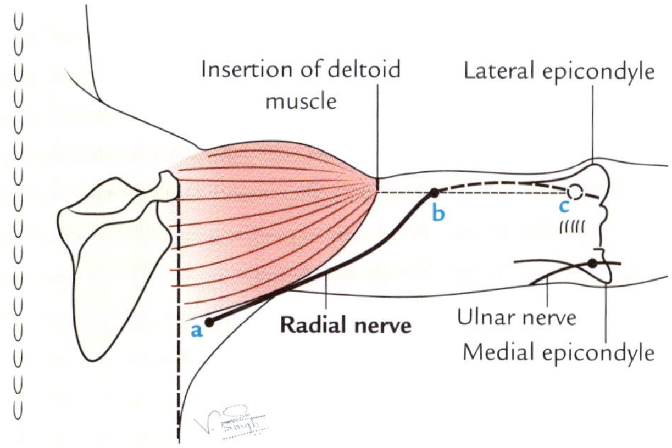

FIG. 14.8 ■ Surface marking of the radial nerve.

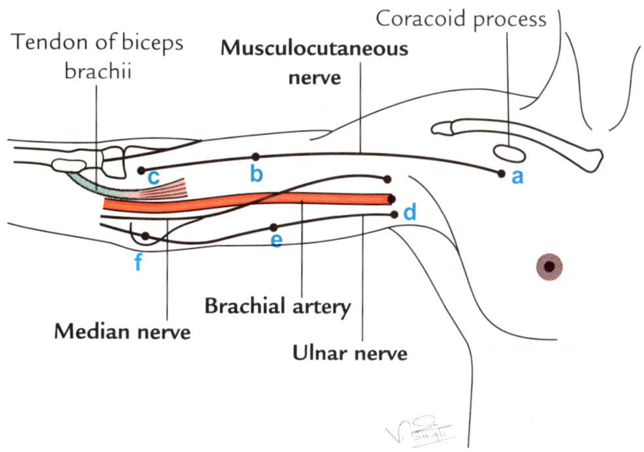

FIG. 14.9 ■ Surface marking of the ulnar, median, and musculocutaneous nerves.

MUSCULOCUTANEOUS NERVE IN THE ARM (FIG. 14.9)

- Mark a point 'a' about 5 cm below the coracoid process.
- Mark a midpoint 'b' on elevation produced by tendon of biceps brachii.
- Mark a point 'c' lateral to the tendon of biceps brachii 2 cm above the level of elbow.

Now the musculocutaneous nerve is marked on the surface by joining these points.

N.B.

Two centimetres above the bend of elbow musculocutaneous nerve pierces the deep fascia to become subcutaneous nerve called *lateral cutaneous nerve of forearm*.

ULNAR NERVE IN THE ARM (FIG. 14.9)

- Mark a point 'd' on the lower limit of lateral wall of axilla, that is at the end of axillary artery.

- Mark a point 'e' on the midpoint of brachial artery/ middle of the medial border of the arm.
- Mark a point 'f' on the back of medial epicondyle on the ulnar nerve which can be rolled here by fingers.

Now the ulnar nerve is marked on the surface by joining these points.

MEDIAN NERVE IN THE ARM (FIG. 14.9)

- Surface mark the brachial artery (see page 184).
- Now mark the median nerve, lateral to the artery in the upper half, and medial to the artery in the lower half. Note nerve crosses in front of artery from lateral to medial side in the middle of the arm.

MEDIAN NERVE IN THE FOREARM (FIG. 14.10)

- Mark a point 'a' in midline at the bend of elbow at the level of neck of radius.
- Mark a point 'b' in front of wrist 1 cm medial to the tendon of flexor carpi radialis (FCR).

Now the median nerve is marked on the surface by joining these points.

N.B.

At the front of wrist, the median nerve projects out laterally from under cover of palmaris longus muscle.

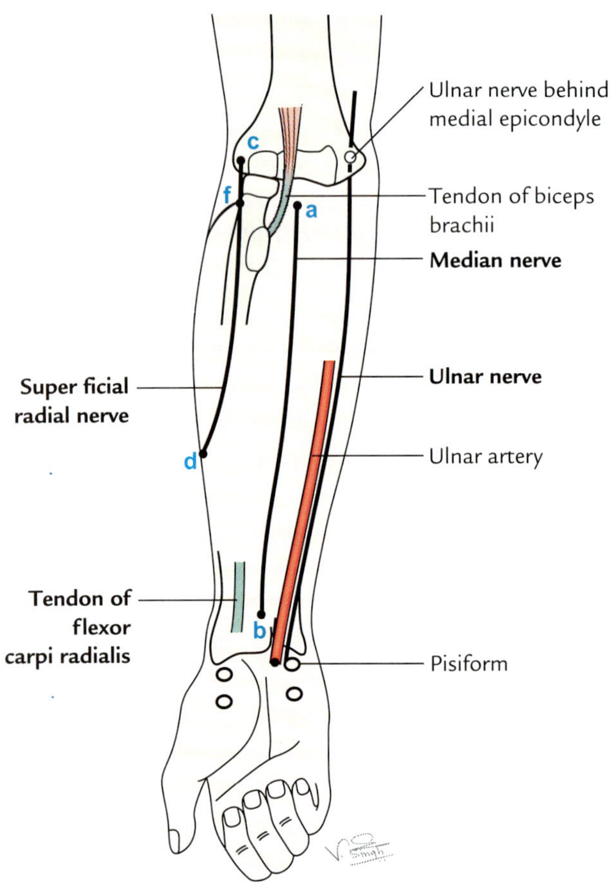

FIG. 14.10 ■ Surface marking of the median, ulnar, and radial nerves in the forearm.

ULNAR NERVE IN THE FOREARM (FIG. 14.10)

- Mark a point on the back of the medial epicondyle of humerus.
- Mark a point just lateral to the pisiform bone.

Now the ulnar nerve is marked on the surface by joining these points. Note in the lower two-thirds of the forearm, the ulnar nerve lies medial to the ulnar artery and lateral to the tendon flexor carpi ulnaris (FCU) (not shown in the figure).

RADIAL NERVE IN THE FOREARM (FIGS. 14.10 AND 14.11)

- Mark a point 'c' 1 cm lateral to the tendon of biceps on just below the lateral epicondyle humerus.
- Mark a point 'd' at the junction of upper two-thirds and lower one-third of the lateral border of the forearm.
- Mark a point 'e' in the distal part of anatomical snuffbox.

Now the radial nerve is marked on the surface by joining these points. Note the course of nerve is vertical in between first two points, and at the second point, the nerve inclines backwards to reach the anatomical snuffbox on the dorsolateral aspect of the hand.

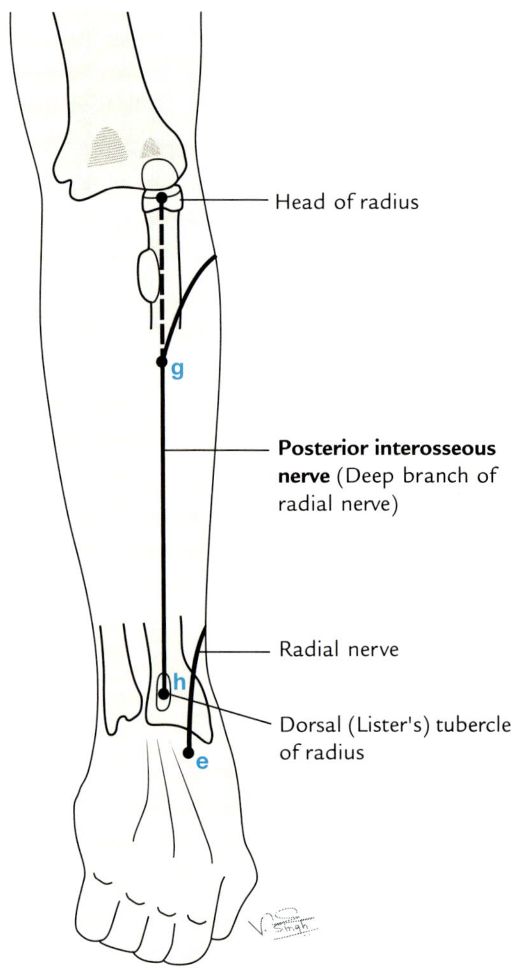

FIG. 14.11 ■ Surface marking of the posterior interosseous nerve.

POSTERIOR INTEROSSEOUS NERVE (DEEP BRANCH OF RADIAL NERVE) (FIG. 14.11)

- Mark a point 'f' just below the level of (front of) lateral epicondyle, 1 cm lateral to the tendon of biceps brachii.
- Mark a point 'g' on the line joining middle of posterior aspect of radial head and dorsal tubercle/Lister's tubercle at the junction of its upper and middle thirds.
- Mark a point 'h' on the back 1 cm medial to the dorsal/Lister's tubercle.

RETINACULA OF WRIST

FLEXOR RETINACULUM

- First mark the pisiform bone, tubercle of scaphoid, hook of hamate, and crest of trapezium.
- Flexor retinaculum is marked by joining above points.
- Upper border is obtained by joining the first points and lower border is obtained by joining the last two points. Upper border is concave upwards and lower border is concave downwards (Fig. 14.5).

EXTENSOR RETINACULUM

- Draw a 2-cm-long line on salient lower part of anterior border of radius above the styloid process.
- Draw a 2-cm-long line from tip of styloid process of ulna along the medial side of carpus (pisiform and triquetral bones).

Extensor retinaculum is marked by these two oblique lines joining the ends above lines (see page 123 and Fig. 9.22).

IDENTIFICATION OF STRUCTURES ON THE FRONT OF DISTAL FOREARM (FIGS. 14.12 AND 14.13)

Tendons of FCU, palmaris longus, and *FCR* are readily identified when wrist is flexed against resistance (Fig. 14.12).

N.B.

(a) Tendon of FCR is located approximately at the junction of lateral and middle thirds of an imaginary line drawn transversely across the distal forearm.

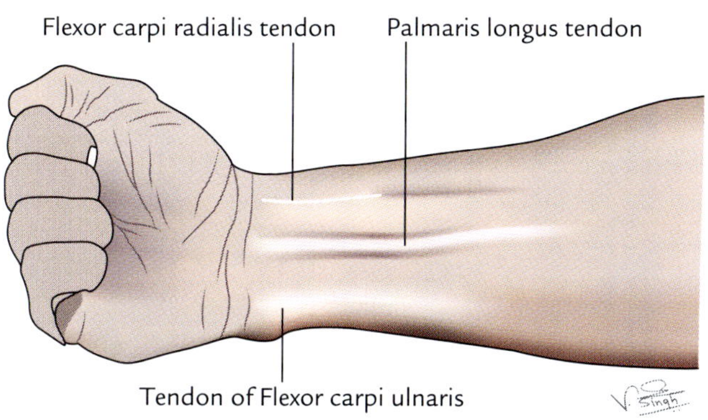

FIG. 14.12 ■ Identification of three tendons (i.e. tendons of flexor carpi ulnaris, palmaris longus, and flexor carpi radialis) in front of distal forearm.

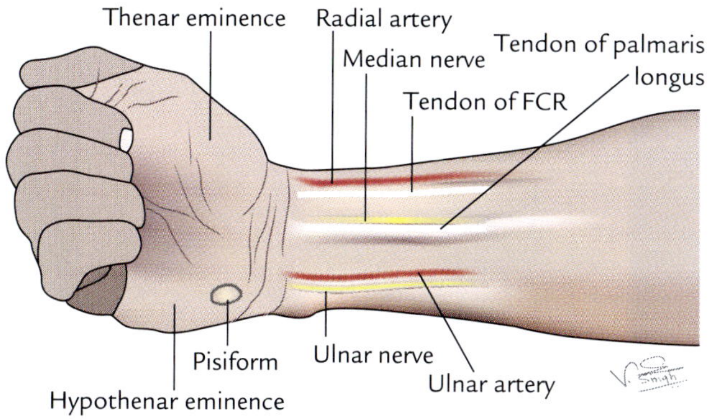

FIG. 14.13 ■ Identification of the arteries and nerves in front of distal forearm.

- ***Tendon of palmaris longus*** lies medial to the tendon of FCR and is most prominent.
- ***Tendon of FCU*** is easily palpated along the medial border of distal forearm and inserts on the pisiform.
- ***Ulnar artery*** lies immediately lateral to tendon of FCU.
- ***Radial artery*** lies immediately lateral to tendon of FCR.
- ***Median nerve*** lies between tendons of FCR and palmaris longus.

PULSE POINTS IN THE UPPER LIMB

The arterial pulse can be felt at following six locations in the upper limb (Fig. 14.14):

1. **Axillary pulse in axilla:** Pulsations of axillary artery can be felt against the lower part of the lateral wall of axilla, lateral to the dome of skin covering the floor of the axilla.
2. **Brachial pulse in midarm:** Pulsations of brachial artery can be felt on medial side of midarm, that is at the level of insertion of coracobrachialis. Here, the artery lies in the cleft between biceps and triceps brachii muscles.

N.B.

This is the site where cuff of blood pressure machine compresses the brachial artery while recording the blood pressure.

3. **Brachial pulse in the cubital fossa:** Pulsations of brachial artery in the cubital fossa are easily felt medial to the tendon of biceps brachii. This is the site where stethoscope is placed to hear the pulse of artery while taking blood pressure.
4. **Radial pulse in distal forearm:** Pulsations of radial artery can be easily felt in front of distal forearm immediately lateral to tendon of FCR and distal to styloid process of radius. It can also be felt in the anatomical snuffbox.

N.B.

It is the most common site for taking a pulse.

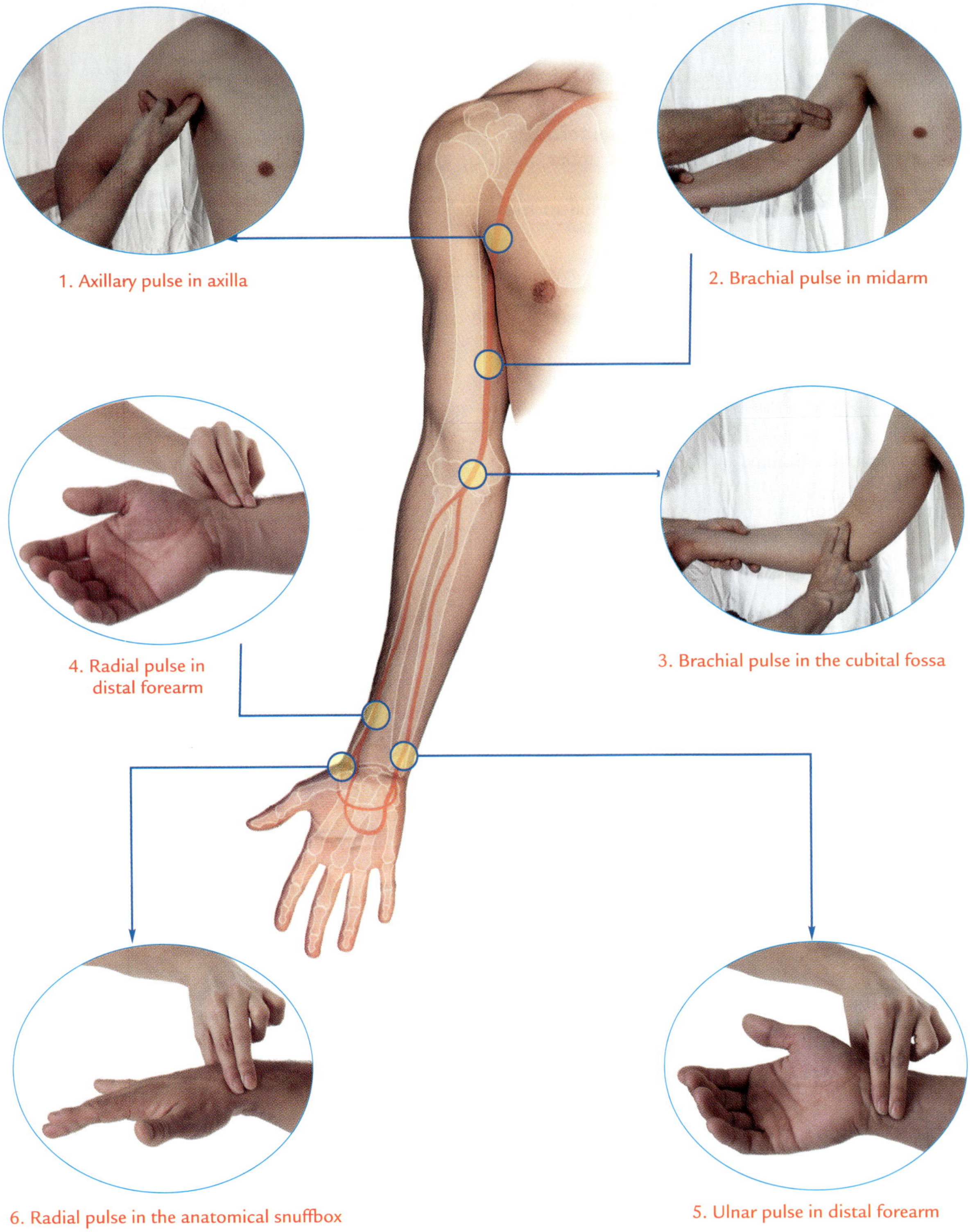

FIG. 14.14 ■ Sites of the pulse points in the upper limb. (*Source: Gray's Anatomy for Students*, 3ed.: Richard L. Drake, Wayne Vogl, Adam W.M. Mitchell, Fig. 7.123, Page 828, Elsevier Inc., 2005.)

5. **Ulnar pulse in the distal forearm:** Here, the pulsations of ulnar artery can be felt immediately lateral to the tendon of FCU.
6. **Radial pulse in the anatomical snuffbox:** Pulsations of radial artery are easily felt as it crosses the floor of anatomical snuffbox to reach the first interosseous space to enter the palm.

N.B.

From site of radial pulse at the distal forearm, the radial artery runs obliquely backwards and forwards to reach the anatomical snuffbox.

SEGMENTAL INNERVATION OF MOVEMENTS OF UPPER LIMB

- Shoulder
  - Abduction C5, 6
  - Adduction C6, 7, 8
  - Lateral rotation C5
  - Medial rotation C6, 7, 8
- Elbow
  - Flexion C5, 6
  - Extension C5, 6
- Radio-ulnar
  - Supination C6
  - Pronation C7
- Wrist
  - Flexion C7, 8
  - Extension C7, 8
- MP joints
  - Adduction T1
  - Abduction T1
- Interphalangeal joints
  - Flexion C7, 8
  - Extension C7, 8

SECTION II

THORAX

CHAPTER

15

Introduction to Thorax

SPECIFIC LEARNING OBJECTIVES

After studying this chapter, the student should be able to:

- Describe the boundaries of thoracic inlet, cavity, and outlet. AN 21.3
- Describe the diaphragm under the following headings: (a) origin, (b) insertion, (c) nerve supply, (d) actions, and (e) applied anatomy.
- Write short notes on: (a) Sibson's fascia, (b) central tendon of diaphragm, and (c) thoracic cage.
- Give the anatomical/embryological basis of: (a) thoracic inlet syndrome and (b) posterolateral hernia of diaphragm (hernia of Bochdalek).
- Enumerate: (a) structures passing through thoracic inlet, and (b) structures passing through major openings of diaphragm.

The thorax (G. thorakos = chest) is the part of body between root of the neck and abdomen. The term chest is used as a synonym of thorax. The thoracic cavity contains lungs and heart—the principal organs of respiration and circulation, respectively.

SURFACE LANDMARKS

The diseases of thoracic viscera are the leading cause of death all over the world. Therefore, surface landmarks of the thorax are extremely important to the physicians in providing reference locations for performing **inspection** (visual observation), **palpation** (feeling with firm pressure), **percussion** (detecting densities through tapping), and **auscultation** (listening sounds with the stethoscope).

BONY LANDMARKS

The bony landmarks of the thoracic wall are as follows (Fig. 15.1):

1. **Suprasternal notch (jugular notch):** It is felt just above the superior border of the manubrium sterni between the proximal medial ends of the two clavicles. It lies at the level of lower border of the body of T2 vertebra. The trachea can be palpated in this notch.
2. **Sternal angle (angle of Louis):** It is felt as a transverse ridge about 5 cm below the suprasternal notch. It marks the angle made between the manubrium and the body of the sternum (the angle between the long axis of manubrium and body of sternum is 163° posteriorly and 17° anteriorly). It lies at the level of intervertebral disc between the T4 and T5 vertebrae. The second rib cartilage articulates on either side with the sternum at this level. Hence, it is used as a surface landmark for counting the ribs (for details see page 205).
3. **Xiphisternal joint:** It can be felt at the apex of infrasternal/subcostal angle formed by the meeting of anterior end of costal margins. The xiphisternal joint lies at the level of the upper border of the body of T9 vertebra.
4. **Costal margin:** It forms the lower boundary of the thorax on each side and is formed by the cartilages of the 7th to 10th ribs and the free ends of 11th and 12th ribs. The lowest point of costal margin is formed by the 10th rib and lies at the level of L3 vertebra.
5. **Subcostal angle:** It is situated at the inferior end of the sternum between the sternal attachments of the seventh costal cartilage.
6. **Thoracic vertebral spines:** The first prominent spine felt at the lower end of nuchal furrow (midline furrow on the back of neck) is the spine of C7 vertebra (vertebra prominens). All the thoracic spines are counted below this level. For reference, the third thoracic spine lies at the level of root of spine of scapula and seventh thoracic spine lies at the level of inferior angle of the scapula.

SOFT TISSUE LANDMARKS

1. **Nipple:** In males, the nipple is usually located in the fourth intercostal space about 4 in (10 cm) from the midsternal line. In females, its position varies considerably.
2. **Apex beat of the heart:** It is lowermost and outermost thrust of cardiac pulsation, which is felt in the left fifth intercostal space 3.5 in (9 cm) from the midsternal line or just medial to the midclavicular line.

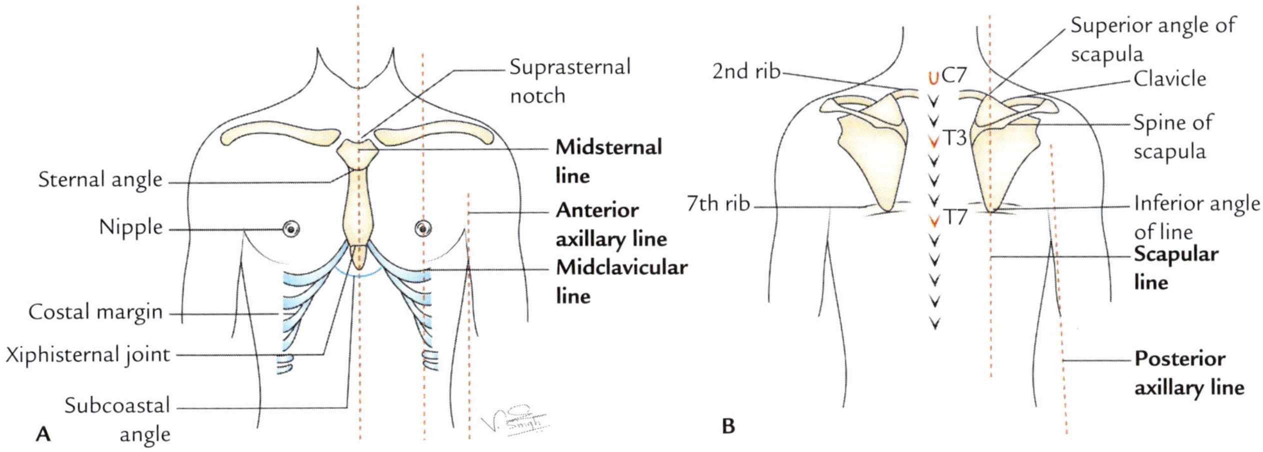

FIG. 15.1 ■ Surface landmarks on the thoracic wall: (**A**) anterior aspect; (**B**) posterior aspect.

LINES OF ORIENTATION (FIG. 15.1)

The following imaginary lines are often used to describe surface locations on the anterior and posterior chest wall.

1. **Midsternal line:** It runs vertically downwards in the median plane on the anterior aspect of the sternum.
2. **Midclavicular line:** It runs vertically downwards from the midpoint of the clavicle to the midinguinal point. It crosses the tip of the ninth costal cartilage.
3. **Anterior axillary line:** It runs vertically downwards from the anterior axillary fold.
4. **Midaxillary line:** It runs vertically downwards from the point in the axilla located between the anterior and posterior axillary folds.
5. **Posterior axillary line:** It runs vertically downwards from the posterior axillary fold.
6. **Scapular line:** It runs vertically downwards on the posterior aspect of the chest passing through the inferior angle of the scapula with arms at the sides of the body.

THORACIC CAGE AN 21.3

The thorax is supported by a skeletal framework called **thoracic cage**. The thoracic cage surrounds and protects the heart and lungs in the thoracic cavity. It provides attachment to muscles of thorax, upper extremities, back, and diaphragm. It is osteocartilaginous and elastic in nature. It is primarily designed for increasing or decreasing the intrathoracic pressure so that air is sucked into lungs during inspiration and expelled from lungs during expiration—an essential mechanism of respiration.

BOUNDARIES OF THORACIC CAVITY (FIG. 15.2)

The **thoracic cage** is formed:

Anteriorly: By sternum (breast bone).

Posteriorly: By 12 thoracic vertebrae and intervening intervertebral discs.

Laterally: By 12 pairs of ribs and associated costal cartilages on each side.

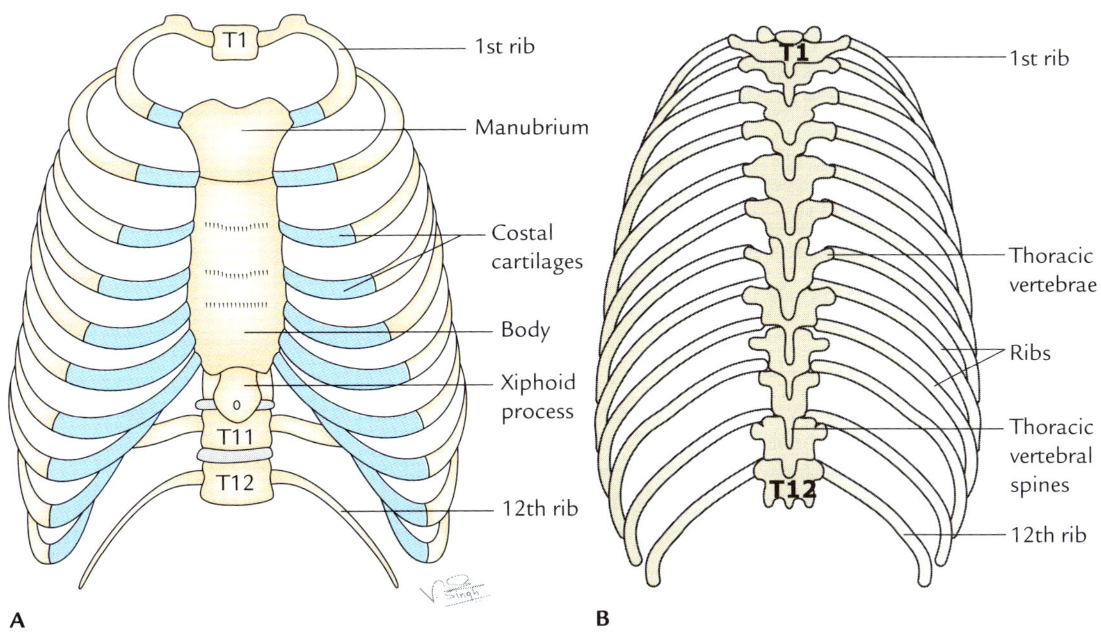

FIG. 15.2 ■ Thoracic cage: (**A**) anterior aspect; (**B**) posterior aspect.

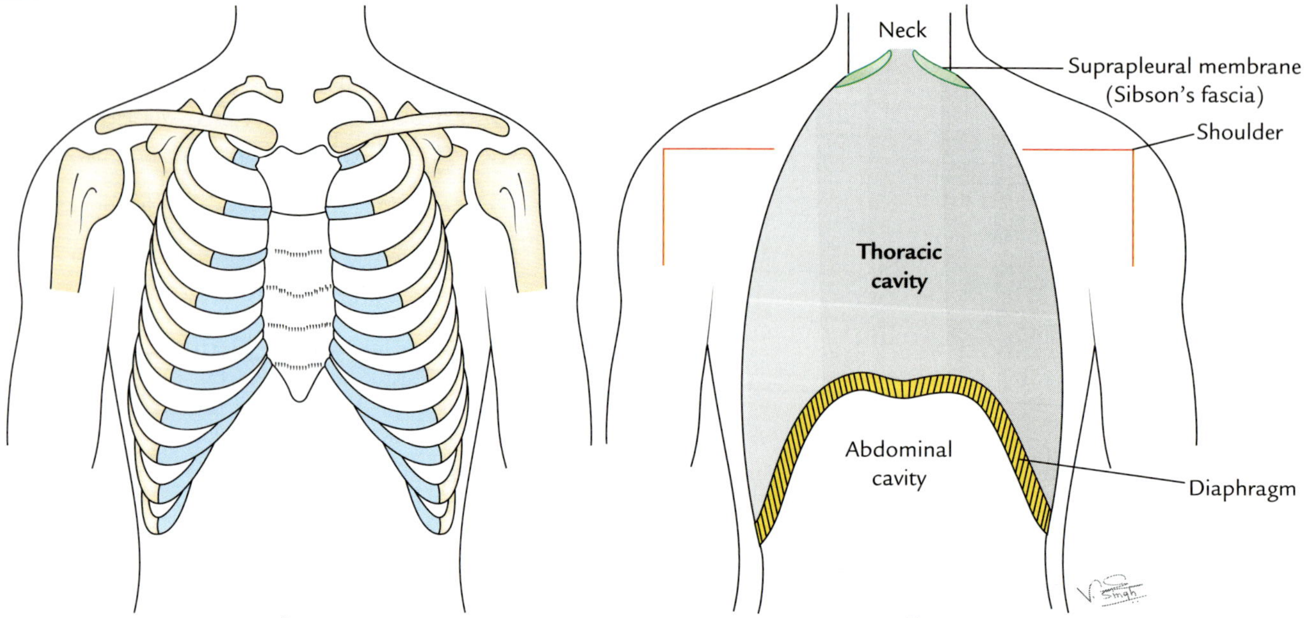

FIG. 15.3 ■ Thoracic cage and thoracic cavity: (**A**) shape of thoracic cage; (**B**) schematic diagram to show how the size of thoracic cavity is reduced by upward projection of the diaphragm and by inward projection of the shoulder.

The **rib cage** is formed by sternum, costal cartilages, and ribs attached to the thoracic vertebrae.

The ribs articulate as follows:

1. *Posteriorly:* All the ribs articulate with the thoracic vertebrae.
2. *Anteriorly:*
   (a) The upper seven ribs (first to seventh) articulate with the side of sternum through their costal cartilages.
   (b) The next three ribs (e.g. eighth to tenth) articulate with each other through their costal cartilages.
   (c) The lower two ribs (e.g. 11th and 12th) do not articulate with any rib and the anterior ends of their costal cartilages are free.

N.B.

The costal cartilages of seventh to tenth ribs form a sloping **costal margin**.

SHAPE (FIG. 15.3)

The thoracic cage and thoracic cavity resembles a truncated cone with its narrow end above and broad end below. The **narrow upper end** is continuous above with root of neck from which it is partly separated on either side by the suprapleural membranes (Sibson's fascia). The **broad lower end** is completely separated from abdominal cavity by the diaphragm, but provides passage to structures like aorta, oesophagus, and inferior vena cava (Fig. 15.3B).

The **diaphragm** is dome shaped with its convexity directed upwards. Thus, the upper abdominal viscera lies within the thoracic cage and are protected by it.

In life, the upper end of thorax appears broad due to the presence of shoulder girdle made up of clavicles and scapulae and associated scapular musculature (Fig. 15.3A).

N.B.

The thoracic cavity is actually much smaller than one assumes because the upper narrow part of thoracic cage appears broad (*vide supra*) and lower broad part of thoracic cage is encroached by the abdominal viscera due to dome-shaped diaphragm.

The thoracic cavity is divided into three compartments: one median and two lateral. The median compartment called mediastinum occupied by heart and structures transporting air (*viz.* trachea), blood (*viz.* great blood vessels), and food (*viz.* oesophagus) and two lateral compartments called right and left pleural cavities enclosing respective lungs.

TRANSVERSE SECTION OF THORAX

In transverse section, the **adult thorax is kidney shaped** with transverse diameter more than the anteroposterior diameter (Fig. 15.4B and C). This is because the ribs are placed obliquely in adults.

In transverse section, the **thorax of infants below the age of 2 years is circular** with equal transverse and anteroposterior diameter (Fig. 15.4A). This is because the ribs are horizontally placed.

The transverse sections of thorax in adult and infant are compared in Table 15.1.

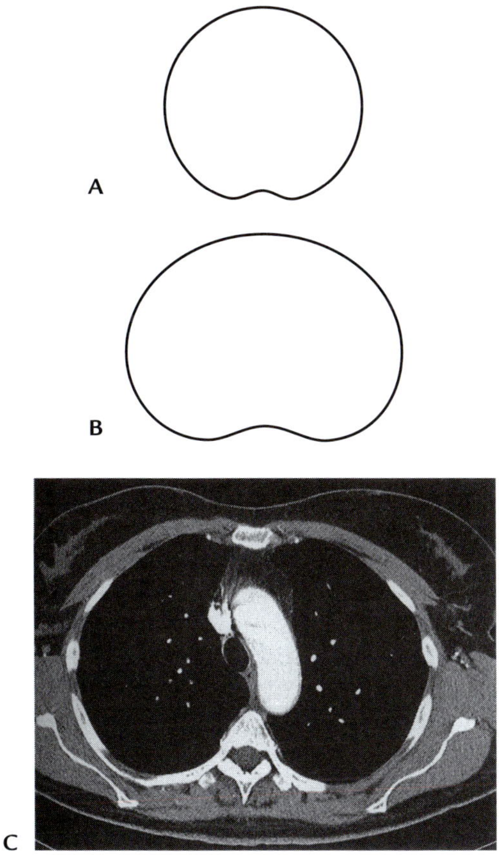

FIG. 15.4 ■ The shape of thoracic cavity as seen in transverse section of thorax: (**A**) in infant; (**B**) in adult; (**C**) transverse section of adult thorax as seen in CT scan.

TABLE 15.1 Comparison of thoracic cavity as seen in transverse sections of the thorax in an adult and infant

Thoracic cavity in adult	Thoracic cavity in infant
Kidney shaped	Circular
Ribs obliquely placed	Ribs horizontally placed
Transverse diameter can be increased by thoracic breathing (hence, respiration is thoracoabdominal)	Transverse diameter cannot be increased by thoracic breathing (hence, respiration is purely abdominal)

CLINICAL CORRELATION

Children are prone to pneumonia: The thorax up to 2 years after birth is circular in cross section. Therefore, the diameter of thorax cannot be increased within the circumference, the length of which remains constant. Therefore, in children up to the age of 2 years, the respiration is almost entirely abdominal.

Consequently, young *children are prone to suffer from pneumonia after abdominal operations*, because they resist breathing (being abdominal) due to pain. As a result, the secretions in the lungs tend to accumulate, which may become infected and cause *pneumonia*.

SUPERIOR THORACIC APERTURE (THORACIC INLET) AN 21.3

The thoracic cavity communicates with the root of the neck through a narrow opening called *superior thoracic aperture* or *thoracic inlet*.

N.B.

The *superior thoracic aperture* is called *thoracic outlet* by the clinicians because important arteries and T1 spinal nerves emerge from thorax through this aperture and enter the neck and upper limbs.

Anatomists refer to the superior thoracic aperture as thoracic inlet because air and food enter the thorax through trachea and oesophagus, respectively.

Boundaries (Fig. 15.5)

Anteriorly: Superior border of manubrium sterni.
Posteriorly: Anterior border of the superior surface of the body of T1 vertebra.
Laterally (on each side): Medial border of first rib and its cartilage.

The upper end of anterior boundary lies 4 cm (1.5 in) below the upper end of posterior boundary because first rib slopes downwards and forwards from its posterior end to anterior end (Fig. 15.6). Therefore, plane of thoracic inlet slopes (directed) downwards and forwards with an obliquity of about 45°. The upper border of manubrium sterni lies at the level of lower border of T2 vertebra (Fig. 15.7).

N.B.

Due to downward and forward inclination of thoracic inlet, the apex of lung with the overlying pleura (called cervical pleura) projects into the root of the neck.

Shape and Dimensions

Shape: Reniform/kidney shaped.
Dimensions: Transverse diameter: 11–12 cm/4.5 in.
Anteroposterior diameter: 5–6 cm/2.5 in.

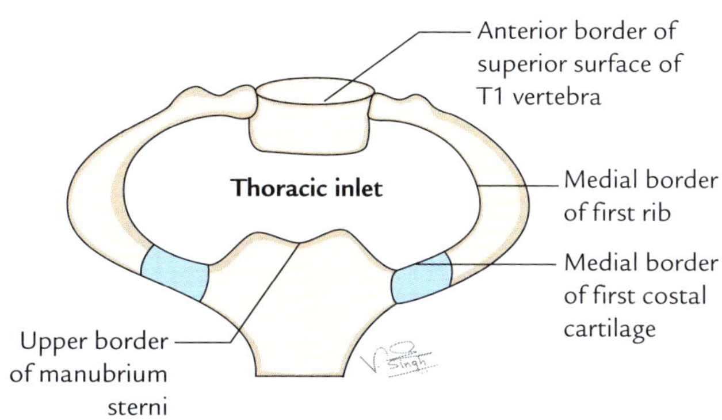

FIG. 15.5 ■ Boundaries of the thoracic inlet.

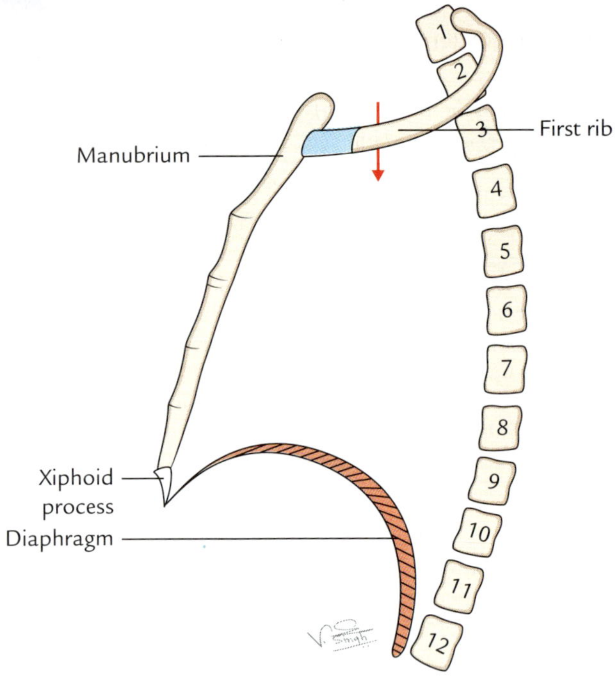

FIG. 15.6 ■ Superior thoracic aperture; arrow (lateral view).

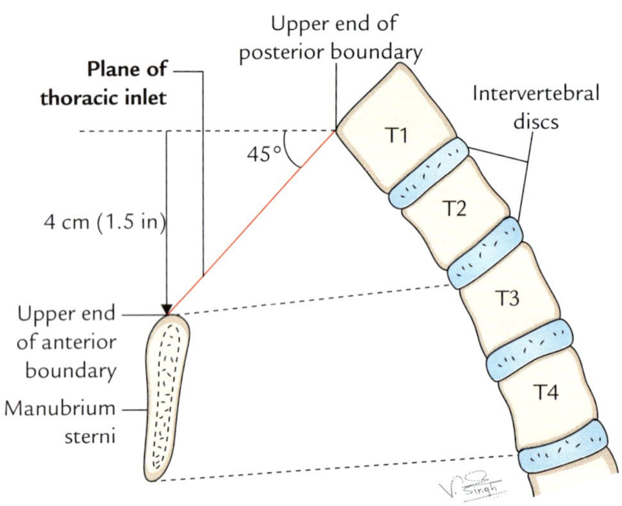

FIG. 15.7 ■ Plane of the thoracic inlet.

DIAPHRAGM OF SUPERIOR THORACIC APERTURE (SUPRAPLEURAL MEMBRANE/ SIBSON'S FASCIA)

The part of thoracic inlet, on either side, is closed by a dense fascial sheet called **suprapleural membrane** or **Sibson's fascia**, or diaphragm of superior thoracic aperture. It is **tent shaped.**

Attachments and Relations (Fig. 15.8)

The apex of Sibson's fascia is attached to the tip of transverse process of C7 vertebra, and its base is attached to the inner border of first rib and its costal cartilage. Its superior surface is related to the subclavian vessels and its inferior surface is related to cervical pleura, covering the apex of the lung.

Functions

The functions of Sibson's fascia are as follows:

1. It protects the underlying cervical pleura, beneath which lies the apex of the lung.
2. It resists the intrathoracic pressure during respiration. As a result, the root of neck is not puffed up and down during respiration.

N.B.

Morphologically, Sibson's fascia represents the spread out degenerated tendon of *scalenus minimus* (or *pleuralis*) *muscle*.

Structures Passing Through Thoracic Inlet (Fig. 15.9)

- Muscles:
  1. Sternohyoid.
  2. Sternothyroid.
  3. Longus cervicis/longus colli.
- Arteries:
  1. Right and left internal thoracic arteries.
  2. Brachiocephalic trunk/artery.
  3. Left common carotid artery.
  4. Left subclavian artery.
  5. Right and left superior intercostal arteries.

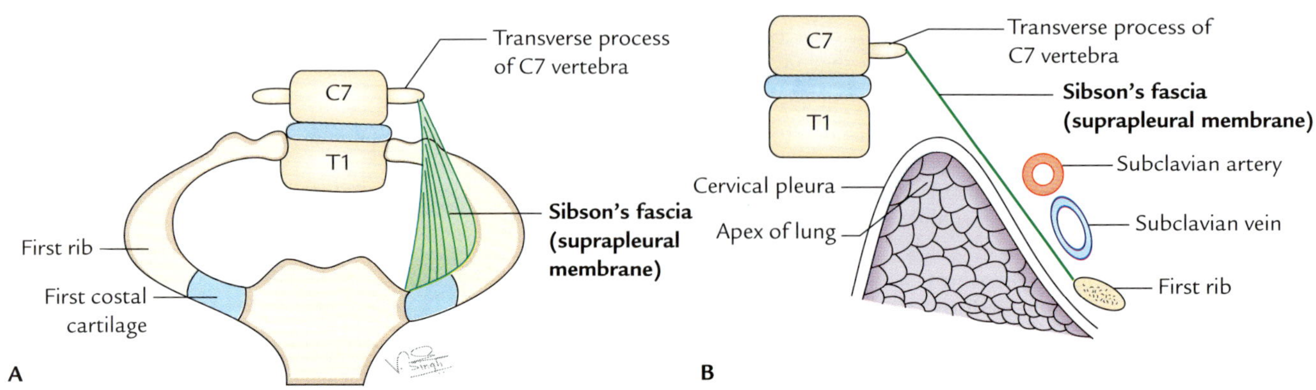

FIG. 15.8 ■ Suprapleural membrane/Sibson's fascia: (**A**) attachments; (**B**) relations.

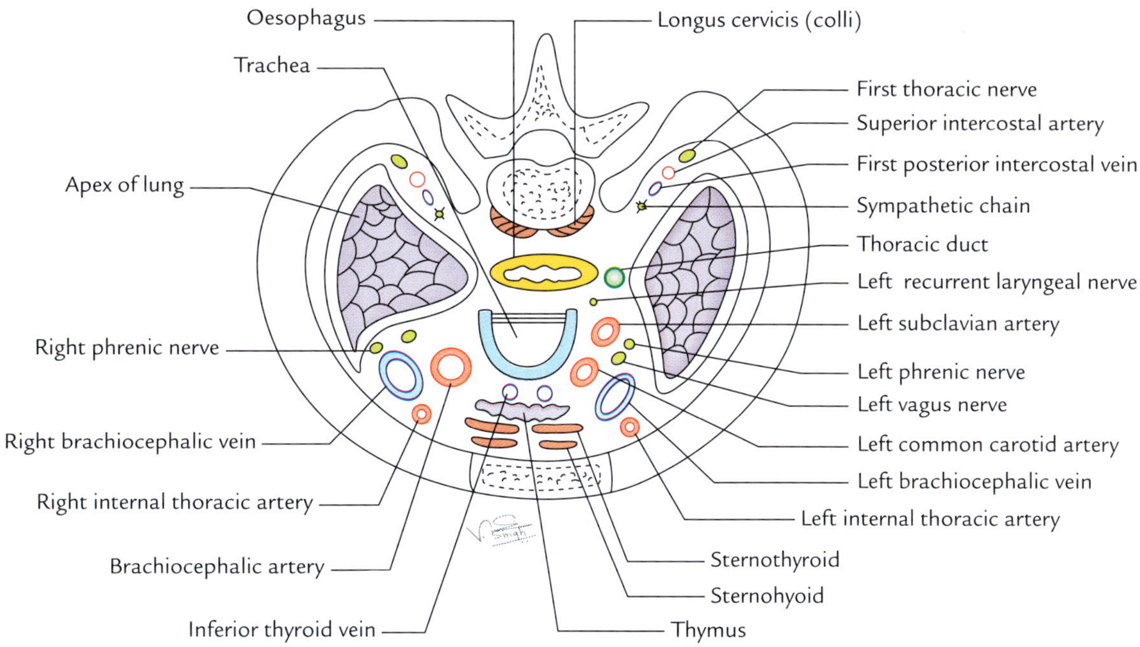

FIG. 15.9 ■ Structures passing through the thoracic inlet.

- Nerves:
  1. Right and left vagus nerves.
  2. Left recurrent laryngeal nerve.
  3. Right and left phrenic nerves.
  4. Right and left first thoracic nerves.
  5. Right and left sympathetic chains.
- Veins:
  1. Right and left brachiocephalic veins.
  2. Right and left first posterior intercostal veins.
  3. Inferior thyroid veins.
- Lymphatics: Thoracic duct.
- Others:
  1. Anterior longitudinal ligament.
  2. Oesophagus.
  3. Trachea.
  4. Right and left domes of cervical pleura, anteriorly.
  5. Apices of right and left lungs, anteriorly.

CLINICAL CORRELATION

Thoracic inlet syndrome: The subclavian artery and lower trunk of the brachial plexus arch over the first rib to pass through gap between scalenus anterior and scalenus medius (scalene triangle). Hence they may be stretched and pushed up by the presence of a congenitally hypertrophied scalenus anterior muscle or a cervical rib. This leads to thoracic inlet syndrome (also called *scalenus anterior syndrome* or *cervical rib syndrome*). It presents the following clinical features:

- Numbness, tingling, and pain along the medial side of forearm and hand, and wasting of small muscles of the hand due to the involvement of lower trunk of brachial plexus (T1).
- There may be ischaemic symptoms in the upper limb such as pallor and coldness of the upper limb, and weak radial pulse due to compression of the subclavian artery.

The clinicians call this syndrome as '***thoracic outlet syndrome***.' For details see page 168, Vol III.

INFERIOR THORACIC APERTURE (THORACIC OUTLET) AN 21.3

The inferior thoracic aperture is broad and surrounds the upper part of the abdominal cavity. The large musculoaponeurotic diaphragm attached to the margins of thoracic outlet separates the thoracic cavity from the abdominal cavity.

Boundaries

Anteriorly: Xiphisternal joint.

Posteriorly: Body of 12th thoracic vertebra.

Laterally (on each side): Costal margin (formed by costal cartilages of 7th to 10th ribs) and 11th and 12th ribs.

DIAPHRAGM OF INFERIOR THORACIC APERTURE (FIG. 15.10)

The thoracic outlet is closed by a large dome-shaped flat muscle called **diaphragm**. Since it separates thoracic cavity from abdominal cavity, it is also termed **thoraco-abdominal diaphragm**.

The diaphragm is the **principal muscle of respiration**. It is dome shaped and consists of peripheral muscular part, and central fibrous part called **central tendon**.

Origin

The origin of the diaphragm is divided into three parts, *viz*.

1. Sternal.
2. Costal.
3. Vertebral.

Sternal part: It consists of two fleshy slips which arise from the posterior surface of the xiphoid process.

Costal part: On each side, it consists of six fleshy slips which arise from the inner surface of lower six ribs near their costal cartilages.

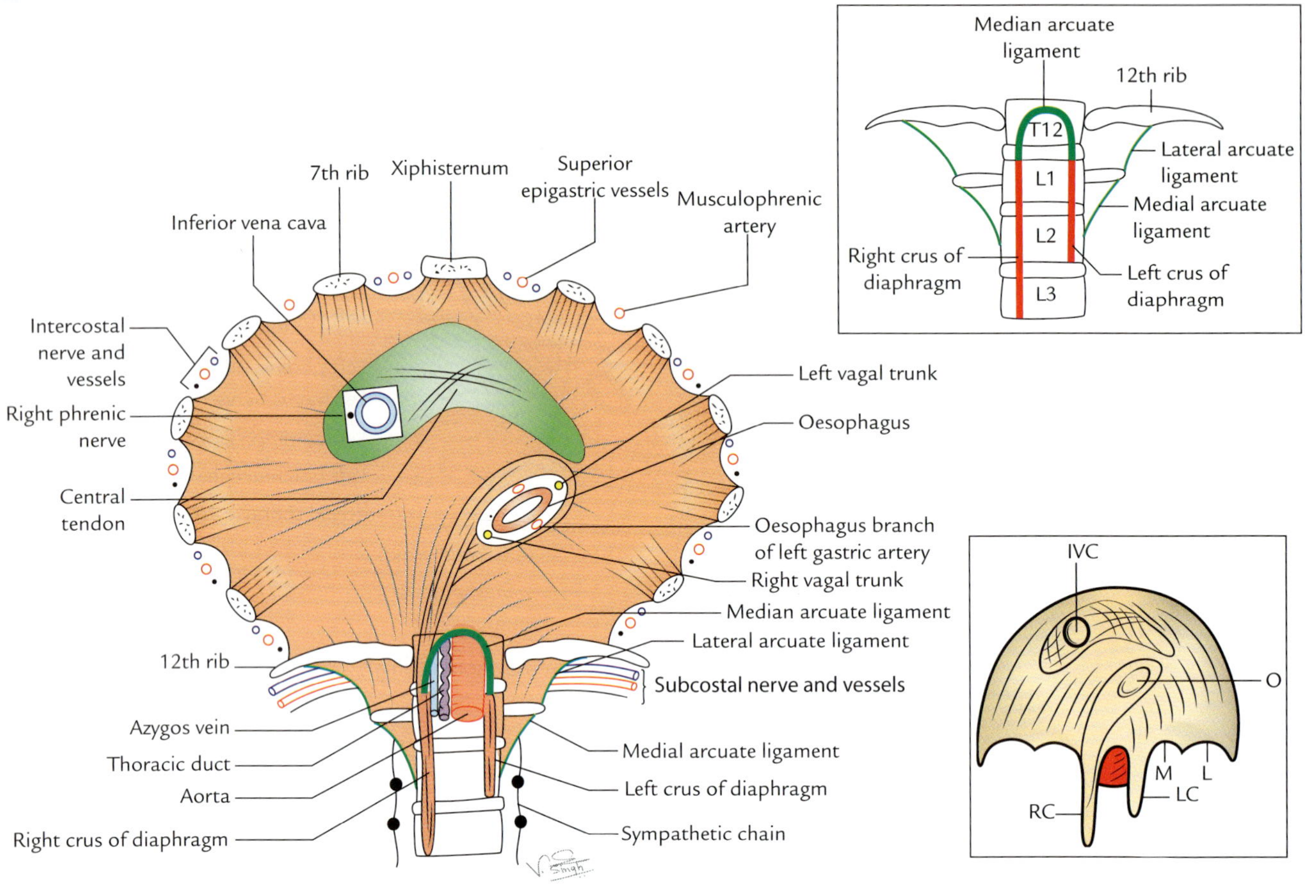

FIG. 15.10 ■ Origin, insertion, and openings of the diaphragm. Figure in the right upper inset shows details of vertebral origin of the diaphragm. While the figure in right lower inset shows simplified figure of dome-shaped diagram (IVC = inferior vena cava, O = oesophagus, RC = right crus of diaphragm, LC = left crus of diaphragm, M = medial lumbocostal arch, L = lateral lumbocostal arch).

Vertebral part: This part arises by means of (a) right and left crura of diaphragm and (b) five arcuate ligaments.

Crura

- *Right crus:* It is a vertical fleshy bundle which arises from the right side of anterior aspects of the upper three lumbar vertebrae and intervening intervertebral discs.
- *Left crus:* It is vertical fleshy bundle which arises from the left side of anterior aspects of upper two lumbar vertebrae and the intervening intervertebral disc.

The medial margins of the crura are tendinous.

Arcuate Ligaments

- **Median arcuate ligament** is an arched fibrous band stretching between the upper ends of two crura.
- **Medial arcuate ligament** is the thickened upper margin of the psoas sheath. It extends from the side of the body of L2 vertebra to the tip of the transverse process of L1 vertebra.
- **Lateral arcuate ligament** is the thickened upper margin of fascia covering the anterior surface of the quadratus lumborum. It extends from the tip of transverse process of L1 vertebra to the 12th rib.

N.B.

The right crus is attached to more number of vertebrae because the right side diaphragm has to contract on the massive liver.

Insertion

From circumferential origin (*vide supra*), the muscle fibres converge towards the central tendon and insert into its margins.

The features of the central tendon are as follows:

1. It is trifoliate in shape having (a) single triangular anterior/central leaflet and two (b and c) tongue-shaped posterior leaflets. It resembles an equilateral triangle. The right posterior leaflet is short and stout, whereas the left posterior leaflet is thin and long.
2. It is inseparably fused with the fibrous pericardium.
3. It is located nearer to the sternum than to the vertebral column.

Surfaces and Relations

The **superior surface** of diaphragm projects on either side as **dome** or **cupola** into the thoracic cavity. Depressed area between the two domes is called **central tendon**. The superior surface is covered by endothoracic fascia and is related to the bases of right and left pleura on the sides and to the fibrous pericardium in the middle.

The **inferior surface** of diaphragm is lined by the diaphragmatic fascia and parietal peritoneum.

- *On the right side it is related to* (a) right lobe of the liver, (b) right kidney, and (c) right suprarenal gland.
- *On the left side it is related to* (a) left lobe of the liver, (b) fundus of stomach, (c) spleen, (d) left kidney, and (e) left suprarenal gland.

Openings of the Diaphragm

The openings of diaphragm are classified into two types: (a) major openings and (b) minor openings.

Major Openings (*Fig. 15.10*)

There are three named major openings, *viz*.

1. *Vena caval opening.*
2. *Oesophageal opening.*
3. *Aortic opening.*

The location, shape, and vertebral levels of these openings are presented in Table 15.2.

The structure passing through three major opening of diaphragm is listed in Table 15.3.

N.B.

Effect of contraction of diaphragm on three major openings:

- Contraction of diaphragm *enlarges the caval opening* to enhance venous return.
- Contraction of diaphragm has a *sphincteric effect on the oesophageal opening* (pinch-cock effect).
- Contraction of diaphragm has *no effect on the aortic opening* because strictly speaking it is outside the diaphragm.

Minor Openings

These are unnamed. Structures passing through these openings are as follows:

1. **Superior epigastric vessels** pass through the gap (*space of Larry*) between the muscular slips arising from xiphoid process and seventh costal cartilage.

TABLE 15.2 Location, shape, and vertebral level of three major openings of the diaphragm

Opening	Location	Shape	Vertebral level
Vena caval opening	In the central tendon slightly to the right of median plane between the central and right posterior leaflets	Quadrangular or square	T8 (body)
Oesophageal opening	Slightly to the left of median plane (the fibres of right crus split around the opening and act like pinch cock)	Oval or elliptical	T10 (body)
Aortic opening	In the midline behind the median arcuate ligament	Circular or round	T12 (lower border of the body)

TABLE 15.3 Structures passing through three major openings of the diaphragm

Opening	Structures passing through
Vena caval opening	• Inferior vena cava • Right phrenic nerve
Oesophageal opening	• Oesophagus • Right and left vagal trunks • Oesophageal branches of left gastric artery
Aortic opening	From right to left these are: - Azygos vein - Thoracic duct - Aorta

2. **Musculophrenic artery** passes through the gap between the slips of origin from seventh to eighth ribs.
3. **Lower five intercostal nerves and vessels** (i.e. 7th to 11th) pass through gaps between the adjoining costal slips.
4. **Subcostal nerves and vessels** pass deep to the lateral arcuate ligament.
5. **Sympathetic chain** passes deep to the medial arcuate ligament.
6. **Greater**, **lesser**, and **least splanchnic nerves** pass by piercing the crus of diaphragm on the corresponding side.
7. **Hemiazygos vein** pierces the left crus of the diaphragm.

Nerve Supply

The diaphragm is supplied by:

(a) Right and left phrenic nerves and
(b) Lower five intercostal and subcostal nerves.

Motor supply: By right and left phrenic nerves.

Sensory supply:

(a) *Central part:* By right and left phrenic nerves.
(b) *Peripheral part:* By lower sixth to tenth intercostal nerves.

The **phrenic nerves** are formed one on either side in the neck from ventral rami of C3–C5. It lies on anterior aspect of scalenus anterior. Then descend vertically deep to subclavian vein into thorax on the side of pericardium to provide an all-important motor supply to the diaphragm—the *key respiratory muscle*.

The detailed distribution is as follows: the *right phrenic nerve* provides motor innervation to the right half of the diaphragm up to the right margin of oesophageal opening, and *left phrenic nerve* provides motor innervation to the left half of the diaphragm up to the left margin of the oesophageal opening.

The phrenic nerves also provide sensory innervation to the central tendon of the diaphragm, and pleura and peritoneum related to it.

The *intercostal nerves* supply the peripheral parts of the diaphragm.

Arterial Supply

The diaphragm is supplied by the following arteries:

1. **Superior phrenic arteries** (also called *phrenic arteries*) from thoracic aorta.
2. **Inferior phrenic arteries,** from the abdominal aorta.
3. **Pericardiophrenic arteries,** from the internal thoracic arteries.
4. **Musculophrenic arteries,** the terminal branches of the internal thoracic arteries.
5. **Superior epigastric arteries,** the terminal branches of the internal thoracic arteries.
6. Lower five intercostal and subcostal arteries from the aorta.

Lymphatic Drainage

The lymph from diaphragm is drained into the following groups of lymph nodes:

1. **Anterior diaphragmatic lymph nodes,** situated behind the xiphoid process.
2. **Posterior diaphragmatic lymph nodes,** situated near the aortic orifice.
3. **Right lateral diaphragmatic nodes,** situated near the caval opening.
4. **Left lateral diaphragmatic nodes,** situated near the oesophageal opening.

Actions of Diaphragm

The diaphragm acts to subserve the following functions:

1. **Muscle of inspiration:** The diaphragm is the main/principal muscle of respiration. When it contracts, it descends and increases the vertical diameter of the thoracic cavity (for details see page 228).
2. **Muscle of abdominal straining:** The contraction of diaphragm along with contraction of muscles of anterior abdominal wall raises the intraabdominal pressure to evacuate the pelvic contents (voluntary expulsive efforts, e.g. micturition, defaecation, vomiting, and parturition).
3. **Muscle of weight lifting:** By taking deep breath and closing the glottis, it is possible to raise the intraabdominal pressure to such an extent that it will help support the vertebral column and prevent its flexion. This assists the postvertebral muscles in lifting the heavy weights.
4. **Thoracomuscular pump:** The descent of diaphragm decreases the intrathoracic pressure and at the same time increases the intraabdominal pressure. This pressure change compresses the inferior vena cava, and consequently its blood is forced upward into the right atrium.
5. **Sphincter of oesophagus:** The fibres of the right crus of diaphragm subserve a sphincteric control over the oesophageal opening.

CLINICAL CORRELATION

- **Diaphragmatic paralysis (paralysis of diaphragm):** The unilateral damage of phrenic nerve leads to *unilateral diaphragmatic paralysis.* The condition is diagnosed during fluoroscopy when an elevated hemidiaphragm is seen on the side of lesion, and showing paradoxical movements. The bilateral damage of phrenic nerves leads to complete diaphragmatic paralysis. It is a serious condition as it may cause respiratory failure.
- **Hiccups:** They occur due to involuntary spasmodic contractions of the diaphragm accompanied by the closure of the glottis. Hiccups normally occur after eating or drinking as a result of gastric irritation.

  The pathological causes of hiccups include diaphragmatic irritation, phrenic nerve irritation, hysteria, and uraemia.

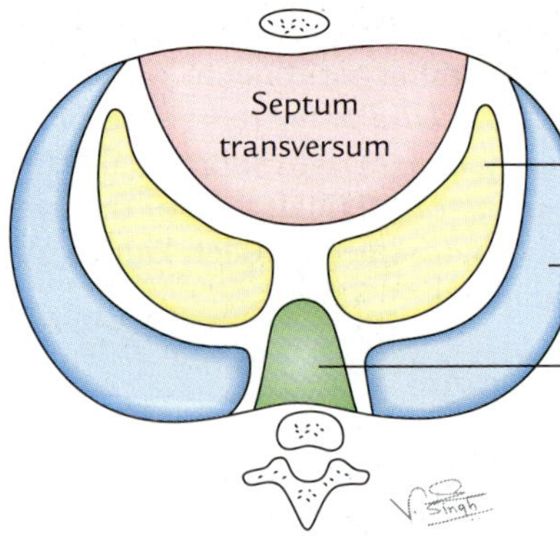

FIG. 15.11 Developmental components (primordia) of the diaphragm.

Development

The diaphragm develops in the region of neck from the following four embryonic structures (primordia) (Fig. 15.11):

1. Septum transversum, ventrally.
2. Pleuroperitoneal membranes at the sides.
3. Dorsal mesentery of oesophagus, dorsally.
4. **Body wall (mesoderm),** peripherally.

Adult Derivatives

- *Central tendon of diaphragm* develops from septum transversum.
- *Domes of diaphragm* develop from pleuroperitoneal membranes.
- *Part of diaphragm around the oesophagus* develops from the dorsal mesentery of oesophagus.
- *Peripheral part of diaphragm* develops from the body wall (mesoderm).

For details of development, refer *Textbook of Clinical Embryology*, 3ed. by Vishram Singh.

N.B.

Descent of diaphragm: The musculature of diaphragm develops from third to fifth cervical myotomes (C3–C5), hence it receives its motor innervations from C3 to C5 spinal segments (i.e. **phrenic nerve**). Later, when diaphragm descends from the neck to its definitive position (i.e. thoracoabdominal junction), its nerve supply is dragged down. This explains the long course of the phrenic nerve.

CLINICAL CORRELATION

Diaphragmatic hernias

- **Congenital:** The various types of congenital diaphragmatic hernias are as follows:
  (a) **Posterolateral hernia** (commonest congenital diaphragmatic hernia; Fig. 15.12): In this condition, there is herniation of abdominal contents into the thoracic cavity, which compress the lung and heart. The herniation occurs through the gap (pleuroperitoneal hiatus) between the costal and vertebral origins of the diaphragm called *foramen of Bochdalek*. The gap remains due to failure of closure of pleuroperitoneal canal. It occurs commonly on the left side (for details see *Clinical and Surgical Anatomy*, 2ed. by Vishram Singh).

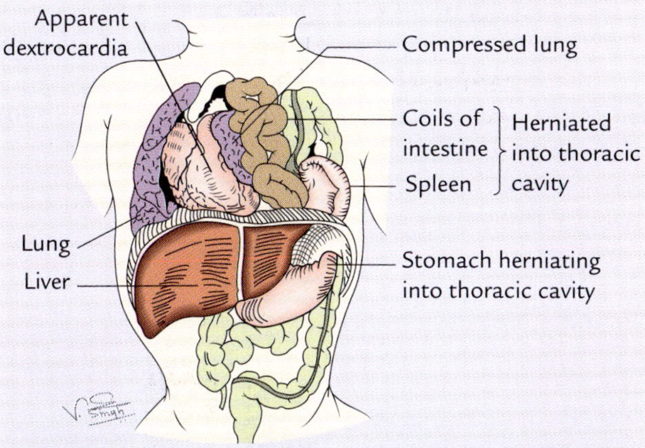

FIG. 15.12 ■ Posterolateral hernia of diaphragm. (*Source: Textbook of Clinical Embryology*: Vishram, Fig. 21.8, Page 229, RELX India Pvt. Ltd., 2022.)

  (b) **Retrosternal hernia:** It occurs through the gap between the muscular slips of origin from xiphisternum and seventh costal cartilage (space of Larry or foramen of Morgagni). It is more common on the right side. Thus hernial sac usually lies between pericardium and right pleura. Usually it causes no symptoms in the infants, but in later age, the patients complain of discomfort and dysphagia (difficulty in swallowing).
  (c) **Paraoesophageal hernia:** In this condition, there is defect in the diaphragm to the right and anterior to the oesophageal opening. The anterior wall of the stomach rolls upwards in the hernial sac through this defect, until it becomes upside down in the thoracic cavity. An important feature of paraoesophageal hernia is that the normal relationship of gastrooesophageal junction in relation to diaphragm is not disturbed.
- **Acquired:** The acquired diaphragmatic hernias may be either traumatic or hiatal (sliding).
  (a) **Traumatic hernia:** It may occur due to an open injury to the diaphragm by the penetrating wounds or closed injury to the diaphragm in road traffic accidents leading to sudden severe increase in the intraabdominal pressure.
  (b) **Hiatal (sliding) hernia** (Fig. 15.13)**:** This is the *commonest of all the internal hernias*. In sliding hernia, the gastrooesophageal junction and cardiac end of stomach slides up into the thoracic cavity, but only anterolateral portion of the herniated stomach is covered by peritoneum, therefore the stomach itself is not within the hernial sac. The hiatal hernia is caused by the weakness of the diaphragmatic muscle surrounding the oesophageal opening and increased intraabdominal pressure. This may cause regurgitation of acid contents of stomach into the oesophagus leading to *peptic oesophagitis*. The patient complains of heart burn. The sliding hernia is usually associated with short oesophagus.

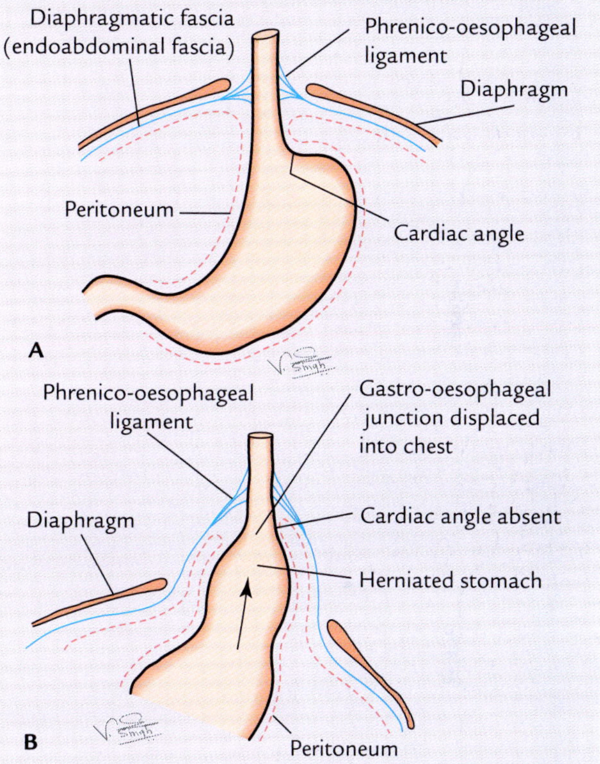

FIG. 15.13 ■ Acquired hiatal (sliding) hernia: (**A**) normal position of stomach; (**B**) herniated stomach.

Golden Facts to Remember

• Principal muscle of respiration	Diaphragm
• Commonest congenital diaphragmatic hernia	Posterolateral hernia of Bochdalek
• Commonest of all the internal hernias	Acquired hiatal (sliding) hernia
• Superior thoracic aperture is called by clinicians as	Thoracic outlet
• Diaphragm receives its motor innervations from C3 to C5 spinal segments (phrenic nerve) because	Diaphragm develops from third to fifth cervical myotomes in the neck

CLINICAL CASE STUDY

A male infant was brought to the hospital having markedly laboured respiration and cyanosis. The heart sounds were displaced and there was an apparent dextrocardia. The left side of the chest was dull (flat) to percussion and had diminished breath sounds. The abdomen was characteristically scaphoid (i.e. boat shaped). The X-ray chest revealed the presence of bowel, spleen, and portions of the liver within thorax. A diagnosis of **congenital posterolateral (Bochdalek) hernia of diaphragm** was made.

Questions

1. Tell the congenital defect of diaphragm that leads to posterolateral hernia of Bochdalek.
2. Posterolateral (Bochdalek) hernia is common on which side—right or left?
3. What are the different types of congenital diaphragmatic hernia?
4. Which is the commonest congenital hernia of the diaphragm? Give its incidence.

Answers

1. Congenital gap between the vertebral and costal origins of the diaphragm due to failure of closure of pleuroperitoneal canal.
2. It is three to five times more common on the left side.
3. (a) Posterolateral hernia, (b) retrosternal hernia, and (c) congenital paraoesophageal hernia or rolling hernia.
4. Posterolateral hernia of Bochdalek. Its incidence is 1:2000 births.

CHAPTER 16

Bones and Joints of the Thorax

SPECIFIC LEARNING OBJECTIVES

After studying this chapter, the student should be able to:

- Identify and describe the salient features of sternum, first rib, and typical thoracic vertebra. AN 21.1
- Enumerate: (a) anatomical events occurring at the sternal angle, (b) structures passing in front of the neck of the first rib, and (c) structures lying behind the manubrium sterni.
- Write short notes on: (a) cervical rib, (b) sternal puncture, and (c) rib fracture.
- Identify and describe the features of atypical ribs; and atypical thoracic vertebrae. AN 21.2
- Enumerate various joints of the thorax. Describe the costovertebral and costotransverse joints in detail.
- Describe type, articular surfaces, and movements of manubriosternal and xiphisternal joints. AN 21.8

BONES OF THE THORAX

The bones of the thorax form the major part of the thoracic cage and provide support and protection to viscera (e.g. heart and lungs) present within the thoracic cavity. The thoracic cage is not static in nature but dynamic as it keeps on moving at its various joints.

The bones of the thorax are:

1. Sternum
2. Twelve pairs of ribs
3. Twelve thoracic vertebrae

STERNUM AN 21.1

The sternum (breast bone; Fig. 16.1A and B) is an elongated flat bone that lies in the anterior median part of the chest wall. It is about 17 cm long.

PARTS

The sternum consists of the following three parts:

1. **Upper part**, the manubrium sterni/episternum
2. **Middle part**, the body/mesosternum
3. **Lower part**, the xiphoid process/metasternum

The sternum resembles a *dagger* or a *small sword* in shape. Its three parts—manubrium, body, and xiphoid-represent the handle, blade, and point of the sword, respectively.

The upper part of the sternum is broad and thick, whereas its lower part is thin and pointed. Its anterior surface is slightly rough and convex, while its posterior surface is smooth and slightly concave.

The manubrium and body of the sternum lie at an angle of 163° to each other, which increases slightly during inspiration and decreases during expiration. The angle between the long axis of the manubrium and the long axis of the body of the sternum is about 17°.

Anatomical Position

In anatomical position, the sternum as a whole is directed downward and inclined slightly forward with its rough convex surface facing anteriorly. Its broad upper end is directed upward and its pointed lower end is directed downward.

FEATURES AND ATTACHMENTS

Manubrium (Episternum; Figs. 16.1 and 16.2)

It is roughly quadrilateral in shape. It lies opposite to the third and fourth thoracic vertebrae. It is the thickest and strongest part of the sternum and presents the following features:

1. Two surfaces—anterior and posterior
2. Four borders—superior, inferior, and lateral (right and left)

The **anterior surface** on each side provides attachment to the sternal head of the sternocleidomastoid and pectoralis major muscles.

The **posterior surface** is smooth and forms the anterior boundary of the superior mediastinum.

- On each side, it provides attachment to two muscles:
  - (a) *sternohyoid* at the level of the clavicular notch and
  - (b) *sternothyroid* at the level of the facet for the first costal cartilage.
- Lower half is related to the arch of aorta.
- Upper half is related to three branches of the arch of aorta, *namely*, brachiocephalic artery, left common carotid artery, left subclavian artery, and left brachiocephalic vein.

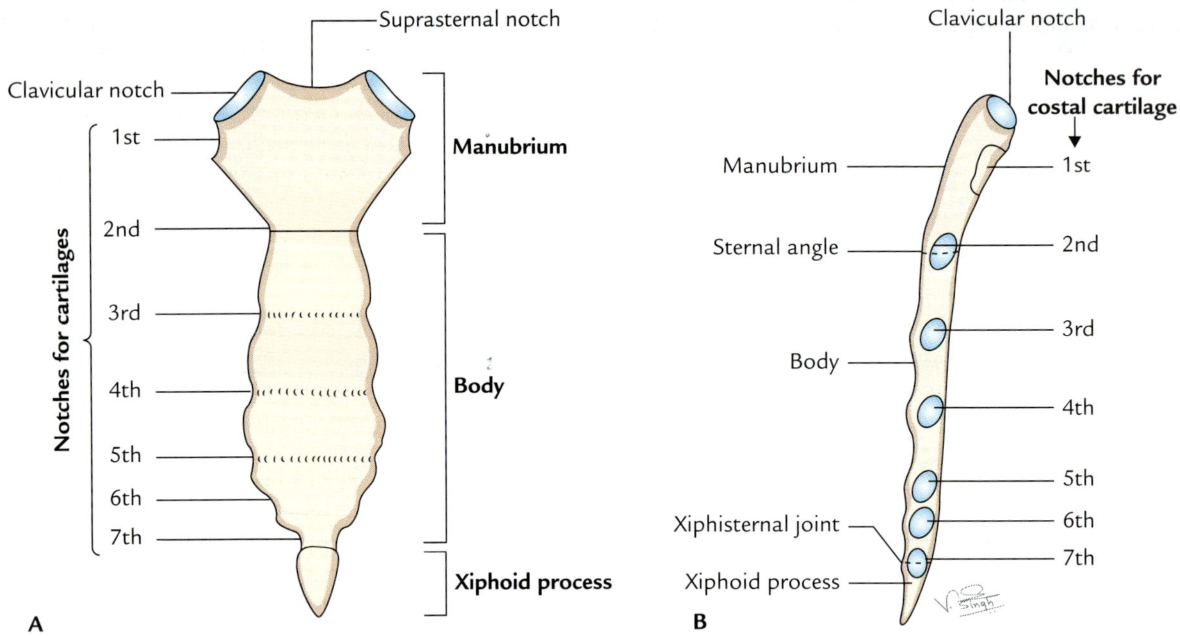

FIG. 16.1 ■ Features of the sternum. (**A**) Anterior aspect and (**B**) lateral aspect.

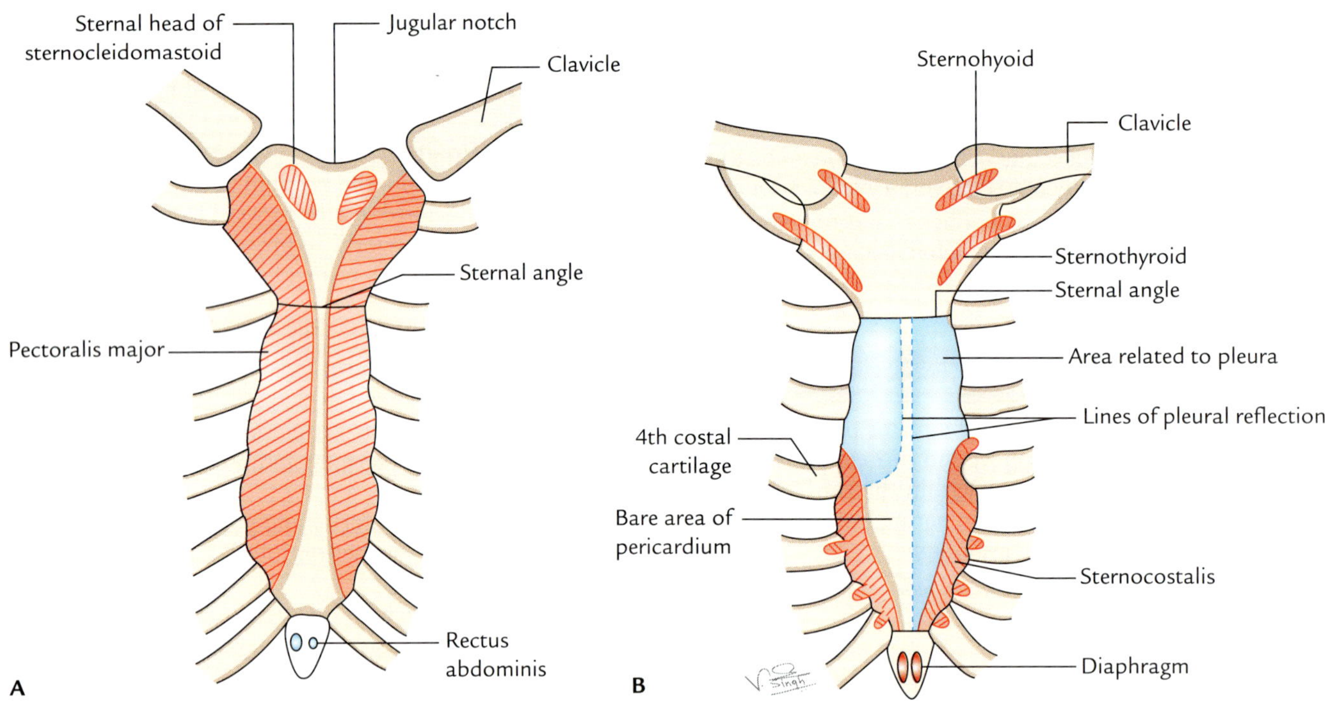

FIG. 16.2 ■ Attachments on the sternum. (**A**) Anterior surface and (**B**) posterior surface.

The **upper border** is thick, rounded, and concave. It presents a notch called the *suprasternal notch* or *jugular notch*.

- It provides attachment to the interclavicular ligament.
- Clavicular notch on either side of the suprasternal notch articulates with the clavicle to form the *sternoclavicular joint (saddle-shaped synovial joint)*.

The **lateral border** presents two articular facets:

- Upper facet articulates with the first costal cartilage to form the primary cartilaginous joint.
- Lower demifacet along with other demifacet in the body of the sternum articulates with the second costal cartilage.

The **lower border** articulates with the upper end of the body of the sternum to form the secondary cartilaginous joint called the *manubriosternal joint*. The manubrium makes a slight angle with the body at this junction called the **sternal angle** or the **angle of Louis**. It is recognized by the presence of a transverse ridge on the anterior aspect of the sternum.

Body (Mesosternum; Figs. 16.1 and 16.2)

The features of the body are as follows:

1. It is longer, narrower, and thinner than the manubrium.
2. It is broadest roughly in the middle, opposite to the articulation of the fifth costal cartilage.
3. Its **upper end** articulates with the manubrium at the sternal angle to form symphysis—the *manubriosternal joint*.
4. Its **lower end** articulates with the xiphoid process to also form the secondary cartilaginous joint (symphysis)—the *xiphisternal joint*.
5. Its **anterior surface** presents three faint transverse ridges, indicating the lines of fusion of four small segments called the **sternebrae**. The anterior surface on each side gives origin to the pectoralis major muscle.
6. Its **posterior surface** is smooth and slightly concave.
   (a) Lower part of the posterior surface gives origin to the *sternocostalis muscle*.
   (b) On the right side of the median plane, the posterior surface is related to the pleura that separates it from the lung.
   (c) On the left side of the median plane, the upper half of the body is related to the pleura and lower half to the pericardium (*bare area of the pericardium*).
7. Its **lateral border** articulates with the 2nd–7th costal cartilages to form synovial joints. (Strictly speaking, the second costal cartilage articulates at the side of the manubriosternal junction and the seventh costal cartilage articulates at the side of the xiphisternal junction.)

Xiphoid Process (Metasternum; Figs. 16.1 and 16.2)

1. It is the lowest and smallest part of the sternum.
2. It varies greatly in size and shape.
3. It may be bifid or perforated.
4. Its **anterior surface** provides insertion to the medial fibres of the rectus abdominis.
5. Its **posterior surface** gives origin to the sternal fibres of the diaphragm.
6. Its **tip** provides attachment to the upper end of the linea alba.

Muscles attached on the posterior and anterior surfaces of the sternum are summarized below:

Muscle attached on the anterior surface of the sternum	Muscles attached on the posterior surface of the sternum
• Sternal head of sternocleidomastoid	• Sternohyoid • Sternothyroid
• Pectoralis major	• Sternocostalis
• Rectus abdominis	• Diaphragm (sternal fibers)

Sternal Angle

The sternal angle can be felt as a transverse ridge on the sternum about 5 cm below the suprasternal notch. *The sternal angle is an important surface bony landmark for many anatomical events that occur at this level.* These are:

- Second costal cartilage articulates, on either side, with the sternum at this level; hence, this level is *used for counting the ribs*.
- It lies at the level of the intervertebral disc between the T4 and T5 vertebrae.
- Horizontal plane passing through this level separates the superior mediastinum from the inferior mediastinum.
- Ascending aorta ends at this level.
- Arch of aorta begins and ends at this level.
- Descending aorta begins at this level.
- Trachea bifurcates into the right and left principal bronchi at this level.
- Upper border of heart lies at this level.
- Azygos vein arches over the root of the right lung to end in the superior vena cava.

CLINICAL CORRELATION

- **Sternal puncture:** ***Manubrium sterni is the preferred site for bone marrow aspiration*** because it is subcutaneous and readily accessible. The bone marrow sample is required for haematological examination. A thick needle is inserted into the upper part of the manubrium to avoid injury to arch of aorta, which lies behind the lower part. Sternal puncture is not advisable in children because in them the plates of the compact bone of the sternum are very thin and if a needle passes through and through the manubrium, it will damage the arch of aorta and its branches, leading to *fatal haemorrhage*.
- **Mid-sternotomy:** To gain access to the mediastinum for surgical operations on heart and great blood vessels, the sternum is often divided in the median plane called *mid-sternotomy*.
- **Funnel chest (pectus excavatum):** It is an abnormal shape of the thoracic cage in which chest is compressed anteroposteriorly and the sternum is pushed backward by the overgrowth of the ribs and may compress the heart.
- **Pigeon chest (pectus carinatum):** It is an abnormal shape of the thoracic cage in which chest is compressed from side to side and the sternum projects forward and downward like a keel of a boat.
- **Sternal fracture:** It is common in automobile accidents; for example when the driver's chest is hit against the steering wheel, the sternum is often fractured at the sternal angle. The backward displacement of fractured fragments may damage aorta, heart, or liver and cause severe bleeding that may prove fatal.

OSSIFICATION

The sternum develops from two vertical cartilaginous plates (**sternal plates**) that fuse in the midline.

The sternum ossifies from **six double (paired) centres,** *namely*,

- One for manubrium
- Four for body, one for each sternebrae
- One for xiphoid process

1. Manubrium: 5th month
2. Body
   - (a) First sternebra: 6th month
   - (b) Second sternebra: 7th month
   - (c) Third sternebra: 8th month
   - (d) Fourth sternebra: 9th month
3. Xiphoid process: 3rd year

} of IUL*

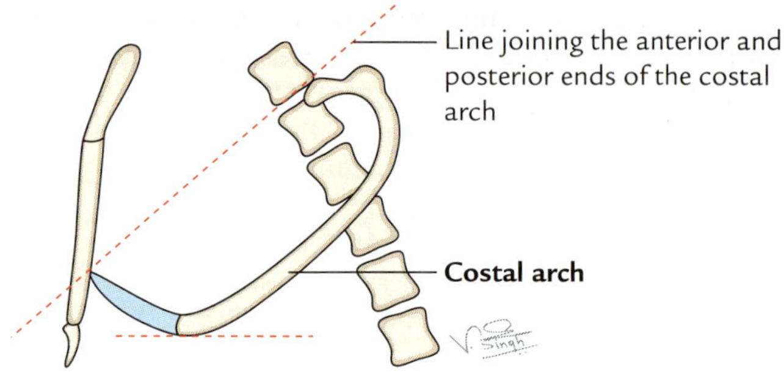

FIG. 16.3 ■ Costal arch (side view).

Appearance

The centres appear in descending order for different parts of the sternum as mentioned above.

Fusion

The fusion occurs as follows:

1. Fusion between sternal plates takes place from below upward. It begins at puberty and is completed by 25 years.
2. The xiphoid process fuses with the body at the age of 40 years.
3. Manubrium does not fuse with the body. As a result, the secondary cartilaginous manubriosternal joint usually persists throughout life. In about 10% individuals, fusion occurs in old age.

CLINICAL CORRELATION

Sternal foramen and cleft sternum: The two sternal plates fuse in the caudocranial direction. Sometimes sternebrae fail to fuse in the midline; as a result, defect occurs in the body of the sternum in the form of *sternal foramen* or *cleft sternum*. The cleft sternum is often associated with ***ectopia cordis***.

RIBS

AN 21.1, AN 21.2

The ribs are flat, ribbon-like, elastic bony arches that extend from thoracic vertebrae posteriorly to the lateral borders of the sternum anteriorly. Their anterior ends are connected to the costal cartilage. The rib along with its costal cartilage constitute the **costa**. The ribs and their costal cartilages form greater part of the thoracic skeleton.

NUMBER

Normally, there are 12 pairs of ribs (but the occurrence of accessory cervical or lumbar rib may increase them to 13 pairs or the absence of 12th rib may reduce them to 11 pairs).

Arrangement and General Outline

1. The ribs are arranged one below the other, and the gaps between the adjacent ribs are called *intercostal spaces*.
2. The length of ribs increases from the first to seventh rib and then gradually decreases; hence, seventh rib is the longest rib.
3. The transverse diameter of the thorax increases progressively from the first to eighth rib; hence, the eighth rib has the greatest lateral projection.
4. The ribs are arranged obliquely, that is their anterior ends lie at the lower level than their posterior ends (Fig. 16.3).
5. The obliquity of ribs increases progressively from the first to ninth rib; hence, the ninth rib is most obliquely placed.
6. The width of ribs is gradually reduced from above downward.

The anterior ends of the first seven ribs are connected to the sternum through their costal cartilages. The cartilages at the anterior ends of the 8th, 9th, and 10th ribs are joined to the next higher cartilage. The anterior ends of the 11th and 12th ribs are free and, therefore, called the floating ribs.

N.B.

- The 10th rib usually have free anterior ends in Japanese.
- The first rib slopes downward along its entire extent.
- The middle of each costal arch (consisting of a rib and its costal cartilage) except the first rib lies at a lower level than a straight line joining the two ends of the costa (Fig. 16.3).

Classification

A. According to Features

1. Typical ribs: 3rd–9th.
2. *Atypical ribs:* 1st, 2nd, 10th, 11th, and 12th.

The typical ribs have the same general features, whereas the atypical ribs have special features and, therefore, can be differentiated from the remaining ribs.

B. According to Relation With the Sternum

1. *True ribs:* 1st–7th (i.e. upper seven ribs)
2. *False ribs:* 8th–12th (i.e. lower five ribs)

True ribs articulate with the sternum anteriorly, whereas **false ribs** do not articulate with the sternum anteriorly.

C. According to Articulation

1. Vertebrosternal ribs: 1st–7th
2. Vertebrochondral ribs: 8th–10th
3. Vertebral (floating) ribs: 11th and 12th

The **vertebrosternal ribs** articulate posteriorly with vertebrae and anteriorly with the sternum.

The **vertebrochondral ribs** articulate posteriorly with vertebrae and anteriorly their cartilages join the cartilage of the higher rib.

*IUL–Intrauterine life.

The **vertebral** or **floating ribs** articulate posteriorly with the vertebrae, but their anterior ends are free but attached to small pieces of hyaline cartilages.

TYPICAL RIBS (FIG. 16.4)

Parts

Each rib has three parts: (a) anterior end, (b) posterior end, and (c) shaft.

The **anterior end** bears a concave depression.

The **posterior end** consists of the head, neck, and tubercle.

The **shaft** is the longest part and extends between the anterior and posterior ends. It is flattened and twisted. It has inner and outer surfaces and upper and lower borders. It is curved with convexity directed outward and bears a costal groove on its inner surface near the lower border. Five centimetres away from tubercle, it abruptly changes its direction; this is called the **angle of the rib.**

Side Determination and Anatomical Position

The side of the rib can be determined by holding it in such a way that its posterior end having a head, neck, and tubercle is directed posteriorly, its concavity faces medially, and its sharp border is directed inferiorly.

In an **anatomical position,** the posterior end is higher and nearer the median plane than the anterior end.

Features and Attachments

Anterior (Costal) End

It bears a small cup-shaped depression that joins the corresponding costal cartilage to form a primary cartilaginous *costochondral joint*.

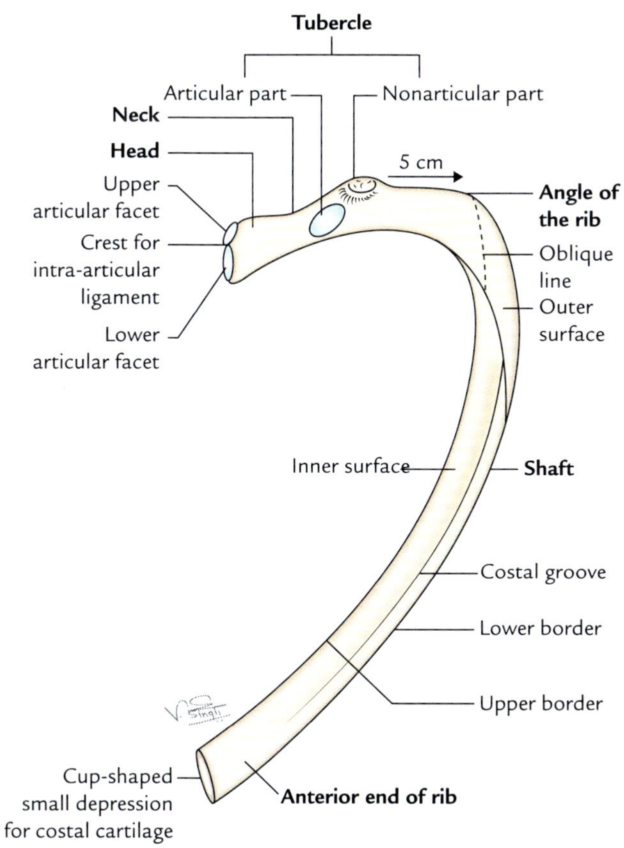

FIG. 16.4 ■ Features of a typical rib.

Posterior End

It presents the head, neck, and tubercle.

Head

It has **two articular facets**: lower and upper.

1. The *lower larger facet* articulates with the body of numerically corresponding vertebra.
2. The *upper smaller facet* articulates with the next higher vertebra.

The crest separating the two articular facets lies opposite to the intervertebral disc.

Neck

1. It lies in front of the transverse process of the corresponding vertebra.
2. It has **two borders**—superior and inferior and **two surfaces**—anterior and posterior.
3. The upper border is sharp crest-like, whereas the lower border is rounded.
4. The posterior surface is rough and pierced by foramina.

Tubercle

1. It is situated on the outer surface of the rib at the junction of the neck and the shaft.
2. It is divided into **two parts**—medial *articular part* and lateral *nonarticular part*. The articular part bears a small oval facet that articulates with the transverse process of the corresponding vertebra. The nonarticular part is rough and provides attachment to ligaments.

Shaft

1. It is thin and flattened.
2. It presents **two surfaces**—outer and inner, **two borders**—upper and lower, and **two angles**—posterior and anterior.

Borders

Superior border

The superior border is thick and rounded and presents the outer and inner lips:

- The *outer lip* gives attachment to the external intercostal muscles.
- The *inner lip* gives attachment to the internal intercostal and intercostalis intimus muscles.

Lower border

The lower border is sharp and forms the lower border of the costal groove and gives origin to the external intercostal muscle.

Surfaces

Outer surface

1. It is smooth and convex and presents **two angles**—posterior and anterior.
   - The posterior angle (generally called only angle) is marked by an oblique ridge.
   - The anterior angle is marked by an indistinct oblique line.

Inner surface

It is smooth and concave. It presents a **costal groove** near its lower border. The costal groove becomes unrecognizable in the anterior part.

- The **costal groove** lodges the intercostal nerve and vessels from above downward, as follows (*Mnemonic:* VAN):
  1. Intercostal **V**ein
  2. Intercostal **A**rtery
  3. Intercostal **N**erve
- The **internal intercostal** muscle is attached to the floor of the groove (intervening between intercostal nerves and vessels and bone).
- The **intercostalis intimus** is attached to the upper border of the costal groove.

N.B.

Three characteristic features of a typical rib:
- It is thin, flat, long and *curved* along its entire extent; and has inner and outer surfaces.
- It is *angulated*, that is presents two bends—one 5 cm in front of the tubercle and one 2 cm behind the anterior end.
- It is *twisted*, on its long axis, so that the two ends of the rib cannot touch the same horizontal plane.

(*Mnemonic:* **CAT**—**C**urve, **A**ngle, and **T**wist).

ATYPICAL RIBS

First Rib (Fig. 16.5) AN 21.1

Distinguishing Features

1. It is shortest, broadest, and most acutely curved.
2. Its shaft is flattened above downward so that it has the upper and lower surfaces, and outer and inner borders.
3. Its head is small, rounded, and bears a single circular articular facet to articulate with the side of the first thoracic vertebra.
4. Its angle and tubercle coincide.
5. It has no costal groove on its lower surface.
6. Its neck is rounded and elongated. It is directed upward, backward, and laterally.
7. Its anterior end is larger and thicker.

N.B.

The shaft of the first rib slopes obliquely downward and forward to its sternal end. It is due to this obliquity that the pulmonary and pleural apices projects into the root of the neck.

Side Determination

Side of the first rib can be determined by holding the rib in such a way that:

(a) its larger end is directed anteriorly and its smaller end is directed posteriorly,
(b) the surface of its shaft having two grooves separated by a ridge is directed superiorly, and
(c) its concave border is directed inward and its convex border is directed outward.

N.B.

Trick for students for side determination of the first rib: Keep the rib on the table top considering its position in your own body. Now note that the rib belongs to the side on which its both ends touch the surface. If the rib is placed on the wrong side, then only its anterior end will be touching the surface.

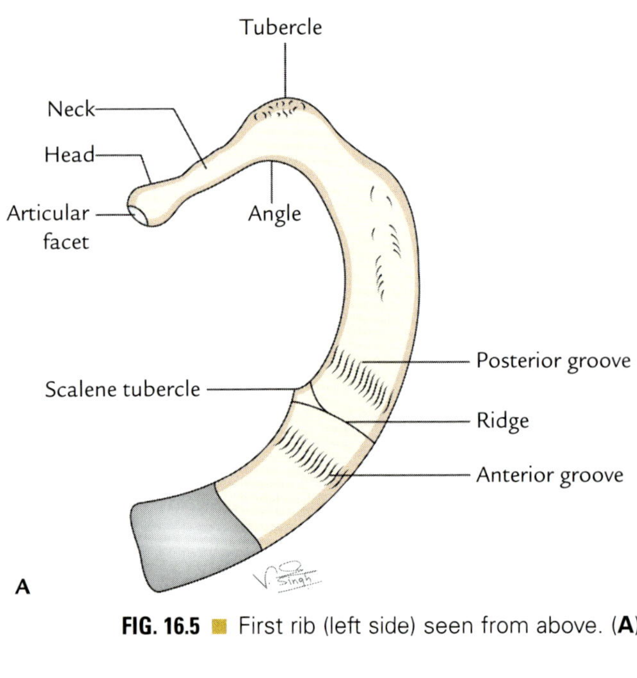

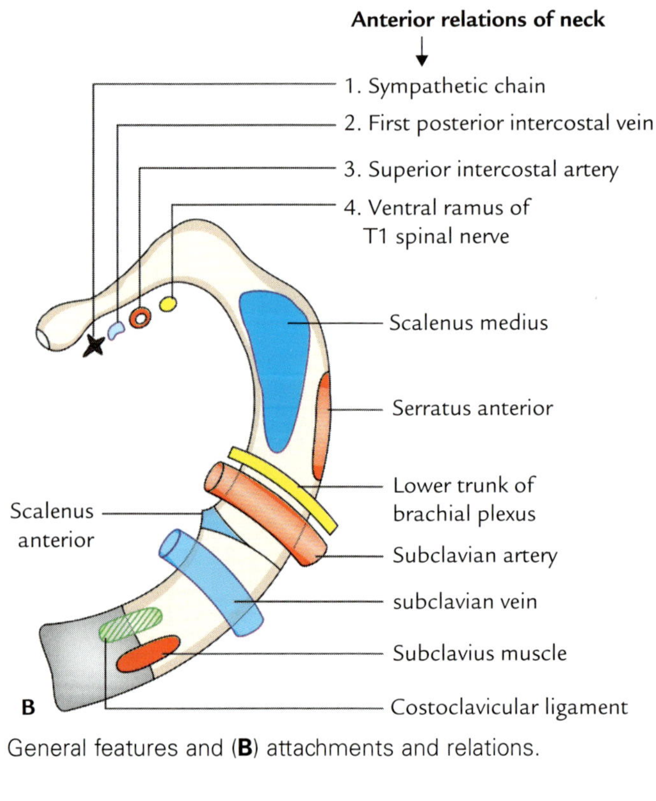

FIG. 16.5 First rib (left side) seen from above. (**A**) General features and (**B**) attachments and relations.

Features and Attachments

Inner border

1. It presents a scalene tubercle about its middle. Tubercle and adjoining part of the upper surface provides attachment to the scalenus anterior muscle.
2. It provides attachment to the Sibson's fascia (suprapleural membrane).

Outer border

It provides origin to the first digitation of serratus anterior about its middle, just behind the groove for the subclavian artery.

Superior (upper) surface

1. It is crossed obliquely by two shallow grooves (anterior and posterior) separated by a slight ridge. The ridge is continuous with the scalene tubercle. The anterior groove lodges subclavian vein, while posterior groove lodges the subclavian artery and lower trunk of the brachial plexus.
2. The area behind the posterior groove up to the costal tubercle provides attachment to the scalenus medius muscle.
3. The area in front of the anterior groove and near the anterior end provides attachment to **subclavius muscle** (anteriorly) and **costoclavicular ligament** (posteriorly).

Lower surface

It is related to the costal pleura.

Neck

1. It is elongated and directed upwards, backwards, and laterally.
2. The following structures form **anterior relations of the neck** from the medial to lateral side:
   (a) Sympathetic **chain**
   (b) First posterior intercostal **v**ein
   (c) Superior intercostal **a**rtery
   (d) Ventral ramus of the first thoracic **n**erve

Memory trick: Chain pulling the **VAN**.

Second Rib (Fig. 16.6)

Distinguishing Features and Attachments

1. Its length is twice to that of the first rib.
2. Its shaft is sharply/highly curved. Angle is slight and located close to tubercle.
3. Its shaft is not twisted; hence, both the ends of the rib touch the table top when placed on it.
4. *Near its middle, the outer convex surface of the shaft presents a* ***rough tuberosity,*** which provides attachment to the serratus anterior muscle (lower part of the first and whole of the second digitation).
5. The *outer surface of the shaft* is convex and *faces more upwards than outward*. The *inner surface of the shaft* is concave and *faces more downwards than inwards*.
6. Posterior part of the internal surface presents a **short costal groove.**
7. The upper border and adjoining part of the upper surface provide attachment to the scalenus posterior and serratus posterior superior muscles.

Tenth Rib

Distinguishing Features

1. It has a single articular facet on its head, which articulates with the body of the corresponding thoracic vertebra.
2. It is slightly shorter than the typical rib.

Eleventh Rib

It is short rib with pointed anterior end.

Distinguishing Features

1. It has a single large, articular facet on its head.
2. It has no neck and no tubercle.

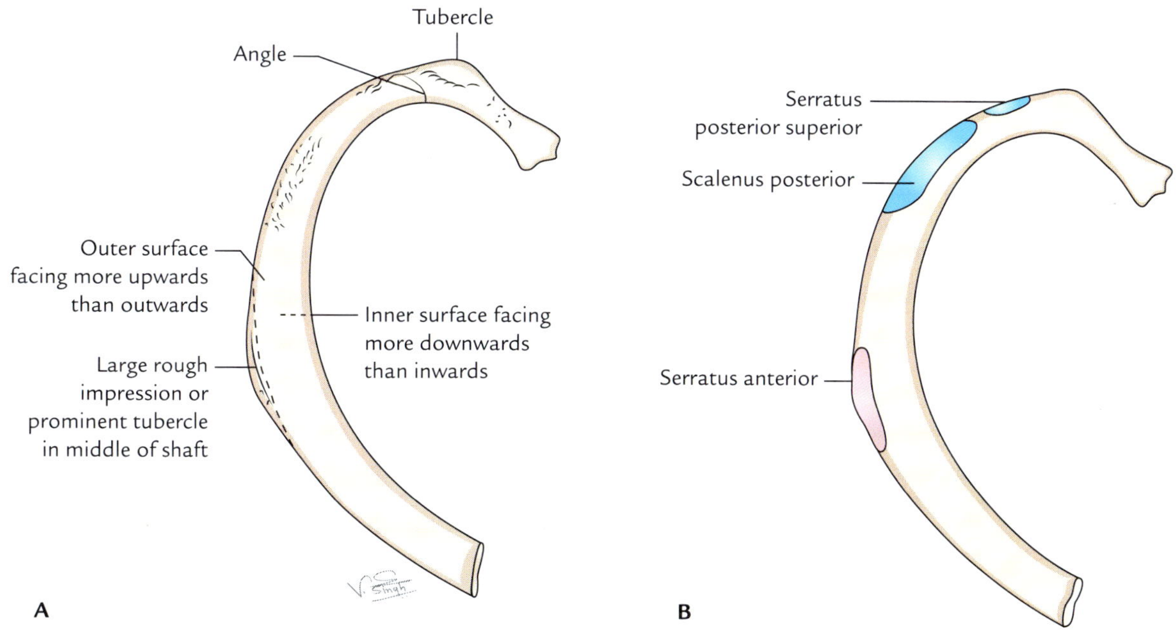

FIG. 16.6 ■ Second rib (right). (**A**) General features and (**B**) attachments.

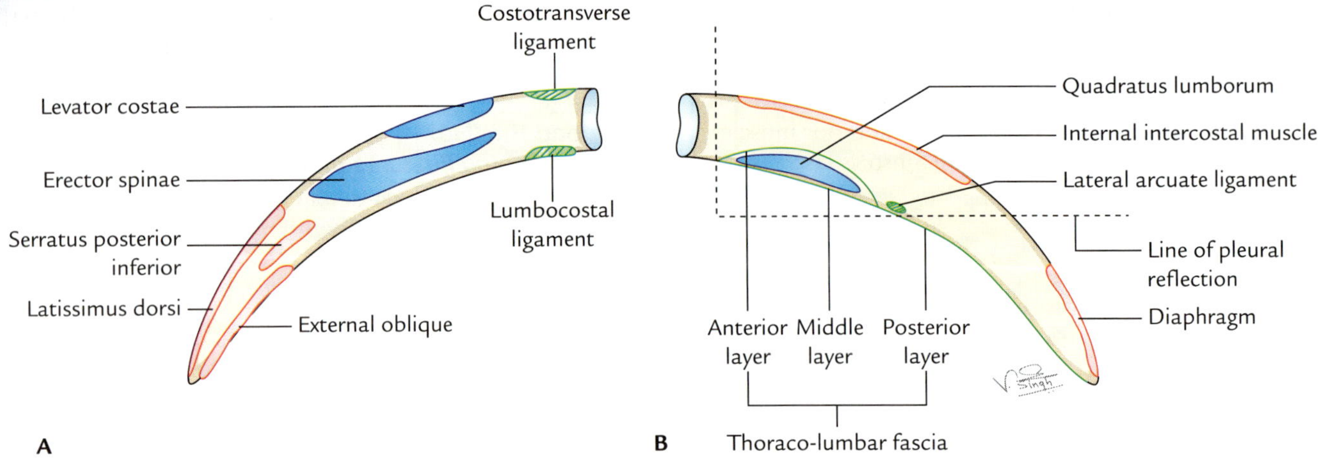

FIG. 16.7 ■ Twelfth rib (right side) showing attachments. (**A**) Outer surface and (**B**) inner surface.

3. Its anterior end is pointed and tipped with the cartilage.
4. It has a slight angle and a shallow costal groove.
5. Its inner surface is directed upward and inward.

Twelfth Rib (Fig. 16.7)

Distinguishing Features

The 12th rib has the same features as the 11th, except that:

1. It has no angle.
2. It has no costal groove.
3. It is much shorter than the 11th.

Side Determination

The side of the 12th rib can be determined by keeping the rib in such a way that:

1. Its pointed anterior end is directed anterolaterally and its broader end posteromedially.
2. Its slightly concave surface faces inward and upward.
3. Its sharper border is directed inferiorly.

Attachments

Outer surface

1. Near the tip, it provides attachment to the latissimus dorsi muscle above and external oblique muscle below.
2. Its medial half provides attachment to the erector spinae muscle.

Inner surface

1. An oblique line crossing the middle of this surface marks the line of *pleural reflection*.
2. Lower part of the medial half provides attachment to the *quadratus lumborum muscle*.
3. Middle two-fourths near the upper border provides attachment to the *internal intercostal muscle*.
4. Upper part of lateral one-fourth near the tip provides attachment to the *diaphragm*.

TABLE 16.1 Atypical features of 11th and 12th ribs

11th rib	12th rib
• Short rib about 6 inches in length	• Much shorter than 11th rib about 5½ inches in length.
• No curvature	• No curvature
• Shaped like a small knife without handle with pointed anterior end	• Shaped like a small knife without handle with pointed anterior end
• Slight angle	• No angle
• Shallow short costal groove	• No costal groove
• Inner surface faces slightly upwards	• Inner surface faces slightly upwards
• Single articular facet on head for numerically corresponding vertebra	• Single articular facet for numerically corresponding vertebra

Lower border

1. Close to the head, it provides attachment to the *lumbocostal ligament*, which stretches from the transverse process of the L1 vertebra.
2. *Lateral arcuate ligament* is attached to it, just lateral to the quadratus lumborum.

Upper border

The upper border provides attachment to the external and internal intercostal muscles.

The atypical features of 11th and 12th ribs are summarized in Table 16.1.

OSSIFICATION

A. **Ossification of Typical Ribs (Table 16.1)**
   - All the typical ribs ossify by four centres:
     (a) *One primary centre* for the shaft near angle.
     (b) *Three secondary centres*: one for head, one for the articular part of the tubercle, and one for the nonarticular part of the tubercle.

- Primary centre appear at the eighth week of IUL.
- Secondary centres of all the ribs appear at puberty.
- Fusion in all the ribs occurs at the age of 20 years.

B **Ossification of Some Atypical Ribs**

- The ***first rib is ossified*** by three centres: one primary centre for the shaft and two secondary centres—one for the head and one for the tubercle.
- ***Eleventh and twelfth ribs are ossified*** by two centres each: one primary centre for the shaft and one secondary centre for the head.

CLINICAL CORRELATION

- **Cervical rib:** The costal element of the C7 vertebra may elongate to form a cervical rib in about 5% individuals. The condition may be unilateral or bilateral. It occurs more often unilaterally and somewhat more frequently on the right side. The cervical rib may have a blind tip or the tip may be connected to the first rib by the fibrous band or cartilage or bone. It may compress the lower trunk of the brachial plexus and subclavian artery to cause thoracic outlet syndrome of clinicians. The compression produces: (a) pain along the medial side of the forearm and hand and (b) disturbance in the circulation of the upper limb, *viz*. feeble radial pulse (for details, see *Clinical and Surgical Anatomy*, 2ed. by Vishram Singh).
- **Lumbar rib (Gorilla rib):** It develops from the costal element of the L1 vertebra. Its incidence is more common than the cervical rib but remains undiagnosed as it usually does not cause symptoms. It may be confused with the fracture of the transverse process of the L1 vertebra.
- **Fracture of rib:** Usually, the middle ribs are involved in the fracture. The rib commonly fractures at its angle (posterior angle) as it is the weakest point.

N.B.

- Fracture of ribs is rare in children as the ribs are elastic in them.
- First two ribs (first and second ribs) are protected by the clavicle and the last two ribs (11th and 12th) are mobile (floating); hence, they are rarely injured.

- **Flail chest (stove in chest):** When ribs are fractured at two sites (e.g. anteriorly and at an angle), the flail chest occurs. The flail segments of ribs are sucked in during inspiration and pushed out during expiration, leading to a clinical condition called *paradoxical respiration*.

THORACIC VERTEBRAE AN 21.1, AN 21.2

There are 12 thoracic vertebrae. They are identified by the presence of costal facet/facets on the sides of their bodies for articulation with the heads of the ribs. These articulations are the characteristic of thoracic vertebrae as they are not found in the cervical, lumbar, and sacral vertebrae. The size of the thoracic vertebrae increases gradually from above downward.

The bodies of the upper thoracic vertebrae gradually changes from the cervical to thoracic type and those of lower from thoracic to lumbar type. Thus, the body of the T1 vertebra is typically cervical in type and that of the T12 vertebra is typically lumbar in type.

N.B.

The presence of the articular facet(s) on the side of the body is the *cardinal feature of the thoracic vertebrae*.

CLASSIFICATION

According to the features, the thoracic vertebrae are classified into two types:

1. Typical: second to eighth
2. Atypical: first and ninth to twelfth

TYPICAL THORACIC VERTEBRAE AN 21.1

Characteristic Features (Fig. 16.8)

1. **Presence of articular facets on each side of the body.**
2. **Body is heart shaped**, particularly in the mid-thoracic region when viewed from above. Its transverse and anteroposterior measurements are almost equal.
3. **Vertebral foramen is circular.**
4. **Spinous processes are long, slender, and angulated downwards.**
5. **Transverse process is prominent and bears an articular facet for articulation with the rib.**
6. **Pedicles** are attached to the upper part of the body, thus making the inferior vertebral notch deeper.

Parts

The thoracic vertebra consists of two parts:

1. Body
2. Vertebral arch

The body and vertebral arch enclose a vertebral foramen in which lies the spinal cord surrounded by its meninges.

Body

1. It is heart shaped, when viewed from above.
2. Its anteroposterior and transverse dimensions are almost equal.
3. On each side, the bodies have two costal facets: superior and inferior.
   - *Superior facet* is larger and situated near the upper border of the body in front of the root of the pedicle.
   - *Inferior facet* is smaller and situated near the lower border in front of the inferior vertebral notch.

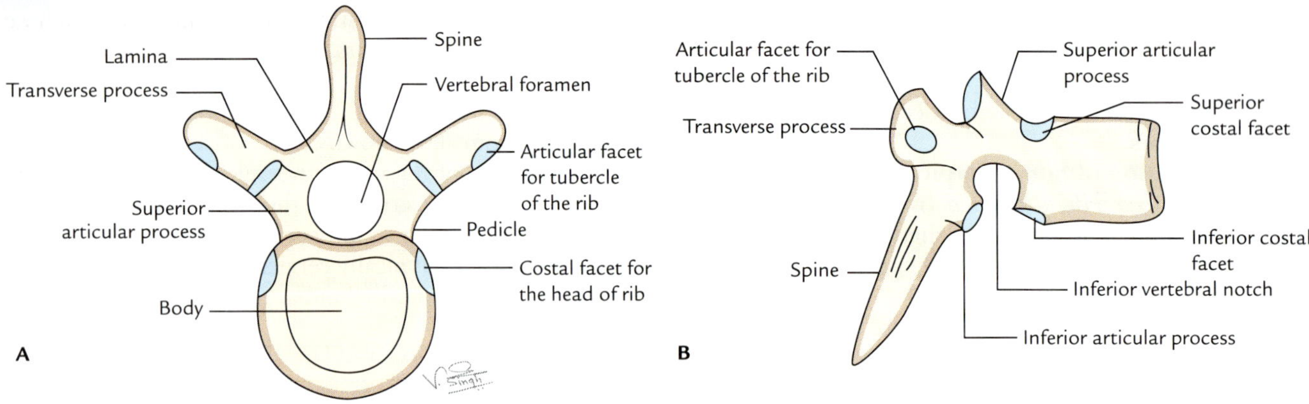

FIG. 16.8 ■ Features of a typical thoracic vertebra. (**A**) Superior view and (**B**) lateral view.

Vertebral Arch

It consists of a pair of pedicles anteriorly and two laminae posteriorly:

- The *pedicles* (right and left) are short rounded bony bars, which project backward and laterally from the posterior aspect of the body.
- The *laminae* (right and left)—each pedicle continues posteromedially as a vertical plate of bone. The laminae of two sides join with each other in the posterior midline.
- The *spinous process* arises in the midline where the two laminae meet posteriorly.
- *Two transverse processes*, one on either side arises from the junction of the pedicle and lamina.
- *Two paired articular processes*, two on each side spring from the lamina, the superior articular process project rather more from pedicle than the lamina, the inferior articular process springs from a lamina.

N.B.

Each vertebra has seven processes: Paired (Rt. and Lt.) transverse processes, paired (Rt. and Lt.) superior articular processes, paired (Rt. and Lt.)—inferior articular processes and a single spinous process.

Features and Attachments

Body

1. The *upper larger costal facet* (actually demifacet) articulates with the head of the numerically corresponding rib.
2. The *lower smaller costal facet* (actually demifacet) articulates with the head of the next lower rib.
3. Anterior and posterior surfaces of the body provide attachment to the anterior and posterior longitudinal ligaments, respectively. These ligaments are attached to both the upper and lower borders of the body.
4. Posterior surface of the body is marked by vascular foramina for *basivertebral veins*, which are covered by the posterior longitudinal ligament.

Pedicles

1. They are attached nearer to the superior border of the body; as a result, the *superior vertebral notch* is shallow and the *inferior vertebral notch* is deep.
2. The deep inferior vertebral notch together with the small superior vertebral notch of the next lower vertebra completes the intervertebral foramen, through which the spinal nerve leaves the vertebral canal.

Laminae

1. They are short, broad, and thick, and they overlap each other from above downward.
2. Their margins provide attachment to the ligamenta flava.

Superior Articular Processes

The articular facets on the superior articular process are directed backward and slightly laterally and articulate with the inferior articular facet of the next higher vertebra.

Inferior Articular Processes

The articular facet on the inferior articular process is flat and faces forward and little downward and medially. It articulates with the superior articular facet of the next lower vertebra.

Transverse Processes

They are large club shaped and projects laterally and slightly backward.

- The facet on the anterior aspect of the tip of the transverse process articulates with the tubercle of the numerically corresponding rib.
- They provide attachments to the ligaments and muscles related to the rib cage and back.

Spine

The spines are directed backward and downward. The spinous processes of the middle four vertebrae (i.e. from fifth to eighth) are very long, vertical, and overlap each other. The spinous processes of the upper four and lower four vertebrae are relatively short and less oblique in direction (Fig. 16.9).

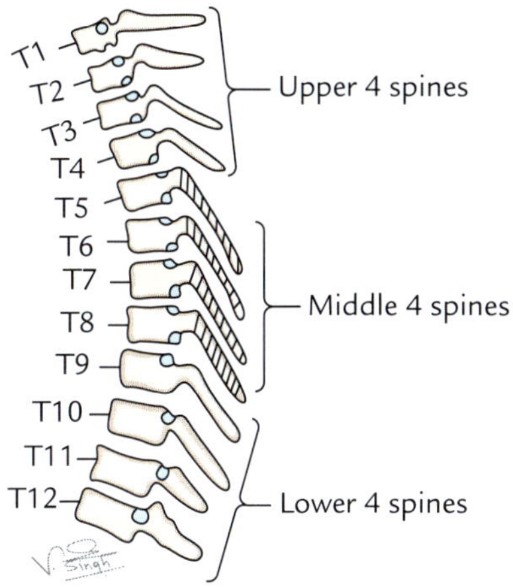

FIG. 16.9 ■ Showing backward and downward inclination of the spinous processes of the thoracic vertebrae.

N.B.

- The spinous process of the T1 vertebra is most prominent and more or less horizontal in its projection and can be palpated at the back of the root of the neck just below the lower end of the median nuchal furrow.
- The spinous process of the T8 vertebra is the longest.

The backward slant decreases. At the 11th vertebra, the spine is directed almost downward. It is termed the **anticlinal vertebra**, below this level spines slant slightly dorsally. The spines provide attachment to the supraspinous and interspinous ligaments.

N.B.

The spines of the middle four thoracic vertebrae are almost vertical.

ATYPICAL THORACIC VERTEBRAE (FIG. 16.10)

AN 21.2

First Thoracic Vertebra

Distinguishing Features

1. The body of vertebra resembles to that of cervical vertebra, *viz.* C7 vertebra.
2. The body is heart shaped. It is narrow anteroposteriorly. Its upper surface is concave from side to side with an upward projecting lip on either sides. The anterior border of the inferior surface projects downward.
3. The **superior costal facet** on the side of the body is **circular** and articulates with the whole of the facet on the head of the first rib.
4. The superior vertebral notches are deep (i.e. clearly seen) as in the cervical vertebra.
5. The **inferior costal facet** on the side of body is half (i.e. **demifacet**) and articulates with the head of the second rib.
6. The spinous process is thick, long, and nearly horizontal.

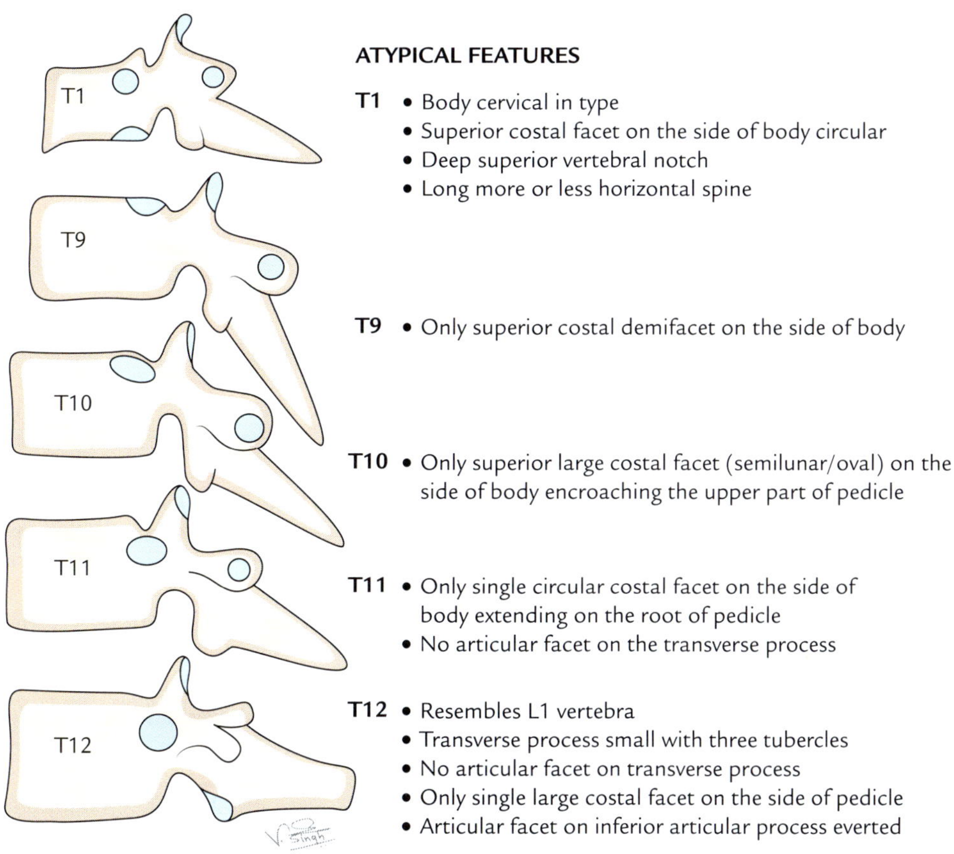

FIG. 16.10 ■ Features of atypical thoracic vertebrae.

Ninth Thoracic Vertebra

Distinguishing Features

1. The lower costal facet on each side of the body is absent.
2. The body on each side possesses only superior costal facet (demifacet) for articulation with the ninth rib.

Tenth Thoracic Vertebra

Distinguishing Features

The body on each side possesses only a single articular facet, which is semilunar or oval for articulation with the 10th rib. The costal facet encroaches on the upper part of the pedicle.

Eleventh Thoracic Vertebra

Distinguishing Features

1. Body on each side possesses a single large circular costal facet for articulation with the head of the 11th rib. The costal facet extends onto the root of the pedicle.
2. Transverse processes are small and do not possesses a costal facet on their tips to articulate with tubercle of 11th rib (as 11th rib has no tubercle).

Twelfth Thoracic Vertebra

Distinguishing Features

1. It is largest and most inferior of the thoracic vertebra.
2. It resembles the first lumbar vertebra.
3. Body on each side possesses a large single costal facet that is more on the lower part of the pedicle than on the body.
4. Transverse process is small and presents three tubercles—superior, middle, and inferior. It has no articular facet (as 12th rib has no tubercle).
   The three tubercles of the transverse process of the 12th thoracic vertebra correspond with the following processes of the lumbar vertebra:
   (a) Superior tubercle corresponds to the *mamillary process* of the lumbar vertebra.
   (b) Middle tubercle corresponds to the true *transverse process* of the lumbar vertebra.
   (c) Inferior tubercle corresponds to the *accessory process* of the lumbar vertebra.
5. Articular facet on inferior articular process everted (lumbar type).

The important distinguishing features of the atypical thoracic vertebrae (i.e. 1st, 9th, 10th, 11th, and 12th) are enumerated in Table 16.2.

N.B.

T12 thoracic vertebra is a hybrid vertebra with anatomical features of both thoracic and lumbar vertebrae.

It is among the most susceptible vertebra to damage from compression and often called as *transition vertebra*, due to its proximity to lumbar vertebra. Partly it possesses features of both thoracic and lumbar vertebrae.

TABLE 16.2 Distinguishing features of atypical thoracic vertebrae **AN 1.2**

Vertebra	Distinguishing features
T1	• Resembles the seventh cervical vertebra • Superior costal facet is circular • Superior vertebral notch is deep and clearly seen
T9	• Presence of only superior demifacet
T10	• Presence of only single large complete costal facet
T11	• Presence of a single large circular costal facet • Absence of an articular facet on the transverse process
T12	• Resembles the first lumbar vertebra • Presence of a single large circular facet extending onto the root of the pedicle • Transverse process presents three tubercles: superior, inferior, and lateral • Articular facet on inferior articular process everted (lumbar type)

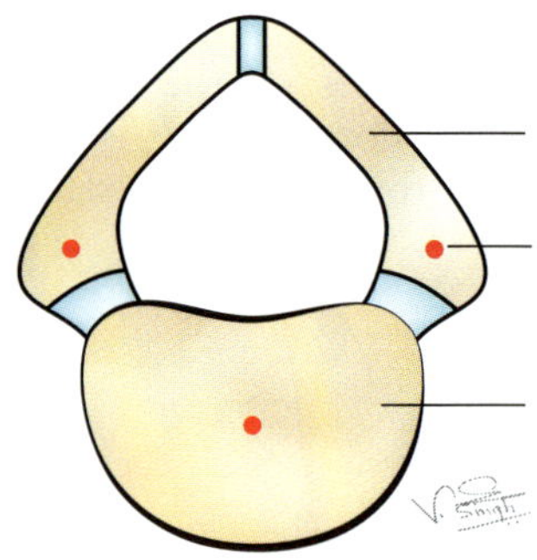

FIG. 16.11 Primary centres of ossification of a typical thoracic vertebra (vertebra at birth consists of 3 bony parts).

Ossification of a Typical Thoracic Vertebra (Fig. 16.11)

It ossifies in cartilage by eight centres, *viz.* three primary and five secondary. The **three primary centres** are one for each half of vertebral arch near root, and one for centrum. They appear around second month (8–9 weeks) of foetal life (Fig. 16.11).

The **five secondary centres**, one for tip of spine, one each for transverse processes and one each for plates of cartilages on upper and lower surfaces of the body.

They appear at about puberty and fuse with the rest of the body by 25th year of age (Fig. 16.12A).

The centres in the upper and lower plates of cartilages on the upper and lower surfaces of the body form a ring of bone around the central cartilaginous plate of the vertebral body (Fig. 16.12B).

Occasionally, the body (centrum) gets ossified by two centres and if one centre fails to develop, it will lead to **hemivertebra**. This may cause scoliosis.

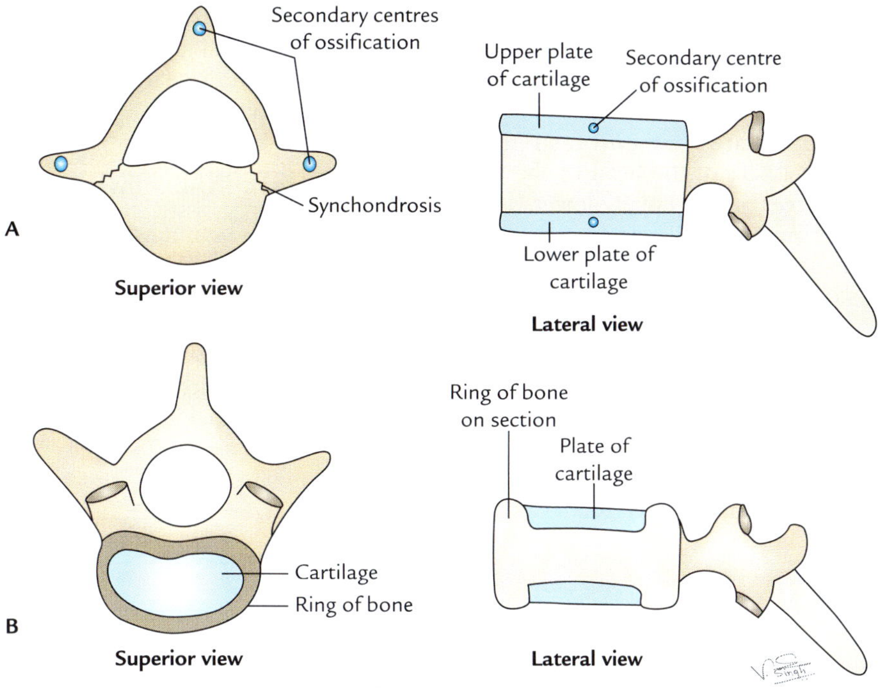

FIG. 16.12 ■ **A.** Secondary centres of ossification of vertebra, **B.** Completely developed vertebra.

N.B.

According to some authorities, the body of vertebra is considered as modified long bone because centrum of vertebral body is comparable to the diaphysis and annular epiphysis to the ends of a long bone.

CLINICAL CORRELATION

Lesions of thoracic spine

(a) **Compression fracture of vertebral bodies:** Due to fixed position for being attached to ribs.
(b) **Metastatic spinal tumours:** Due to spread of cancer cells from breast and prostate.
(c) **Tuberculosis/cold abscess:** Is most common in lower thoracic and upper lumbar vertebrae.
(d) **Scoliosis of thoracic spine:** An abnormal lateral curvature of spine
(e) **Kyphosis:** Is an excessive curvature of thoracic spine, that is forward bending of the back.

COSTAL CARTILAGES

The costal cartilages are made up of the hyaline cartilage and are mainly responsible for providing elasticity and mobility to the chest wall.

First to seventh cartilages connect the respective ribs with the lateral border of the sternum and they increase in length from first to seventh.

Eighth to tenth cartilages at their anterior ends are connected with the lower border of the cartilage above and there is a gradual decrease in length from 8th to 10th.

Eleventh and twelfth cartilages end in free pointed extremities.

JOINTS OF THE THORAX

The joints of the thorax are as follows:

1. Costovertebral
2. Costotransverse
3. Costochondral
4. Interchondral
5. Manubriosternal
6. Intervertebral

COSTOVERTEBRAL JOINTS AN 21.8

These joints are formed by the articulation of articular facets on the head of the ribs and costal facets on the bodies of the thoracic vertebrae (Fig. 16.13).

The head of the typical rib articulates with the body of the numerically corresponding vertebra and also with the body of the next higher vertebra.

TYPE

Synovial type of plane joint.

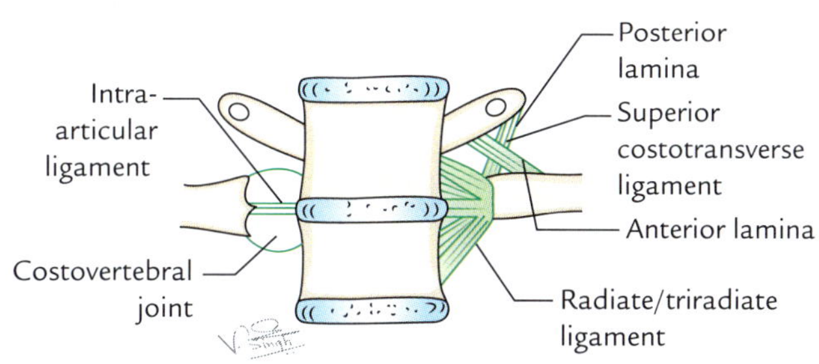

FIG. 16.13 ■ Costovertebral joint.

Ligaments

1. **Capsular ligament (joint capsule):** It is the fibrous capsule that covers/encloses the joint and is attached to the articular margins.
2. **Radiate ligament/triradiate ligament:** It stretches from the anterior aspect of the head of the rib and divides into three bands: upper, lower, and middle. The upper and lower bands are attached to the sides of the upper and lower vertebrae. The middle band (also called the *intraarticular ligament*) gets attached to the intervertebral disc.
3. **Intraarticular ligament:** It stretches from the crest between the two articular facets on the head of the rib to the intervertebral disc and divides the joint cavity into two parts.

The 1st, 10th, 11th, and 12th ribs articulate with the bodies of the numerically corresponding vertebrae.

N.B.

Costovertebral joint of typical ribs has two joint cavities and those of the atypical ribs have a single joint cavity.

COSTOTRANSVERSE JOINTS (FIG. 16.14) AN 21.8

The tubercle articulates with the transverse process of the numerically corresponding vertebra to form a synovial joint. It is absent in the 11th and 12th ribs.

TYPE

Plane type of synovial joint.

LIGAMENTS

1. **Capsular ligament (joint capsule):** It is a thin fibrous sac enclosing the joint.
2. **Superior costotransverse ligament:** It has two layers—anterior and posterior. The anterior layer stretches between the crest of the rib and the lower aspect of the transverse process of the vertebra above. The posterior layer stretches between the posterior aspects of the neck to the transverse process above.
3. **Inferior costotransverse ligament:** It extends from the posterior aspect of the neck of the rib to the transverse process of its own vertebra.
4. **Lateral transverse ligament:** It stretches between the nonarticular parts of the tubercle to the tip of the transverse process.

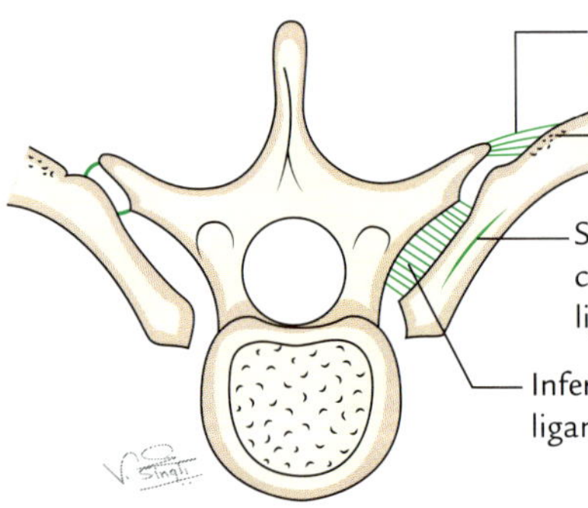

FIG. 16.14 ■ Costotransverse joint.

COSTOCHONDRAL JOINTS AN 21.10

The costochondral joints are primary cartilaginous joints between the anterior end of the rib and its cartilage. They permit no movements.

CHONDROSTERNAL JOINTS

These are joints between the medial ends of the first to seventh costal cartilages and the lateral border of the sternum. They are often termed by clinicians as *sternocostal joints.*

(First chondrosternal joint is primary cartilaginous joint synchondrosis) and does not permit any movement.

Second to seventh costal cartilages articulate with the sternum by synovial joints. Each joint has a single cavity, except the second costosternal joint where the cavity is divided into two parts.

N.B.

The costal cartilage of the first rib is united with manubrium sterni by a plate of fibrocartilage and hence it is not a typical primary cartilaginous joint (synchondrosis).

INTERCHONDRAL JOINTS AN 21.10

In the interchondral joint, 7th–9th costal cartilages come into contact with one another and articulate with each other by the number of ***small synovial joints***. At some sites, they are also united by ligaments. The union between the 9th and 10th costal cartilages is usually ligamentous.

MANUBRIOSTERNAL JOINT AN 21.8

The manubriosternal joint is formed between the lower end of the manubrium sterni and the upper end of the body of the sternum.

It is a secondary cartilaginous joint (symphysis) between the manubrium and the body of the sternum. It permits slight sliding movements of the body of the sternum on the manubrium during respiration.

N.B.

The *manubriosternal joint* is not a typical symphysis because as a rule, bones taking part in the formation of a symphysis do not undergo bony union, but in many individuals, after 30 years of age, bony union does take place between the manubrium and the body of sternum.

XIPHISTERNAL JOINT AN 21.8

It is a ***primary cartilaginous joint between body and xiphoid process***. The cartilage within the joint ossifies in old age.

INTERVERTEBRAL JOINTS AN 21.8

The intervertebral joints are formed

(a) between the bodies of the vertebrae and
(b) between the articular processes of the vertebra.

JOINTS BETWEEN THE BODIES OF THE VERTEBRAE

These are secondary cartilaginous joint. The inferior and superior surfaces of the adjacent vertebral bodies are covered by thin plates of hyaline cartilages, which in turn are united by the fibrocartilaginous intervertebral disc. The disc consists of an outer rim by fibrocartilage—*the annulus fibrosus* and a central core of gelatinous substance—the *nucleus pulposus*. These joints are held together by the anterior and posterior longitudinal ligaments of the vertebral column (for details, see *General Anatomy with Systemic Anatomy, Radiological Anatomy, Medical Genetics, 4ed.* by Vishram Singh).

JOINTS BETWEEN THE ARTICULAR PROCESSES

The joints between the superior and inferior articular processes of the adjacent vertebrae are called **facet** (*zygapophysial*) *joints*. They are plane type of synovial joints and permit gliding movements. The zygapophysial joints of the thoracic vertebrae are directed vertically. This limits flexion and extension but facilitates rotation. The rotation is greatly facilitated because the articular process of the thoracic vertebrae is set on an arc (Fig. 16.15). The ligaments are a joint capsule that encloses the articular surfaces. The accessory ligaments are: (a) ligamenta flava between the laminae of the adjacent vertebrae, (b) supraspinous, (c) interspinous, and (d) intertransverse ligaments.

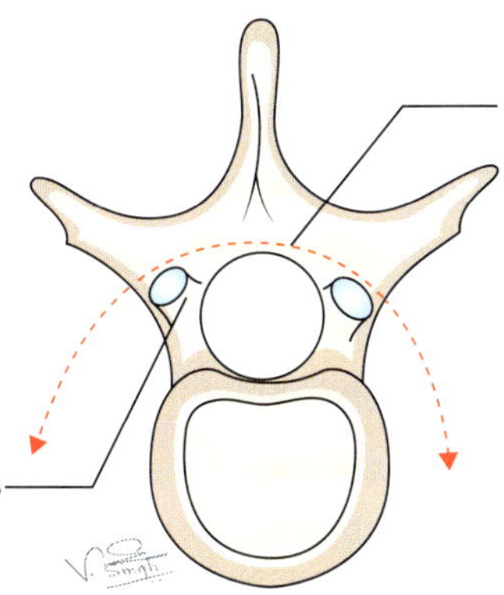

FIG. 16.15 The articular processes of the thoracic vertebra are set on an arc.

Movements

The movements of the flexion and extension are best permitted in the cervical and the lumbar regions, while the rotatory movements are best seen in the thoracic region.

Golden Facts to Remember

• Thickest and strongest part of the sternum	Manubrium sterni
• Most preferred site of bone marrow aspiration in adults	Manubrium sterni
• Most important surface bony landmark of thoracic cage	Sternal angle
• Widest and most curved rib	First
• Narrowest and smallest rib	Twelfth
• Longest rib	Seventh
• Most laterally projecting rib	Eighth
• Most oblique rib	Ninth
• Commonest accessory rib	Lumbar rib
• Gorilla rib	Lumbar rib
• Race in which anterior ends of 10th ribs are usually free	Japanese
• Smallest and most variable part of the sternum	Xiphoid process
• Thoracic vertebra with the smallest body	T3 vertebra
• Thoracic vertebra with the longest spine	T8 vertebra
• Anticlinal vertebra	T11 vertebra
• All the sternocostal joints are plane synovial joints except	First sternocostal joint which is primary cartilaginous joint (synchondrosis)
• Most susceptible vertebra for damage due to compression	T12 vertebra

CLINICAL CASE STUDY

A 25-year-old final year medical student told his Professor of Anatomy that he often feels pain in his right upper limb and his radial pulse becomes feeble, especially during exercise. He also told that sometimes he feels pain that radiates along the medial side of his forearm and hand. On examination, the professor noted a bony swelling in the root of the neck on the right side. X-ray of the neck revealed normal cervical spine. **Chest X-ray, however, revealed the presence of cervical rib on the right side**. The student was referred to an orthopaedic surgeon who after physical examination and seeing reports advised the student to have his cervical rib removed; otherwise, the vascular problem would worsen.

Questions

1. What is cervical rib?
2. Which structures are likely to be compressed by the cervical rib?
3. What complication could occur if the cervical rib is not removed?

Answers

1. The elongation of the costal element of the transverse process of the seventh cervical vertebra.
2. (a) Subclavian artery and (b) lower trunk of the brachial plexus.
3. The cervical rib causes angulation of the subclavian artery over the first rib. Left untreated, a clot tends to form distal to the kinked vessel and portions of the clot (emboli) may enter the circulation of the upper limb, which may block one of the digital arteries in the hand and cause *gangrene of* finger *tips*. The prolonged compression of the lower trunk brachial plexus (C8 and T1) may cause wasting of the most of the small muscles of the hand.

CHAPTER 17

Thoracic Wall, Intercostal Muscles and the Mechanism of Respiration

SPECIFIC LEARNING OBJECTIVES

After studying this chapter, the student should be able to:

- Describe the extent, attachment, direction of fibres, nerve supply, and actions of intercostal muscles. AN 21.4
- Describe the types and mechanism of respiration. AN 21.9
- Give the anatomical basis of: (a) sites of eruption of cold abscess on body wall, (b) internal mammary artery (IMA) graft, and (c) intercostal nerve block.
- Describe the origin, course, relations, and branches of a typical intercostal nerve. AN 21.5
- Mention on the origin, course, relations, and branches of: (a) typical intercostal nerve and (b) superior intercostal artery and subcostal artery. AN 21.7
- Write short notes on: (a) intercostal space and (b) internal thoracic artery.

The **thoracic wall proper** is formed by the **thoracic cage and muscles** that extend between the ribs called intercostal muscles (intrinsic muscles of thoracic wall). However, thoracic wall is liberally covered all over by the extrinsic muscles. The thoracic cage is described in detail in Chapter 15, page 193.

COVERINGS OF THE THORACIC WALL AN 21.4

The thoracic wall is covered from superficial to deep by:

1. Skin
2. Superficial fascia
3. Deep fascia
4. Muscles

Skin: The skin covering the thoracic wall is thin on its anterior aspect and thick on its back aspect. The distribution of hair is variable and depends on the age, sex, and race.

Cutaneous nerves: The cutaneous innervation in front of the thorax is provided by the cutaneous branches of the anterior primary rami of the thoracic spinal nerves (T2–T6) in sequence from above downward by the T2 at the level of the second rib to the T6 at the level of the xiphoid process. The skin above the level of the second rib is supplied by the anterior primary ramus of C4 via supraclavicular nerves.

N.B.

- The anterior rami of C5-T1 innervate the skin of the upper limb.
- The cutaneous innervation on the back of the thorax (on either side of the midline for about 5 cm) is provided by the posterior rami of the thoracic spinal nerves.

Superficial fascia: The superficial fascia is denser on the posterior aspect of the chest to sustain the pressure of the body when lying in the supine position. The superficial fascia on the front of the chest contains breast (mammary gland), which is rudimentary in males and well developed in adult females. The breast is described in detail in Chapter 3.

Deep fascia: The deep fascia is thin and ill defined (except in the pectoral region) to allow the free movement of the thoracic wall during breathing.

Muscles: The thoracic wall is liberally covered by the following extrinsic muscles:

1. **Muscles of the upper limb:**
   (a) Pectoralis major and pectoralis minor muscles cover the front of the thoracic wall.
   (b) Serratus anterior covers the side of the thoracic wall.
2. **Muscles of abdomen:** Rectus abdominis and external oblique cover the lower part of the front of the thoracic wall.
3. **Muscles of back:**
   (a) Trapezius and latissimus dorsi
   (b) Levator scapulae, rhomboideus major and minor
   (c) Serratus posterior superior, and serratus posterior inferior
   (d) Erector spinae

N.B.

- The thoracic wall is more or less completely covered by extrinsic muscles except in the anterior and posterior median lines.
- On the back, the thoracic wall is thinly covered by musculature in the region of triangle of auscultation (see pages 61 and 64).

INTERCOSTAL (INTRINSIC) MUSCLES OF THE THORACIC WALL (FIGS. 17.1–17.3) AN 21.4

The intrinsic muscles of the thoracic wall are called intercostal muscles. They are arranged in three layers from superficial to deep. These are as follows (Fig. 17.1A):

1. ***External intercostal muscle*** (superficial layer)
2. ***Internal intercostal muscle*** (intermediate layer)
3. ***Transversus thoracis muscle*** (deep layer)

The muscle layer is lined by the **endothoracic fascia**, which in turn is lined by the parietal pleura.

These three layers of muscles are comparable to the three layers of muscles in the anterior abdominal wall.

The intercostal nerve and vessels form a neurovascular bundle which lie between the intermediate and deep layers (neurovascular plane).

N.B.

In addition to the above-mentioned three intrinsic muscles, there is another set of muscles called *levatores costarum*.

External Intercostal Muscle (11 Pairs)

Extent: Each muscle extends in the intercostal space from *tubercle of the rib* behind to the *costochondral junction*

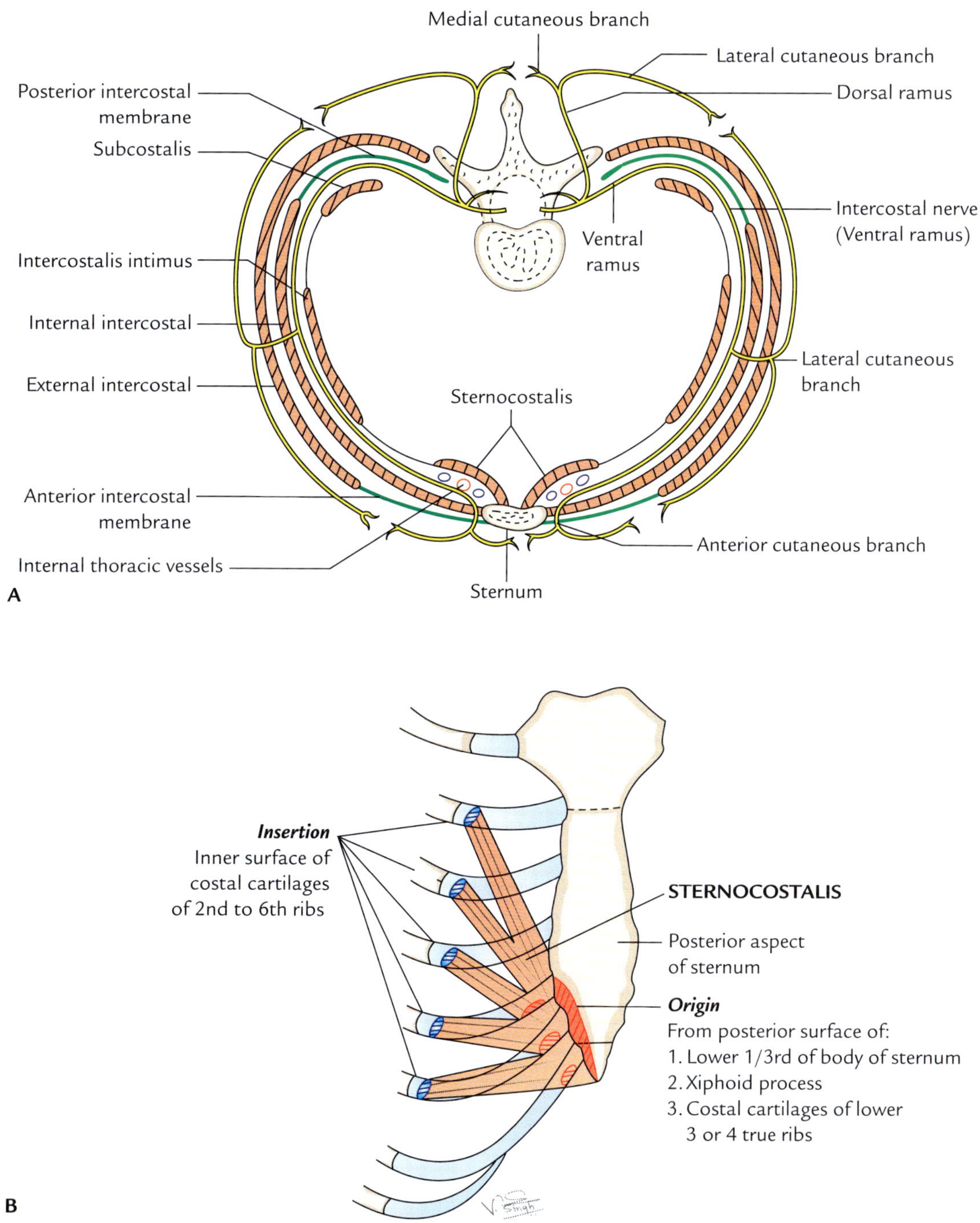

FIG. 17.1 ■ Intrinsic muscles of the thoracic wall. (**A**) Layers of intrinsic muscles and course and branches of typical intercostal nerve and (**B**) the origin and insertion of the sternocostalis muscle.

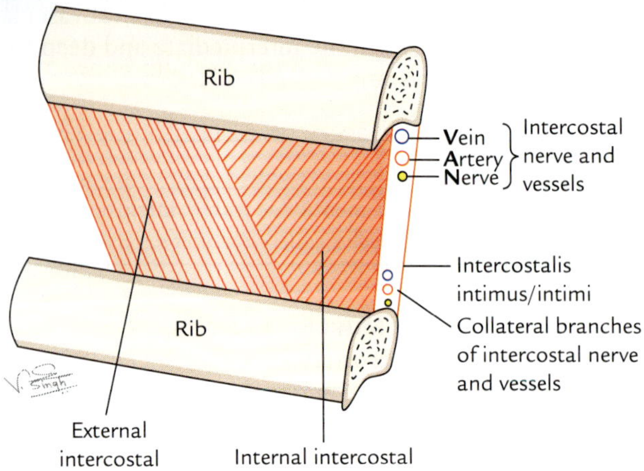

FIG. 17.2 ■ Contents of the intercostal space as seen in dissection.

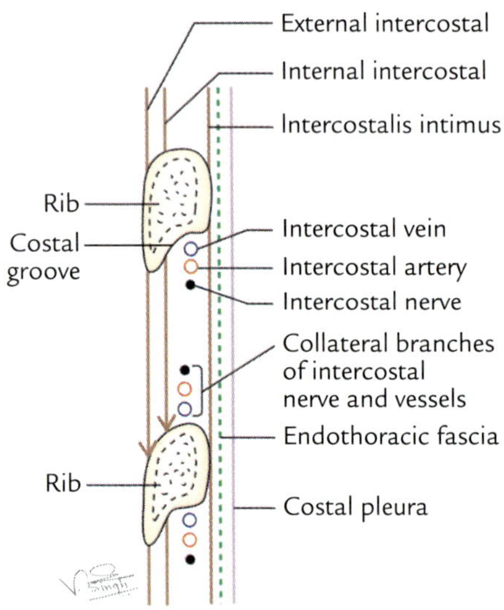

FIG. 17.3 ■ Contents of the intercostal space as seen in the vertical section.

in front, where it is replaced by *anterior intercostal membrane*.

Origin and insertion: It arises from the lower border of the rib above and inserts into the outer lip of the upper border of rib below.

Direction of fibres: The fibres of the external intercostal muscle are directed downward, forward, and medially (*in the posterior part, however, the fibres are directed downward and laterally*).

Nerve supply: By intercostal nerve of the same space.

Actions: The external intercostal muscles elevate the ribs during inspiration.

Internal Intercostal Muscle (11 Pairs)

Extent: Each muscle extends in the intercostal space from the lateral border of sternum in front to the angle of rib behind, where it is replaced by the *posterior intercostal membrane*.

Origin and insertion: It arises from the floor of the costal groove of the upper rib and inserts into the inner lip of the upper border of the rib below.

Direction of fibres: Its fibres are directed downward, backward, and laterally (i.e. at right angle to those of external intercostal muscle).

Nerve supply: By intercostal nerve of the same space.

Actions: The internal intercostal muscles elevate the ribs during inspiration.

Transversus Thoracis Muscle

The transversus thoracis muscle is divided into the following three parts:

1. Intercostalis intimus
2. Subcostalis
3. Sternocostalis

Intercostalis Intimus (11 Pairs)

Extent: It occupies the middle two-fourth of the intercostal space.

Origin and insertion: It arises from the inner surface of the rib above (upper border of costal groove) and inserts on to the inner surface of the rib below.

Direction of fibres: It is the same as those of internal intercostal muscles.

Nerve supply: By intercostal nerve of the same space.

Actions: The intercostal intimi muscles elevate the ribs during inspiration.

N.B.

Intercostal muscles depress the ribs during **forced expiration**.

Subcostalis Muscles (Total Number Variable)

The subcostalis muscles lie in the same plane as the intercostalis intimus in the posterior part of the intercostal space. It intervenes between the intercostal nerve and vessels, and pleura.

Origin and insertion: It arises from the inner surface of the rib near the angle and inserts on the inner surface of the second or third rib below.

Direction of fibres: It is the same as that of the internal intercostal muscle.

Nerve supply: By intercostal nerves.

Actions: Depressor of the ribs.

Sternocostalis (*Fig. 17.1B*)

The sternocostalis muscle one on either side is situated on the inner aspect of front of the chest wall (behind the sternum and costal cartilages) occupying the anterior part of the upper intercostal spaces, except the first space. The sternocostalis muscle intervenes between the anterior end of the intercostal nerves and the pleura.

Origin: It arises from (a) lower one-third of the posterior surface of the body of sternum, (b) posterior surface of the xiphoid process of the sternum, and (c) posterior surface of the costal cartilages of lower three or four ribs.

Insertion: The fibres diverge upward and laterally as slips to be inserted into the lower border and inner surfaces of the costal cartilages of second to sixth ribs.

Nerve supply: By intercostal nerves.

Action: It draws down the costal cartilages in which it is inserted.

The origin insertion, extent, direction of fibres, nerve supply, and actions of intrinsic muscles of thorax are given in Table 17.1.

INTERCOSTAL SPACES (FIGS. 17.2 AND 17.3)

The spaces between the two adjacent ribs (and their costal cartilages) are known as *intercostal spaces*. Thus there are 11 intercostal spaces on either side.

Each typical intercostal space is directed downward and forward. It is narrow towards vertebral column and broad towards sternum. Its widest part being at costochondral junction.

The third to sixth spaces are called **typical intercostal spaces** because the blood and nerve supply of third to sixth intercostal spaces is confined only to the thorax.

TYPICAL INTERCOSTAL SPACE

Boundaries

Superior: Sharp lower margin of the upper rib and its cartilage.

Inferior: Blunt upper margin of the lower rib and its cartilage.

Anterior: Lateral border of the sternum between the costal notches.

Posterior: Body of the corresponding thoracic vertebra.

CONTENTS OF A TYPICAL INTERCOSTAL SPACE

Each space contains the following structures (Fig. 17.3):

1. Three intercostal muscles (from outside inward), viz.
   (a) External intercostal
   (b) Internal intercostal
   (c) Innermost intercostal (intercostalis intimus)
2. Intercostal nerve
3. Intercostal arteries, one posterior and two anterior
4. Intercostal veins, one posterior and two anterior
5. Intercostal lymph vessels and lymph nodes

N.B.

- *Plane of neurovascular bundle in the intercostal space*: The neurovascular bundle consisting of the intercostal nerve and vessels lies between the internal intercostal and innermost intercostal muscles, that is, between the intermediate and deep layers of intercostal muscles.

TABLE 17.1 **Intrinsic muscles of the thoracic wall**

Muscle	Origin	Insertion	Extent	Direction of fibres	Nerve supply	Actions
1. External intercostal	Lower border of rib above	Outer lip of upper border of rib below	From costochondral junction to tubercle of rib (anteriorly it continues *as anterior intercostal membrane*)	Downward, forward, and medially	Intercostal nerve of the same space	Elevates the rib during inspiration
2. Internal intercostal	Floor of the costal groove of the rib above	Inner lip of upper border of rib below	From lateral border of sternum to the angle of rib (posteriorly it continues as *posterior intercostal membrane*)	Downward, backward, and laterally	Intercostal nerve of same space	Elevates the rib during inspiration
3. Transversus thoracis						
(a) Intercostalis intimus	Inner surface of rib above	Inner surface of rib below	Confined to the middle 2/4th of the intercostal space	Downward, backward, and laterally	Intercostal nerve of same space	Elevates the rib during inspiration
(b) Subcostalis	Inner surface of rib near angle	Inner surface of second or third ribs below	Confined to posterior parts of lower spaces only	Downward, backward, and laterally	Intercostal nerves	Depressor of ribs
(c) Sternocostalis	• Lower one-third of the posterior surface of the body of sternum • Posterior surface of xiphoid process • Posterior surface of costal cartilages of lower three or four ribs near sternum	Costal cartilages second to sixth ribs	Anterior part of upper spaces except the first space	Upward and laterally	Intercostal nerves	Draws second to sixth cartilages downward

They are arranged in the following order from above downward:

1. Intercostal **v**ein
2. Intercostal **a**rtery
3. Intercostal **n**erve

(*Mnemonic:* VAN.)

- *Intercostal muscles:* The intercostal muscles are a group of muscles that are present in the intercostal space and help form and move the chest wall.

  The following muscles constitute intercostal muscles:
  1. External intercostal muscle
  2. Internal intercostal muscle
  3. Innermost intercostal muscle (intercostalis intimi)

  Nerve supply: By intercostal nerves.

  The intercostal muscles are described in detail on pages 219–221.

Actions

The actions of intercostal muscles are as follows:

1. They act as strong supports for the rib preventing their separation.
2. **They act** during respiration.
   - *External intercostal muscles* elevate the ribs during inspiration. *Internal intercostal and intercostal intimi* also elevate the ribs during forced inspiration.
   - They pull down the rib cage and push air out of lungs.

INTERCOSTAL NERVES **AN 21.5**

The 12 pairs of thoracic spinal nerves supply the thoracic wall. As soon as they leave the intervertebral foramina, they divide into anterior and posterior rami (Fig. 17.4).

The anterior primary rami of upper 11 thoracic spinal nerves (T1–T11) are called **intercostal nerves** as they course through the intercostal spaces. The anterior primary ramus of the 12th thoracic spinal nerve runs in the abdominal wall below the 12th rib; hence, it is called the **subcostal nerve**.

N.B.

Unique features: The intercostal nerves are the anterior primary rami of thoracic spinal nerves. They are segmental in character unlike the anterior primary rami from other regions of the spinal cord that form nerve plexuses, namely, cervical, brachial, lumbar, and sacral.

Classification

The intercostal nerves are classified into the following two groups:

1. Typical intercostal nerves (3rd−6th)
2. Atypical intercostal nerves (1st, 2nd, 7th−11th)

The **typical intercostal nerves** are those that remain confined to their own intercostal spaces.

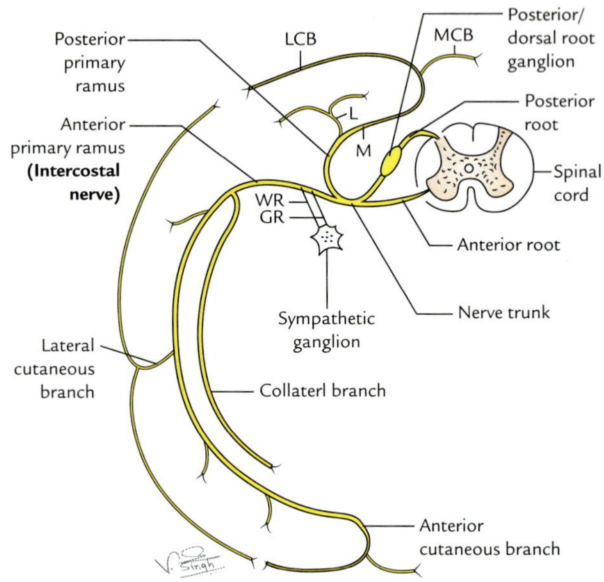

FIG. 17.4 ■ Typical thoracic spinal nerve (GR = grey rami communicantes, WR = white rami communicantes, L = lateral muscular branch, M = medial sensory branch, MCB = medial cutaneous branch, LCB = lateral cutaneous branch).

The **atypical spinal nerves** extend beyond the thoracic wall and partly or entirely supply the other regions.

TYPICAL INTERCOSTAL NERVE

Course and Relations (Fig. 17.4)

The typical intercostal nerve is the *anterior primary ramus of the typical thoracic spinal nerve*. After its origin, it turns laterally behind the sympathetic trunk and then enters into the **intercostal space** between the parietal pleura and posterior intercostal membrane. It then enters the **costal groove** of the corresponding rib to course laterally and forwards.

In the costal groove, it comes into relation with the corresponding intercostal vessels and forms the **neurovascular bundle** of the intercostal space.

In the intercostal space, vein, artery, and nerve lie in that order from above downward (Fig. 17.2).

Near the sternal end of the intercostal space, the intercostal nerve crosses in front of the internal thoracic artery. Then it pierces internal intercostal muscle, anterior intercostal membrane, and pectoralis major muscle to terminate as the **anterior cutaneous nerve**.

N.B.

- In the posterior part of the intercostal space, the intercostal nerve lies between the pleura and posterior intercostal membrane.
- In the remaining greater part of the intercostal space, it lies between the internal intercostal and intercostalis intimus muscles.

Branches (Fig. 17.4)

1. **Rami communicantes:** Each nerve communicates with the corresponding thoracic sympathetic ganglion by white and grey rami communicantes.

2. **Muscular branches:** These are small slender branches from the nerve, which supply intercostal muscles and serratus posterior, superior and inferior.
3. **Collateral branch:** It arises in the posterior part of the intercostal space near the angle of the rib and runs in the lower part of the space along the upper border of the rib below in the same neurovascular plane. It supplies intercostal muscles, parietal pleura, and periosteum of the rib.
4. **Lateral cutaneous branch:** It arises in the posterior part of the intercostal space near the angle of the rib and accompanies the main nerve for some distance, then pierces the muscles of the lateral thoracic wall along the midaxillary line. It divides into anterior and posterior branches to supply the skin on the lateral thoracic wall.
5. **Anterior cutaneous branch:** It is the terminal branch of the nerve, which emerges on the side of the sternum. It divides into medial and lateral branches and supplies the skin on the front of the thoracic wall.

ATYPICAL INTERCOSTAL NERVES AN 21.7

The atypical intercostal nerves are as follows:

1. **First intercostal nerve:** The greater part of this nerve joins the ventral ramus C8 spinal nerve to form lower trunk of the brachial plexus. The remaining part of the nerve is very small and it lacks both lateral and anterior cutaneous branches.
2. **Second intercostal nerve:** Its lateral cutaneous branch is called **intercostobrachial nerve**. It courses across the axilla and joins the medial cutaneous branch of the arm. The intercostobrachial nerve supplies the skin of the floor of the axilla and upper part of the medial side of the arm. *In coronary arterial disease, the cardiac pain is referred along this nerve to the medial side of the arm.*
3. **Seventh to eleventh intercostal nerves:** These nerves leave the corresponding intercostal spaces to enter into the anterior abdominal wall; hence, they are called **thoraco-abdominal nerves**. These nerves supply intercostal muscles of the corresponding intercostal spaces. In addition, they supply:
   (a) muscles of anterior abdominal wall, for example, external oblique, internal oblique, transverse abdominis, and rectus abdominis muscles, and
   (b) skin and parietal peritoneum covering the outer and inner surfaces of the abdominal wall, respectively.

CLINICAL CORRELATION

- **Root pain/girdle pain:** Irritation of intercostal nerves caused by the diseases of thoracic vertebrae produces severe pain, which is referred around the trunk along the cutaneous distribution of the affected nerve. It is termed *root pain* or *girdle pain*.
- **Sites of eruption of cold abscess on the body wall:** Pus from the tuberculous thoracic vertebra/vertebrae (*Pott's disease*) tends to track along the neurovascular plane of the space and may point at three sites of emergence of cutaneous branches of the thoracic spinal nerve, viz. (a) just lateral to the sternum, (b) in the midaxillary line, and (c) lateral to the erector spinae muscle (Fig. 17.5).
- **Herpes zoster:** In *herpes zoster* (*shingles*) involving the thoracic spinal ganglia, the cutaneous vesicles appear in

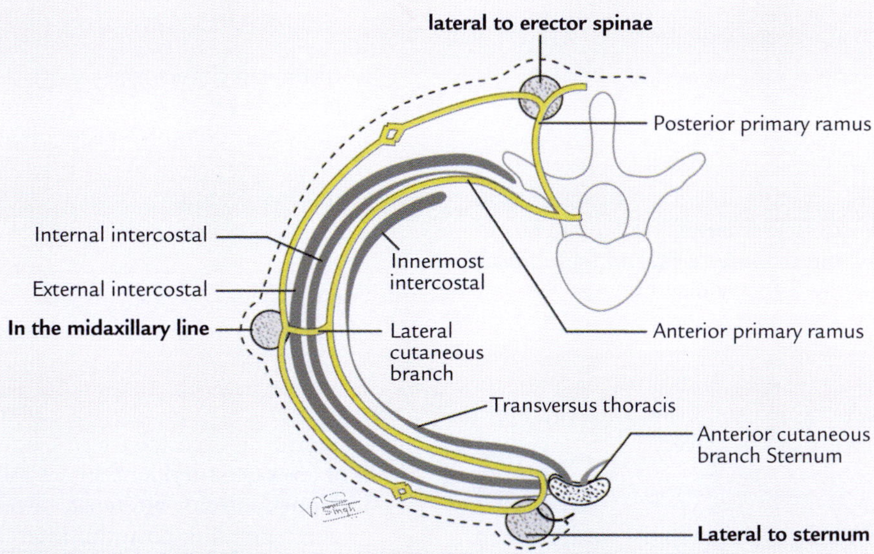

FIG. 17.5 ■ Sites of eruption of tuberculous cold abscess on the body wall. (*Source: Clinical and Surgical Anatomy,* 2ed.: Vishram Singh. Fig. 3.1, Page 104, Elsevier, 2007.)

the dermatomal area of the distribution of the intercostal nerve. It is an extremely painful condition.
- **Intercostal nerve block** is given to produce local anaesthesia in one or more intercostal spaces by injecting the anaesthetic agent around the nerve trunk near its origin, that is, just lateral to the vertebra.
- **Thoracotomy:** The *conventional thoracotomy* (*postero-lateral*) is performed along the sixth rib. The neurovascular bundle is protected from injury by lifting the periosteum of the rib.
- Considering the position of neurovascular bundle in the intercostal space, it is safe to insert the needle, a little above the upper border of the rib below.

INTERCOSTAL ARTERIES AN 21.6

The thoracic wall has rich blood supply. It is provided by the posterior and anterior intercostal arteries.

Each intercostal space contains one posterior and two anterior intercostal arteries (upper and lower).

POSTERIOR INTERCOSTAL ARTERIES AN 21.6

There are 11 pairs of posterior intercostal arteries, one in each space. They supply the greater part of the intercostal spaces (Fig. 17.6).

Origin

1. The first and second posterior intercostal arteries are the branches of the superior intercostal artery—a branch of the costocervical trunk.
2. The 3rd–11th posterior intercostal arteries arise directly from the descending thoracic aorta (Fig. 17.6A).

Course and Relations

In Front of the Vertebral Column (Fig. 17.6B)

- The right posterior intercostal arteries are longer than the left because the descending aorta lies on the left side of the front of the vertebral column. They pass behind the oesophagus, thoracic duct, azygos vein, and sympathetic chain but in front of the anterior aspect of vertebral body.
- The left posterior intercostal arteries are shorter and pass behind the hemiazygos vein and sympathetic chain, but in front of the side of the vertebral body.

In the Intercostal Space

In the intercostal space, the posterior intercostal artery lies between the intercostal vein above and the intercostal nerve below. The neurovascular bundle in the intercostal space lies between the internal intercostal and intercostalis intimus muscles.

Termination

Each posterior intercostal artery ends at the level of the costochondral junction by anastomosing with the upper anterior intercostal artery of the space.

Branches

1. **Dorsal branch:** It supplies the spinal cord, vertebra and muscles, and skin of the back.
2. **Collateral branch:** It arises near the angle of the rib and runs forward along the upper border of the rib below and ends by anastomosing with the lower anterior intercostal artery.
3. **Muscular branches:** They supply intercostal, pectoral, and serratus anterior muscles.
4. **Lateral cutaneous branch:** It closely follows the lateral cutaneous branch of the intercostal nerve.
5. **Mammary branches (external mammary arteries):** They arise from posterior intercostal arteries of the second, third, and fourth intercostal spaces and supply the breast/mammary gland.
6. **Right bronchial artery:** It arises from right third posterior intercostal artery.

CLINICAL CORRELATION

- **Paracentesis thoracis:** During *paracentesis thoracis* (aspiration of fluid from pleural cavity), the needle should never be inserted medial to the angle of the rib to avoid injury to the posterior intercostal artery, as it crosses the space obliquely from below upward (for details, see page 222).
- **Coarctation of aorta:** In *coarctation of aorta* (narrowing of the arch of aorta), the posterior intercostal arteries are markedly enlarged and cause notching of the ribs, particularly in their posterior parts.

ANTERIOR INTERCOSTAL ARTERIES AN 21.6

There are two intercostal arteries in each intercostal space. They are present in the upper nine intercostal spaces only.

Origin

1. In first to sixth spaces, they arise from the *internal thoracic artery*.
2. In seventh to ninth spaces, they arise from the *musculophrenic artery*, one of the terminal branches of internal mammary artery.

N.B.

The 10th and 11th intercostal spaces do not extend forward enough to have anterior intercostal arteries.

Termination

The anterior intercostal arteries are short and end at the level of costochondral junction as follows:

1. Upper anterior intercostal artery anastomoses with corresponding posterior intercostal artery.
2. Lower anterior intercostal artery anastomoses with the collateral branch of the corresponding posterior intercostal artery.

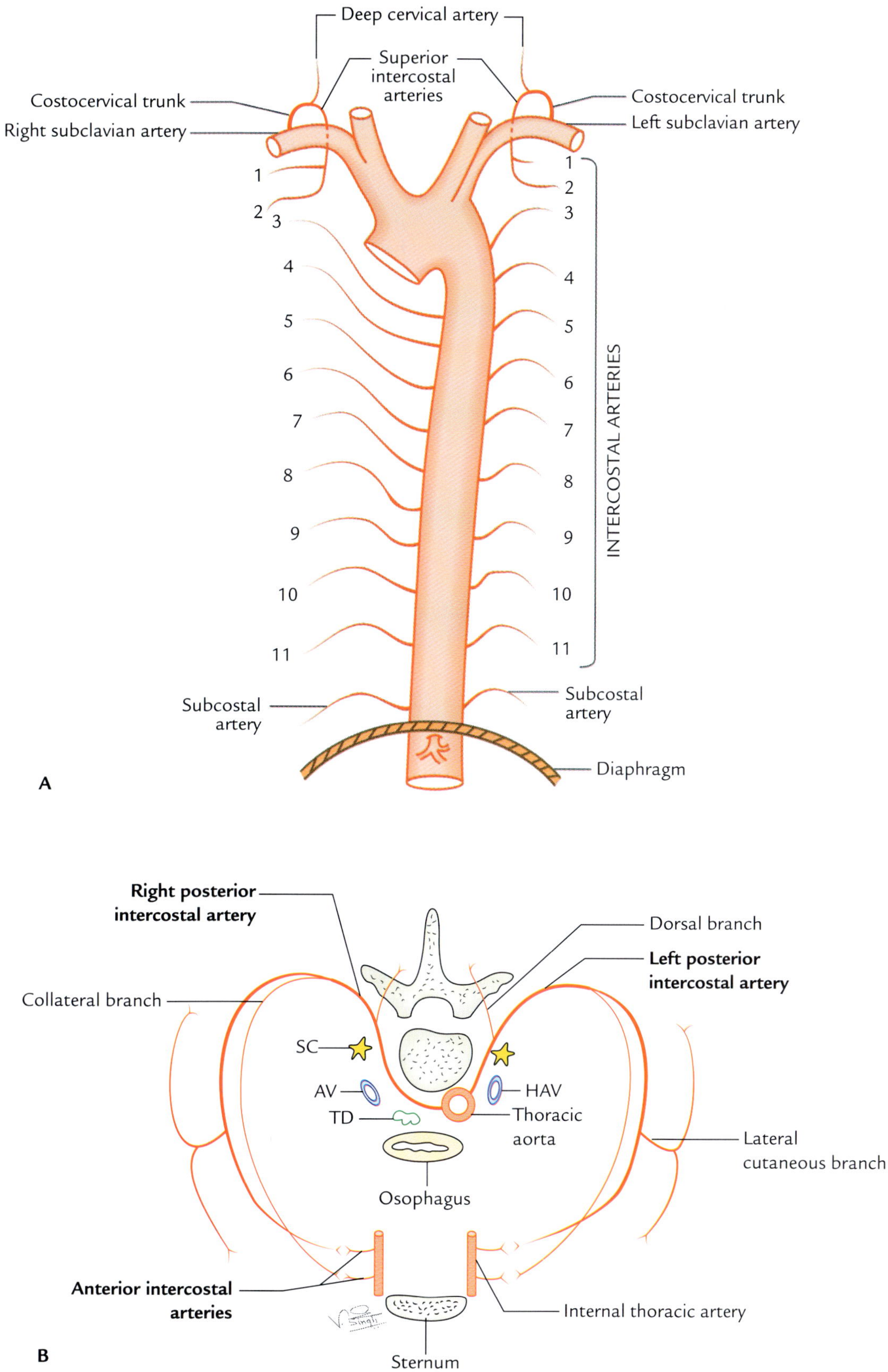

FIG. 17.6 ■ Posterior intercostal arteries. (**A**) Origin and (**B**) course and relations (SC = sympathetic chain, AV = azygos vein, TD = thoracic duct, HAV = hemiazygos vein).

INTERCOSTAL VEINS

The number of intercostal veins corresponds with the number of intercostal arteries, that is, each intercostal space contains two anterior intercostal veins and one posterior intercostal vein. Their tributaries correspond to the branches of the arteries.

ANTERIOR INTERCOSTAL VEINS AN 21.6

1. They are present only in the upper nine spaces.
2. *Each space contains two anterior intercostal veins* and accompanies the anterior intercostal arteries.

Termination

1. Veins of upper six spaces end in the internal thoracic vein.
2. Veins of seventh, eighth, and ninth spaces end in the musculophrenic vein.

POSTERIOR INTERCOSTAL VEINS AN 21.6

1. They are present in all the spaces.
2. *Each space contains only one posterior intercostal vein.*
3. Each vein accompanies the posterior intercostal artery.
4. Its tributaries correspond to the branches of posterior intercostal artery.

Termination (Fig. 17.7)

The mode of drainage (termination) of posterior intercostal veins differs on the right and left sides. For details see Table 17.2.

The right subcostal vein joins the right ascending lumbar vein to form *azygos vein*. While left subcostal vein joints left ascending lumbar vein to form *hemiazygos vein*. The 5th to 8th left posterior intercostal veins join to form *accessory hemiazygos vein*. Azygos, hemiazygos and accessory hemiazygos veins lie on either side of thoracic vertebral column.

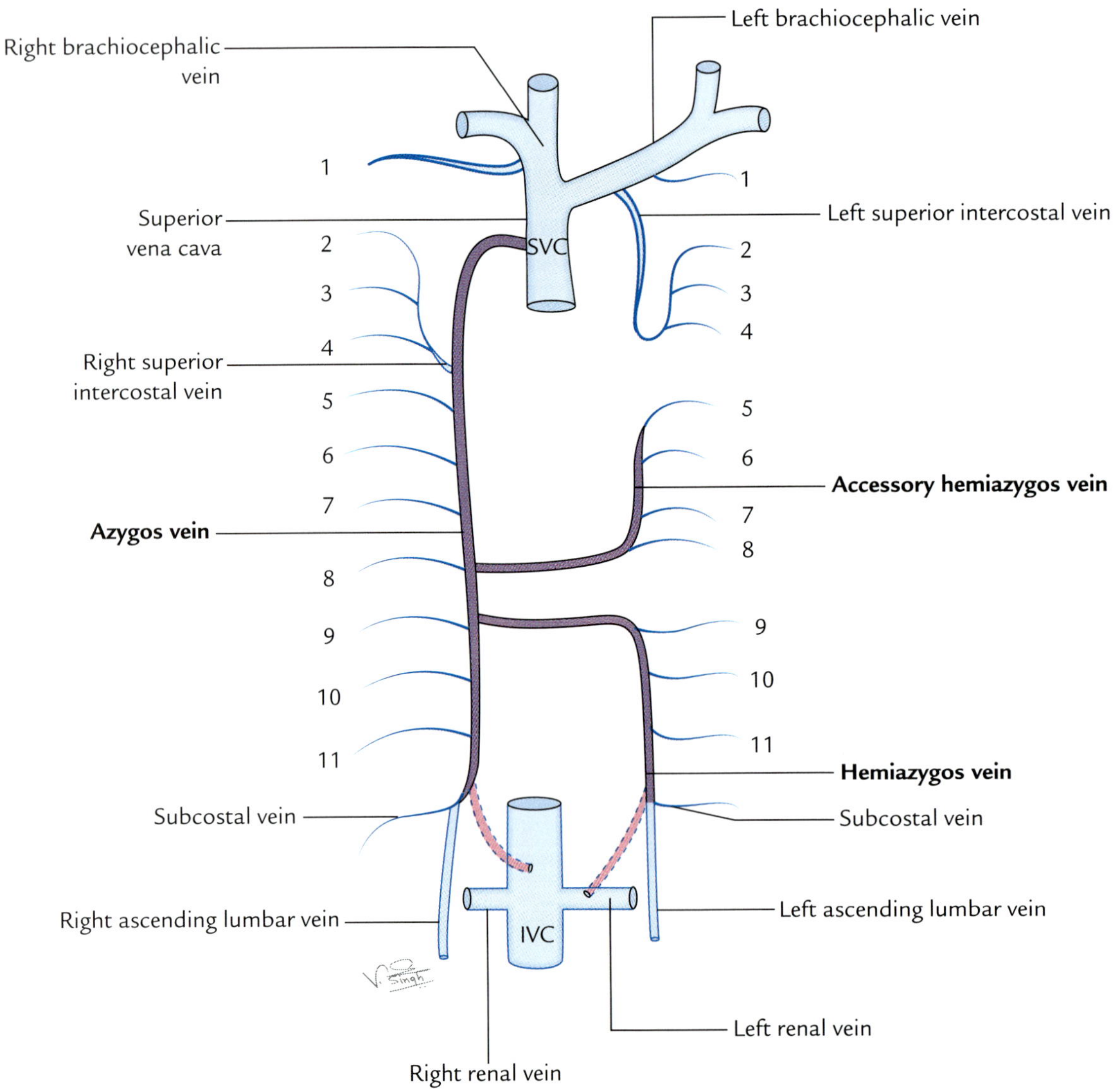

FIG. 17.7 ■ Drainage of posterior intercostal veins. Note that posterior intercostal veins are numbered 1–11 from above downward. Note azygos vein is connecting IVC and SVC with each other. The azygos, hemiazygos, and accessory hemiazygos veins are coloured violet (SVC = superior vena cava, IVC = inferior vena cava).

TABLE 17.2 **The mode of termination of right and left posterior intercostal veins**

Right posterior intercostal veins	Left posterior intercostal veins
1st (highest) drains into the right brachiocephalic vein	1st (highest) drains into the left brachiocephalic vein
2nd, 3rd and 4th join to form the *right superior intercostal vein*, which in turn drains into the azygos vein	2nd, 3rd and 4th join to form the *left superior intercostal vein*, which in turn drains into left brachiocephalic vein
5th to 8th drain into the azygos vein	5th to 8th drain into the accessory hemiazygos vein
9th to 11th drain into azygos vein	9th to 11th drain into the hemiazygos vein

INTERCOSTAL LYMPH VESSELS AND LYMPH NODES

LYMPH VESSELS

1. Lymph vessels from skin of anterior chest wall pass into the *anterior axillary lymph nodes*.
2. Lymph vessels from skin of posterior chest wall pass into the *posterior axillary lymph nodes*.
3. The lymph vessels from the anterior parts of the spaces drain into anterior intercostal/internal mammary lymph nodes. The efferent from these nodes unites with those of tracheobronchial and brachiocephalic nodes to form the bronchomediastinal trunk, which drains into right lymphatic duct on the right side and thoracic duct on the left side.
4. The lymph vessels from the posterior parts of the spaces drain into posterior intercostal nodes. The efferent from the posterior intercostal nodes of lower four spaces unites to form a slender lymph trunk, which descends and drains into the *cisterna chyli*. The efferent from posterior intercostal nodes of upper spaces drains into the right lymphatic duct on the right side and thoracic duct on the left side.

LYMPH NODES

1. Posterior intercostal nodes.
2. Anterior intercostal/internal mammary (parasternal) nodes.

The posterior intercostal nodes are located in the posterior part of the intercostal spaces on the necks of the ribs.

The anterior intercostal nodes lie along the course of internal thoracic (mammary) artery.

INTERNAL THORACIC ARTERY (FIG. 17.8)

There are two internal thoracic arteries, right and left, situated deep to anterior chest wall, one on either side of sternum.

Origin

The *internal thoracic artery* (also called *internal mammary artery*) arises from the first part of the subclavian artery (lower surface), about 2.5 cm above the medial end of the clavicle, opposite to the origin of the thyrocervical trunk.

Course and Termination

The internal thoracic artery descends behind the medial end of the clavicle and upper six costal cartilages, about 1 cm away from the lateral margin of the sternum. It ends in the sixth intercostal space by dividing into *superior epigastric* and *musculophrenic arteries*.

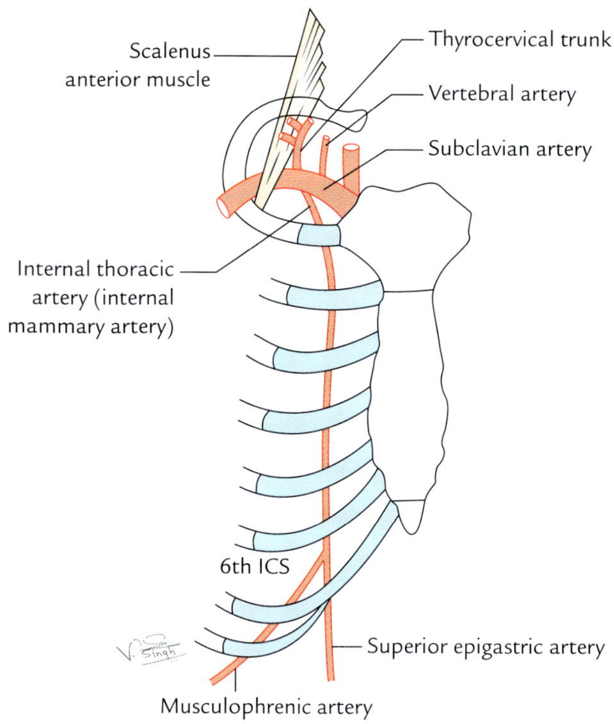

FIG. 17.8 Origin, course, and termination of internal thoracic artery (ICS = intercostal space).

Relations

Anteriorly: From above downward, it is related to the following:

- Medial end of the clavicle
- Internal jugular vein
- Brachiocephalic vein
- Phrenic nerve
- Pectoralis major
- Upper six costal cartilages
- External intercostal membranes
- Internal intercostal muscles
- Upper six intercostal nerves

Posteriorly:

- Above the second costal cartilage, it is related to endothoracic fascia and pleura.
- Below the second costal cartilage, it is related to sternocostalis muscle, which intervenes between the artery and the endothoracic fascia and pleura.

N.B.

The internal mammary artery is accompanied by two venae comitantes, which unite at the level of third costal cartilage to form the *internal thoracic* (*mammary*) vein, which runs upward along the medial side of the artery to terminate into the brachiocephalic vein at the root of the neck.

Branches

1. **Pericardiophrenic artery:** It arises in the root of the neck above the first costal cartilage, and descends along with phrenic nerve to the diaphragm. It supplies pericardium and pleura.
2. **Mediastinal branches:** They are small inconstant twigs, which supply connective tissue, thymus, and front of the pericardium.
3. **Anterior intercostal arteries:** They are two for each of the upper six intercostal spaces.
4. **Perforating branches:** They accompany the anterior cutaneous branches of intercostal nerves. In females, the perforating branches of second, third, and fourth intercostal spaces are quite large and supply the breast.
5. **Superior epigastric artery:** It runs downwards behind the seventh costal cartilage between the sternal and first costal slips of diaphragm to enter the rectus sheath where it ends by anastomosing with the inferior epigastric artery. It supplies anterior body wall from xiphoid process to the umbilicus.
6. **Musculophrenic artery:** It runs downward and laterally behind the seventh, eighth, and ninth costal cartilages, and gives two anterior intercostal arteries to each of the seventh, eighth, and ninth intercostal spaces. It pierces the diaphragm near the ninth costal cartilage to reach under surface. It supplies diaphragm and muscles of the anterior abdominal wall.

CLINICAL CORRELATION

Role of internal mammary artery in the treatment of coronary heart diseases:

- The *internal thoracic artery* is sometimes used to treat coronary heart disease. When the segment of coronary artery is blocked by atherosclerosis (mostly), the diseased arterial segment is bypassed by inserting a graft. The graft most commonly used is taken from great saphenous vein of the leg. In some patients, the myocardium is revascularized by mobilizing the internal thoracic artery and joining its distal cut end to the coronary artery distal to the diseased segment.

  The **internal mammary artery graft (IMA graft)** is preferred over grafts from other vessels because IMA graft lasts long. Recently, it has been found that internal mammary arteries are less prone to develop atherosclerosis because of their histological peculiarity. The walls of these arteries contain only elastic tissue and the cells of their endothelial lining secrete some chemicals, which prevents atherosclerosis. The left internal mammary artery is preferred over the right internal mammary artery because it is easier to access it.
- Earlier the *internal thoracic artery* was used to be ligated in the third intercostal space in order to reinforce the blood supply to the heart by diverting blood from this artery to its *pericardiophrenic branch*. This procedure is now obsolete.

TYPES OF RESPIRATION AN 21.9

The respiration consists of two alternate phases of (a) inspiration and (b) expiration, which are associated with alternate increase and decrease in the volume of thoracic cavity, respectively. During inspiration, the air is taken in (*inhaled*) and during expiration, the air is taken out (*exhaled*).

Rate of Respiration

The average rate of respiration is 18 per minute in normal resting state of an adult. It is faster in children and slower in the elderly.

MECHANICS OF RESPIRATION

INSPIRATION

Normally the pressure within thoracic cavity is less than that of atmospheric pressure.

During inspiration the volume of thoracic cavity increases, which creates further negative intrathoracic pressure, and consequently air is sucked into the lungs.

An **increase in the capacity** of the thoracic cavity occurs **vertically**, **anteroposteriorly**, and **transversely** (i.e. side to side) by different mechanisms.

Vertical Diameter

Increase in vertical diameter occurs due to contraction of diaphragm.

Theoretically, the vertical diameter of the thoracic cavity can increase if the roof of the thoracic cavity is raised or its floor lowered or both. The roof of the thoracic cavity is formed by a **tough suprapleural membrane**, which is fixed, and hence cannot move up and down.

However, the floor of the thoracic cavity is formed by the freely movable diaphragm. Thus, when the diaphragm contracts, its central tendon descends, and its domes are flattened. As a result, there is an increase in the vertical diameter of the thoracic cavity (Fig. 17.9).

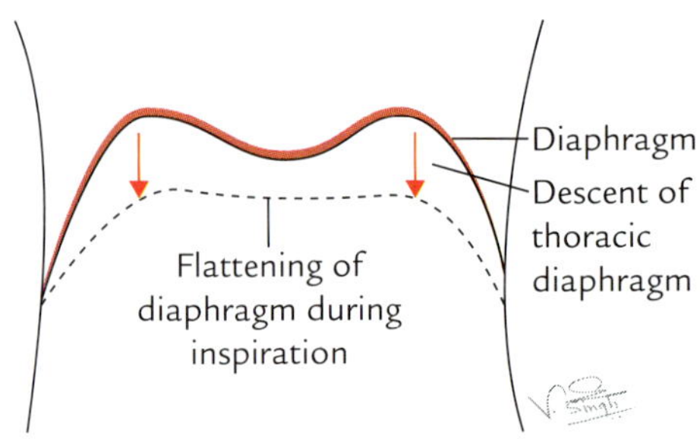

FIG. 17.9 ■ Increase in the vertical diameter of the thoracic cavity due to the descent of the diaphragm.

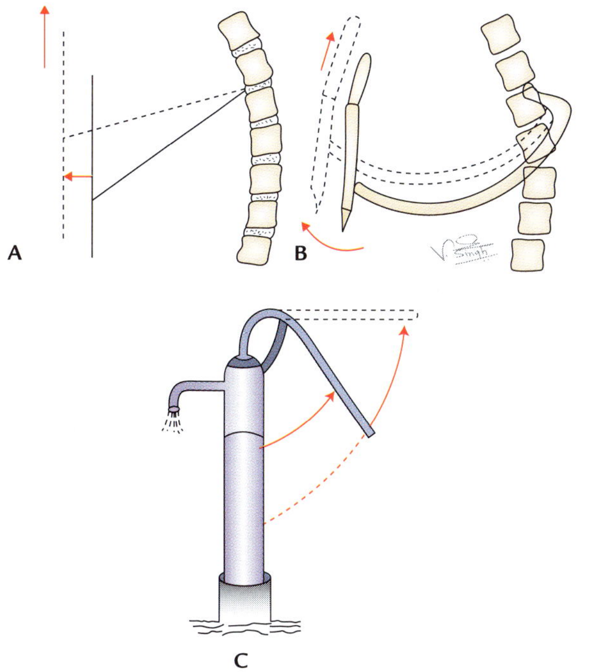

FIG. 17.10 Increase in the anteroposterior diameter of the thoracic cavity due to forward and upward movements of sternum. (**A**) Idealized representation. (**B**) Actual movement of sternum. (**C**) Real pump showing movement of its handle.

Anteroposterior Diameter

An increase in the anteroposterior diameter of the thoracic cavity occurs when *sternum moves forward and upward due to elevation of vertebrosternal ribs by contraction of external intercostal muscles*. It is called **pump-handle movement** (Fig. 17.10).

Each rib acts as a lever, the fulcrum of which lies just lateral to the tubercle of the rib. Thus, two arms of lever are greatly disproportional; for example, the posterior arm is very short and anterior arm is very long. Thus, slight movement at the vertebral end of the rib is greatly magnified at the anterior end of the rib (Fig. 17.11).

Since anterior ends of the ribs are at a lower level than their posterior ends, during elevation of the ribs, when their anterior ends move upward and forward, they carry with them the sternum. (This movement occurs mostly in vertebrosternal ribs.) Consequently, the anteroposterior diameter of the thoracic cavity is increased. This movement is termed **pump-handle movement** because sternum moves up and down like a handle of pump during respiration (Fig. 17.11).

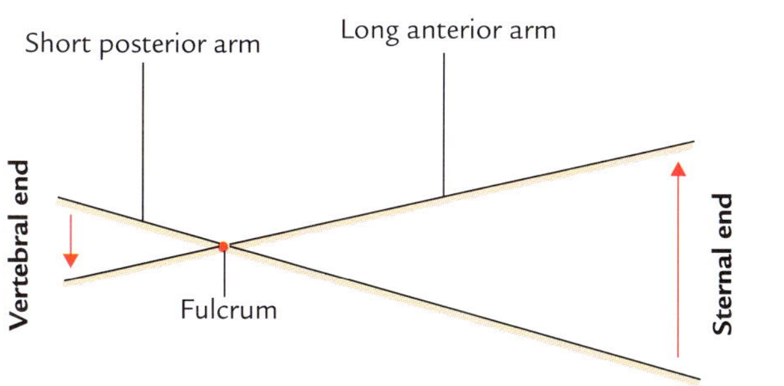

FIG. 17.11 Mechanism of increase in the anteroposterior diameter of the thoracic cavity. This is because the ribs act as levers with fulcrum just lateral to the tubercle.

Transverse Diameter

The increase in transverse diameter of thoracic cavity occurs due to elevation of vertebrochondral ribs by *contraction of external intercostal muscles*. It is called as a bucket handle movement.

The middle of the shaft of the ribs lies at the lower level than the plane passing through its two ends (anterior and posterior; Fig. 15.12). This arrangement resembles a **bucket handle**. Therefore, during the elevation of the ribs, the shafts of the ribs move outwards like the bucket handle—**bucket-handle movement**. This causes increase in the transverse diameter of the thoracic cavity (Fig. 17.12). The axis of movement passes from the tubercle of the rib to the middle of the sternum.

The bucket-handle movement is produced by vertebrochondral ribs.

The main factors responsible for increase in various diameters of the thoracic cavity are summarized in Table 17.3.

EXPIRATION

The expiration is the passive process brought about by:

(a) elastic recoil of the alveoli of the lungs,
(b) relaxation of the intercostal muscles and the diaphragm,
(c) increase in the tone of the muscles of the anterior abdominal wall.

TYPES OF RESPIRATION (BREATHING)

The respiration is classified into the following three types:

1. Quiet respiration
2. Deep respiration
3. Forced respiration

In **quiet respiration**, the movements are normal as described above.

In **deep respiration**, movements described for quiet respiration are increased. The first rib is elevated by scalene and sternocleidomastoid muscles.

In **forced respiration**, all movements are exaggerated. The scapula is fixed and elevated by trapezius, levator scapulae, rhomboideus major, and rhomboideus minor muscles, so that pectoral muscles and serratus anterior can raise the ribs.

The muscles acting during different types of respiration (i.e. respiratory muscles) are enumerated in Table 17.4.

> **CLINICAL CORRELATION**
>
> **Posture of patient during asthmatic attack:** During asthmatic attack (characterized by breathlessness/difficulty in breathing), the patient is most comfortable in sitting up, leaning forwards, and fixing the arms on the bed/table. This is because in the sitting position, the diaphragm is at its lowest level, allowing maximum ventilation. The fixation of arms fixes the scapulae, so that the pectoral muscles and serratus anterior may act on the ribs which they elevate.

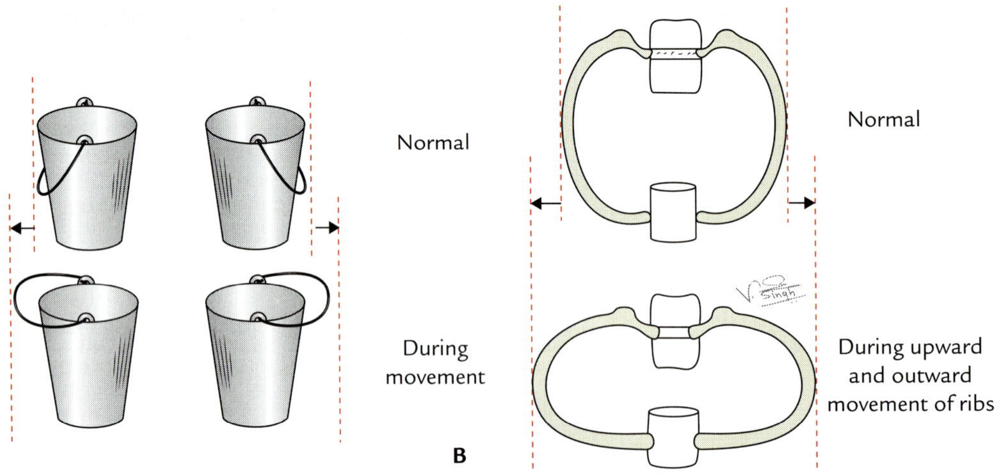

FIG. 17.12 ■ Increase in the transverse diameter of the thoracic cavity due to bucket-handle movements of vertebrochondral rib. (**A**) Idealized representation. (**B**) Actual movements of the ribs.

TABLE 17.3 Factors responsible for the increase in various diameters of the thoracic cavity during inspiration

Diameter	Factors responsible for increase
Vertical	Descent (contraction) of the diaphragm
Anteroposterior	**Pump-handle movement** of the sternum (brought about by the elevation of vertebrosternal ribs)
Transverse	**Bucket-handle movement** of the vertebrochondral ribs

TABLE 17.4 Muscles acting during different types of respiration

Type of respiration	Inspiration (elevation of ribs)	Expiration (depression of ribs)
Quiet respiration	• External intercostal muscles • Diaphragm	• Passive • No muscles
Deep respiration	• External intercostal muscles • Scalene muscles • Sternocleidomastoid • Levatores costarum • Serratus posterior superior • Diaphragm	• Passive • No muscles
Forced respiration	• All the muscles involved in deep inspiration (*vide supra*) • Levator scapulae • Trapezius • Rhomboids • Pectoral muscles • Serratus anterior	• Quadratus lumborum • Internal intercostal muscles • Transversus thoracis • Serratus posterior inferior

Golden Facts to Remember

• Anterior primary rami of all the thoracic spinal nerves are intercostal nerves *except*	Anterior primary ramus of the T12 spinal nerve which is a *subcostal nerve*
• Main movement to increase the anteroposterior diameter of the thoracic cavity	*Pump-handle movement* of sternum brought about by the elevation of vertebrosternal ribs (second to sixth ribs)
• Main movement to increase the transverse diameter of the thoracic cavity	*Bucket-handle movement* of vertebrochondral ribs
• Main factor responsible for increase of vertical diameter of the thoracic cavity	Contraction of the diaphragm
• Position of body in which diaphragm lies at the highest level	Supine position
• Position of body in which diaphragm lies at the lowest level	Sitting position
• Principal muscle of respiration • Muscle of weight lifting	} Diaphragm

CLINICAL CASE STUDY

A 55-year-old patient came to the hospital with complaints of weakness, loss of weight, and pain on the back of chest. On examination, tenderness was noted on percussion, in the region of thoracic spine. Small bulges were also seen on the surface of the chest at three sites: (a) lateral to the sternum, (b) in the midaxillary line, and (c) lateral to the erector spinae muscle. The X-ray of thoracic spine revealed *collapse of vertebral bodies* of T5 and T6 vertebrae and a *perispinal soft tissue shadow*. He was diagnosed as a case of **Pott's disease**.

Questions

1. What is Pott's disease?
2. What is the cause of perispinal soft tissue shadow?
3. Mention the anatomical basis of small bulges noted on the surface of the chest wall (*vide supra*).

Answers

1. Tuberculosis of spine (i.e. vertebrae).
2. Perispinal abscess.
3. The pus from the region of tubercular spine (**cold abscess**) tracks around the thoracic wall along the plane of neurovascular bundle and points on the surface of the chest at the sites of exit of cutaneous branches of the intercostal nerve, that is (a) lateral to the erect spinae muscle, (b) in the midaxillary line, and (c) just lateral to the sternum.

CHAPTER

18 Pleural Cavities

SPECIFIC LEARNING OBJECTIVES

After studying this chapter, the student should be able to:

- Mention the extent of pleura and describe pleural recesses and their applied anatomy. AN 24.1
- Mention the blood supply, lymphatic drainage, and nerve supply of pleura. AN 24.1
- Describe the boundaries and contents of the superior, anterior, middle, and posterior mediastinum. AN 21.11
- Write short notes on: (a) pleura, (b) pleural recesses, (c) pulmonary ligament, and (d) paracentesis thoracis.
- Enumerate sites where the pleura extends beyond the thoracic cage.
- Give the anatomical basis of: (a) pleural effusion, (b) pneumothorax, and (c) referred pain of the pleura.
- Enumerate differences between the parietal and visceral pleurae.

The thoracic cavity is divided into three compartments (Fig. 18.1A): right lateral compartment, left lateral compartment, and middle compartment. Each lateral compartment is occupied by a lung enclosed in the serous sac called the **pleural cavity** (Fig. 18.1B). The middle compartment contains, essentially, all the thoracic structures except lungs, such as the heart with its pericardium, great blood vessels that leave or enter the heart, structures that traverse the thorax to enter the abdomen in passing from the neck to the abdomen or from the abdomen to the neck such as oesophagus, vagus nerves, phrenic nerves, and thoracic duct.

The mass of tissues and organs occupying the middle compartment forms a mobile septum—**mediastinum** that completely separates the two pleural cavities.

PLEURAL CAVITIES

Each lung is enclosed in a serous sac that consists of two continuous serous membranes: the **visceral pleura** and the **parietal pleura**. The visceral pleura invests all the surfaces of the lung forming its shiny outer surface of lung, whereas the parietal pleura lines the pulmonary cavity (i.e. thoracic wall and mediastinum; Fig. 18.1B).

The space between the visceral and parietal pleurae is called the **pleural cavity**.

A little description of development of lung makes it easier to understand the relationship of the lung and pleura.

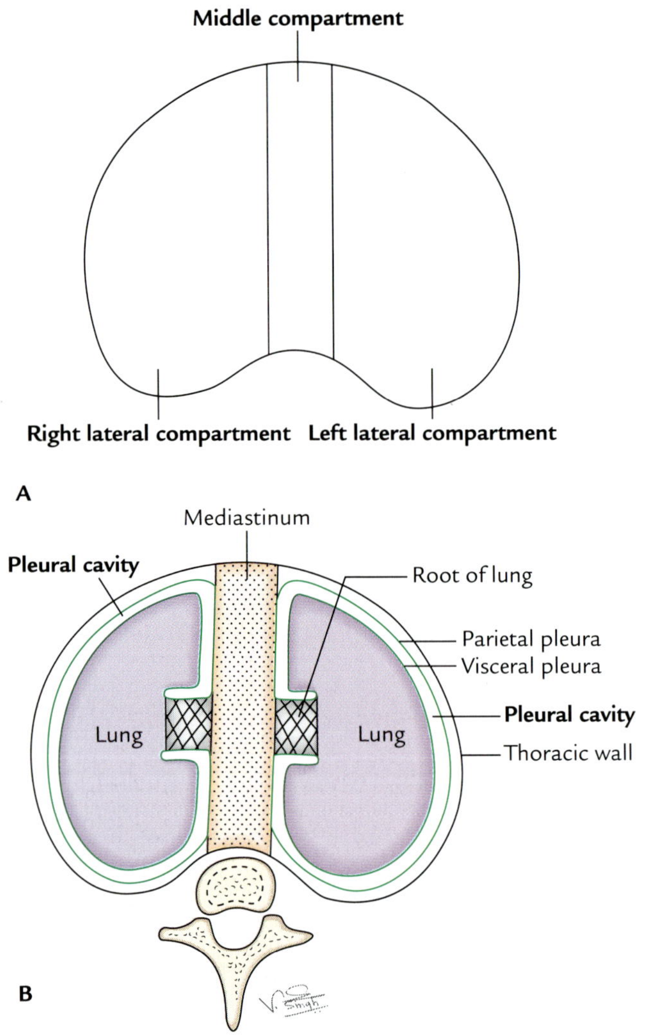

FIG. 18.1 ■ Compartments of the thoracic cavity. (**A**) Empty compartments and (**B**) lateral compartments occupied by lung enclosed in the serous sac (pleural sac).

During early embryonic life, each lateral compartment of the thoracic cavity is occupied by a closed serous sac, which is invaginated from the medial side by developing the lung (Fig. 18.2). As a result of this invagination, it is converted into a double-layered sac. The outer layer is called the **parietal pleura** and the inner layer is called the **visceral pleura**. The visceral pleura is continuous with the parietal pleura at the root of the lung. The parietal and visceral layers are separated from each other by a slit-like potential space called the **pleural cavity**. The pleural cavity is normally filled with a thin film of tissue fluid that lubricates the adjoining surfaces of the pleura and allows them to move on each other without friction.

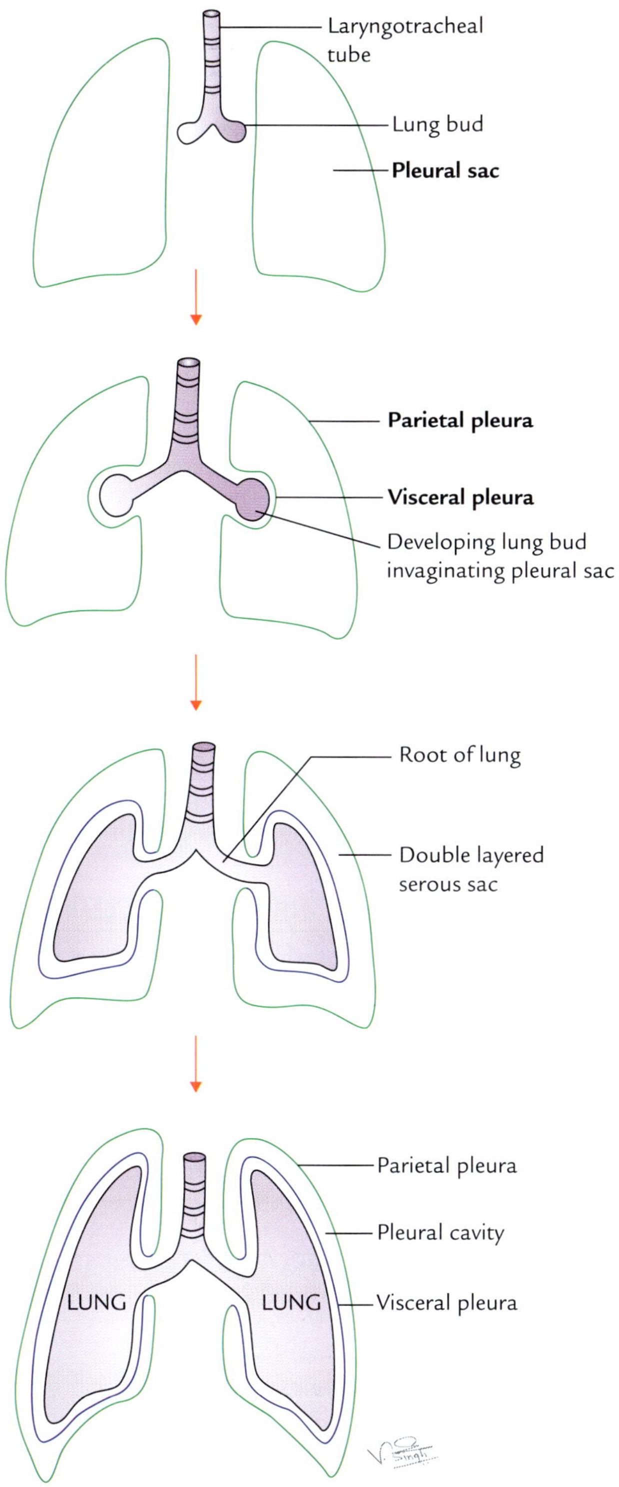

FIG. 18.2 ■ Invagination of developing lungs into the closed serous sacs.

The two layers become continuous with each other by means of a **cuff of the pleura**, which surrounds the root of the lung consisting of structures entering and leaving the lung at the hilum of the lung, such as principal bronchi and pulmonary vessels. To allow the movement of the principal bronchi and pulmonary vessels during respiration, the cuff of pleura hangs down as loose triangular fold called **pulmonary ligament**. The pulmonary ligament extends from the root of the lung as far down as the diaphragm between the lung and the mediastinum.

PLEURA **AN 24.1**

The pleura like peritoneum is a serous membrane lined by the flattened epithelium (mesothelium). On each side, it invests the lung and lines the thoracic cavity. The epithelium lining this membrane secretes a watery lubricant—the **serous fluid**.

LAYERS OF THE PLEURA

The pleura consists of two layers: (a) visceral pleura and (b) parietal pleura. The moistened space between the two layers is called the *pleural cavity (vide supra)*.

Visceral Pleura (Pulmonary Pleura)

The visceral pleura completely covers the surface of the lung except at the hilum and along the attachment of the pulmonary ligament. It also extends into the depths of the fissures of the lungs. It is firmly adherent to the lung surface and cannot be separated from it.

Parietal Pleura

The parietal pleura is thicker than the visceral pleura and it lines the walls of the pulmonary cavity.

The parietal pleura is like a half cone (Fig. 18.3). It lines the costae (thoracic wall), diaphragm, lateral surface of the mediastinum, and Sibson's fascia (cervical diaphragm).

Subdivisions of Parietal Pleura

For the purpose of description, it is customary to divide parietal pleura, according to the surface, which it lines, covers, or the region in which it lies. Thus, the parietal pleura is divided into the following four parts (Fig. 18.4):

1. Costal pleura
2. Diaphragmatic pleura
3. Mediastinal pleura
4. Cervical pleura

Costal pleura: It lines the inner surface of the thoracic wall (consisting of ribs, costal cartilages, and intercostal spaces) to which it is loosely attached by a thin layer of the loose areolar tissue called **endothoracic fascia**. In living beings, endothoracic fascia is easily separable from the thoracic wall.

Diaphragmatic pleura: It covers the superior surface of the diaphragm. In quiet respiration, the costal and

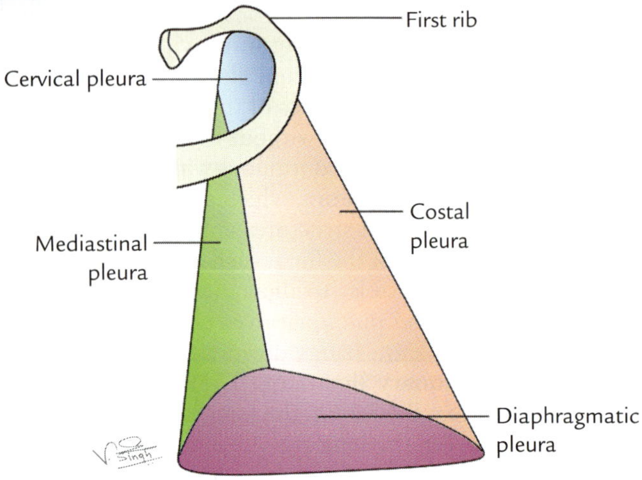

FIG. 18.3 ■ Subdivisions of parietal pleura.

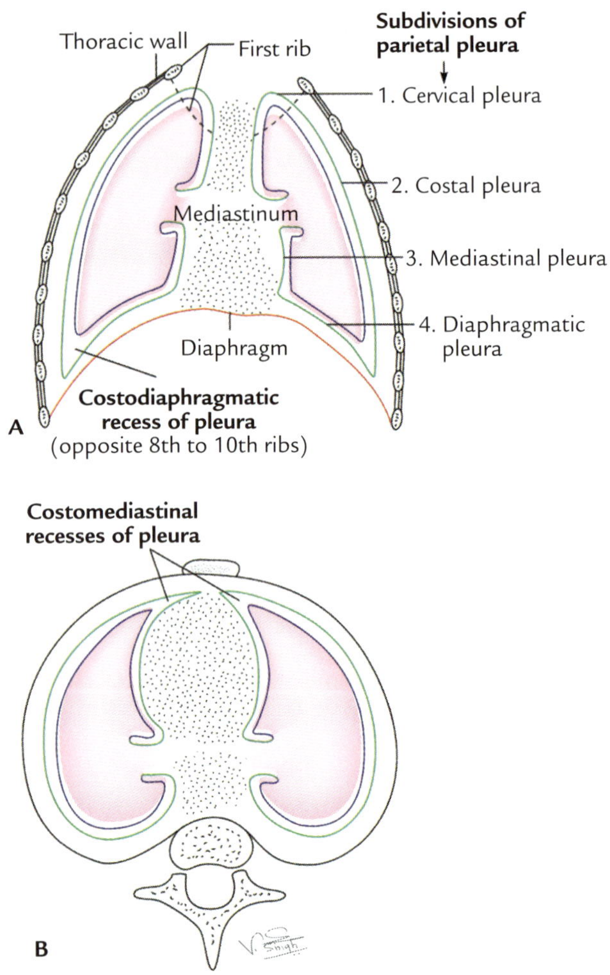

FIG. 18.4 ■ Reflection of the pleura as seen in (**A**) vertical section of the thoracic cavity and (**B**) transverse section of the thoracic cavity.

diaphragmatic pleurae are in opposition to each other below the inferior border of the lung.

Mediastinal pleura: It lines the corresponding surface of the mediastinum and forms its lateral boundary. It is reflected as a cuff over the root of the lung and becomes continuous with the visceral pleura.

Cervical pleura: It is the dome of the parietal pleura, which covers the apex of lung. It extends into the root of the neck about 1 in (2.5 cm) above the medial end of the clavicle and 2 in (5 cm) above the first costal cartilage. It is called **cupola** and covers the apex of the lung. Therefore, utmost caution should be taken while penetrating this area with an anaesthetic needle. It is covered by the **suprapleural membrane**.

Relations of the cervical pleura: The relations of the cervical pleura are as follows:

Anteriorly: Subclavian artery and scalenus anterior muscle.
Posteriorly: Neck of the first rib and structures passing in front of it (see pages 208–209).
Laterally: Scalenus medius muscle.
Medially: Great vessels of the neck.

PULMONARY LIGAMENT

The pleura surrounds the root of the lung similar to the cuff (sleeve) of the jacket around the wrist (Fig. 18.4A). It extends down as a fold called the **pulmonary ligament**. The pulmonary ligament (Fig. 18.5) extends from the root of the lung as far down as the diaphragm between the lung and the mediastinum. The fold is filled with the loose areolar tissue and contains few lymphatics.

Functions

The functions of pulmonary ligaments are as follows:

1. It provides a *dead space* into which the pulmonary veins can expand during increased venous return as during exercise.
2. It allows the descent of the root of the lung with the descent of the diaphragm during inspiration. As a result, the apex of the lung comes down from the tough suprapleural membrane, leaving an empty space below the membrane. Now, the apex of the lung can expand into this empty space.

SURFACE MARKINGS OF THE PARIETAL PLEURA

The **surface marking of the visceral pleura** corresponds with the surface marking of lungs as it is closely applied on their surfaces. Hence it is described with that of the lung on page 245.

The following text deals with **surface marking of the parietal pleura** (Fig. 18.6).

The knowledge of reflection of the parietal pleura on the surface of the chest wall is of great importance while carrying out various medical and surgical procedures.

Parts of the Parietal Pleura (Figs. 18.3 and 18.4)

The parietal pleura is divided into four parts:

- Cervical pleura
- Mediastinal pleura
- Diaphragmatic pleura
- Costal pleura

The reflection of the parietal pleura can be marked on the surface by the following lines:

1. **Cervical pleura:** It is marked by a curved line (with convexity directed upward) drawn from the

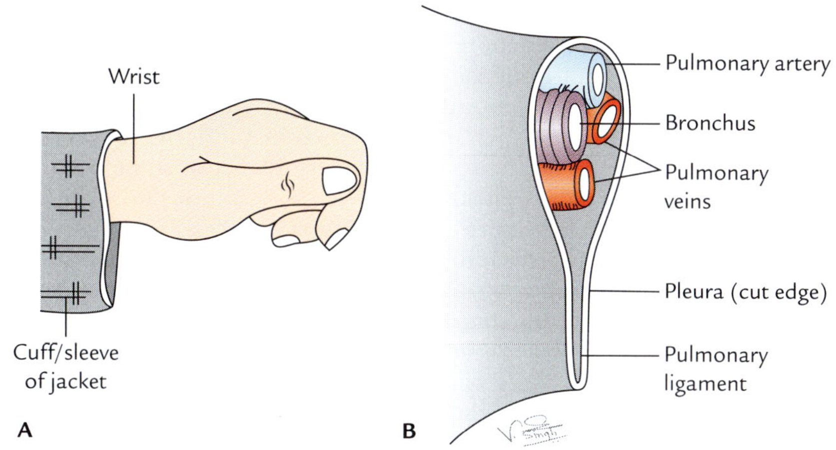

FIG. 18.5 ■ Root of the lung and pulmonary ligament. (**A**) Cuff (sleeve) of the jacket around wrist simulating the pulmonary ligament and (**B**) structures forming the root of the lung.

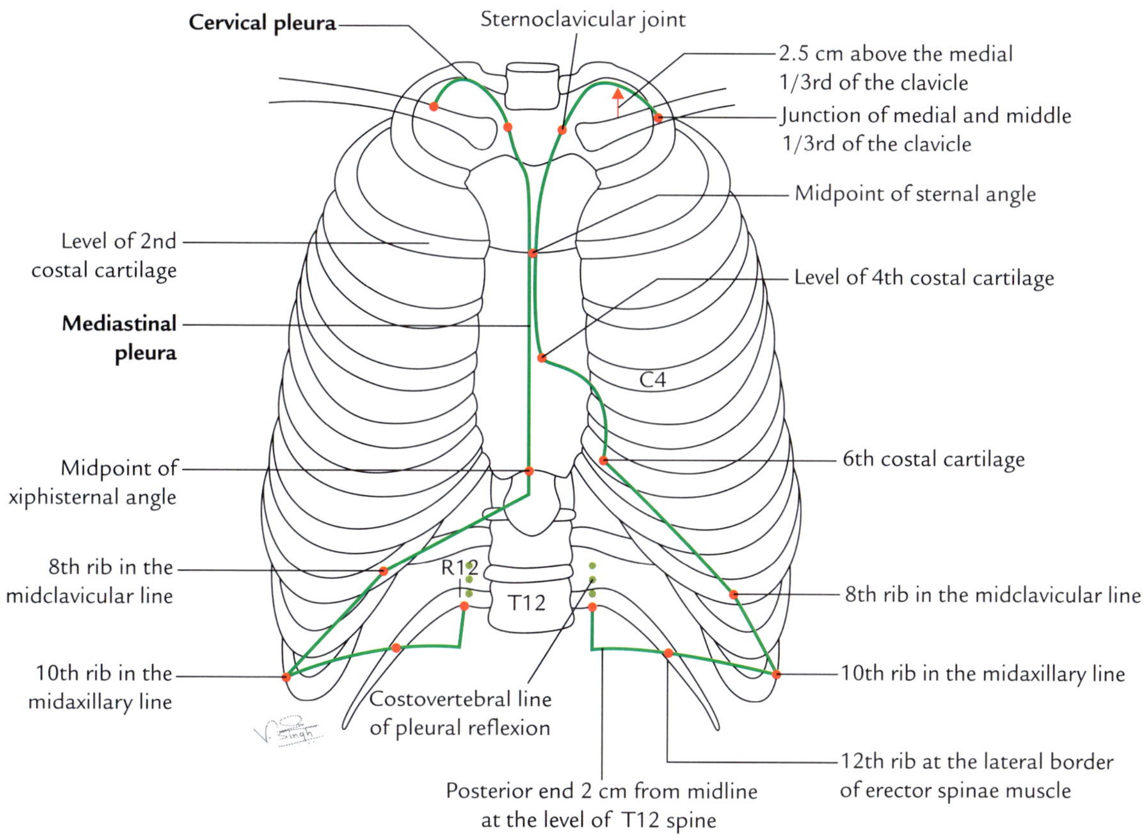

FIG. 18.6 ■ Schematic diagram showing the lines of pleural reflection (C4 = 4th costal cartilage, R12 = 12th rib, T12 = 12th thoracic vertebra, BA = bare area of heart).

sternoclavicular joint to the junction of the medial third and the middle third of the clavicle. The summit of the dome of the pleura lies 1 in (2.5 cm) above the medial one-third of the clavicle. It covers the apex of the lung.

2. **Mediastinal pleura:** It is marked by *anterior (costomediastinal) line of pleural reflection*. It differs on the two sides:
   (a) **On the right side**, it extends downward and medially from the right sternoclavicular joint to the midpoint of the sternal angle, and then descends vertically up to the midpoint of the xiphisternal joint.
   (b) **On the left side**, it extends downward and medially from the left sternoclavicular joint to the midpoint of the sternal angle, then descends vertically only up to the level of the fourth costal cartilage. It then arches outward to reach the lateral margin of the sternum and runs downward a short distance lateral to this margin to reach the sixth costal cartilage, about 3 cm from the midline, leaving a part of pericardium directly in contact with the anterior chest wall (**bare area of the heart**).

3. **Diaphragmatic pleura:** It is marked by **inferior (costodiaphragmatic) line of pleural reflection:** It passes laterally around the chest wall from the lower limit of the anterior line of pleural reflection. It differs slightly on two sides:
   (a) **On the right side**, the line of reflection starts from the xiphisternal joint or behind the xiphoid process and crosses the 8th rib in the midclavicular line, 10th rib in the midaxillary line, and 12th rib at the lateral border of the erector spinae muscle, 2 cm lateral to the spine of the T12 vertebra.
   (b) **On the left side**, the line of reflection starts at the level of the sixth costal cartilage, about 2 cm lateral to the midline. Thereafter, it follows the same course as on the right side.

   Posterior (costovertebral) line of pleural reflection: It ascends from the end of the inferior line, 2 cm lateral to the T12 spine along the vertebral column to the point, 2 cm lateral to the spine of the C7 vertebra. The costal pleura becomes the mediastinal pleura along this line.
4. **Costal pleura:** It lines the thoracic wall from which it is separated by endothoracic fascia – a layer of loose areolar tissue.

N.B.

The inferior margin of the lung passes more horizontally than the inferior margin of the pleura. Consequently, it crosses the 6th rib in the midclavicular line, 8th rib in the midaxillary line, and 10th rib at the lateral border of the erector spine.

The ribs crossed by the inferior margin of the lung and pleura in the *midclavicular line*, *midaxillary line*, and *lateral* to the *erector spine* are compared below:

Inferior margin of lung: 6th rib, 8th rib, and 10th rib
Inferior margin of pleura: 8th rib, 10th rib, and 12th rib

RECESSES OF THE PLEURA

Normally, the space between the parietal pleura and visceral pleura is only a potential space and is filled with thin film of the serous fluid. However, in areas of pleural reflection on to the diaphragm and mediastinum, the space between the parietal and visceral pleurae is greatly expanded. These expanded regions of the pleural cavity are called **pleural recesses** (Fig. 18.4). They are essential for lung expansion during deep inspiration. Thus, *pleural recesses serve as reserve spaces of the pleural cavity for the lungs to expand during deep inspiration.* The recesses of the pleura are as follows:

1. **Costodiaphragmatic recesses** (right and left)
2. **Costomediastinal recesses** (right and left)

N.B.

In addition to the above recesses of the pleura, there are three more small recesses, namely,

- ***Right and left retro-oesophageal recesses***
  These are formed by the reflection of the mediastinal pleura behind the oesophagus. Each recess is thought to be occupied by a part of the lung and contributes to the retrocardiac space seen in the radiographs of the chest.
- ***Infracardiac recess***
  It is a small recess of the right pleural sac that sometimes extends beneath the inferior vena cava.

Costodiaphragmatic recess (Fig. 18.4A): It is located inferiorly between the costal and diaphragmatic pleurae. Vertically, it measures about 5 cm and lies opposite to the 8th–10th ribs along the midaxillary line. The costodiaphragmatic recesses are the most dependent parts of the pleural cavities; hence, the fluid of pleural effusion is first collected at these sites.

Costomediastinal recess (Fig. 18.4B): It is located anteriorly between the costal and mediastinal pleurae and lies between the sternum and costal cartilages. The right costomediastinal recess is possibly occupied by the anterior margin of the right lung even during quiet breathing. The left costomediastinal recess is large due to the presence of the cardiac notch in the left lung. Its location can be confirmed clinically by percussion (tapping) of the chest wall. As one moves during tapping from the area of the underlying lung tissue to the area of the left costomediastinal recess unoccupied by the lung tissue, a change in tone, from resonant to dull, is noticed. This is called the area of superficial cardiac dullness.

CLINICAL CORRELATION

Radiological appearance of pleural effusion: When a small quantity of fluid is accumulated in the costodiaphragmatic recess (pleural effusion), the costodiaphragmatic angle is obliterated (widening of the angle) (Fig. 18.7). It is seen as a radiopaque shadow with a fluid line in chest X-ray. This may be the first indication of pleural effusion. Therefore, recesses of pleura are examined routinely in the chest radiographs.

The costodiaphragmatic recess lies opposite to 8th–10th ribs in midaxillary line.

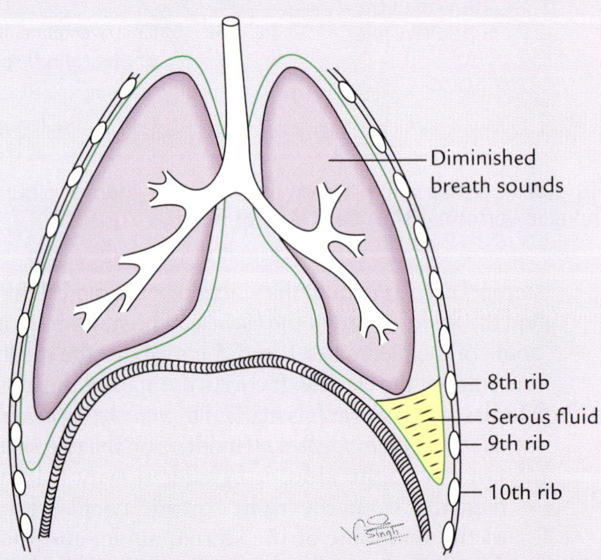

FIG. 18.7 Pleural effusion. Serous fluid in costodiaphragmatic recess.

- **Sites of the extension of the pleura beyond the thoracic cage:** There are five sites where the pleura extends beyond the thoracic cage. These sites are as follows:
  1. On either side in the root of the neck (as domes of the pleura).
  2. In the right xiphicostal/costoxiphoid angle.
  3. On either side in the costovertebral angles.

  The pleura can be punctured inadvertently at these sites during surgical procedures.

NERVE SUPPLY OF THE PLEURA

The **parietal pleura** develops from the somatopleuric layer of the lateral plate of mesoderm; hence, it is supplied by the somatic nerves and is sensitive to pain:

- Costal and peripheral parts of the diaphragmatic pleura are supplied by the *intercostal nerves.*
- Mediastinal and central parts of the diaphragmatic pleura are supplied by the *phrenic nerve.*

The **visceral pleura** develops from the splanchnopleuric layer of the lateral plate of the mesoderm; hence, it is supplied by the autonomic (sympathetic) nerves (T2–T5) and is insensitive to pain.

CLINICAL CORRELATION

Referred pain of the pleura: The pain from the central diaphragmatic pleura and the mediastinal pleura is referred to the neck or the shoulder through phrenic nerves (C3–C5) because the skin at these sites has the same segmental supply through the supraclavicular nerves (C3–C5).

BLOOD SUPPLY AND LYMPHATIC DRAINAGE OF THE PLEURA

Blood supply of the parietal pleura is the same as that of the thoracic wall and the blood supply of the visceral (pulmonary) pleura is the same as that of the lung.

Table 18.1 enumerates the differences between the parietal and visceral pleurae.

TABLE 18.1 Differences between the parietal and visceral pleurae

Parietal pleura	Visceral pleura
Lines the thoracic wall and mediastinum	Covers the surface of the lung
Develops from the somatopleuric mesoderm	Develops from the splanchnopleuric mesoderm
Innervated by the somatic nerves	Innervated by the autonomic nerves
Sensitive to pain	Insensitive to pain
Blood supply and lymphatic drainage are the same as that of the thoracic wall	Blood supply and lymphatic drainage are the same as that of the lung

CLINICAL CORRELATION

- **Pleurisy or pleuritis:** It is the inflammation of the parietal pleura. Clinically it presents as pain, which is aggravated by respiratory movements and radiates to the thoracic and abdominal walls. It is commonly caused by *pulmonary tuberculosis*. The pleural surface becomes rough due to the accumulation of inflammatory exudate. Due to the roughening of the pleural surfaces, friction occurs between the two layers of the pleura during respiratory movements. Thus, *pleural rub* can be heard with a stethoscope on the surface of the chest wall during inspiration and expiration.
- The collection of the serous fluid, air, blood, and pus in the pleural cavity is termed ***hydrothorax*** (pleural effusion), **pneumothorax, haemothorax**, and **pyothorax (empyema)**, respectively.
- **Pleural effusion** (Fig. 18.7)**:** Normally, the pleural cavity contains only 5–10 mL of clear fluid that lubricates the pleural surfaces to allow their smooth movements without friction. The excessive accumulation of fluid in the pleural cavity is called *pleural effusion*. It usually occurs due to the inflammation of the pleura. The pleural effusion leads to the decreased expansion of the lung on the side of effusion. **Clinically it can be detected with decreased breath sounds and dullness on percussion on the site of effusion.**
- **Thoracocentesis/pleural tap:** It is a procedure by which an excess fluid is aspirated from the pleural cavity. It is performed with the patient in sitting position. Usually, **the needle is inserted in the sixth intercostal space in the midaxillary line**. The needle is inserted into the lower part of the intercostal space along the upper border of the rib to avoid injury to the intercostal nerve and vessels. The pleural fluid is located by percussion or real-time ultrasound. **The needle passes in succession through skin, superficial fascia, serratus anterior, intercostal muscles, endothoracic fascia, and parietal pleura to reach the pleural cavity.**
- **Pneumothorax** (Fig. 18.8)**:** Accumulation of air in the pleural cavity is called *pneumothorax*.
  - *Spontaneous pneumothorax*: As the name suggests, under this condition, air enters the pleural cavity

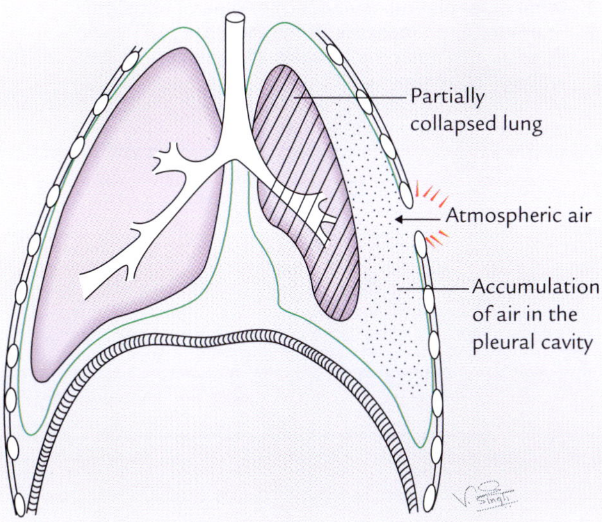

FIG. 18.8 Pneumothorax.

suddenly due to the rupture of emphysematous bullae of the lung.
- *Open pneumothorax*: This condition occurs due to stab wounds on the thoracic wall piercing the pleurae, leading to the communication of air in the pleural cavity with the outside (atmospheric) air. Consequently, each time when the patient inspires, the air is sucked into the pleural cavity. Sometimes the clothing and the layers of the thoracic wall combine to form a valve so that air enters through the wound during inspiration, but cannot exit through it. In these circumstances, air pressure builds up continuously in the pleural cavity on the wounded side, which pushes the mediastinum to the opposite (healthy) side. This is called *tension pneumothorax*. The tension pneumothorax is characterized by (a) the collapse of the lung on the affected side and (b) the compression of the lung on the healthy side.

- **Reffered pain of pleura**
  - The *central part of diaphragmatic pleura and mediastinal pleura* are innervated by phrenic nerves (C4). Hence, irritation of central pleura causes referred pain on to the tip of shoulders, *viz.* pain in left shoulder due to splenic rupture (Kehr's sign) and pain in right shoulder due to cholecystitis.
  - The *peripheral part of diaphragmatic pleura and costal pleura* are innervated by intercostal nerves. Hence, irritation of these regions cause referred pain in thoracic and abdominal walls.

Golden Facts to Remember

• Most dependent part of the pleural cavity	Costodiaphragmatic recess
• Most preferred site for the pleural aspiration	Midaxillary line in the sixth intercostal space
• Nerve providing sensory innervation to the parietal pleura overlying the right dome of the diaphragm	Right phrenic nerve
• Area of superficial cardiac dullness	Area on the front of the chest left to the sternum between the fourth and sixth costal cartilages
• Key structures present in mediastinum	Heart and structures transporting air, blood, and food

CLINICAL CASE STUDY

A 30-year-old female visited the hospital and complained that she had been feeling severe pain on the right side of her chest for the past two weeks and has little difficulty in breathing. She also told that pain often radiated to the anterior abdominal wall. On auscultation, the doctor noticed the absence of breath sounds over the inferior lobe of her right lung. The X-ray of the chest PA view revealed blunting of the right costodiaphragmatic angle and the line of the fluid level. She was diagnosed as a case of **pleural effusion**.

Questions

1. What is (a) pleural cavity and (b) pleural effusion?
2. Enumerate the recesses of the pleura.
3. What is the anatomical basis of radiation of pain to the anterior abdominal wall?
4. Mention the (a) cause of pleural effusion and (b) site where pleural fluid accumulates first.

Answers

1. (a) Potential space between the parietal and visceral layers of the pleura. (b) Accumulation of the serous fluid in the pleural cavity.
2. Right and left costomediastinal recesses and the right and left costodiaphragmatic recesses.
3. The peripheral part of the diaphragmatic pleura and costal pleura are supplied by intercostal nerves. The lower five intercostal nerves also supply the skin and muscle of the anterior abdominal wall. Hence, pain is often referred to the anterior abdominal wall.
4. (a) Inflammation of the pleura (i.e. pleuritis). (b) Costodiaphragmatic recess being the most dependent.

Lungs (Pulmones)

CHAPTER 19

SPECIFIC LEARNING OBJECTIVES

After studying this chapter, the student should be able to:

- Describe the external features of lungs and discuss the relationship of structures, in its hilum. AN 24.2
- Mention the blood supply, lymphatic drainage, and nerve supply of lungs. AN 24.5
- Describe bronchopulmonary segments in detail and discuss their clinical significance. AN 24.3
- Give the brief account of: (a) comparison of the right and left lungs, and (b) relation of mediastinal surfaces of the right and left lungs.
- Write short notes on: (a) carina of trachea, (b) root of lung, and (c) pulmonary ligament.
- Surface marking of lung and pleura. AN 25.9
- Give the anatomical/embryological basis of:
  - (a) Azygos lobe.
  - (b) Hilar shadows of the lung in a radiograph.
  - (c) Metastasis of bronchogenic carcinoma.
  - (d) Segmental resection of the lung.
  - (e) Postural drainage of lung abscess.

The **lungs** or **pulmones** are the principal organs of respiration. The two lungs (right and left) are situated in the thoracic cavity, one on either side of the mediastinum enclosed by the pleural sac. The main function of lungs is to oxygenate the blood, that is the exchange of O_2 and CO_2 between inspired air and blood.

Each lung is large conical/pyramidal shaped with its base resting on the diaphragm and its apex extending into the root of the neck. The right lung is larger and heavier than the left lung. The right lung weighs about 700 g and left lung about 650 g. The right lung has three lobes and the left lung has two lobes. The lobes are separated from each other by deep fissures. They are supplied by lobar bronchi (Fig. 19.1).

The lungs are attached to the trachea and heart by principal bronchi and pulmonary vessels, respectively.

The lungs of newborn babies and those who live in a clean environment are rosy pink in colour, but lungs of those living in polluted areas or those who are smokers are brown or black in colour, with mottled appearance due to inhaled carbon particles.

In the adults, the lungs are spongy in texture and crepitate on touch due to the presence of air in their alveoli. They float in water. In foetus and stillborn children, the lungs are solid and do not crepitate on touch due to the absence of air in their alveoli. They sink in water.

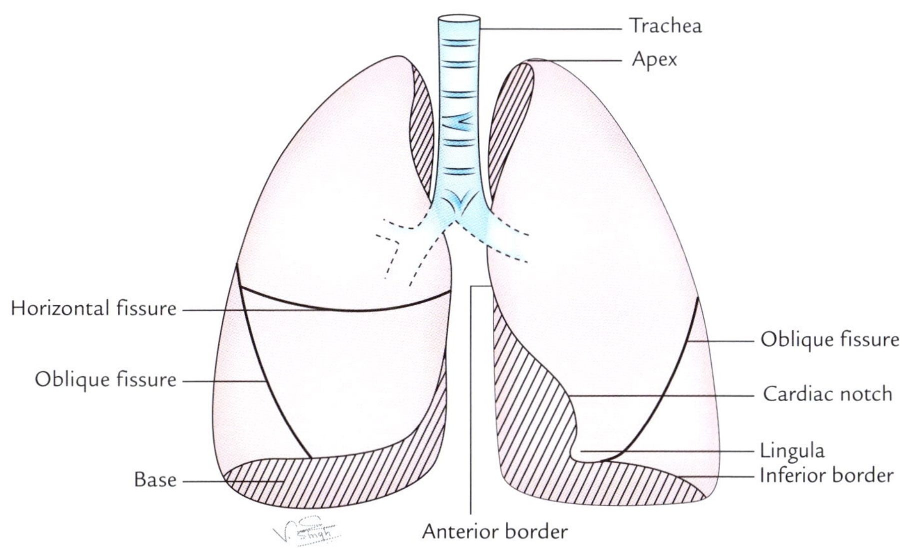

FIG. 19.1 ■ Trachea and lungs as seen from the front.

EXTERNAL FEATURES AN 24.2

Each lung presents the following features (Figs. 19.1 and 19.2):

1. Apex
2. Base
3. Three borders (anterior, posterior, and inferior)
4. Two surfaces (costal and medial)

Anatomical position and side determination

The side of the lung can be determined by holding the lung in such a way that:

(a) its conical end (*apex*) is directed upward and its broader end (*base*) is directed downward,

(b) its convex surface (*costal surface*) is directed outward and its flat medial surface presenting hilum is directed inward,

(c) its thin margin (*anterior margin*) should face forward and its rounded border (*posterior border*) should face backward.

N.B.

The side should not be determined by the number of fissures and lobes as they are variable.

The external features are discussed in detail in the following text.

APEX

The apex is rounded/blunt superior end of the lung. It extends into the root of the neck about 3 cm superior to the anterior end of the first rib and 2.5 cm above the medial one-third of the clavicle. It is covered by the cervical pleura and suprapleural membrane.

Relations

Anterior: (a) Subclavian artery, (b) internal thoracic artery, and (c) scalenus anterior.

Posterior: Neck of the first rib and structures in front of it, for example (a) ventral ramus of the first thoracic nerve, (b) superior intercostal artery, (c) first posterior intercostal vein, and (d) sympathetic chain (stellate ganglion).

N.B.

- All the structures related to the apex are separated from it by the suprapleural membrane.
- The apex is grooved by the subclavian artery on the medial side and on the front.

CLINICAL CORRELATION

Pancoast syndrome: It occurs due to the involvement of structures related to the posterior aspect of the apex of the lung by the cancer of the lung apex.

Clinical features

- Pain along the medial side of the forearm and hand, and wasting of small muscles of the hand due to the involvement of ventral ramus of T1.
- *Horner's syndrome*, due to the involvement of the sympathetic chain.
- Erosion of the first rib.

N.B.

Cancer of lung apex may spread to involve neighbouring structures, such as subclavian or brachiocephalic vein, subclavian artery, phrenic nerve causing the following signs and symptoms:

- Venous engorgement and oedema in the neck, face, and arm due to the involvement of subclavian and brachiocephalic veins.
- Diminished brachial and/or radial pulse due to compression of subclavian artery.
- Paralysis of haemidiaphragm due to the infiltration of the phrenic nerve.

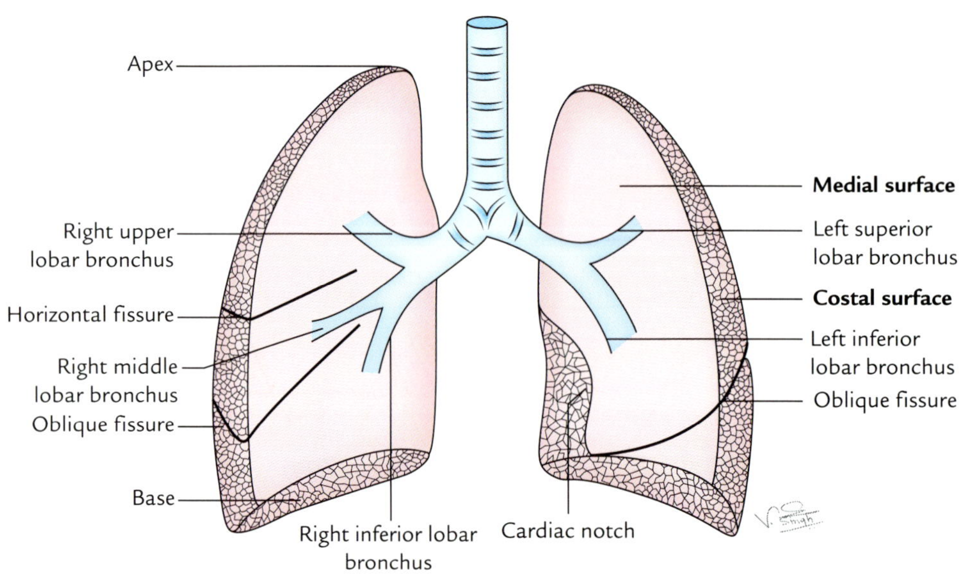

FIG. 19.2 ■ Lobes of the lung with lobar bronchi.

BASE (DIAPHRAGMATIC SURFACE)

The base is a lower semilunar concave surface that rests on the dome of the diaphragm; hence, it is also sometimes called the *diaphragmatic surface*.

Relations

On the right side, the lung is separated from the liver by the right dome of the diaphragm, and on the left side, the left lung is separated from the spleen and fundus of stomach by the left dome of the diaphragm.

N.B.

The base of the right lung is deeper (i.e. more concave) because the right dome of the diaphragm rises to the more superior level due to the presence of the liver underneath it.

BORDERS

The borders of the lungs are as follows:

1. **Anterior border:** It is thin and shorter than the posterior border. The anterior border of the right lung is vertical. The anterior border of the left lung presents a wide **cardiac notch**, which is occupied by the heart and pericardium. In this region, the heart and pericardium are uncovered by the lung. Hence, this region is responsible for an **area of superficial cardiac dullness**. Below the cardiac notch, it presents a tongue-shaped projection called **lingula**.
2. **Posterior border:** It is thick and rounded. It extends from the spine of the C7 vertebra to the spine of the T10 vertebra.
3. **Inferior border:** It is semilunar in shape and separates the base (also called diaphragmatic surface) from the costal and medial surfaces.

SURFACES

The surfaces of the lungs are diaphragmatic (base), costal and medial.

Diaphragmatic Surface

Described above.

Costal Surface

It is large, smooth, and convex. It is covered by the visceral pleura. It is in contact with costal pleura.

Relations

It is related to the lateral thoracic wall. (In an embalmed and hardened lung, the costal surface presents impressions of the ribs.)

The number of ribs related to this surface is as follows:

- Upper six ribs in the midclavicular line.
- Upper eight ribs in the midaxillary line.
- Upper ten ribs in the scapular line.

Medial Surface

It is divided into two parts: (a) small posterior **vertebral part** and (b) large anterior **mediastinal part**.

Relations

The **vertebral part** is related to the vertebral column, posterior intercostal vessels, and greater and lesser splanchnic nerves.

The **mediastinal part** presents a hilum, and it is related to mediastinal structures such as heart, great blood vessels, and nerves. Since the right and left surfaces of the mediastinum consists of different structures. The relations of the mediastinal surface of the two lungs differ because structures forming the right and left surfaces of the mediastinum differ. To understand the relations of the mediastinal surfaces of the lungs, the students are advised to know the structures forming the right and left surfaces of the mediastinum.

Structures forming the right surface of the mediastinum (Fig. 19.3A):

1. The right mediastinal surface is mainly consists of the right atrium.
2. Above the right atrium are present the superior vena cava and right brachiocephalic vein.
3. Behind these structures are present the trachea and oesophagus.
4. The azygos vein, a large venous channel, runs upward along the side of the vertebral column and arches over the root of the right lung to terminate into the superior vena cava.
5. Three neural structures, namely (a) right phrenic nerve, (b) right vagus nerve, and (c) right sympathetic chain.
   - The **phrenic nerve** runs to the diaphragm passing superficial to three venous structures from above downward: (i) superior vena cava, (ii) right atrium, and (iii) inferior vena cava. This course is in front of the root of the lung.
   - The **vagus nerve** lies against the right side of the trachea and travels behind the lung root. Here it breaks up into branches to take part in the formation of the posterior pulmonary plexus and oesophageal plexus.
   - The **sympathetic trunk** runs in the paravertebral gutter. The splanchnic nerves leave its lower half, run medially, and pierce the crura of the diaphragm to reach the abdomen.

Structures forming the left surface of the mediastinum (Fig. 19.3B):

1. The left ventricle and aorta are the main structures forming the left surface of the mediastinum.
2. Aorta ascends at first, arches over the left lung root, and then descends behind the lung root.
3. Three greet vessels (brachiocephalic trunk, left common carotid artery, and left subclavian artery) arise from the aortic arch and ascend up to reach the root of the neck.
4. The oesophagus as it descends through the thorax shifts to the left behind the heart and gently crosses the line of the descending aorta.
5. Three neural structures, namely (a) left phrenic nerve, (b) left vagus nerve, and (c) left sympathetic chain.
   - The **left phrenic nerve** crosses the aortic (left) side, passes in front of the lung root, and runs down superficial to the left ventricle to reach the diaphragm.
   - The **left vagus nerve** is held away from the trachea by the aortic arch. Here it gives the recurrent

TABLE 19.1 Relations of the mediastinal surfaces of the right and left lungs

Mediastinal surface of the right lung	Mediastinal surface of the left lung
Right atrium	Left ventricle
Superior and inferior vena cavae	—
Arch of azygos vein	Arch of aorta and descending thoracic aorta
Right brachiocephalic vein	Left subclavian and left common carotid arteries
Oesophagus and trachea	Oesophagus and thoracic duct
Three neural structures • Right phrenic nerve • Right vagus nerve • Right sympathetic chain	Four neural structures • Left phrenic nerve • Left vagus nerve • Left recurrent laryngeal nerve • Left sympathetic chain

laryngeal branch, which hooks under the aortic arch, ascends up into the tracheoesophageal groove. Below the aortic arch, the vagus nerve runs behind the lung root and breaks up into posterior pulmonary and oesophageal branches.
- The position of the **sympathetic trunk** and **splanchnic nerves** is similar to those of the right side.

The relations of the mediastinal surfaces of the right and left lungs are given in Table 19.1 and shown in Figs. 19.3 and 19.4.

The impressions produced by mediastinal structures on the medial surfaces of lungs are shown in Figs. 19.5 and 19.6.

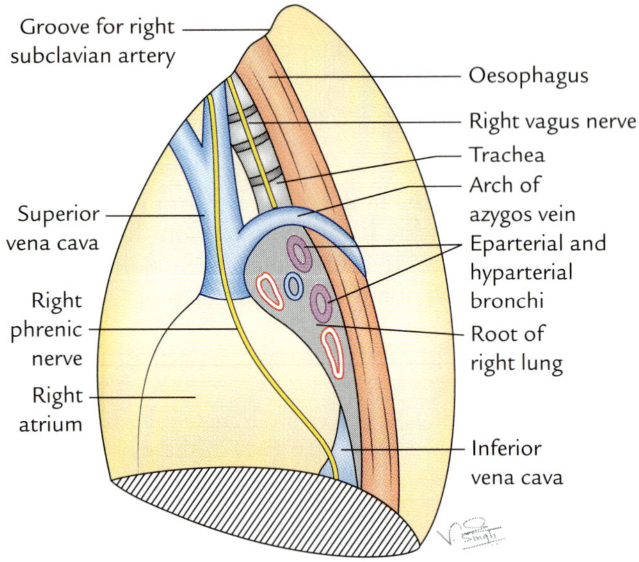

FIG. 19.3 Structures related to the mediastinal surface of the right lung and producing impressions on this surface.

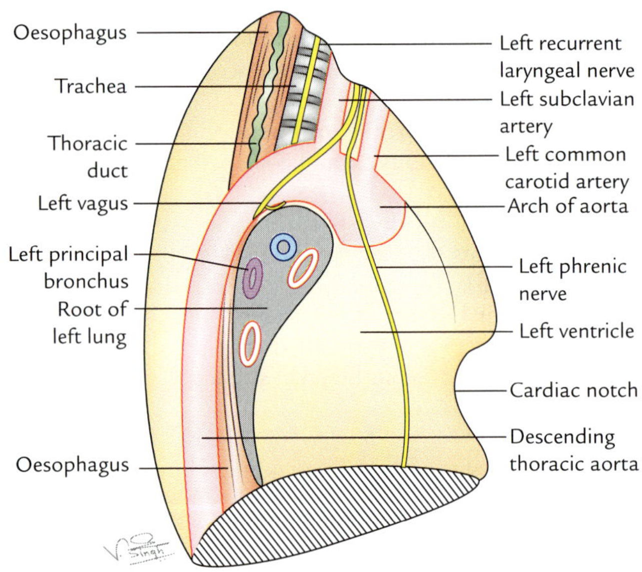

FIG. 19.4 Structures related to the mediastinal surface of the left lung and producing impression on this surface.

LOBES AND FISSURES

The **right lung is divided into three lobes**: superior, middle, and inferior by two fissures—(a) an oblique fissure and (b) a horizontal fissure (Figs. 19.1 and 19.2).

The **left lung is divided into two lobes**: (a) superior and (b) inferior by an oblique fissure.

1. **Oblique fissure:** A long oblique fissure runs obliquely downward and forward crossing the posterior border about 6 cm (2 in) below the apex and the inferior border about 7.5 cm (3 in) lateral to the midline. It separates the superior and middle lobes from the inferior lobe.
2. **Horizontal fissure:** A short horizontal fissure is present only in the right lung. It starts from the oblique fissure at the midaxillary line and runs horizontally forward to the anterior border of the lung. It separates the superior and middle lobes.

The **oblique fissure** in the left lung runs obliquely downward and forward crossing the posterior border about 6 cm below the apex and the inferior border almost at its apex. It separates the superior lobe from the inferior lobe.

N.B.

- The *oblique fissure* acts as a plane of cleavage so that during inspiration, the upper part of the lung expands forward and laterally, whereas the lower part of the lung expands downward and backward.
- In X-ray chest posteroanterior (PA) view, the horizontal fissure is visible in 60% of the cases. The oblique fissure is usually visible in the X-ray chest lateral view.
- Oblique fissure of the left lung is more vertical than that of the right lung.

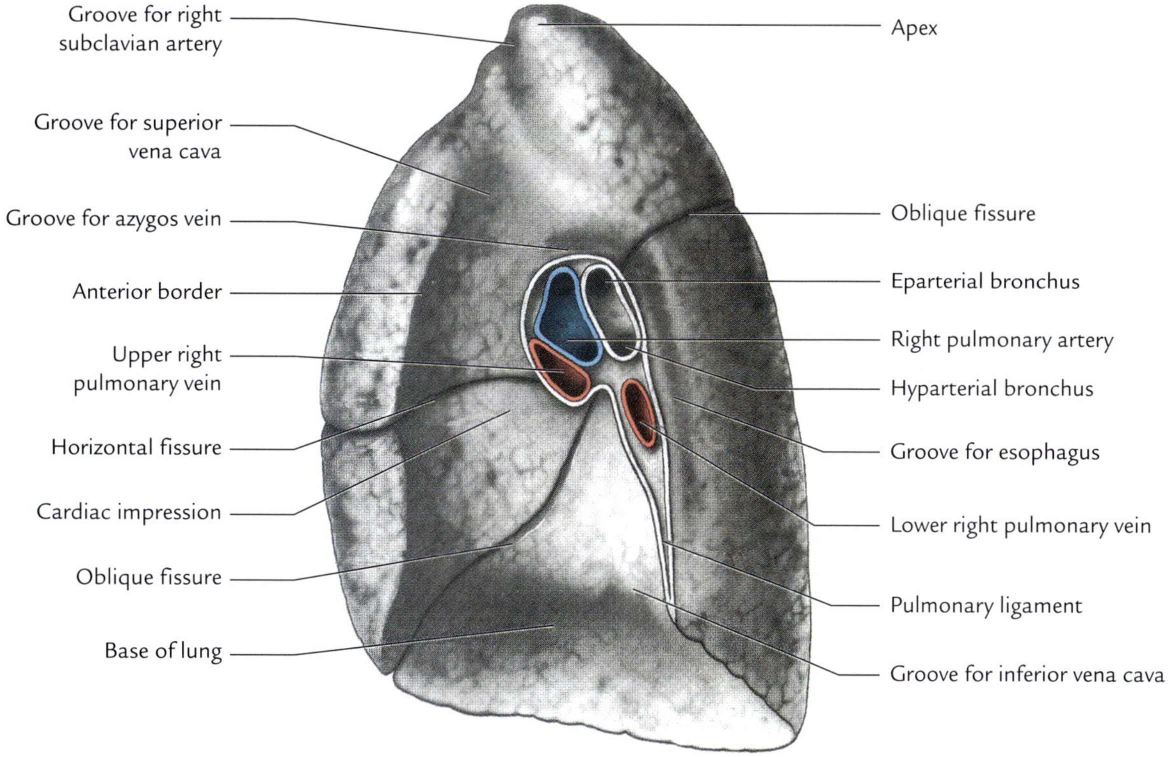

FIG. 19.5 ■ The impressions produced by mediastinal structures on the medial surface of the right lung (*Source*: *Gray's Anatomy: The Anatomical Basis of Clinical Practice*, 39th ed.: Susan Standring (Editor-in-Chief). Fig. 63.6, Page 1066, Elsevier Ltd. 2005.)

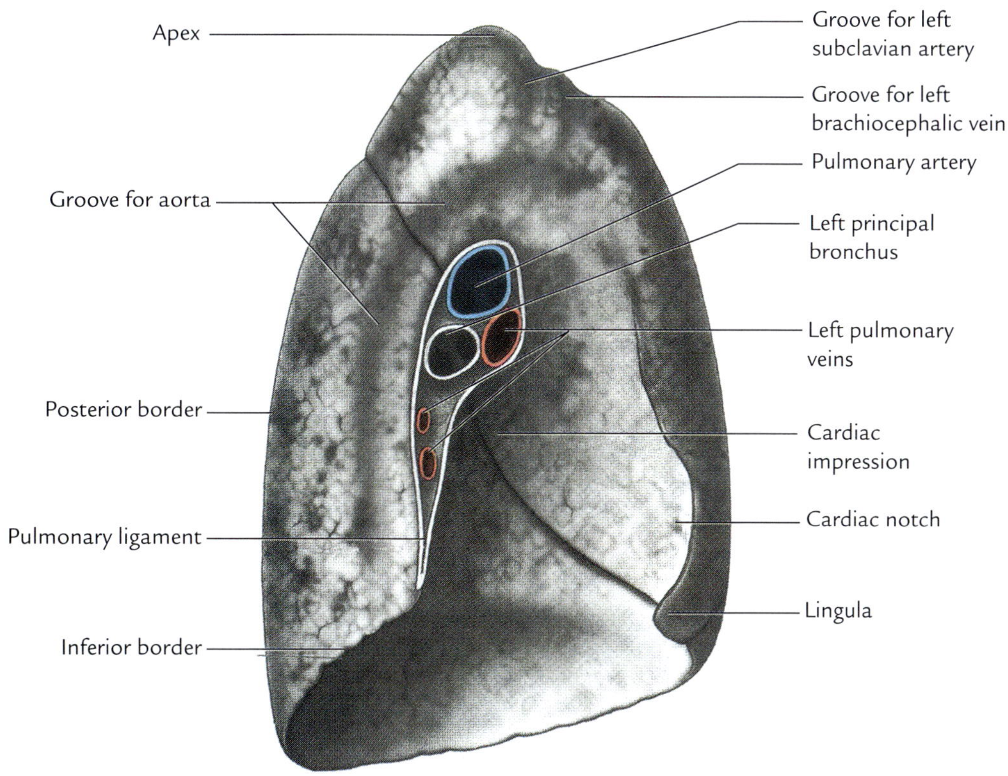

FIG. 19.6 ■ The impressions produced by mediastinal structures on the medial surface of the left lung (*Source*: *Gray's Anatomy: The Anatomical Basis of Clinical Practice*, 39th ed.: Susan Standring (Editor-in-Chief), Fig. 63.7, Page 1067, Elsevier Ltd. 2005.)

CLINICAL CORRELATION

- **Identification of the completeness of the fissure:** It is important before performing lobectomy (i.e. the removal of the lobe of the lung because individuals with incomplete fissures are more prone to develop postoperative air leakage than those with complete fissures).
- **Accessory lobes and fissures**
  - ***Lobe of the azygos vein*** (Fig. 19.7): Sometimes the medial part of the superior lobe is partially separated by a fissure of variable length, which contains the terminal part of the azygos vein, enclosed in the free margin of a mesentery derived from the mediastinal pleura. This is termed the *lobe of azygos vein*. It varies in size and sometimes includes the apex of the lung.
  - A left horizontal fissure is a normal variant found in 10% of the individuals.

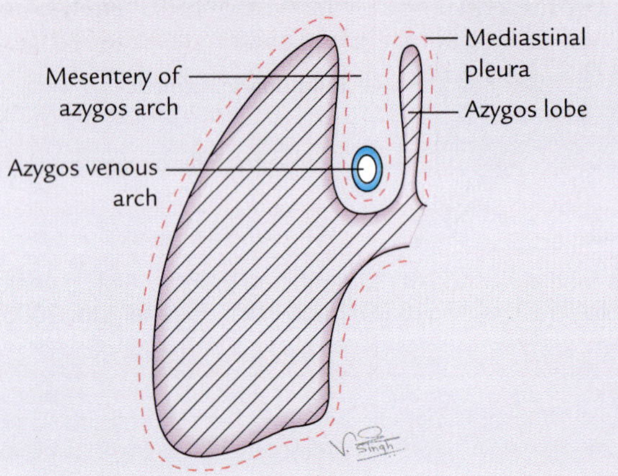

FIG. 19.7 Formation of the azygos lobe of the lung.

ROOT OF THE LUNG AN 24.2

EXTERNAL FEATURES

The root of the lung is a short broad pedicle connecting the medial surface of the lung with the mediastinum. It consists of structures entering and leaving the lung at the hilum.

The **hilum** is the area on the mediastinal surface of the lung through which structures enter or leave the lung.

The root of the lung is surrounded by a tubular sheath derived from the mediastinal pleura.

COMPONENTS

The root of the lung consists of the following structures:

1. Principal bronchus in the left lung, and eparterial and hyparterial bronchi in the right lung
2. Pulmonary artery
3. Pulmonary veins (two in number)
4. Bronchial arteries (one on the right side and two on the left side)
5. Bronchial veins
6. Lymphatics of the lung
7. Anterior and posterior pulmonary plexuses of the nerves

N.B.

The root of the lung lies opposite to the bodies of the T5, T6, and T7 vertebrae.

RELATIONSHIP OF STRUCTURES IN THE ROOT OF THE LUNG AT THE HILUM

The roots of the right and left lungs are similar but not identical.

The arrangement of structures in the roots of the lungs is as follows (Fig. 19.8):

1. **From before backward** (it is more or less similar on two sides):
   (a) Pulmonary vein (superior pulmonary vein)
   (b) Pulmonary artery
   (c) Bronchus (left principal bronchus on the left side, whereas eparterial and hyparterial bronchi on the right side).
   Mnemonic: **VAB** (**V**ein, **A**rtery, and **B**ronchus).
2. **From above downward**, it differs on two sides as follows:

Right side	Left side
(a) Eparterial **b**ronchus	(a) Pulmonary **a**rtery
(b) Pulmonary **a**rtery	(b) Left principal **b**ronchus
(c) Hyparterial **b**ronchus	(c) Inferior pulmonary **v**ein
(d) Inferior pulmonary **v**ein	

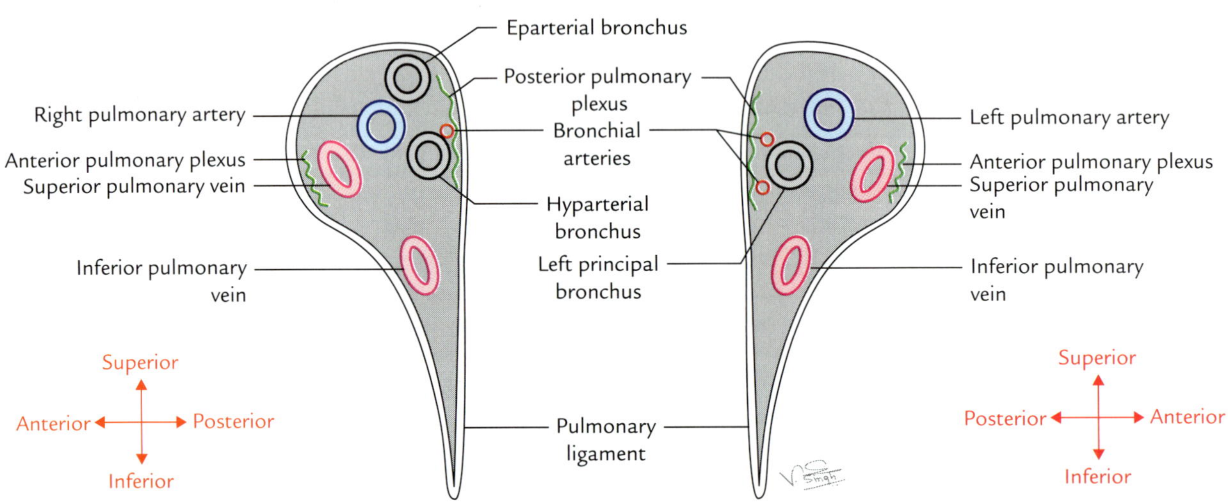

FIG. 19.8 Arrangement of structures in the roots of the right and left lungs seen in a section.

N.B.

The difference in the arrangement of structures from above downward on the two sides is because right principal bronchus before entering the lung at hilum divides into two lobar bronchi, the upper lobar bronchus passes above the pulmonary artery (**eparterial bronchus**) and lower lobar bronchus passes below the pulmonary artery (**hyparterial bronchus**).

RELATIONS OF THE ROOT OF THE LUNG

Anterior:
- Phrenic nerve
- Anterior pulmonary plexus
- Superior vena cava (on the right side only)

Posterior:
- Vagus nerve
- Posterior pulmonary plexus
- Descending thoracic aorta (on the left side only)

Superior:
- Arch of the azygos vein (on the right side only)
- Arch of the aorta (on the left side only).

Inferior:
- Pulmonary ligament.

CLINICAL CORRELATION

Hilar shadow in chest radiograph: In the X-ray chest PA view, the root of each lung casts a radiopaque shadow called the **hilar shadow** in the middle of medial one-third of the lung field. The shadow, in fact, is *cast by pulmonary vessels when seen end on*. The enlargements of bronchopulmonary lymph nodes (hilar lymph nodes) increase the density of the hilar shadows.

The differences between the right and left lungs are given in Table 19.2.

SURFACE MARKINGS OF LUNGS

1. **Apex:** It coincides with the cervical part of the parietal pleura/cervical pleura (for details, see page 234).
2. **Margins:** The lung margins approximately coincide with those of the costal pleura (see page 233), except at the following points (Fig. 19.9):
   (a) ***Anterior border:*** The anterior border of the left lung has a distinct notch (the cardiac notch), which passes laterally behind the fourth and fifth intercostal spaces.

TABLE 19.2 **Differences between the right and left lungs**

	Right lung	Left lung
Size and shape	Larger, shorter, and broader	Smaller, longer, and narrower
Weight	700 g	650 g
Lobes	Three (upper, middle, and lower)	Two lobes (upper and lower)
Fissure	Two (horizontal and oblique)	One (oblique)
Anterior border	Straight	Presents a cardiac notch
Hilum	Two bronchi (eparterial and hyparterial)	One bronchus (left principal bronchus)

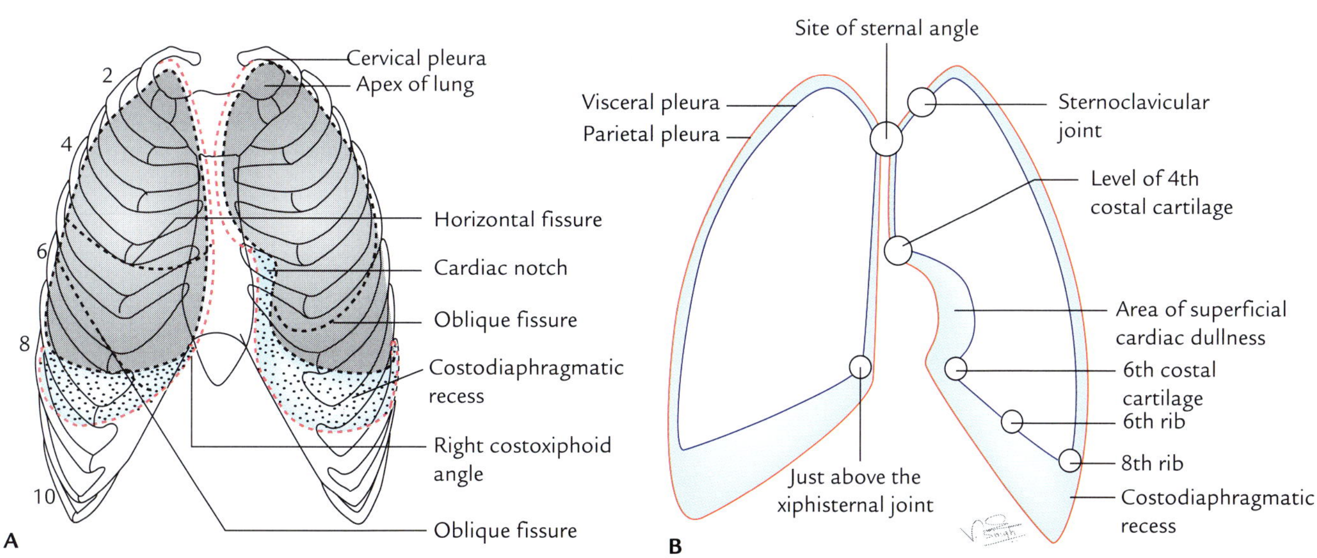

FIG. 19.9 ■ Surface markings of the lung and pleura on the front. (**A**) The relationship of the lung and pleurae in the thoracic cage and (**B**) outlines of the lung and pleura. Note that the outline of the lung is shown by the blue line and that of the pleura by the red line.

(b) ***Lower border:*** The lower border of each lung is two-rib spaces higher than the lower border of the costal pleura. Thus, it lies along the line, which cuts
  (i) sixth rib in the midclavicular line,
  (ii) eighth rib in the midaxillary line, and
  (iii) tenth rib at the lateral border of erector spinae and ends 2 cm lateral to the spine of the T10 vertebra.

(c) ***Posterior border:*** Its lower end ends at the level of spine of the T10 vertebra.

3. **Fissures**
  (a) The ***oblique fissure*** is marked by a line drawn obliquely downward and outward from 1 in (2.5 cm) lateral to the T5 spine to the sixth costal cartilage about 1½ in (4 cm) from the midline.
  In clinical practice, ask the patients to abduct the shoulder to its full extent; the line of the oblique fissure in this position corresponds to the medial border of the rotated scapula.
  (b) The ***transverse fissure*** is marked by a line drawn horizontally along the fourth costal cartilage and meets the oblique fissure where the latter crosses the fifth rib.

CLINICAL CORRELATION

Auscultation of lungs: Visual perception of lungs from the surface for listening lung sounds (Fig. 19.10). During auscultation of lung sounds, it is of utmost importance for the clinicians to visualize the lungs from the surface of chest wall as follows:

- ***Anteriorly:*** The right side of the chest primarily presents the upper and middle lobes separated by the horizontal fissure at about the fifth rib in the midaxillary line to the fourth rib at the sternum. The left side of the chest primarily presents the upper lobe, which is separated from the lower lobe by oblique fissure, extending from the fifth rib in the midaxillary line to the sixth rib at the midclavicular line.
- ***Posteriorly:*** Except for apices, the posterior aspect of chest on either side primarily presents the lower lobe, extending from the spinous process of the T3–T10 vertebrae.
- ***Right lateral:*** The lung lies deep to the area extending from the axilla to the level of the seventh or eighth rib. The upper lobe is demarcated at the level of the fifth rib in the midaxillary line and the sixth rib in the midclavicular line.
- ***Left lateral:*** The lung lies deep to the area extending from the axilla to the seventh or eighth rib. The upper lobe is demarcated at the level of the fifth rib in the midaxillary line and the sixth rib in the midclavicular line.

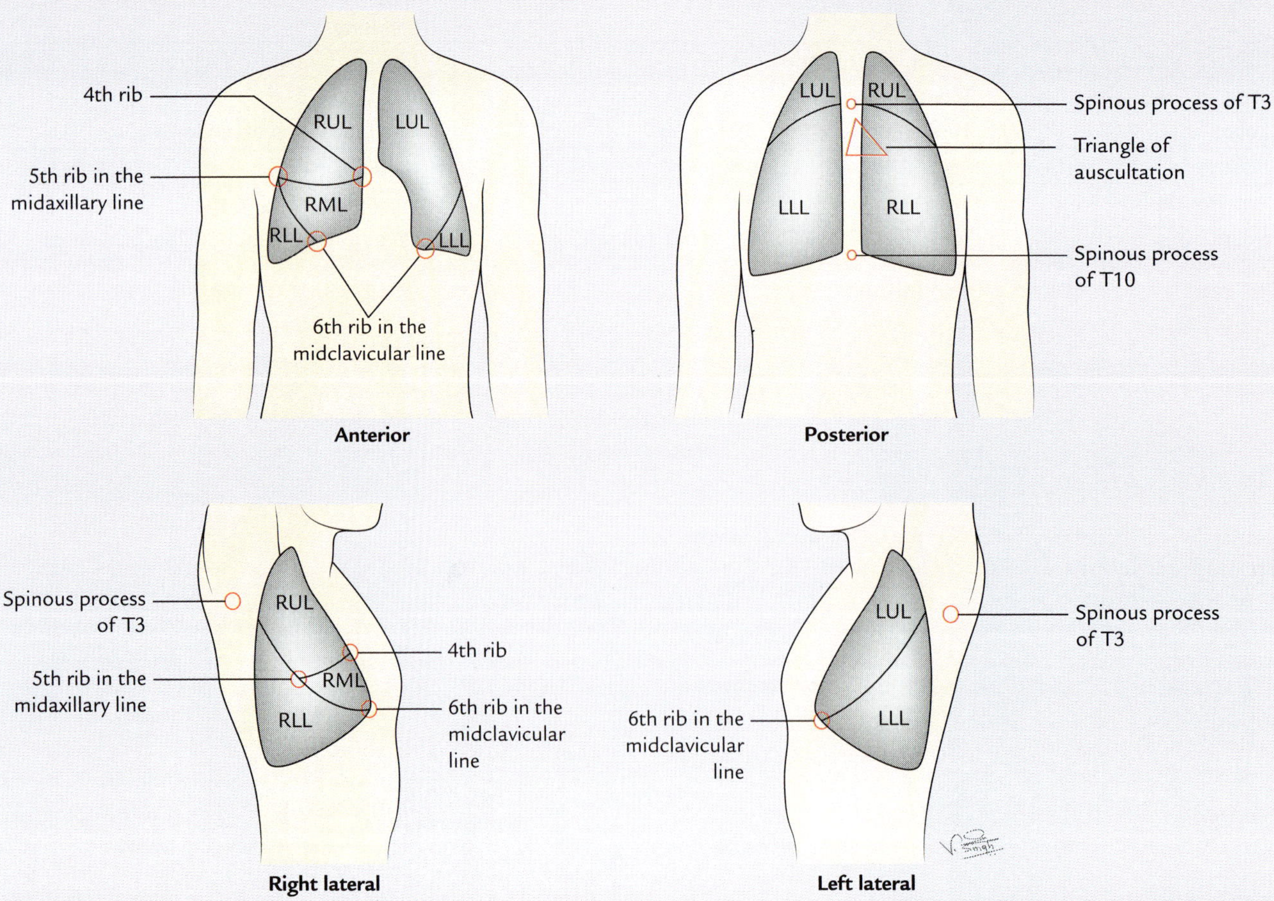

FIG. 19.10 ■ Surface projection of different lobes of lungs (RUL = right upper lobe, LUL = left upper lobe, RML = right middle lobe, RLL = right lower lobe, LLL = left lower lobe).

N.B.

Key points to remember during the auscultation of lungs:

- The superior lobe of the right lung is audible above the fourth rib.
- The middle lobe of the right lung is audible between the fourth and the sixth ribs anteriorly.
- The lower lobes of both lungs are audible below the sixth rib on the front.
- The inferior lobes of the right and left lungs are best examined on the back, especially in the region of the triangle of auscultation.

INTERNAL STRUCTURE OF LUNG

The lung is mainly made up of the **intrapulmonary bronchial tree**, which is concerned with the conduction of air to and fro from the lung, and **pulmonary units**, which are concerned with the gaseous exchange within the lung (for the detailed structure, see textbooks on Histology).

BRONCHIAL TREE AN 24.2

The bronchial tree (also called respiratory tree) consists of the bronchi (*primary*, *secondary* and *tertiary*) and **bronchioles** (**terminal** and **respiratory**).

The primary, secondary and tertiary bronchi are also called the *principal*, *lobar*, and *segmental bronchi*, respectively (Fig. 19.11).

Functions of bronchial tree

- To provide a passageway for air to move into and out of each lung.
- To trap debris and pathogens by its mucous lining.
- To send atmospheric air into pulmonary units for exchange of gases to take place.

The *respiratory bronchioles* aerate pulmonary units.

The various components of *bronchial tree* and *pulmonary unit* are described in the following text.

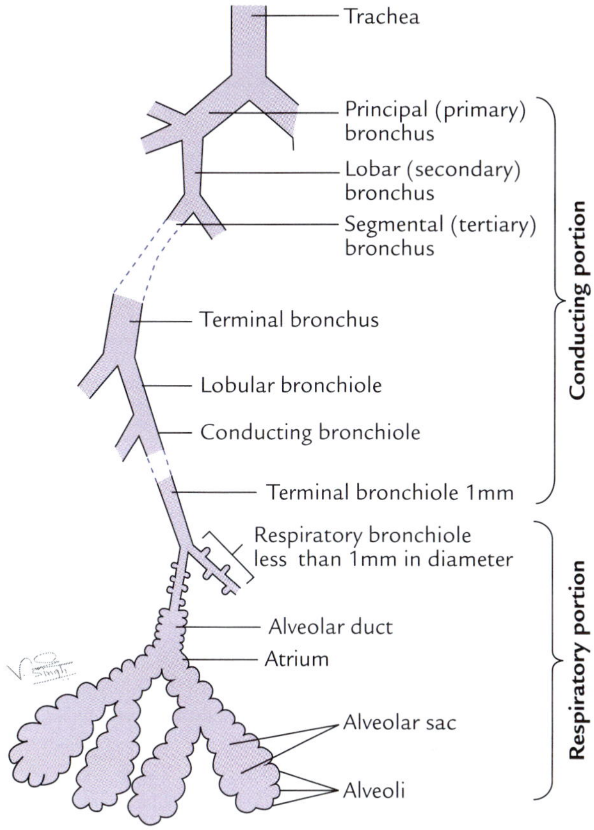

FIG. 19.11 Bronchial tree.

Principal Bronchi

The trachea divides outside the lungs, at the level of the lower border of the T4 vertebra, into two primary (principal) bronchi-right and left for the right lung and left lung, respectively (Figs. 19.12 and 19.13):

As seen in bronchoscopy, lower end of trachea divides at *carina* (a keel-like ridge) into right and left principal bronchi (Fig. 19.14).

1. **Right principal bronchus** is shorter, wider, and more vertical. It is about 1 in (2.5 cm) long and lies more or less in line with the trachea.
2. **Left principal bronchus** is narrower, longer, and more horizontal than the right. It is about 2 in (5 cm) long and does not lie in line with the trachea.

The long axis of the right principal bronchus deviates about 25° from the long axis of the trachea, whereas the long axis of the left principal deviates about 45° from the long axis of the trachea.

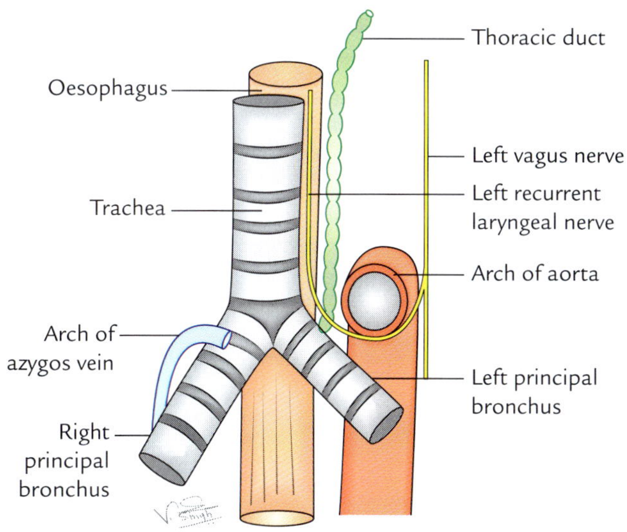

FIG. 19.12 Relation of the principal bronchi.

The left principal bronchus passes to the left below the arch of the aorta and in front of the oesophagus.

The differences between the right and left principal bronchi are summarized in Table 19.3.

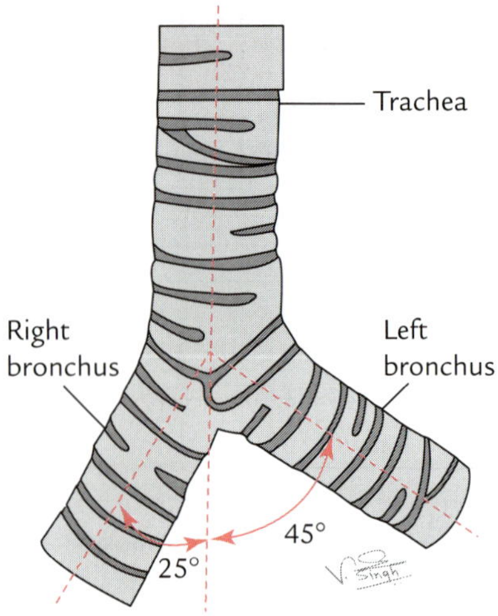

FIG. 19.13 ■ Trachea and principal bronchi.

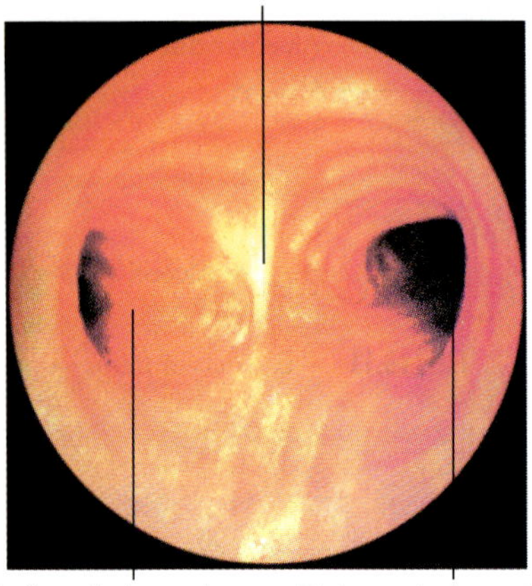

FIG. 19.14 ■ Lower end of the trachea and its main branches as seen on bronchoscopy. (*Source: Gray's Anatomy for Students*: Richard L. Drake, Wayne Vogl, Adam W.M. Mitchell., Fig. 3.48A, Page 151, Elsevier Inc. 2005.)

TABLE 19.3 Differences between right and left principal bronchi

Right principal bronchus	Left principal bronchus
• Shorter and wider (2.5 cm long)	• Longer and narrower (5 cm long)
• More vertical	• More horizontal
• Lies more or less in line with the tracheal lumen	• Does not lie in line with the tracheal lumen
• Forms an angle of 25° with the midline of trachea	• Forms an angle of 45° with the midline of trachea

CLINICAL CORRELATION

- **Aspiration of the foreign body into the right principal bronchus:** The inhaled foreign bodies usually enter in the right principal bronchus because it is shorter, wider, and in line with the trachea. Since the inhaled foreign particles tend to enter in the right principal bronchus, hence in the right lung. As a result, lung abscess occurs more commonly in the right lung.
- **Bronchoscopy (Fig. 19.14):** It is a procedure, in which a flexible, fibre-optic bronchoscope is introduced in the trachea to visualize the interior of the trachea and bronchi. The **carina**, a keel-like median ridge at the bifurcation of the trachea into two principal bronchi is an important landmark visible through the bronchoscope. The widening and distortion of the angle between the principal bronchi (distorting the position of carina) seen in bronchoscopy is a serious prognostic sign, since it usually indicates the carcinomatous involvement of tracheobronchial lymph nodes. The carina of the trachea is also a very sensitive area for cough reflex.
- **Bronchogenic carcinoma:** It is the commonest cancer in the males, especially in chronic cigarette smokers. It usually arises from epithelial lining of the bronchi and forms well-circumscribed gray white mass in the lung. The presence of the circular shadow (popularly called *coin shadow*) in plain X-ray chest (PA view) may be the only finding in an otherwise asymptomatic patient.
- **Metastasis:** The bronchogenic carcinoma may spread (metastasis) to brain by both arterial and venous routes as follows:
  - ***Arterial route***
    Lung capillaries → pulmonary vein → left atrium → left ventricle → aorta → internal carotid and vertebral arteries → brain
  - ***Venous route***
    Bronchial veins → azygos vein → external vertebral venous plexus → internal vertebral venous plexus → cranial dural venous sinuses → brain.

LOBAR BRONCHI

The **right principal bronchus** gives rise to its first branch–*superior lobar bronchus* before it enters the lung. Then enters the right lung through its hilum and divides into *middle and inferior lobar bronchi*, one for each **middle** and **inferior** lobes of the right lung. The **left principal bronchus** on entering the lung divides into two lobar bronchi **superior** and **inferior** one for each lobe of the left lung.

TERTIARY (SEGMENTAL) BRONCHI

Each lobar bronchus divides into segmental (tertiary) bronchi, one for each bronchopulmonary segment (Fig. 19.19).

(a) **On the right side:** These are:
- ***Superior lobar bronchus*** gives rise to three bronchopulmonary segments: **A**pical, **P**osterior, and **A**nterior.
  Mnemonic: **A P**ublic **A**pathy.
- ***Middle lobar bronchus*** gives rise to **M**edial and **L**ateral bronchopulmonary segments (easy to remember: **M**iddle **L**obe: **M**edial and **L**ateral).
- ***Inferior lobar bronchus*** gives to **S**uperior, **M**edial basal, **A**nterior basal, **L**ateral basal, and **P**osterior basal.
  Mnemonic: **S**eed **M**akes **A**nother **L**ittle **P**lant.

(b) **On the left side:** These are:
- ***Superior lobar bronchus*** gives rise to five bronchopulmonary segments: **A**pical, **P**osterior and **A**nterior, **S**uperior lingular and **I**nferior lingular.

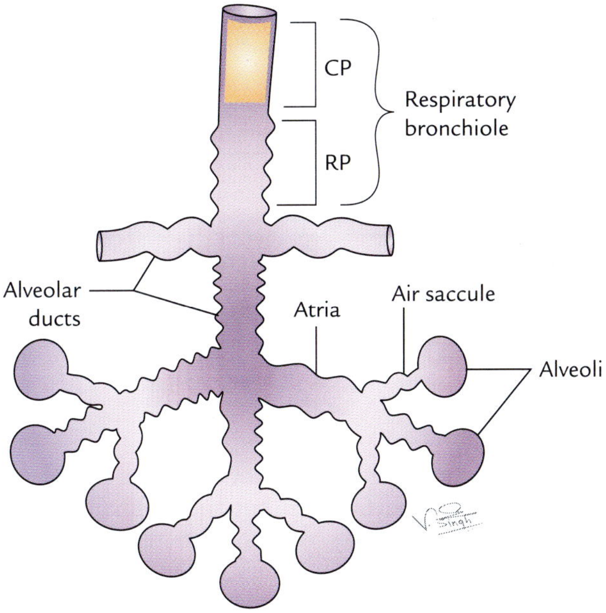

FIG. 19.15 Pulmonary unit (CP = conducting portion of respiratory bronchiole, RP = respiratory portion of respiratory bronchiole).

Mnemonic: **A** **P**ublic **A**pathy **S**een **I**n political leaders after elections.

- **Inferior lobar bronchus** gives rise to five bronchopulmonary segments, *viz.* **S**uperior, **M**edial basal, **A**nterior basal, **L**ateral basal, and **P**osterior basal.

These can be remembered in a way similar to right lobe.

The segmental bronchi divide repeatedly to form very small bronchi called **terminal bronchioles** (about 1 mm in diameter). The terminal bronchioles give off ***respiratory bronchioles*** (less than 1 mm in diameter), which lack cartilage in their walls, hence mainly made up of smooth muscle.

Each **respiratory bronchiole** aerates a small portion of the lung called **pulmonary units**, which is concerned with **gaseous exchange** within the lung.

PULMONARY UNITS

Each pulmonary unit consists of (Fig. 19.15):

(a) **alveolar ducts**
(b) **atria**
(c) **air saccules, and**
(d) **alveoli**

N.B.

- **The respiratory bronchiole represents the transitional zone/part between the conducting and respiratory portions of the respiratory system.**
- **The alveoli are specialized sac-like structures** that form greater part of the lungs. They are the main sites for the gaseous exchange of oxygen and carbon dioxide between the inspired air and blood.

CLINICAL CORRELATION

Emphysema: Under this condition, alveoli of lungs are damaged by chemicals released by pollutants. Clinically, it presents as the shortness of breath and the chest appears barrel shaped in the chest radiograph.

ARTERIAL SUPPLY OF THE LUNGS AN 24.5

The lungs have dual blood supply, that is they are supplied by two sets of arteries, namely,

1. Bronchial arteries
2. Pulmonary arteries

This dual blood supply to lungs is functionally different.

BRONCHIAL ARTERIES

The bronchial arteries supply **oxygenated blood and nutrition to the bronchial tree associated pulmonary tissue and visceral pleura.**

The right lung is supplied by one bronchial artery, which arises from the right third posterior intercostal artery or from the upper-left bronchial artery.

The left lung is supplied by two bronchial arteries, which arise from the descending thoracic aorta.

PULMONARY ARTERIES

The pulmonary arteries supply **deoxygenated blood to the lungs for oxygenation**. Once the blood is oxygenated, it brought back to heart by four pulmonary veins. There is one pulmonary artery for each lung. They are the branches of the pulmonary trunk.

The right and left pulmonary arteries lie anterior to the principal (primary) bronchi as they enter the hilum of their respective lungs. The right pulmonary artery is crossed superiorly by the arch of the azygos vein, whereas the left pulmonary artery lies inferior to the arch of the aorta, at the level of the T5 vertebra. The pulmonary arteries divide into lobar branches in the hilum and subsequently divide into the terminal/segmental branches. The segmental branches branch successively corresponding with the segmental branches of the bronchial tree (Fig. 19.16).

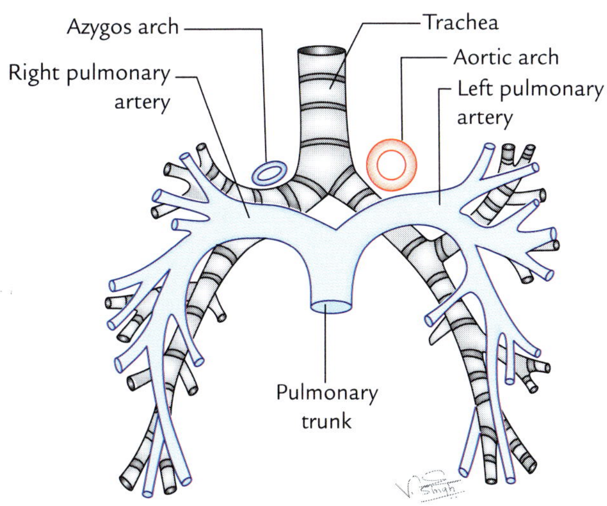

FIG. 19.16 Relationship of the pulmonary arteries to bronchi.

VENOUS DRAINAGE OF LUNGS

The venous blood from lungs is also drained by two sets of veins, namely,

1. Bronchial veins
2. Pulmonary veins

Bronchial veins: The bronchial veins drain the deoxygenated blood from the bronchial tree and pulmonary tissue. There are two bronchial veins on each side:

- The right bronchial veins drain into the azygos veins.
- The left bronchial veins drain into the hemiazygos vein or the left superior intercostal vein.

Pulmonary veins: The pulmonary veins drain the oxygenated blood from the lungs. There are four pulmonary veins, two on each side.

The pulmonary veins do not accompany the pulmonary arteries. The tributaries of the pulmonary veins are intersegmental, while branches of the pulmonary arteries are segmental in distribution.

CLINICAL CORRELATION

If pulmonary veins are obstructed, the oxygenated blood from lungs is drained by *bronchial veins.*

N.B.

- All the veins in the body drain deoxygenated blood except pulmonary veins, which drain the oxygenated blood from the lungs.
- All the arteries of the body supply oxygenated blood except pulmonary arteries, which supply deoxygenated blood to the lungs.
- The bronchial arteries provide nutrition to the bronchial tree, as far as the respiratory bronchioles, that is nonrespiratory portions of the lungs.
- The respiratory portions of the lungs are nourished by pulmonary capillary beds and atmospheric air in the alveoli.

LYMPHATIC DRAINAGE AN 24.5

The lymphatic drainage of the lung is clinically important because lung cancer spreads by the lymphatic path.

The lymph from the lung is drained by two sets of lymph vessels (Fig. 19.17):

1. Superficial vessels
2. Deep vessels

Superficial lymph vessels: These vessels drain the peripheral lung tissue lying beneath the visceral pleura. They form the **superficial (subpleural) plexus** beneath the visceral pleura. The vessels from the plexus pass around the borders and margins of the fissures of the lung to reach the hilum where they drain into the **bronchopulmonary (hilar) lymph nodes**.

Deep lymph vessels: These vessels drain the bronchial tree, pulmonary vessels, and connective tissue septa and form the **deep plexus**. The vessels from the deep plexus run along the bronchi and pulmonary vessels toward the hilum of the lung passing through **pulmonary lymph nodes** located within the lung substance, and finally drain into **bronchopulmonary (hilar) lymph nodes**.

Thus, both superficial and deep lymphatic plexuses drain into bronchopulmonary (hilar) lymph nodes. From hilar lymph nodes, the lymph is drained into the superior and inferior ***tracheobronchial lymph nodes*** located superior and inferior to the bifurcation of the trachea,

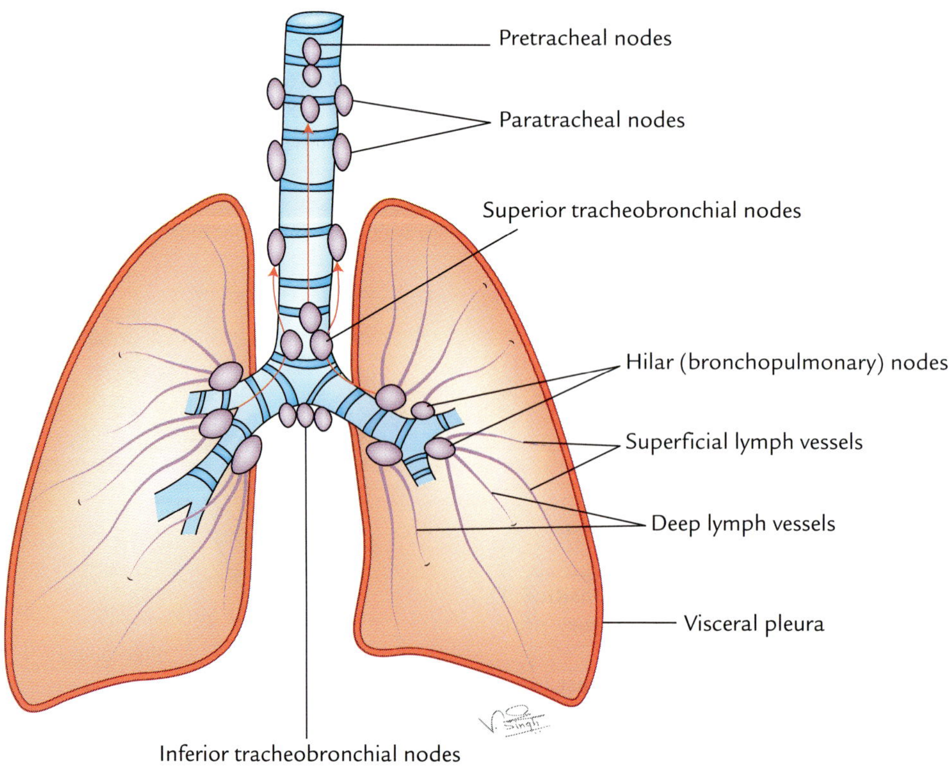

FIG. 19.17 Lymphatic drainage of the lungs.

respectively. These nodes in turn drain into pre and paratracheal lymph nodes and right and left bronchomediastinal lymph trunk, which finally drain into the right lymphatic duct and the thoracic duct on the right and left sides, respectively.

N.B.

All the lymph from the lung is drained into *tracheobronchial lymph nodes* (located at the tracheal bifurcation), which in turn drain into *bronchomediastinal lymph nodes*.

NERVE SUPPLY AN 24.5

The lung is supplied by both parasympathetic and sympathetic nerve fibres:

The **parasympathetic fibres** are derived from the vagus nerve and **sympathetic fibres** are derived from the T2 to T5 spinal segments. Both provide motor supply to the bronchial muscles and secretomotor supply to the mucous glands of the bronchial tree.

The **parasympathetic fibres** cause bronchoconstriction/bronchospasm, vasodilatation, and increased mucous secretion. The **sympathetic fibres** cause bronchodilatation, vasoconstriction, and decreased mucous secretion.

The afferent impulse arising from the bronchial mucous membrane and stretch receptors in the alveolar walls pass to the central nervous system through both sympathetic and parasympathetic fibres.

CLINICAL CORRELATION

- **Bronchial asthma:** It is a common disease of the respiratory system. It occurs due to bronchospasm (spasm of smooth muscle in the wall of bronchioles) that reduces the diameter of the bronchioles. As a result, the patient has great difficulty during expiration, although inspiration is accomplished normally. The airflow is further impeded due to the presence of excessive mucous, which the patient is unable to clear because an effective cough cannot be produced. Clinically, the asthma is characterized by (a) difficulty in breathing (dyspnoea) and (b) wheezing. The sympathomimetic drugs such as epinephrine cause bronchodilatation and relieve from the bronchial asthma/difficulty in breathing.

N.B.

The distal portion of bronchial tree has no cartilage in its wall. Its wall is made up of only smooth muscles, hence its lumen gets blocked by bronchospasm.

- **Bronchiectasis:** It is a clinical condition in which bronchi and bronchioles are dilated permanently as a result of chronic necrotizing infection. They become filled with pus leading to airway obstruction. The basal segments of the lower lobe are prone to this condition.
- **Aspiration pneumonia:** In supine position, aspirated material usually enters into superior (apical) segment of the lower lobe, especially on the right side for it is the most dependent segment in this position. It leads to the collection of secretions that may obstruct the bronchus, leading to the collapse of the superior segment of the lower lobe (*atelectasis*) and *pneumonia*.
- **Pulmonary embolism:** It is blockage of a pulmonary artery by thrombus, fat, and air.

  Thrombus usually arises from distant veins, *viz.* blood clots travel to the lungs from deep veins of leg.

  Fat following a bone fracture when fat surrounding the bone enters in broken vessels.

  Air (trapped air bubbles in vessel lumen) following a canulation in the neck region.

  Effect: Reduced lung perfusion leading to decreased blood oxygenation.

  Clinical features: Dyspnoea, chest pain, tachypnoea, cough and haemoptysis, cyanosis.

BRONCHOPULMONARY SEGMENTS AN 24.3

The bronchopulmonary segments are well-defined, wedge-shaped sectors of the lung, which are aerated by tertiary (segmental) bronchi (Fig. 19.18).

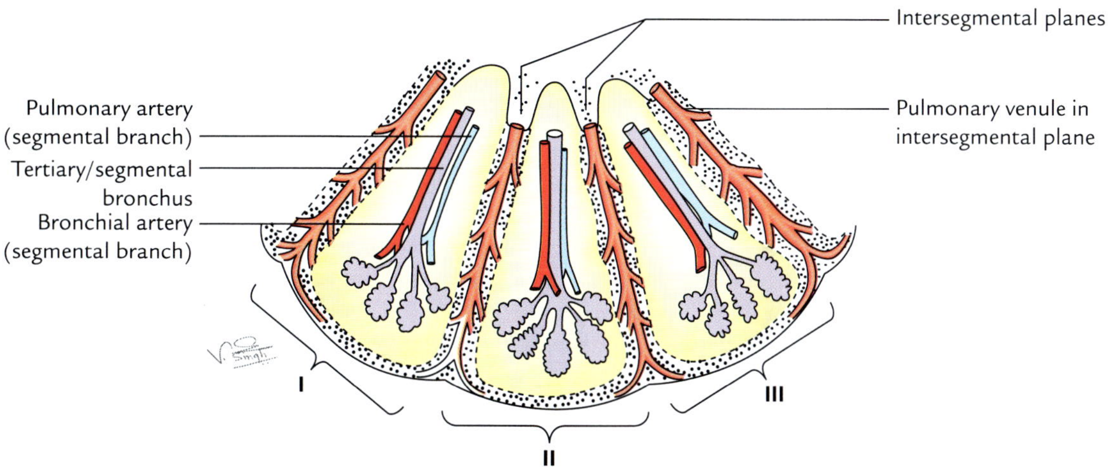

FIG. 19.18 Schematic diagram showing three bronchopulmonary segments (I, II, and III). Note each bronchopulmonary segment is supplied by independent segmental bronchus and segmental arteries (tributaries of the pulmonary and bronchial arteries).

Characteristic features:

1. It is a subdivision of the lobe of the lung.
2. It is pyramidal in shape with the apex directed toward the hilum and base toward the surface of the lung.
3. It is surrounded by the connective tissue.
4. It is aerated by the segmental (tertiary) bronchus.
5. Each segment has its own artery, a segmental branch of the pulmonary artery.
6. Each segment has its own lymphatic drainage and autonomic nerve supply.
7. Drained by intersegmental veins (tributaries of pulmonary veins).
8. Surgically resectable.

Thus, bronchopulmonary segments are the smallest well-defined independent anatomical, functional, and surgical units of the lungs. Therefore, they can be isolated and removed without affecting adjacent regions.

N.B.

The segmental veins (the tributaries of pulmonary veins) run in the intersegmental planes of the connective tissue.

NUMBER AND NOMENCLATURE OF BRONCHOPULMONARY SEGMENTS

The number of bronchopulmonary segments vary among different books by different authors. It may vary from 8–10 in each lung. But in this book, the number is given according to one accepted by the *International Congress of Anatomists* (1960) (Figs. 19.19–19.21).

According to this each lung contains 10 bronchopulmonary segments.

The segmental bronchi are given their numbers as listed in Table 19.4. The lobar bronchi are also shown in Figures 19.19–19.21.

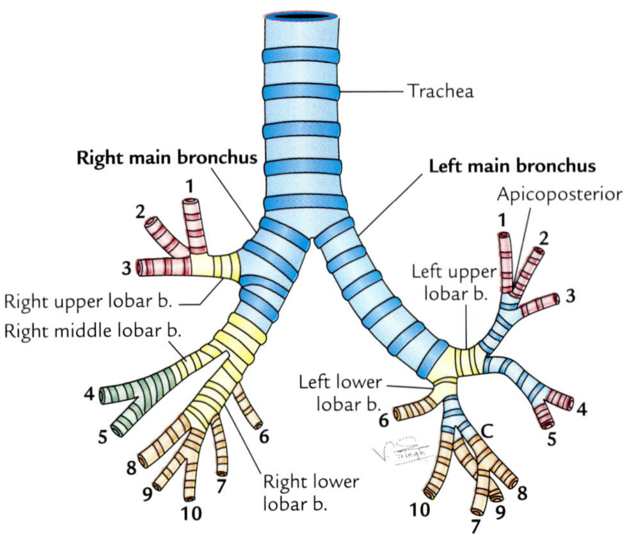

FIG. 19.19 ■ Segmental bronchi of lungs. The main, lobar, and segmental bronchi are also shown (C = Common stem of seven and eight segmental bronchi).

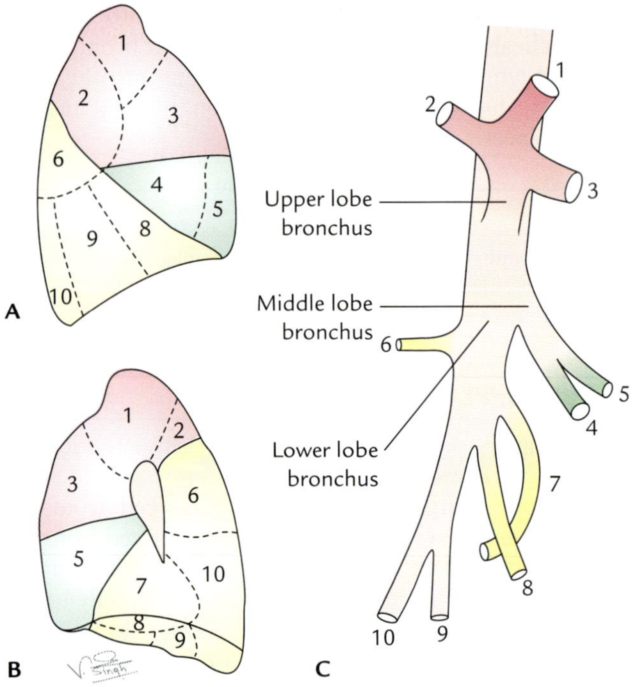

FIG. 19.20 ■ Bronchopulmonary segments of the right lung as seen on (**A**) lateral aspect, (**B**) medial aspect, and (**C**) lobar and segmental bronchi.

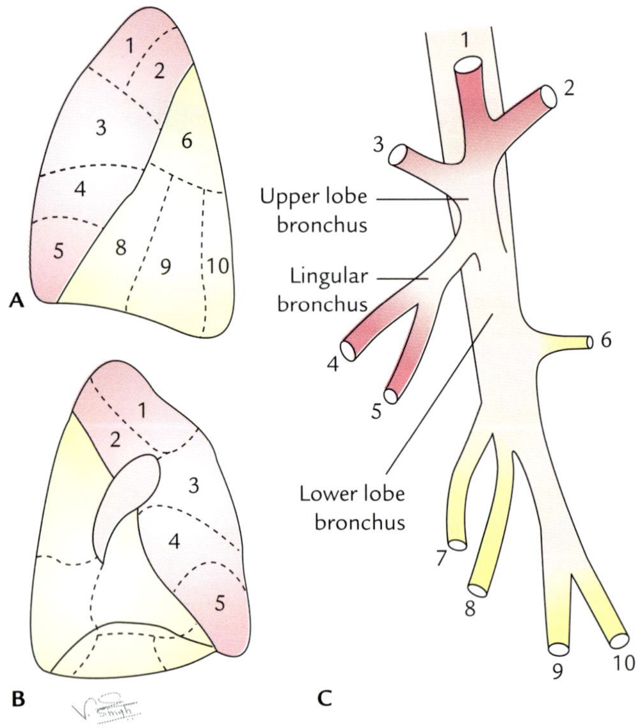

FIG. 19.21 ■ Bronchopulmonary segments of the left lung as seen on (**A**) lateral aspect, (**B**) medial aspect, and (**C**) lobar and segmental bronchi.

There are 10 segments in each lung. They are named and numbered in Table 19.4. The bronchopulmonary segments of the right and left lungs are shown in Figs. 19.20 and 19.21, respectively.

TABLE 19.4 Bronchopulmonary segments

Lung	Lobes	Segments
Right lung	• **Superior**	1. Apical
		2. Posterior
		3. Anterior
	• **Middle**	4. Lateral
		5. Medial
	• **Inferior**	6. Superior (apical)
		7. Medial basal
		8. Anterior basal
		9. Lateral basal
		10. Posterior basal
Left lung	• **Superior**	1. Apical
		2. Posterior
		3. Anterior
		4. Superior lingular
		5. Inferior lingular
	• **Inferior**	6. Superior (apical)
		7. Medial basal
		8. Anterior basal
		9. Lateral basal
		10. Posterior basal

N.B.

In left lung, apical and posterior segments in upper lobe fuse to form *apico-posterior segment*.

Similarly in inferior lobe of left lung, anterior basal and medial basal segments often fuse to form *anteromedial basal segment*.

CLINICAL CORRELATION

- **Aspiration of material in supine position:** In both lungs, the apical segment of the lower lobe is supplied by the segmental bronchus no. 6, which is the highest bronchus to arise from the posterior aspect of the bronchial tree. Hence, material aspirated in supine position from the comatose patient tend to gravitate into the **superior segment of the lower lobe**, usually of the right lung.
- **Segmental resection of the lung:** The knowledge of the bronchopulmonary segments has led to the advancement in conservative **lung surgery**. Since each segment is an independent functional unit, having its own bronchovascular supply and potential planes of separation exist between the segments. Localized chronic disease, such as tuberculosis, bronchiectasis, or benign neoplasm is restricted to one segment; it is, therefore, possible to dissect out and remove the diseased segment leaving the surrounding tissue intact. This procedure is called *segmental resection*.

N.B.

- During segmental dissection, it is important not to ligate intersegmental veins as they will interfere with the venous drainage of the surrounding healthy segments.
- Segmental resection is most often carried out in bronchiectasis.

Golden Facts to Remember

• Components of tracheobronchial tree	Trachea, bronchi, and bronchioles
• Commonest cancer of the lung	Bronchogenic carcinoma
• Commonest type of bronchogenic carcinoma	Adenocarcinoma
• Lung most commonly affected by bronchogenic carcinoma	Right lung
• Commonest site of pulmonary tuberculosis	Apical regions of the lungs
• Most common site of lung abscess	Right lower lobe
• Bronchopulmonary segment most commonly involved in aspiration pneumonia	Superior segment of the lower lobe of the right lung
• Inhaled particles mostly enters into	Right principal bronchus
• Commonest site where the aspirated material enters when the person is sitting/standing/lying in supine position	Right inferior lobe
• Number of alveoli in both lungs	About 300 million
• Smallest resectable unit of the lung	Bronchopulmonary segment
• Principal function of the lungs	Exchange of O_2 and CO_2 between inspired air and blood in lung capillaries

CLINICAL CASE STUDY

A heavy smoker, 60-year-old male, visited the hospital and complained that he lost 10 kg of his weight in past three months and has persistent cough with the blood-stained sputum. He also noticed the loss of sweating on the right side of his face. On physical examination, the doctors found partial ptosis and constriction of pupil in his right eye.

X-ray chest (PA view) revealed a radiopaque shadow in the apical region of the right lung. Biopsy revealed malignancy. **A diagnosis of malignancy of the apex of the lung was made.**

Questions

1. Enumerate the posterior relations of the apex of the lung.
2. Mention the anatomical basis of loss of sweating in the right half of the face, and partial ptosis and constriction (meiosis) of the right eye.
3. What is the bronchopulmonary segment?
4. Which is the most dependent bronchopulmonary segment in supine position?

Answers

1. From medial to lateral, these are: (a) sympathetic chain, (b) highest intercostal vein, (c) superior intercostal artery, and (d) ventral ramus of the first thoracic (T1) spinal nerve.
2. Involvement of the right sympathetic chain (causing Horner's syndrome).
3. Pyramid-shaped segment of the lung lobe aerated by the tertiary bronchus. It is the smallest resectable unit of the lung.
4. Apical (superior) segment of the lower lobe.

Mediastinum

CHAPTER 20

SPECIFIC LEARNING OBJECTIVES

After studying this chapter, the student should be able to:

- Define mediastinum. Give its boundaries and main contents.
- Describe the boundaries and contents of the superior, anterior, middle, and posterior mediastinum. AN 21.11
- Enumerate the subdivision of the mediastinum as seen in a chest radiograph.
- Give the anatomical basis of: (a) mediastinal syndrome, (b) mediastinal shift, and (c) extension of pus in posterior mediastinum from the neck.

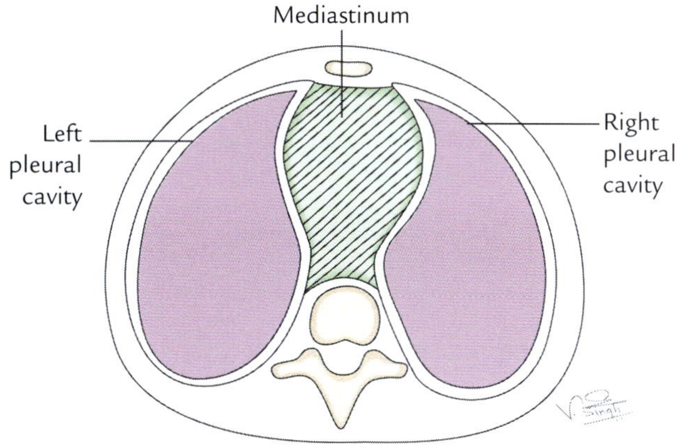

FIG. 20.1 Cross section of the thorax showing the position of the mediastinum.

MEDIASTINUM

The mediastinum (L. middle septum) is the median septum of the thoracic cavity between the two pleural cavities. It consists of all the viscera and structures of the thoracic cavity (e.g. heart and its great blood vessels, oesophagus, trachea and principal bronchi, aorta, mediastinal lymph nodes, etc.) except the lungs. The mediastinum occupies the central compartment of the thoracic cavity. Thus strictly speaking, it is a broad central partition which separates the two laterally placed pleural cavities (Fig. 20.1). It is covered on either side by the mediastinal pleura.

BOUNDARIES (FIGS. 20.2 AND 20.4) AN 21.11

Anterior: Sternum.
Posterior: Vertebral column (bodies of thoracic vertebrae and intervening intervertebral discs).
Superior: Superior thoracic aperture.
Inferior: Diaphragm.
On each side: Mediastinal pleura.

N.B.

The **mediastinum** is not a rigid structure as observed by the students in the cadaver (embalmed dead body). In a living individual, mediastinum is a highly mobile septum because it consists primarily of hollow visceral structures bound together by loose connective tissue, often infiltrated with fat.

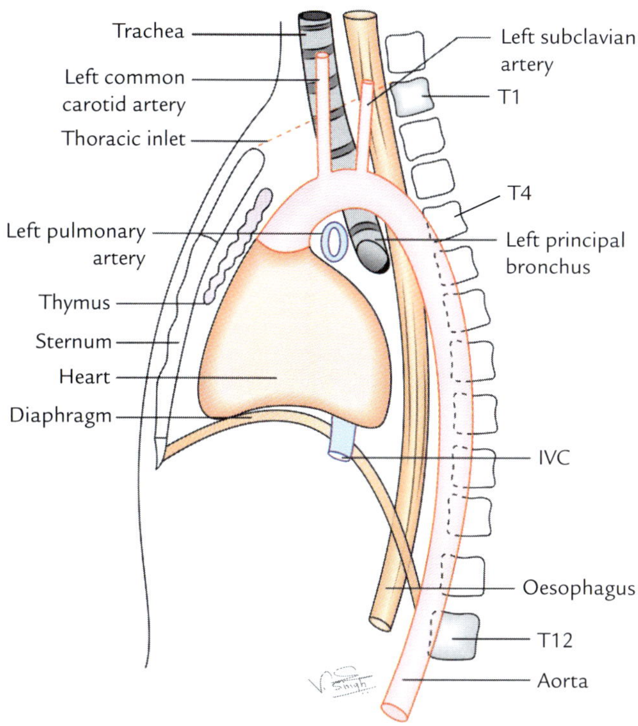

FIG. 20.2 Boundaries and contents of the mediastinum. Note that all the mediastinal structures are not depicted (IVC = inferior vena cava).

CONTENTS

The major contents of the mediastinum are (Fig. 20.2):

1. Thymus
2. Heart and great vessels enclosed in the pericardial sac
3. Ascending aorta, arch of aorta and descending aorta with their branches
4. Tracheal bifurcation
5. Superior vena cava
6. Azygos vein
7. Oesophagus
8. Thoracic duct
9. Neural structures, such as sympathetic trunks, vagus nerves, and phrenic nerves
10. Lymph nodes

LATERAL SURFACES OF MEDIASTINUM

The structures forming the right and left lateral surfaces of the mediastinum are shown in Fig. 20.3.

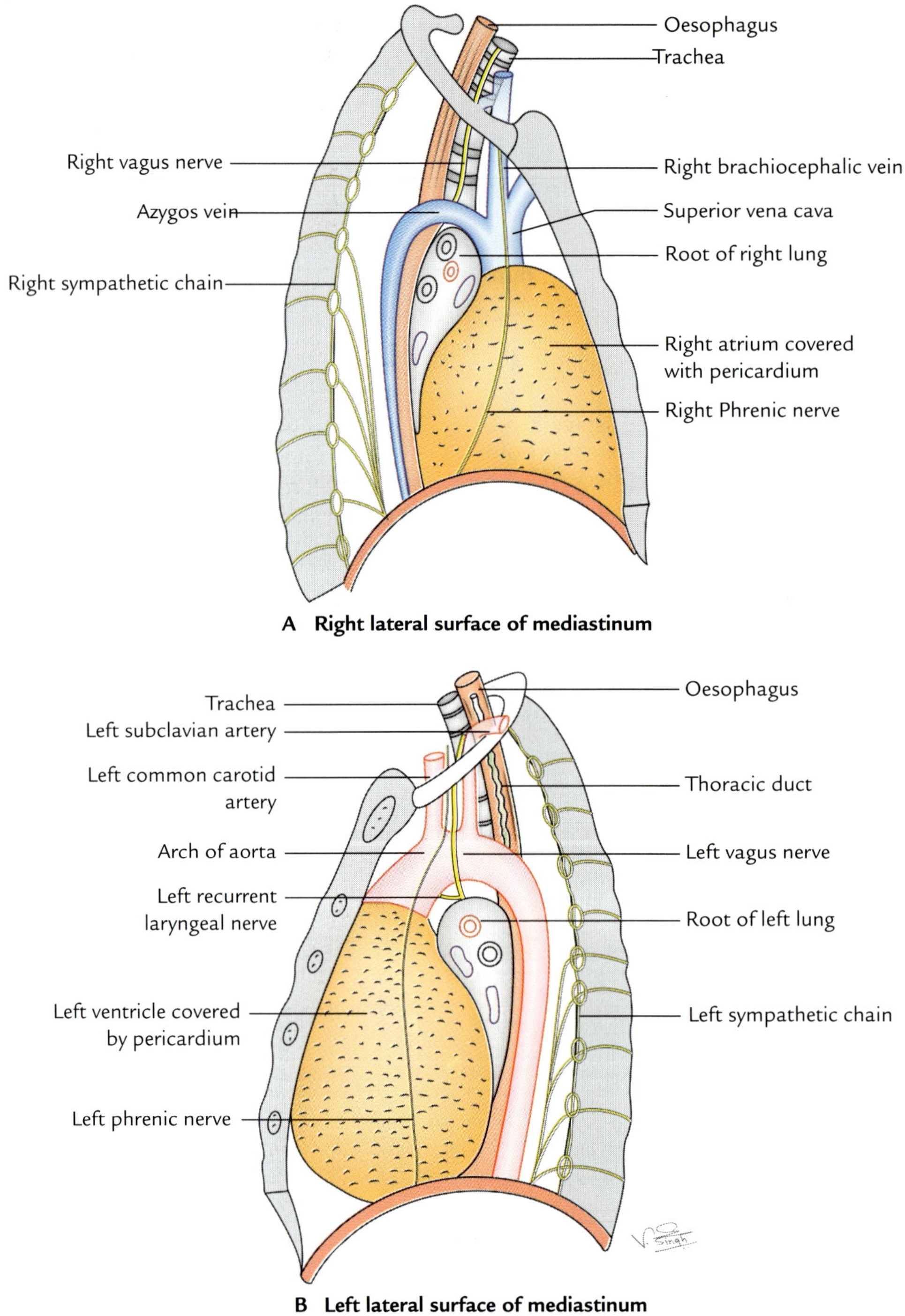

FIG. 20.3 ■ Mediastinal structure as seen from its lateral aspect in the sagittal section of the thorax. (**A**) Right side and (**B**) left side.

DIVISIONS

For the purpose of description and organization of structures, the mediastinum is artificially divided into two parts: (a) superior mediastinum and (b) inferior mediastinum by an imaginary plane (transverse thoracic plane) passing through the sternal angle anteriorly, and the lower border of the body of the fourth thoracic (T4) vertebra/intervertebral disc between T4 and T5 vertebrae posteriorly.

The inferior mediastinum is further subdivided into three parts by the pericardium (enclosing heart). The part in front of the pericardium is called the **anterior mediastinum**, and the part behind the pericardium is called the **posterior mediastinum**. The pericardium and its contents (heart and roots of its great vessels) constitute the **middle mediastinum** (Fig. 20.4).

The divisions and subdivisions of the mediastinum are shown in Flowchart 20.1.

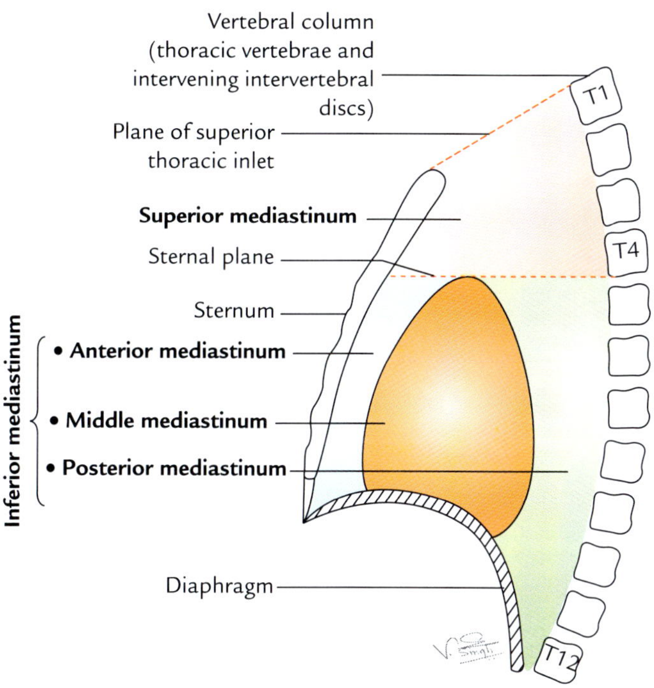

FIG. 20.4 ■ Divisions of the mediastinum.

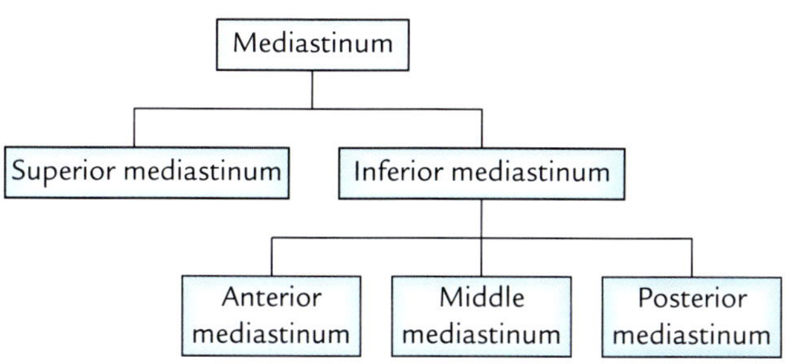

FLOWCHART 20.1 ■ Divisions and subdivisions of the mediastinum.

CLINICAL CORRELATION

- **Visualization of the subdivisions of the mediastinum in a chest radiograph:** The subdivisions of the mediastinum are well visualized in the lateral view of the X-ray of chest (Fig. 20.5).
- The shadow above the sternal plane represents the *superior mediastinum*.
- The subdivisions of the *inferior mediastinum* are demarcated as follows:
  (a) **cardiac shadow** above the anterior part of the diaphragm represents the *middle mediastinum*;
  (b) **retrosternal shadow** in front of the cardiac shadow represents the *anterior mediastinum*;
  (c) **retrocardiac shadow** between the cardiac shadow and the shadow of the vertebral column represents the *posterior mediastinum*.

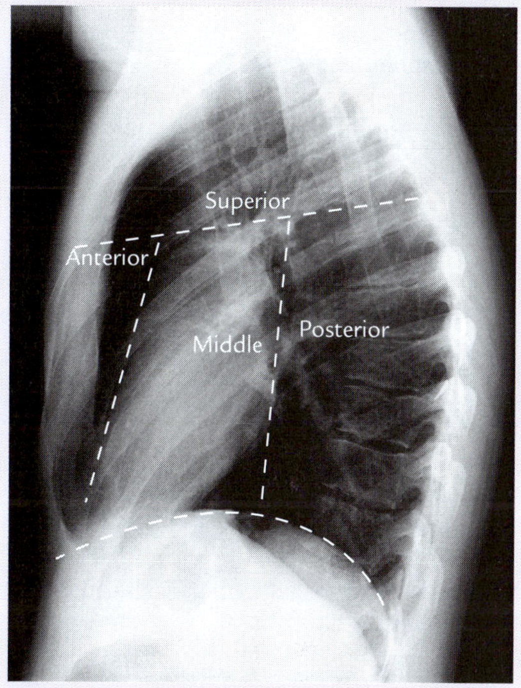

FIG. 20.5 ■ Parts of the mediastinum demonstrated on a chest radiograph (lateral view). (*Source*: *Integrated Anatomy*. David J.A. Heylings, Roy A.J. Spence, Barry E. Kelly, Fig. 4.13, p. 99, Elsevier Limited, 2007.)

SUPERIOR MEDIASTINUM

Boundaries (Fig. 20.4)

Anterior: Manubrium sterni.
Posterior: Bodies of the upper four thoracic vertebrae.
Superior: Plane of the superior thoracic aperture.
Inferior: An imaginary plane passing through the sternal angle in front and the lower border of the body of the fourth thoracic vertebra behind (transverse thoracic plane).
On each side (lateral): Mediastinal pleura.

Contents (Figs. 20.6 and 20.7)

1. Arteries
   (a) Arch of aorta
   (b) Brachiocephalic artery
   (c) Left common carotid artery
   (d) Left subclavian artery
2. Veins
   (a) Right and left brachiocephalic veins
   (b) Upper half of the SVC
   (c) Left superior intercostal vein
   (d) Arch of azygos vein
3. Nerves
   (a) Phrenic nerves (right and left)
   (b) Vagus nerves (right and left)
   (c) Sympathetic trunks and cardiac nerves (right and left)
   (d) Left recurrent laryngeal nerve
4. Lymphoid organs and lymphatics
   (a) Thymus
   (b) Thoracic duct
   (c) Lymph nodes
5. Tubes
   (a) Trachea
   (b) Oesophagus
6. Muscles
   (a) Sternohyoid
   (b) Sternothyroid
   (c) Longus colli

N.B.

For the purpose of orientation during surgery, the major structures of the superior mediastinum are arranged in the following order from anterior to posterior:
- Thymus
- Large veins
- Large arteries
- Trachea
- Oesophagus and thoracic duct
- Sympathetic trunks

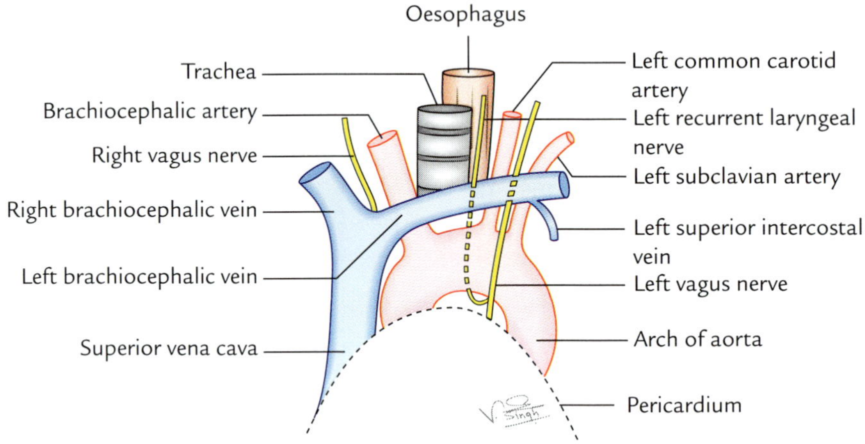

FIG. 20.6 ■ Arrangement of structures in the superior mediastinum as seen in dissection. Note that great veins are anterior to the great arteries.

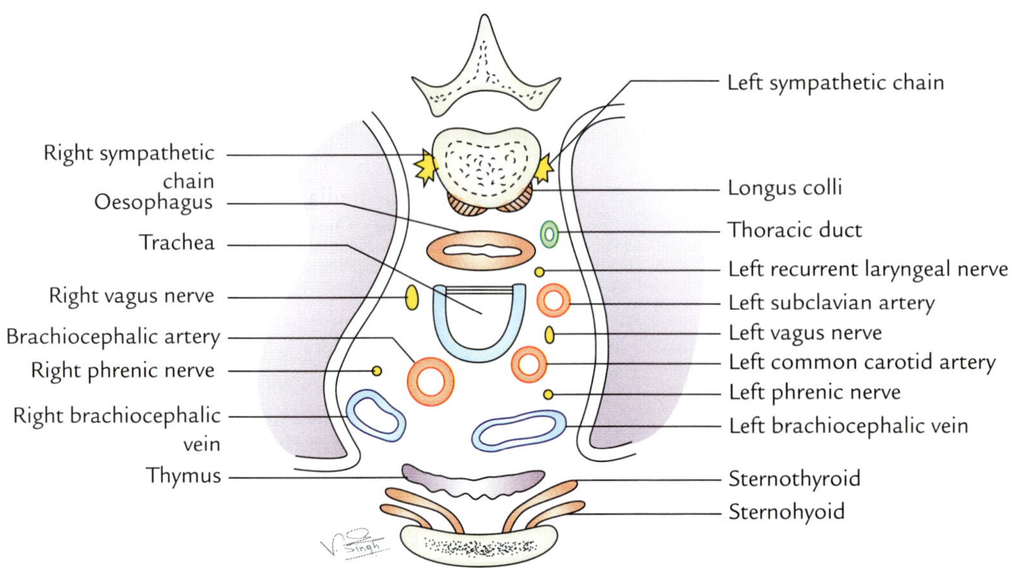

FIG. 20.7 ■ Transverse section of the superior mediastinum showing the arrangement of its contents (seen from above).

CLINICAL CORRELATION

Potential dead space in the superior mediastinum: In the superior mediastinum, all large veins (SVC, right and left brachiocephalic veins) are on the right side and all the large arteries (arch of aorta and its three branches) are on the left side. Consequently, during increased blood flow, the large veins expand enormously, while the large arteries do not expand at all. This is because there is sufficient dead space on the right side. It is into this space that tumours of the mediastinum tend to project.

ANTERIOR MEDIASTINUM

BOUNDARIES (Fig. 20.4)

Anterior: Body of sternum
Posterior: Pericardium enclosing heart
Superior: Transverse thoracic plane separating the superior and inferior mediastinum
Inferior: Diaphragm
On each side: Mediastinal pleura

CONTENTS

1. Loose areolar tissue
2. Superior and inferior *sternopericardial ligaments* stretching between the sternum and pericardium
3. Three or four lymph nodes and lymphatics
4. Mediastinal branches of internal thoracic (mammary) arteries
5. Lower portion of thymus (in children)

CLINICAL CORRELATION

Spread of infection from neck to anterior mediastinum: The *anterior mediastinum* is a very narrow space. It is continuous through the superior mediastinum with the pretracheal space of the neck. Therefore, neck infection in pretracheal space may spread into the anterior mediastinum.

MIDDLE MEDIASTINUM

Boundaries (Fig. 20.4)

Anterior: Anterior mediastinum
Posterior: Posterior mediastinum
Superior: Superior mediastinum
Inferior: Diaphragm

Contents (Fig. 20.8)

1. Heart
2. Pericardium
3. Arteries:
   (a) Ascending aorta
   (b) Pulmonary trunk dividing into two pulmonary arteries
   (c) Pericardiophrenic arteries

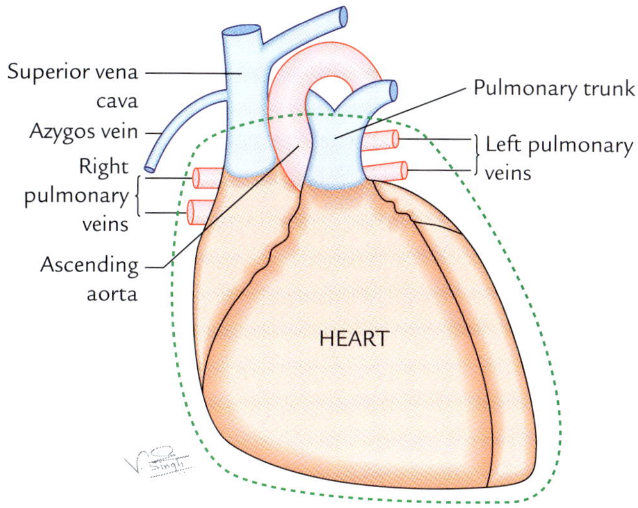

FIG. 20.8 ■ Main contents of the middle mediastinum.

4. Veins:
   (a) SVC (lower half)
   (b) Pulmonary veins (right and left)
5. Nerves:
   (a) Phrenic nerves
   (b) Deep cardiac plexus
6. Lymph nodes:
   (a) Tracheobronchial lymph nodes
7. Tubes:
   (a) Bifurcation of trachea
   (b) Right and left principal bronchi

N.B.

The main contents of the middle mediastinum are pericardium and its contents (e.g. the heart and roots of its great vessels).

POSTERIOR MEDIASTINUM

Boundaries (Fig. 20.4)

Anterior: (a) Pericardium and its contents, (b) bifurcation of the trachea, and (c) pulmonary vessels
Posterior: Bodies of the lower eight thoracic vertebrae and intervening intervertebral discs
Superior: Transverse thoracic plane separating the superior mediastinum from the inferior mediastinum
Inferior: Diaphragm
On each side (lateral): Mediastinal pleura

Contents (Fig. 20.9)

1. Oesophagus
2. Thoracic duct
3. Descending thoracic aorta and its branches
4. Azygos, hemiazygos, and accessory hemiazygos veins
5. Vagus nerves as anterior and posterior oesophageal plexuses
6. Sympathetic trunks and splanchnic nerves
7. Posterior mediastinal lymph nodes

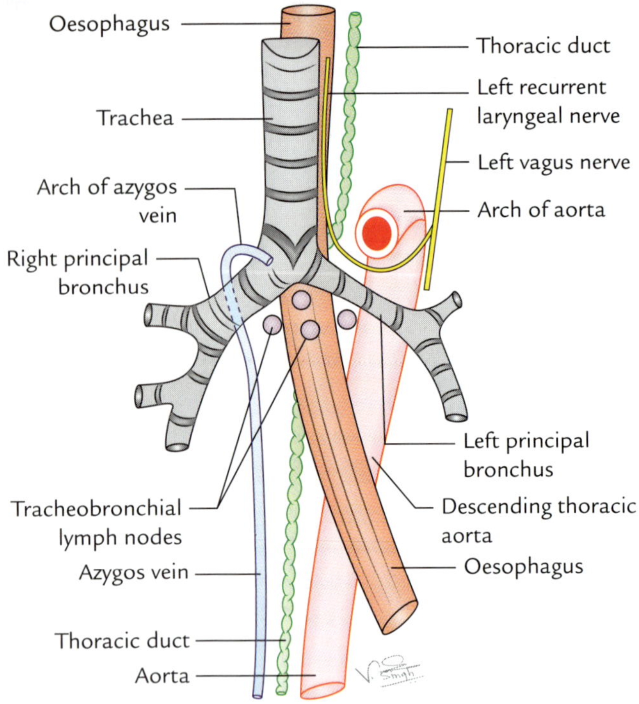

FIG. 20.9 ■ Anterior view of the oesophagus trachea bronchi and aorta. Note that the arch of aorta arches over the left bronchus and azygos vein arches over the right bronchus.

CLINICAL CORRELATION

- **Mediastinitis:** It is the inflammation of the loose connective tissue of the mediastinum. The fascial spaces of the neck (e.g. pretracheal and retropharyngeal spaces) extend below into the mediastinum within the thoracic cavity. Therefore, deep infections of the neck may readily spread into the thoracic cavity causing *mediastinitis*.
- **Subcutaneous emphysema at the root of neck:** The structures that make up the mediastinum are embedded in the loose connective tissue that is continuous with the loose connective tissue of the root of the neck. Therefore, in *oesophageal perforations* caused by penetrating wounds, air escapes into the connective tissue spaces of the mediastinum and may ascend beneath the fascia to the root of the neck, producing *subcutaneous emphysema*.
- **Mediastinal syndrome:** The compression of mediastinal structures by any growth such as tumour or cyst gives rise to a group of signs and symptoms, producing a clinical condition called *mediastinal syndrome*.

  The common causes of mediastinal syndrome are bronchogenic carcinoma, aneurysm of aorta, enlargement of mediastinal lymph nodes in Hodgkin disease.

  The clinical features of mediastinal syndrome are as follows:
  (a) *engorgement of veins* in the upper half of the body: due to obstruction of SVC,
  (b) *dyspnoea* (difficulty in breathing): due to the compression of trachea,
  (c) *dysphagia* (difficulty in swallowing): due to the compression of oesophagus,
  (d) *dysphonia* (hoarseness of voice): due to the compression of the left recurrent laryngeal nerve, and
  (e) erosion of bodies of the thoracic vertebrae: due to pressure on the vertebral column.
- **Widening of the mediastinum:** The widening of the mediastinum is often observed in chest radiographs. It can occur due to a number of reasons such as
  (a) haemorrhage into the mediastinum from lacerated great vessels (aorta, SVC) following trauma, for example, head-on collision,
  (b) massive enlargement of the mediastinal lymph nodes due to cancer of lymphoid tissue, *namely*, malignant lymphoma, and
  (c) enlargement (hypertrophy) of the heart due to congestive heart failure (CHF). It is the common cause of widening of the inferior mediastinum.
- **Mediastinal shift:** The mediastinal shift is common in the lung and pleural pathology. The mediastinum shifts to the affected (diseased) side due to an appreciable reduction in the lung volume and decrease in intrapleural pressure—as in *collapse of lung* and *atelectasis*. The mediastinum shifts to the healthy side when the intrapleural pressure is appreciably high on the affected side—as in *pneumothorax* and *hydrothorax*.

  Mediastinal shift indicates lung pathology. The mediastinal shift can be detected by palpating the trachea in the suprasternal notch.
- **Extension of pus into the posterior mediastinum from the neck:** The posterior mediastinum is continuous through superior mediastinum with spaces in the neck between the pretracheal and prevertebral layers of the deep cervical fascia, such as retropharyngeal space. Therefore, pus from the neck can extend into the posterior mediastinum.
- **Extension of pus into the thighs from the posterior mediastinum:** The psoas sheath communicates with the posterior mediastinum by a funnel-shaped orifice. Therefore, pus from the posterior mediastinum can easily enter the psoas sheath and track down into the thighs in the region of the femoral triangle.

Golden Facts to Remember

• Mediastinum contains all the thoracic viscera except	Lungs
• Largest structure of the mediastinum	Heart
• Commonest cause of the widening of the inferior mediastinum	Enlargement (hypertrophy) of the heart
• Mediastinum is a dynamic, pliable, and movable septum	Because structures forming it are hollow, fluid- or air-filled and bound together by the loose connective tissue
• Compartment of the thoracic cavity occupied by the mediastinum	Central compartment
• Common cause of mediastinal shift to the diseased side	Collapse of lung and atelectasis
• Common cause of mediastinal shift to the healthy side	Pneumothorax/ hydrothorax

CLINICAL CASE STUDY

A 60-year-old male visited the hospital and complained that he (a) has noticed alternation in his voice, (b) has lost 15 kg weight, and (c) has persistent cough with blood-stained sputum. On asking, he told that he is a chronic smoker and smokes 20–30 cigarettes per day. The X-ray chest revealed a large well-circumscribed radiopaque shadow in the hilar region of his right lung and the widening of the mediastinum. A diagnosis of **bronchogenic carcinoma** was made.

Questions

1. bronchogenic carcinoma is common in males or females? Mention the incidence of death.
2. Occurrence of bronchogenic carcinoma is more common in the right lung as compared to the left lung. What is its anatomical basis?
3. What is the cause of hoarseness of the voice?
4. Mention the anatomical basis of metastasis of bronchogenic carcinoma to brain and bones.

Answers

1. It is common in males and accounts for about one-third of all cancer deaths in men.
2. Because the right bronchial tree is more exposed to the carcinogens, for example, cigarette smoke, tarry particles from roads as right bronchus is wider and lies in line with the trachea.
3. The bronchogenic carcinoma spreads rapidly to tracheobronchial and bronchomediastinal lymph nodes and involves the recurrent laryngeal nerve, leading to the hoarseness of voice.
4. Through blood vessels (i.e. haematogenous spread) (for details, please refer *Clinical and Surgical Anatomy*, 2nd edition, by Vishram Singh).

CHAPTER

21

Pericardium and Heart

SPECIFIC LEARNING OBJECTIVES

After studying this chapter, the student should be able to:

- Describe the subdivisions, sinuses, blood supply and nerve supply of pericardium. AN 22.1
- Describe the arterial supply of the heart in detail and discuss its clinical significance.
- Describe the origin, course, and branches of coronary arteries. AN 22.3
- Write short notes on: (a) transverse sinus of the pericardium, (b) oblique sinus of the pericardium, (c) venous drainage of the heart, and (d) interior of the right atrium.
- Describe the external and internal features of each chamber of heart. AN 22.2
- Describe the fibrous skeleton of the heart. AN 22.6
- Describe the anatomical basis of ischaemic heart disease. AN 22.4
- Give the anatomical basis of: (a) angina pectoris and (b) myocardial infarction.
- Describe the formation, course, tributaries, and termination of coronary sinus. AN 22.5
- Surface marking of heart borders, apex beat, and surface projection of valves of heart. AN 25.9

PERICARDIUM

The pericardium (G. around heart) is a fibroserous sac that encloses the heart and the roots of its great blood vessels. The pericardium lies within the middle mediastinum, posterior to the body of the sternum and second to sixth costal cartilages and anterior to the middle four thoracic vertebrae (i.e. from T5 to T8).

The functions of the pericardium are as follows:

(a) It restricts the excessive movements of the heart.
(b) It serves as a lubricated container in which the heart can contract and relax smoothly.
(c) It limits the cardiac distension.

SUBDIVISIONS AN 22.1

The pericardium consists of two components:

(a) An outer single-layered fibrous sac called the fibrous pericardium and
(b) An inner double-layered serous sac called the serous pericardium.

A little description of embryology makes it easier to understand the formation of the different layers of the pericardium.

The heart and great vessels lie inside the fibrous sac and invaginate the serous sac from behind during development. As a result, the external surface of the heart and internal surface of the fibrous pericardium are covered by a layer of the serous pericardium. The layer covering the surface of the heart is called the visceral pericardium or epicardium, and the layer covering the inner aspect of the fibrous pericardium is called the parietal pericardium. The intervening potential space between the two serous layers is called the pericardial cavity (Fig. 21.1).

The pericardium, thus, consists of three layers (Fig. 21.2). From outside to inward, these are as follows:

1. The fibrous layer of the pericardium.
2. The parietal layer of the serous pericardium.

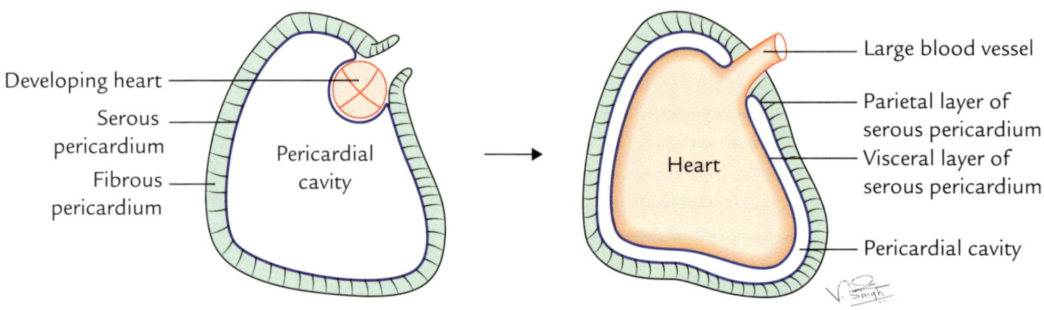

FIG. 21.1 ■ Development of the different layers of the pericardium.

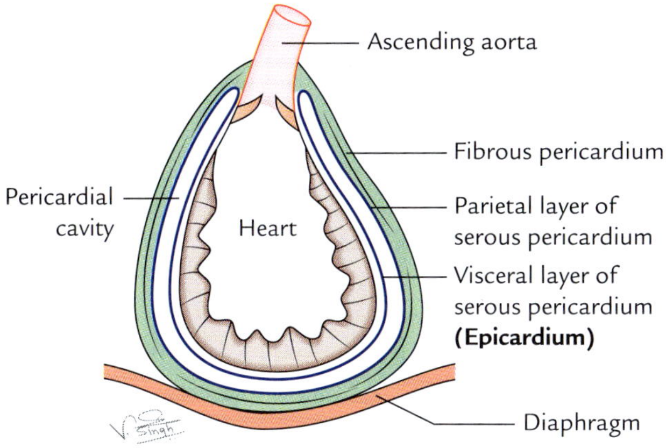

FIG. 21.2 ■ Layers of the pericardium.

3. The visceral layer of the serous pericardium (epicardium).

FIBROUS PERICARDIUM

The fibrous pericardium is a strong fibrous sac that supports the delicate parietal layer of the serous pericardium with which it is firmly adherent.

Features

The features of the fibrous pericardium are as follows:

1. It is conical in shape.
2. Its apex is blunt and fused with the outer coats of the roots of great blood vessels (e.g. ascending aorta, pulmonary trunk, SVC).
3. Its base is broad and blended with the central tendon of the diaphragm.
4. Anteriorly, it is connected to the posterior aspect of the body of sternum by the *superior and inferior sternopericardial ligaments*.
5. Posteriorly, it is related to principal bronchi, oesophagus, and descending thoracic aorta.
6. On each side, it is related to phrenic nerves and pericardiophrenic vessels.

N.B.

In quadrupeds, the fibrous pericardium is separated from the diaphragm by the *serous infracardiac bursa*.

SEROUS PERICARDIUM

The serous pericardium is a thin serous membrane lined by the mesothelium. It is double layered: the outer layer is called the **parietal layer** and the inner layer is called the **visceral layer**.

The outer layer lines the fibrous pericardium and is reflected around the roots of great blood vessels to become continuous with the visceral layer of the pericardium. It is called the **parietal pericardium**.

The inner layer is closely applied to the heart except along the cardiac grooves, where it is separated from the heart by blood vessels. It is called the **visceral pericardium or epicardium**.

TABLE 21.1 **Differences between the parietal and visceral pericardium**

Parietal pericardium	Visceral pericardium (epicardium)
It is adherent to the fibrous pericardium	It is adherent to the myocardium of the heart
It develops from the somatopleuric mesoderm	It develops from the splanchnopleuric mesoderm
It is innervated by the somatic nerve fibres	It is innervated by the autonomic nerve fibres
It is sensitive to pain	It is insensitive to pain

N.B.

The two layers of the serous pericardium are continuous with each other at the roots of great blood vessels [e.g. ascending aorta, pulmonary trunk, superior vena cava (SVC), and inferior vena cava (IVC) and the superior and inferior pulmonary veins] where the pericardial sac was invaginated by the developing heart.

The differences between the parietal and visceral pericardium are listed in Table 21.1.

PERICARDIAL CAVITY

The slit-like potential space between the parietal and visceral layers of the serous pericardium is termed pericardial cavity. Normally, it contains a thin film of serous fluid (about 50 mL) called the pericardial fluid that lubricates the opposed surfaces to avoid friction during the movements of the heart.

The following structures are invested by the serous pericardium:

1. Heart with its vessels and nerves
2. Ascending aorta
3. Pulmonary trunk
4. SVC (lower half)
5. IVC (terminal part)
6. Pulmonary veins (terminal parts)

SINUSES OF PERICARDIUM AN 22.1

There are two sinuses between the parietal and visceral layers of serous pericardium (Figs. 21.3 and 21.4):

1. Transverse sinus
2. Oblique sinus

They are formed due to the reflection of the visceral layer of the serous pericardium around great vessels of the heart.

The visceral pericardium (epicardium) at the roots of great blood vessels is arranged into tubes: (a) arterial tube and (b) venous tube. The *arterial tube* encloses the ascending aorta and pulmonary trunk (*arterial end of the heart tube*). The *venous tube* encloses the SVC and IVC, and four pulmonary veins (*venous end of the heart tube*).

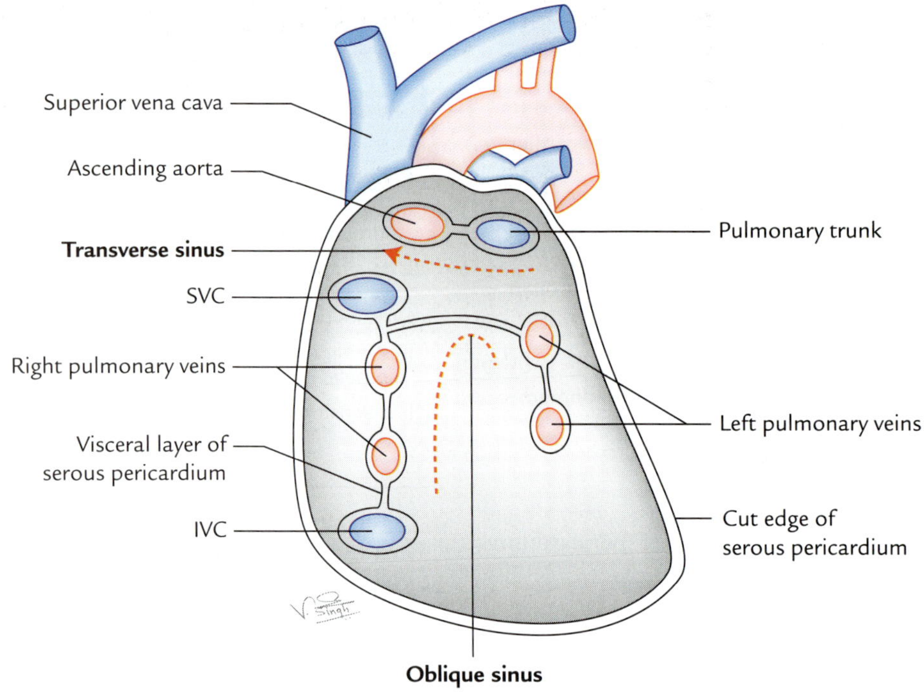

FIG. 21.3 ■ Interior of the serous pericardial sac after the section of the large vessels and the removal of the heart showing transverse and oblique pericardial sinuses (SVC = superior vena cava, IVC = inferior vena cava).

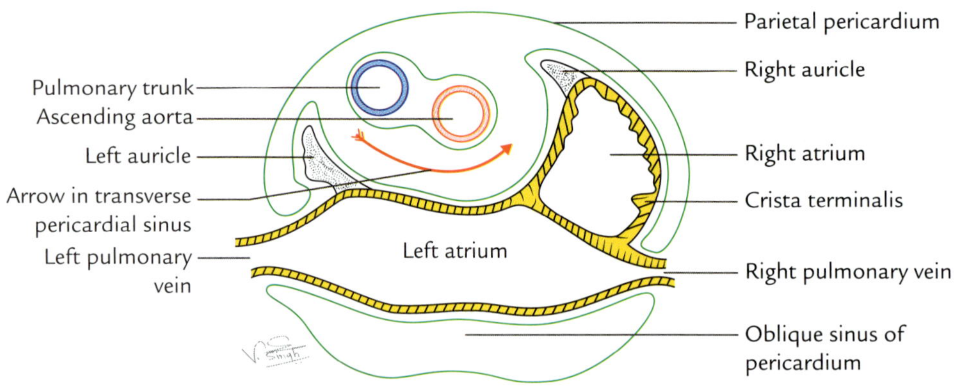

FIG. 21.4 ■ Cross section of the heart through the atria showing the reflection of the pericardium and the formation of the transverse and oblique pericardial sinuses. Note that the left atrium lies behind the pulmonary trunk and aorta, from which it is separated by the transverse sinus of the pericardium.

Transverse Sinus of Pericardium

It is a transverse recess behind the ascending aorta and pulmonary trunk and in front of the SVC and superior pulmonary veins. It develops due to the degeneration of the *dorsal mesocardium*.

It is a horizontal passage between the two pericardial tubes. On each side, it communicates with the general pericardial cavity.

Oblique Pericardial Sinus

It is a recess of the serous pericardium behind the base of the heart (actually left atrium). It is enclosed by a 'J-shaped' sheath of the visceral layer of the serous pericardium enclosing six veins (i.e. two vena cavae and four pulmonary veins).

The oblique sinus is akin to a lesser sac behind the stomach and develops as a result of the absorption of four pulmonary veins into the left atrium. The oblique sinus permits the distension of the left atrium during the return of oxygenated blood in it from the lungs.

Boundaries

Oblique sinus of the pericardium is bounded in the following ways:

Anteriorly: By the left atrium.

Posteriorly: By the parietal pericardium.

On right side: By the reflection of the visceral pericardium along the right pulmonary veins, SVC and IVC.

On the left side: By the reflection of the visceral pericardium along the left pulmonary veins.

Superiorly: By the reflection of the visceral pericardium along the right and left superior pulmonary veins.

Inferiorly: It is open.

CLINICAL CORRELATION

Surgical significance of transverse pericardial sinus: During cardiac surgery, after the pericardial sac is opened anteriorly, a finger is passed through the transverse sinus of the pericardium, posterior to the aorta, and pulmonary trunk (Fig. 21.5).

A temporary ligature is passed through the transverse sinus around the aorta and pulmonary trunk. The tubes of the heart—lung machine are inserted into these vessels and the ligature is tightened.

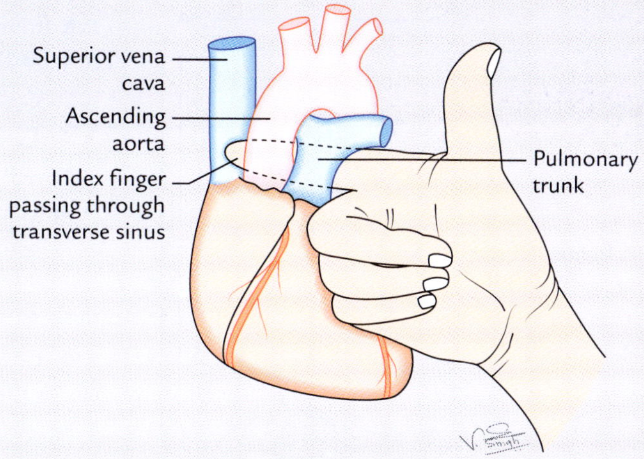

FIG. 21.5 ■ Finger passing through the transverse pericardial sinus.

Arterial Supply AN 22.1

The *fibrous pericardium* and the *parietal layer of seorus pericardium* are supplied by the branches of the following arteries:

1. Internal thoracic artery
2. Musculophrenic arteries
3. Descending thoracic aorta

The *visceral layer* of the serous pericardium is supplied by the coronary arteries.

Nerve Supply AN 22.1

1. The fibrous pericardium and the parietal layer of the serous pericardium are supplied by the phrenic nerves (somatic nerve fibres).
2. The visceral layer of the serous pericardium is supplied by the branches of sympathetic trunks and vagus nerves (autonomic nerve fibres). Thus, the fibrous pericardium and the parietal layer of the serous pericardium are sensitive to pain, whereas the visceral layer of the pericardium is insensitive to pain. Consequently, pain of pericarditis originates from the parietal pericardium.

CLINICAL CORRELATION

- **Pericarditis and cardiac tamponade:** The inflammation of the serous pericardium is called *pericarditis* that causes the accumulation of the serous fluid in the pericardial cavity, the *pericardial effusion*. The excessive accumulation of the serous fluid in the pericardial cavity may compress the thin-walled atria and interfere with the filling of the heart during diastole and consequently the cardiac output is diminished. This condition is clinically termed *cardiac tamponade*.

  The *pericarditis* is the terminal event in the uremia.
- **Pericardiocentesis:** Excessive pericardial fluid can be aspirated from the pericardial cavity by two routes:
  - *Sternal approach*: The needle is inserted through the left fifth or sixth intercostal space immediately adjacent to the sternum.
  - *Subxiphoid approach*: The needle is inserted in the left costoxiphoid angle and passed in an upward and backward direction at an angle of 45° to the skin.
- **Pericardial friction rub:** The roughening of the parietal and visceral layers of the serous pericardium by inflammatory exudate can cause friction between the two layers called the *pericardial friction rub* that can be felt on palpation and heard through the stethoscope.

HEART AN 22.2

Functionally, the heart is made up of two muscular pumps: the right and left (Fig. 21.6). The right pump consists of the right atrium and right ventricle, while the left pump consists of the left atrium and left ventricle. The right pump is responsible for pulmonary circulation and the left pump is responsible for systemic circulation as follows:

- The right atrium receives deoxygenated blood from the whole body through the superior and inferior venae cavae. The blood flows from the right atrium into the right ventricle through the *right AV orifice*. The blood is prevented from regurgitating back to the atrium by means of the *right AV valve*. The right ventricle contracts and propels the blood into the

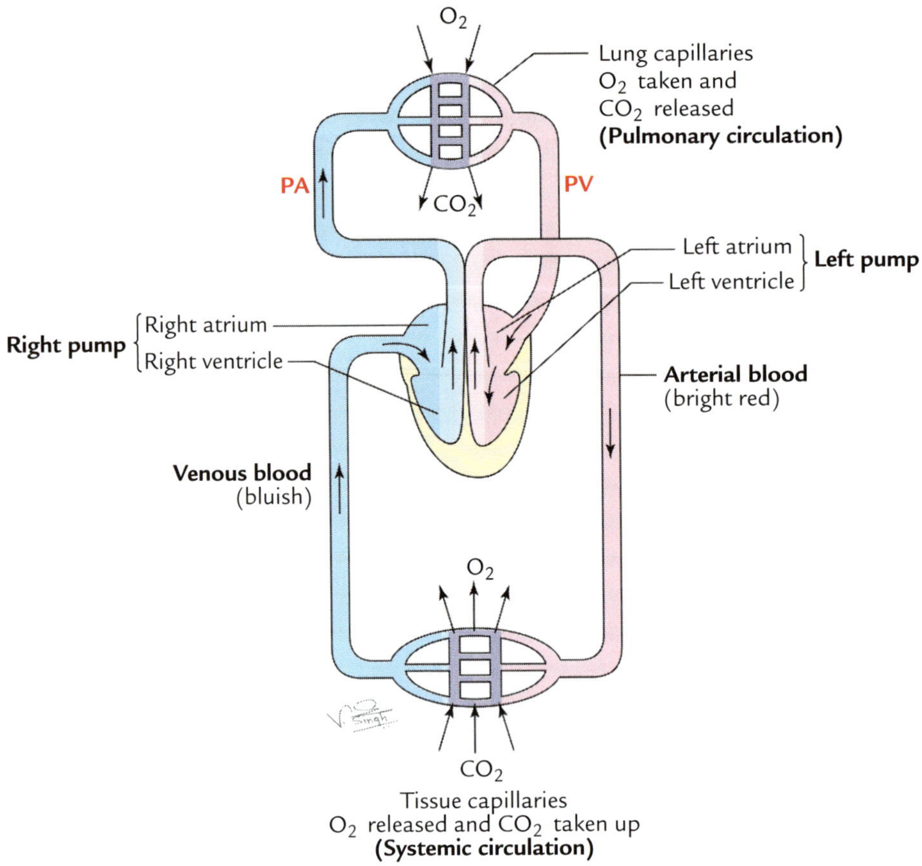

FIG. 21.6 ■ Heart as double pump (PA = pulmonary artery, PV = pulmonary vein).

pulmonary trunk, pulmonary arteries, and finally into the lung where blood is oxygenated (*pulmonary circulation*).

- The left atrium receives the oxygenated blood from lungs through four pulmonary veins. The blood from the left atrium flows into the left ventricle through the *left AV orifice*. The blood is prevented from regurgitating back to the atrium by means of the *left AV valve*. The left ventricle strongly contracts and propels the blood into the ascending aorta and then into the systemic circulation.

N.B.

The right ventricle is required to pump the blood through a relatively low-resistance vascular bed, whereas the left ventricle is required to pump the blood through a relatively high-resistance peripheral vascular bed.

The muscular wall of the left ventricle is, therefore, much thicker than that of the right ventricle.

MORPHOLOGY

The heart (syn. Gk. *Kardia/Cardia*; L. *Cor/Cordis*) is a hollow muscular organ situated in the middle mediastinum of the thoracic cavity, enclosed in the pericardium. I t is somewhat pyramidal in shape and placed obliquely behind the sternum and adjoining parts of costal cartilages so that one-third of the heart is to the right of the median plane and two-thirds of it is to the left of the median plane.

The heart consists of four chambers—right atrium and right ventricle, and left atrium and left ventricle. On the surface, the atria are separated from the ventricles by the atrioventricular (AV) groove (also called the *coronary sulcus*) and ventricles from each other by interventricular grooves.

SHAPE AND MEASUREMENTS

Shape: Pyramidal or conical.
Measurements:
Length = 12 cm.
Width = 9 cm.
Weight = 300 g in males; 250 g in females.

N.B.

The heart is slightly larger than one's own clenched fist.

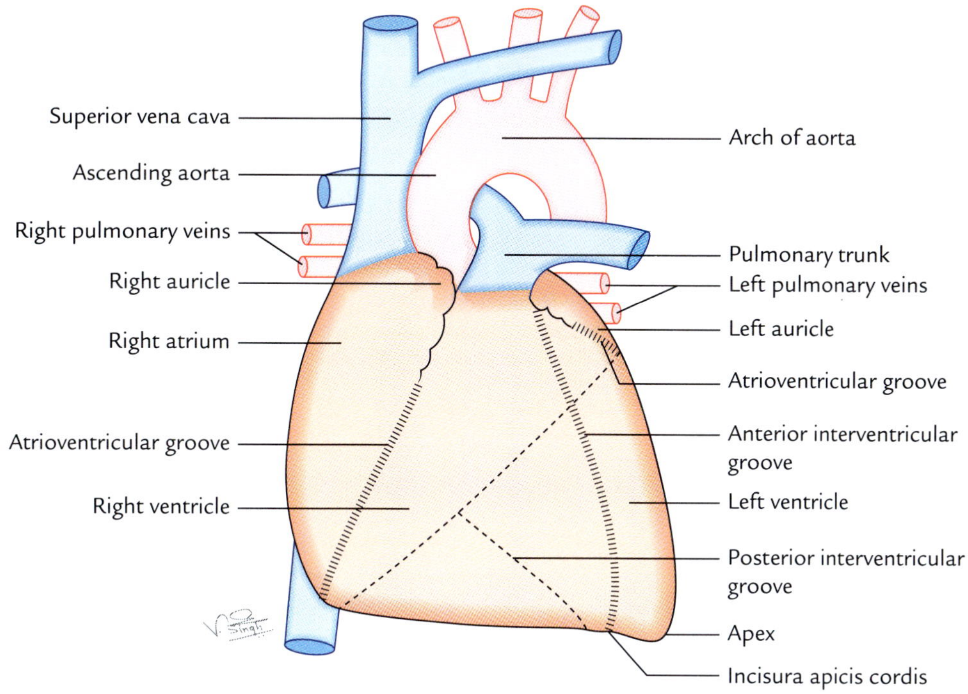

FIG. 21.7 ■ Anterior aspect (sternocostal surface) of the heart. Note that the most of the sternocostal surface is formed by the right atrium and the right ventricle.

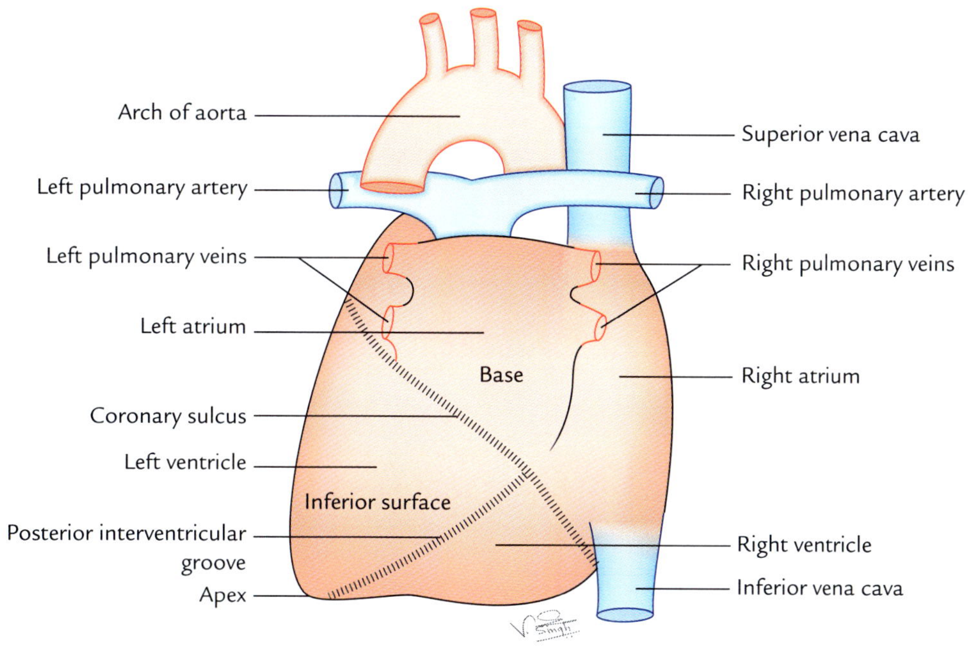

FIG. 21.8 ■ Posterior aspect of the heart.

EXTERNAL FEATURES

AN 22.2

The heart presents the following external features (Figs. 21.7 and 21.8):

1. Apex.
2. Base: posterior surface.
3. Five surfaces: posterior, sternocostal, diaphragmatic, left, and right.
4. Four borders: right, left, upper, and inferior.

Apex of the Heart

The apex of the heart is a conical area formed by left ventricle. It is directed downward and forward, and to the left. It lies at the level of the left fifth intercostal space, 3.5 in (9 cm) from the midline and just medial to the midclavicular line.

CLINICAL CORRELATION

Apex beat: It is the outermost and lowermost thrusts of the cardiac contraction (during ventricular systole) felt on the front of the chest or it is the point of the maximum cardiac impulse (**PMCI**). Normally, the apex beat is felt as a light tap in left fifth intercostal space in the midclavicular line.

In infants, the heart is positioned more horizontally so that the apex of the heart lies in the third or fourth left intercostal space and consequently the **apex beat in children up to 7 years of age is felt in the third or fourth intercostal space just lateral to the midclavicular line.**

N.B.

Normally, the apex of the heart is on the left side and the apex beat is felt on the left side (fifth intercostal space), but sometimes the heart is malpositioned with the apex on the right side. This condition is called ***dextrocardia***. It may be associated with the complete reversal of thoracic and abdominal viscera, a condition called *situs inversus*.

Base of the Heart

The base (or posterior surface) of the heart is formed by two atria, mainly by the left atrium. Strictly speaking, two-thirds of the base is formed by the posterior surface of the left atrium and one-third by the posterior surface of the right atrium. It is directed backward and to the right (i.e. opposite to the apex).

Characteristic features of the base are as follows:

1. It lies opposite to the apex.
2. It lies in front of the middle four thoracic vertebrae (i.e. T5–T8) in the lying-down position and descends one vertebra in the erect posture (T6–T9).
3. The base is separated from the vertebral column by the oblique pericardial sinus, oesophagus, and aorta.

N.B.

Clinically, base is the upper border of the heart where great blood vessels (SVC, ascending aorta, and pulmonary trunk) are attached.

Surfaces of the Heart

The heart has the following five surfaces:

1. Posterior surface
2. Sternocostal (anterior)
3. Diaphragmatic (inferior)
4. Left surface
5. Right surface

Posterior surface: It has been already described above under heading base of heart.

Sternocostal surface: It is formed mainly by the right atrium and right ventricle, which are separated from each other by the anterior part of the AV groove. The sternocostal surface is also partly formed by the left auricle and left ventricle. The right ventricle is separated from the left ventricle by the anterior interventricular groove.

N.B.

- The left atrium is hidden on the front by the ascending aorta and the pulmonary trunk.
- The part of the sternocostal surface is uncovered by the left lung (cardiac notch) forming an *area of superficial cardiac dullness*.

Diaphragmatic surface: This surface is flat and rests on the central tendon of the diaphragm. It is formed by the left and right ventricles that are separated from each other by the posterior interventricular groove. The left ventricle forms the left two-thirds of this surface and right ventricle forms only the right one-third of this surface.

Left surface: It is formed mainly by the left ventricle and partly by the left atrium and auricle. It is directed upward, backward, and to the left.

Right surface: It is rounded and formed by right atrial wall.

Borders of the Heart

The heart has the following four borders:

1. Right border
2. Left border
3. Inferior border
4. Upper border

Right border: It is more or less vertical and is formed by the right atrium. It extends from the right side of the opening of SVC to that of IVC and separates the base from the sternocostal surface.

Left border: It is curved and oblique. It is formed mainly by the left ventricle and partly by the left auricle. It extends from the left auricle to the apex of the heart and separates sternocostal and left surfaces.

Inferior border: It is nearly horizontal and extends from the opening of IVC to the apex of the heart. It is formed by the right ventricle. The right atrium also forms a part of this border. The inferior border separates the sternocostal surface from the diaphragmatic surface. Near the apex it presents a notch called *incisura apicis cordis*.

Upper border: It is slightly oblique and is formed by the right and left atria, mainly by the latter. The upper border is obscured from the view on the sternocostal surface because the ascending aorta and pulmonary trunk lie in front of it. On the surface of the body, it can be marked by a line joining a point on the lower border of the second left costal cartilage, 1.5 in from the median plane to a point on the upper border of third right costal cartilage, 1 in away from the median plane.

CLINICAL CORRELATION AN 25.7

Cardiac shadow in a chest radiograph (Fig. 21.9): In an X-ray of the chest, PA view, the term cardiac shadow is used for the *mediastinal shadow*. The left border of the cardiac shadow, from above downward, is formed by the aortic arch, pulmonary trunk, left auricle, and left ventricle. The right border from above downward is formed by SVC and the right atrium.

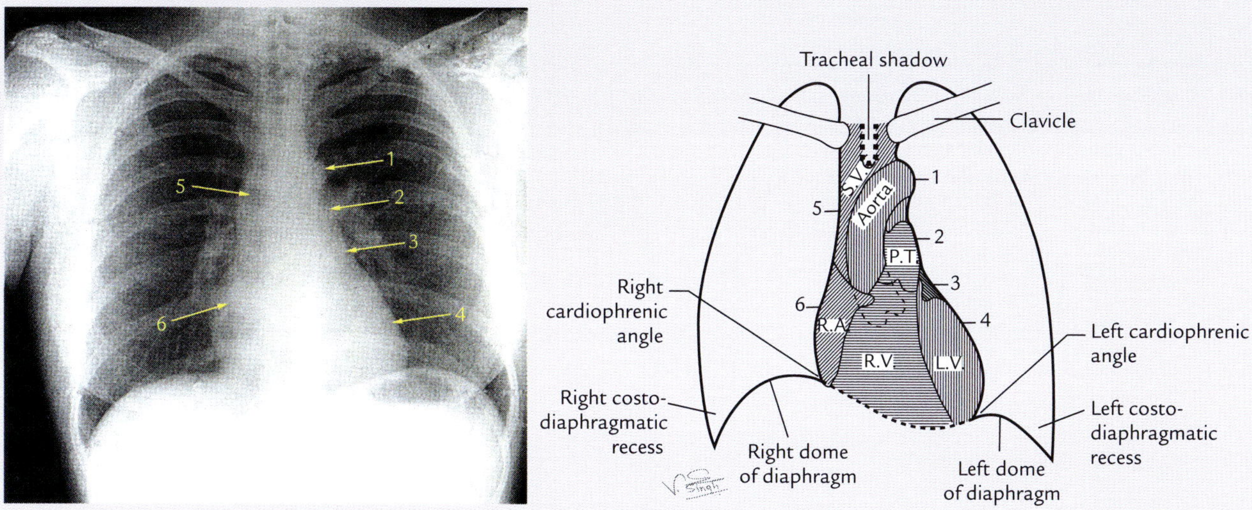

A B

FIG. 21.9 ■ X-ray chest PA view. (**A**) Actual radiograph and (**B**) tracing of the cardiac shadow (1 = aortic knuckle, 2 = pulmonary conus, 3 = left auricle, 4 = left ventricle, 5 = superior vena cava, 6 = right atrium). (*Source*: (A) *Integrated Anatomy:* David J.A. Heylings, Roy A.J. Spence, Barry E. Kelly, Fig. 4.1, p. 94, Elsevier Limited, 2007. (B) *Clinical and Surgical Anatomy*, 2e d.: Vishram Singh, Fig. 3.19, p. 137, Elsevier, 2007.)

Demarcation of Chambers of the Heart on the Surface

On the surface, the chambers of the heart are demarcated or delineated from each other by the following three sulci/grooves (Figs. 21.7 and 21.8):

1. Coronary sulcus (AV groove)
2. Anterior interventricular sulcus
3. Posterior interventricular sulcus

Coronary sulcus (AV groove): It encircles the heart and separates the atria from the ventricles. It is deficient anteriorly due to the root of the pulmonary trunk.

The AV groove is divided into the anterior and posterior parts.

The anterior part consists of the right and left halves.

The right anterior part of the AV groove runs downward and to the right between the right atrium and right ventricle and lodges the right coronary artery.

The left anterior part of the AV groove intervenes between the left auricle and left ventricle. It lodges the circumflex branch of the left coronary artery.

The posterior part of the AV groove intervenes between the base and the diaphragmatic surface of the heart. It lodges *coronary sinus*.

Anterior and posterior interventricular sulci: They separate the right and left ventricles. The anterior interventricular sulcus is on the sternocostal surface of the heart and lodges the anterior interventricular artery and the great cardiac vein. The posterior interventricular groove is on the diaphragmatic surface and lodges the posterior interventricular artery and the middle cardiac vein.

N.B.

The meeting point of the interatrial groove, posterior interventricular groove, and posterior part of the AV groove is termed **crux of the heart**.

CHAMBERS OF THE HEART

The heart consists of four chambers, *namely*:

1. Right atrium
2. Right ventricle
3. Left atrium
4. Left ventricle

The two atrial chambers are separated from each other by a vertical septum—the interatrial septum and the two ventricular chambers are separated from each other by a vertical septum—the interventricular septum.

The right atrium communicates with the right ventricle through the *right AV orifice*, which is guarded by three cusps.

The left atrium communicates with the left ventricle through the *left AV orifice*, which is guarded by two cusps.

The walls of the chambers of the heart are made up of the cardiac muscle—the myocardium, which is covered externally by the serous membrane—the *epicardium* and lined internally by endothelium—the *endocardium*.

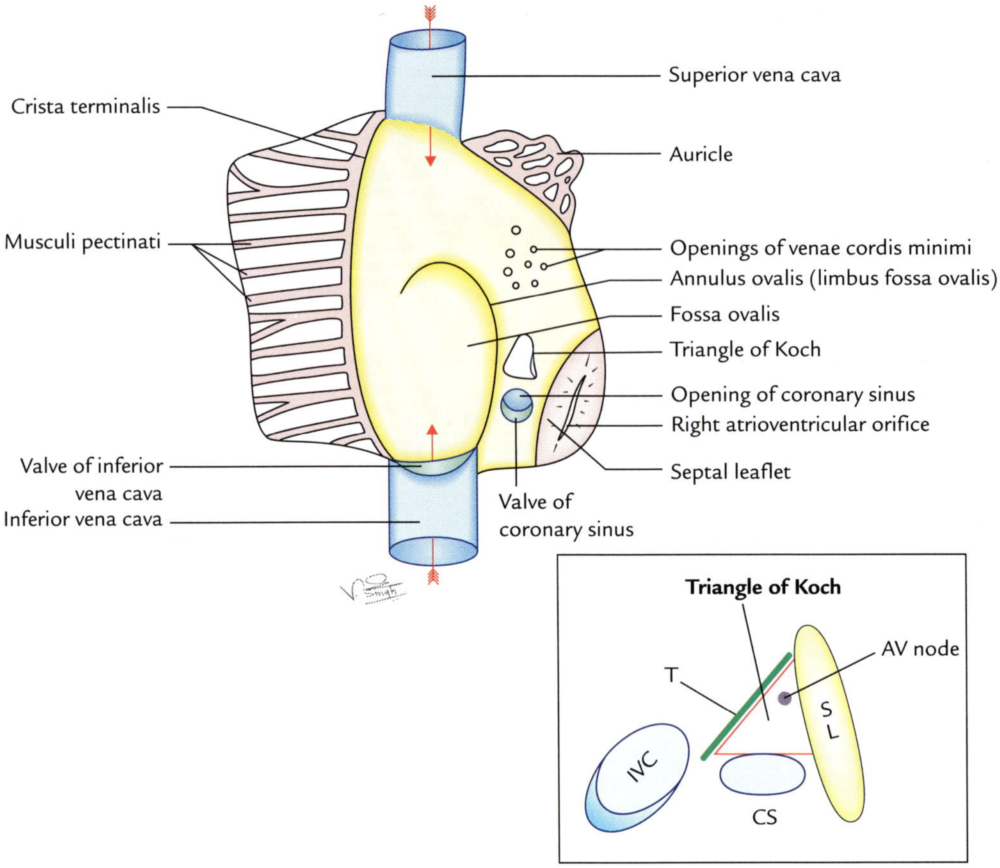

FIG. 21.10 ■ Interior of the right atrium. Figure in the inset on right and below shows boundaries of Koch's triangle (SL = septal leaflet of right AV valve, CS = coronary sinus, T = tendon of Todaro, IVC = inferior vena cava).

The atria are thin walled as compared to the ventricles and have little contractile power.

RIGHT ATRIUM

The right atrium is somewhat a quadrilateral chamber situated behind and to the right side of the right ventricle. It consists of a main cavity and a small outpouching called auricle.

External Features

1. The right atrium is elongated vertically and receives SVC at its upper end and the IVC at its lower end.
2. The upper anterior part is prolonged to the left to form the right auricular appendage, the *right auricle*. The margins of the auricle are notched. The right auricle overlaps the roots of the ascending aorta completely and infundibulum of the right ventricle partly.
3. A shallow vertical groove called sulcus terminalis extends along the right border between the SVC and IVC. The upper part of the sulcus contains the *sinuatrial (SA) node*. Internally, it corresponds to crista terminalis.
4. The vertical right AV groove lodges the right coronary artery and the small cardiac vein.

Internal Features

AN 22.2

The interior of the right atrium is divided into three parts (Fig. 21.10): (a) *Smooth posterior part*—the sinus venarum and (b) *rough anterior part*—the atrium proper and (c) *septal wall*. The first two parts are separated from each other by crista terminalis. The differences between these two parts are enumerated in Table 21.2.

(a) **Smooth posterior part:** It is derived from right horn of the sinus venosus and presents the following features:

i. ***Opening of SVC at the upper end.*** It opens at the upper end of right atrium and has no valve. It returns the blood to heart from the upper half of the body.

ii. ***Opening of IVC at the lower end.*** It is guarded by a rudimentary semilunar valve of IVC or

TABLE 21.2 Differences between the smooth and rough parts of the right atrium

Smooth part (sinus venarum)	Rough part (atrium proper)
Developmentally, it is derived from the right horn of the sinus venosus	Developmentally, it is derived from the primitive atrium
All the venous channels *except* anterior cardiac veins open into this part (e.g. SVC, IVC, coronary sinus, and venae cordis minimi)	Presents a series of transverse ridges, the *musculi pectinati*, which arise from the *crista terminalis* and run forward towards the auricle. The interior of the auricle presents the reticular sponge-like network of the muscular ridges

Eustachian valve. During embryonic life, this valve guides the blood of IVC to the left atrium through forearm ovale.

iii. ***Opening of coronary sinus*** between the opening of IVC and right atrioventricular orifice. It is guarded by the *valve of coronary sinus* or *Thebesian valve*.

iv. ***Openings of venae cordis minimi***: These are small veins present in the wall of all four chambers of heart which open into right atrium through small foramina.

v. ***Intervenous tubercle (of Lower):*** It is a faint projection on the posterior wall of atrium just below the opening of SVC. During embryonic life, it directs the blood of SVC to the right ventricle.

(b) **Rough anterior part**: It is derived from primitive atrial chamber and presents the following features:

i. ***Crista terminalis***, a smooth muscular ridge that extends from SVC above to the IVC below. Externally it corresponds to **sulcus terminalis**.

ii. ***Musculi pectinati***: These are transverse muscular ridges which arise from crista terminalis and run forwards and downwards towards the right atrioventricular orifice, giving the appearance of the teeth of a comb.

iii. ***Reticular network in the auricle*** formed by the interconnection of muscular ridges.

(c) **Septal wall of the right atrium**, that is right surface of interatrial septum: Developmentally, it is derived from the septum primum and septum secundum; and presents the following features:

i. ***Fossa ovalis***, a shallow oval/saucer-shaped depression in the lower part, formed by the septum primum. It represents the site of the foramen ovale in the foetus.

ii. ***Annulus ovalis/limbus fossa ovalis*** forms the distinct upper and lateral margin of the fossa ovalis. It represents the free edge of the *septum secundum*. Inferiorly, the annulus ovalis is continuous with the left end of the valve of IVC.

iii. ***Triangle of Koch***, a triangular area bounded in front by the base of the septal leaflet of the tricuspid valve, behind by anterior margin of the opening of the coronary sinus and above by the tendon of Todaro—a subendocardial ridge. The AV node lies in the apex of triangle (Fig. 21.10, inset).

iv. ***Torus aorticus***, an elevation in the anterosuperior part of the septum produced due to bulging of the right posterior (noncoronary) sinus of the ascending aorta.

v. ***Remains of foramen*** ovale, rare.

CLINICAL CORRELATION

The sponge-like interior of the **right auricle** prevents the free flow of blood and, thus, favours the **formation of the thrombus**. The thrombi may dislodge during auricular fibrillation and may cause pulmonary embolism.

N.B.

- *Opening into the right atrium:* There are a number of openings in the right atrium. These are as follows (Fig. 21.10): ***Opening of SVC, opening of IVC, opening of coronary sinus, right AV orifice (largest opening)***, **and** ***many small orifices of small veins.***
- A very small projection called intervenous tubercle (of Lower) is scarcely visible on the posterior wall of the right atrium just below the opening of SVC. During embryonic life, it directs the blood of SVC to the right ventricle.

RIGHT VENTRICLE

The right ventricle is the thick-walled triangular chamber of the heart that communicates with the right atrium through the *right AV orifice* and with the pulmonary trunk through the *pulmonary orifice*.

External Features

1. It forms the most of the *sternocostal surface* and small part of the *diaphragmatic surface* of the heart. It also forms the inferior border.
2. It is separated from the right atrium by a more or less vertical anterior part of the coronary sulcus/AV groove.

Internal Features (Fig. 21.11) **AN 22.2**

1. The interior of the right ventricle consists of two parts: (a) a large, lower rough inflowing part and (b) a small upper outflowing part, the infundibulum. The two parts are separated from each other by a muscular ridge, the supraventricular crest (infundibuloventricular crest). The differences of two parts are enumerated in Table 21.3.
2. The cavity of the right ventricle is flattened by the forward bulge of the interventricular septum. In the transverse section, it is crescent shaped (Fig. 21.13).
3. The wall of the right ventricle is thinner than that of the left ventricle (ratio 1:3).

Trabeculae Carneae of the Right Ventricular Chamber

These are muscular projections that give the ventricular chamber a sponge-like appearance.

Types of Trabeculae Carneae

Trabeculae carneae are of three types: (a) *ridges* (fixed elevations), (b) *bridges* (only ends are fixed, the central part is free), and (c) *pillars* (base is fixed to the ventricular wall and the apex is free).

Papillary muscles

These represent the pillars of the trabeculae carneae. The papillary muscles project inward. Their bases are attached to the ventricular wall and their apices are connected by thread-like fibrous cords (the chordae tendinae) to the cusps of the tricuspid valve.

There are three papillary muscles in the right ventricle: (a) anterior, (b) posterior (inferior), and (c) septal. The anterior is largest, posterior is small, and septal is usually

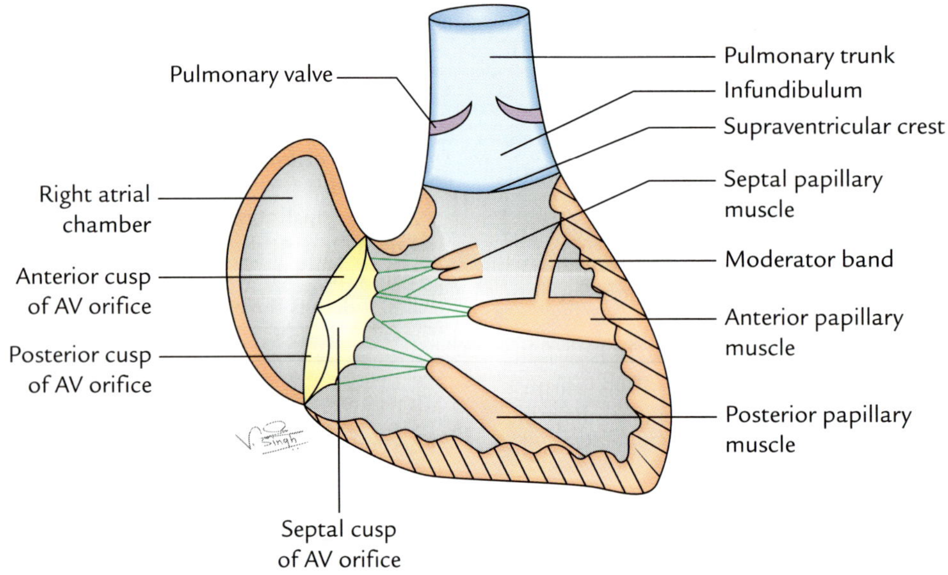

FIG. 21.11 ■ Main features in the interior of right ventricle (AV = atrioventricular).

TABLE 21.3 Differences of inflowing and outflowing parts of the right ventricle

Inflowing lower part	Outflowing upper part
It develops from the primitive ventricle	It develops from the bulbus cordis
It is large in size and lies below the supraventricular crest	It is small in size and lies above the supraventricular crest
It is rough due to the presence of the muscular ridges—the *trabeculae carneae*. It forms most of the right ventricular chamber	It is smooth and forms upper 1 in conical part of the right ventricular chamber—the infundibulum, which gives rise to the pulmonary trunk

divided into two or three nipples. The papillary muscles of the right ventricle are attached to the cusps of the tricuspid valve.

Moderator band (septomarginal trabeculum)

It is a thick muscular ridge extending from the ventricular septum to the base of the anterior papillary muscle, across the ventricular cavity. It conveys the *right branch of the AV bundle* (*bundle of His*), a part of conducting a system of the heart. It prevents the over distension of the right ventricle.

LEFT ATRIUM

External Features

1. It is a thin-walled quadrangular chamber situated posteriorly behind and to the left side of the right atrium. It forms a greater part (left two-thirds) of the base of the heart.
2. Its upper end is prolonged anteriorly to form the left auricle, which overlaps the infundibulum of the right ventricle.
3. Behind the left atrium lies: (a) an oblique sinus of the pericardial cavity and (b) the fibrous pericardium, which separates it from the oesophagus.

Internal Features

AN 22.2

1. The interior of the left atrium is smooth, but the left auricle possesses muscular ridges in the form of the reticulum.
2. The anterior wall of the left atrial cavity presents fossa lunata.

Openings in the Left Atrium

Openings in the left atrium are as follows:

1. Openings of four pulmonary veins in its posterior wall, two on each side. They have no valves.
2. Number of small openings of venae cordis minimae.
3. Left AV orifice. It is guarded by the mitral valve.

LEFT VENTRICLE

The left ventricle is a thick-walled triangular chamber of the heart that communicates with the left atrium through the *left AV orifice* and with the ascending aorta through the *aortic orifice*. The walls of the left ventricle are three times thicker than that of the right ventricle.

External Features

The left ventricle forms the (a) apex of the heart, (b) small part of the sternocostal surface, (c) most of the (left two-thirds) diaphragmatic surface, and (d) most of the left border of the heart.

Internal Features

AN 22.2

The interior of the left ventricle is divided into two parts (Fig. 21.12): (a) a large lower rough inflowing part and (b) a small upper smooth outflowing part—the aortic vestibule.

The differences between these two parts are enumerated in Table 21.4.

The cavity of the left ventricle is circular in cross section because the interventricular septum bulges into the right ventricle.

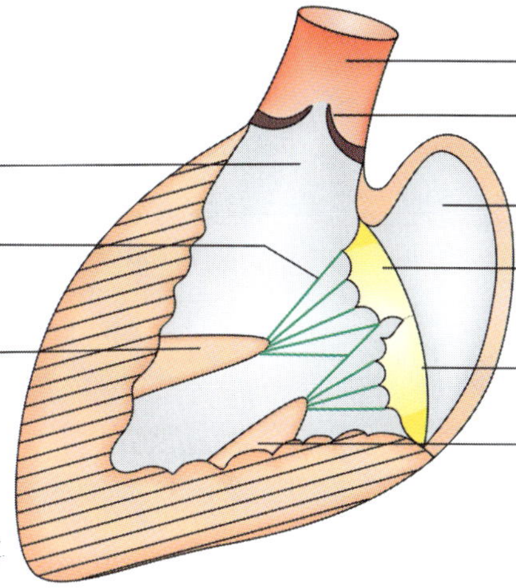

FIG. 21.12 ■ Main features in the interior of the left ventricle.

TABLE 21.4 Differences between the inflowing and outflowing parts of the left ventricle

Inflowing part	Outflowing part
It develops from the primitive ventricle	It develops from the bulbus cordis
It lies below the aortic vestibule	It lies between the membranous part of the interventricular septum and the anterior cusp of the mitral valve
It is rough due to the presence of the trabeculae carneae and forms most of the left ventricular chamber	It is smooth and forms a smooth small upper part—the aortic vestibule, which gives rise to the ascending aorta

Trabeculae Carneae of the Left Ventricle

The trabeculae carneae of the left ventricle are similar to those of the right ventricle but are well developed and present two large papillary muscles (anterior and posterior) and no moderator band. The papillary muscles of the left ventricle are attached to the cusps of the mitral valve by the *chordae tendinae*.

Openings in the Left Ventricle

The openings in the left ventricle are as follows:

1. Left AV orifice
2. Aortic orifice

The main features as seen in the transverse section through the ventricles are shown in Fig. 21.13.

The main differences between the right and left ventricles are listed in Table 21.5.

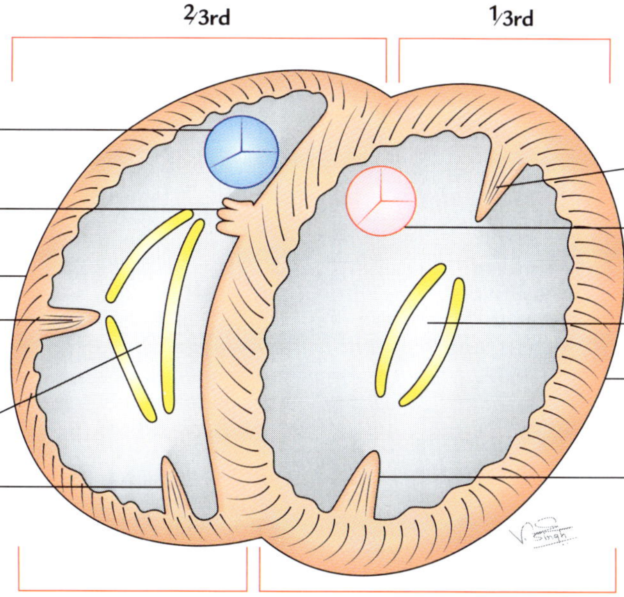

FIG. 21.13 ■ Transverse section across the ventricles of the heart. Note the difference in the thickness of the wall and shape of the right and left ventricular cavities.

TABLE 21.5 Differences between the right and left ventricles

Right ventricle	Left ventricle
Receives deoxygenated blood from the right atrium and pumps it to the lungs through the pulmonary trunk	Receives oxygenated blood from the left atrium and pumps it to the whole body through the aorta
Wall of the right ventricle is thinner than that of the left ventricle (ratio 1:3)	Wall of the left ventricle is thicker than that of the right ventricle (ratio 3:1)
Possesses three papillary muscles (anterior, posterior, and septal)	Possesses two papillary muscles (anterior and posterior)
Moderator band present	Moderator band absent
Cavity of the right ventricle is crescentic in shape in the cross section	Cavity of the left ventricle is circular in shape in the cross section

VALVES OF THE HEART

There are two pairs of valves in the heart (Fig. 21.14): (a) a pair of AV valves and (b) a pair of semilunar valves.

The valves prevent regurgitation of the blood.

ATRIOVENTRICULAR VALVES

The right and left atria communicate with the right and left ventricles through the right and left AV orifices, respectively. The right and left AV orifices are guarded by the right and left AV valves, respectively.

- **Right AV valve (also known as the tricuspid valve):** As the name indicates, it has three cusps—anterior, posterior, and septal which lie against the three walls of the ventricle. The tricuspid orifice can admit the tips of three fingers.
- **Left AV valve (also known as the bicuspid/mitral valve)**: As the name indicates, it has two cusps—a larger anterior/aortic cusp and a smaller posterior cusp. The mitral/bicuspid orifice can admit the tips of two fingers.

Structure

The AV valves are made up of two components (Fig. 21.15):

1. A fibrous ring
2. Cusps

The fibrous rings surround the orifice. The cusps are formed by the fold of the endocardium, enclosing some connective tissue within it. Each cusp has an attached and free margin and atrial and ventricular surfaces. The atrial surfaces are smooth. The ventricular surfaces and free margins are rough and provide attachment to the chordae tendinae. As discussed earlier, the chordae tendinae connect the apices of papillary muscles with margins and ventricular surfaces of the cusps. *The chordae tendinae of each papillary muscle are attached to the contiguous halves of the two cusps.*

The valves are closed during ventricular systole. The papillary muscles shorten and chordae tendinae are pulled upon to prevent the eversion of the cusps of the A. V. valves due to the increased intraventricular pressure.

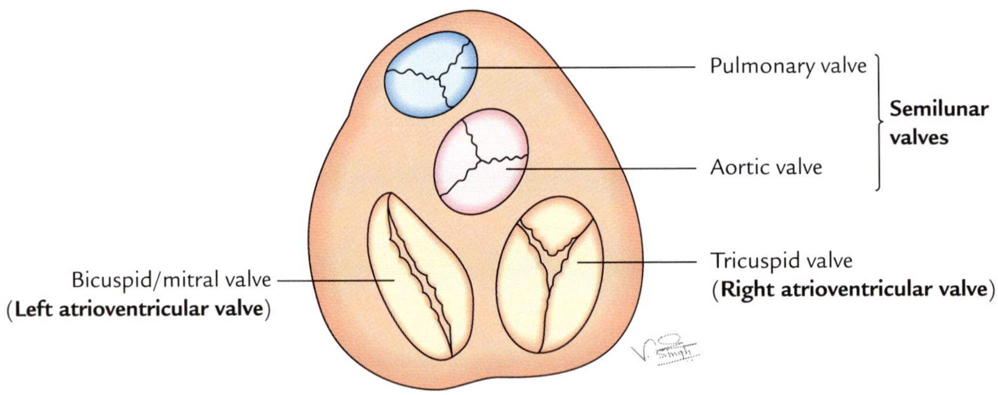

FIG. 21.14 ■ The valves of the heart.

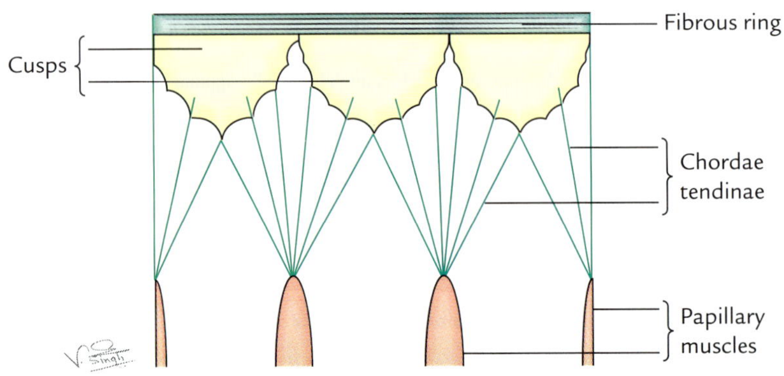

FIG. 21.15 ■ Right atrioventricular (tricuspid) valve spread out to show its structure.

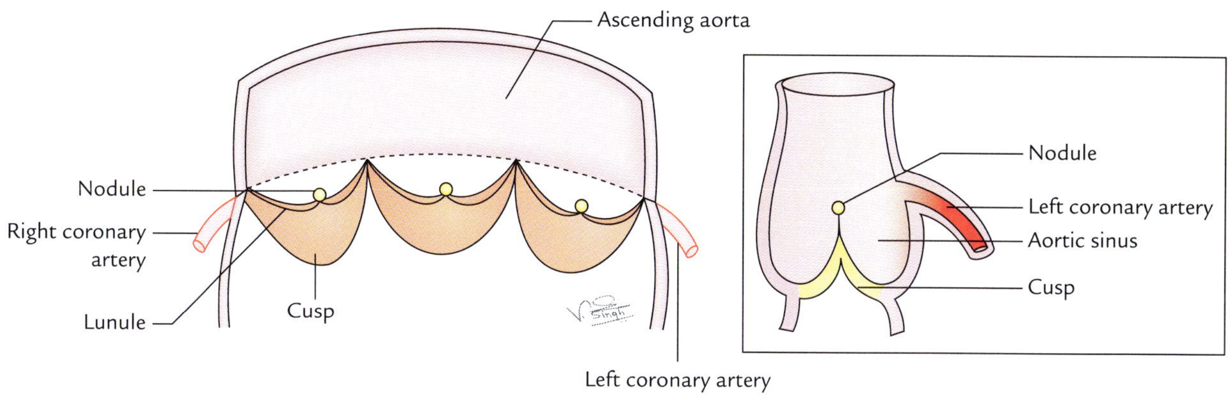

FIG. 21.16 ■ Structure of the aortic valve. Note that it consists of three semilunar cusps. Each cusp has a fibrous nodule at the midpoint of its free edge. The thickened crescentic edge on each side of nodule is the lunule (L. luna = moon). The inset on the right side shows the aortic sinus and the origin of the coronary artery.

N.B.

- The nutrition to the fibrous ring and basal one-third of cusps is provided by the blood vessels.
- The nutrition to the distal two-thirds of the cusps is provided directly by the blood within the chambers of the heart.
- The cusps of the mitral valve are smaller but thicker than those of the tricuspid valve.

CLINICAL CORRELATION

Role of the papillary muscles in acute cardiac failure: The papillary muscles prevent the prolapse of AV valves into the atria during ventricular systole. The rupture of a papillary muscle, following an adjacent myocardial infarction (MI), will allow the prolapse of the affected cusp to occur into the atrium at each systole. This will consequently lead to **acute cardiac failure**.

SEMILUNAR VALVES

The right and left ventricles pump out blood through the pulmonary and aortic orifices, respectively. Each of these orifices is guarded by three semilunar cusps; hence, they are called the *semilunar valves* (Fig. 21.16). Both aortic and pulmonary valves are similar to each other in structure and functions.

Each valve has three cusps that are attached directly to the wall of the aorta/pulmonary trunk.

The cusps form small pockets with their mouths directed upward towards the lumen of great vessels. Each cusp has a fibrous nodule at the midpoint of its free edge. On each side of the nodule, the thickened crescentic edge is called the lunule that extends up to the base. When the valve is closed, the nodules meet in the centre.

The cusps of semilunar valves are open and stretched during ventricular systole and closed during ventricular diastole to prevent the regurgitation of the blood into the ventricle.

N.B.

- No chordae tendinae or papillary muscles are associated with semilunar valves. The attachment of the sides of cusps to the arterial (aortic or pulmonary) wall prevents the regurgitation of blood.
- Opposite to the cusps, the roots of the pulmonary trunk and ascending aorta present three dilatations called sinuses. The blood in these sinuses prevents the cusps from sticking to the wall of great vessels. The anterior aortic sinus gives origin to the right coronary artery and left posterior aortic sinus gives origin to the left coronary artery.

Positions of Cusps in the Pulmonary and Aortic Valves

The positions of cusps of pulmonary valves are: (a) right anterior, (b) left anterior, and (c) posterior.

The positions of cusps of the aortic valve are just opposite to those of the pulmonary valve. They are: (a) right posterior, (b) left posterior, and (c) anterior.

The aortic sinuses are also named accordingly, that is right posterior aortic sinus, left posterior aortic sinus, and anterior aortic sinus. The right coronary artery arises from the anterior aortic sinus and left coronary from the left posterior aortic sinus. Since no coronary artery arises from the right posterior aortic sinus, it is referred to by some anatomists as *noncoronary sinus*.

N.B.

Embryologically, the **pulmonary valve** has anterior, right and left cusps, whereas the **aortic valve** has posterior, right and left cusps (Fig. 21.17). Thus, the left coronary artery arises from the left aortic sinus, the right coronary artery from the right aortic sinus, and no artery arises from the posterior aortic sinus (noncoronary sinus).

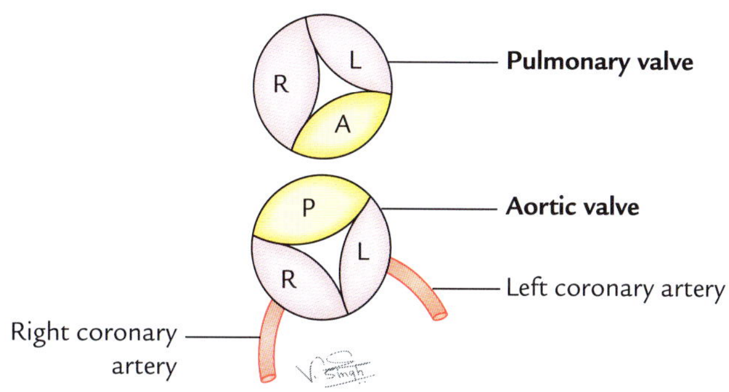

FIG. 21.17 ■ Embryological position of cusps in the pulmonary and aortic valves (P = posterior, A = anterior, R = right, L = left).

CLINICAL CORRELATION

- **Murmurs:** The abnormal heart sounds are called murmurs. They are produced due to the regurgitation of blood heard when the valves are either stenosed or when the valves are not closed properly (leading to regurgitation).
  - In aortic and pulmonary stenosis, the murmur is heard during systole and in insufficiency of these valves they are heard during diastole.
  - In stenosis of mitral and tricuspid valves, the murmurs are heard during diastole and in their insufficiency during systole.
- **Mitral stenosis (narrowing of mitral orifice):** It is most common in young age. Usually, there is a *history* of rheumatic fever in the childhood in these cases. This leads to the rise in the left atrial pressure and enlargement of the left atrium, which may press on the oesophagus.

  Clinically, the features of mitral stenosis will be as follows:
  1. Shortness of breath (dyspnoea)
  2. Dysphagia (difficulty in swallowing)
  3. Hoarseness of voice (Ortner's syndrome)
- **Tricuspid stenosis:** In tricuspid stenosis, blood flow from the right atrium to the right ventricle is reduced. *The* elevation of the right atrial pressure leads to systemic venous congestion and right heart failure.
- **Aortic stenosis:** In aortic stenosis, the accumulation of blood in the left ventricle causes its *dilatation* and hypertrophy. There is low cardiac output which may manifest as syncope (fainting) on exertion.
- **Pulmonary stenosis:** It is almost always congenital, usually a part of Fallot's tetralogy. It leads to the hypertrophy of the right ventricle.

HEART SOUNDS

The two sounds are produced by the heart: the first heart sound is produced by the closure of the AV (tricuspid and mitral) valves and the second heart sound is produced by the closure of the semilunar (aortic and pulmonary) valves. These sounds are heard by the clinicians by auscultation with a stethoscope. The first and second heart sounds are heard as 'LUB' and 'DUB', respectively.

SURFACE MARKINGS OF THE CARDIAC VALVES AND AUSCULTATORY AREAS

The sounds produced by the closure of valves of the heart are best heard not directly over the location of the valve but at areas situated some distance away from the valve in the direction of blood flow through them.

The pulmonary, aortic, mitral, and tricuspid valves are located posterior to the sternum on an oblique line joining the third left costal cartilage to the sixth right costal cartilage (Fig. 21.18).

The position of valves on the surface of the chest and sites of their auscultatory areas are given in Table 21.6 and shown in Fig. 21.18.

N.B.

Blood tends to carry the sound in the direction of its flow; consequently, the auscultatory area is located superficial to the vessel or chamber through which the blood passes and is in direct line with the valve orifice.

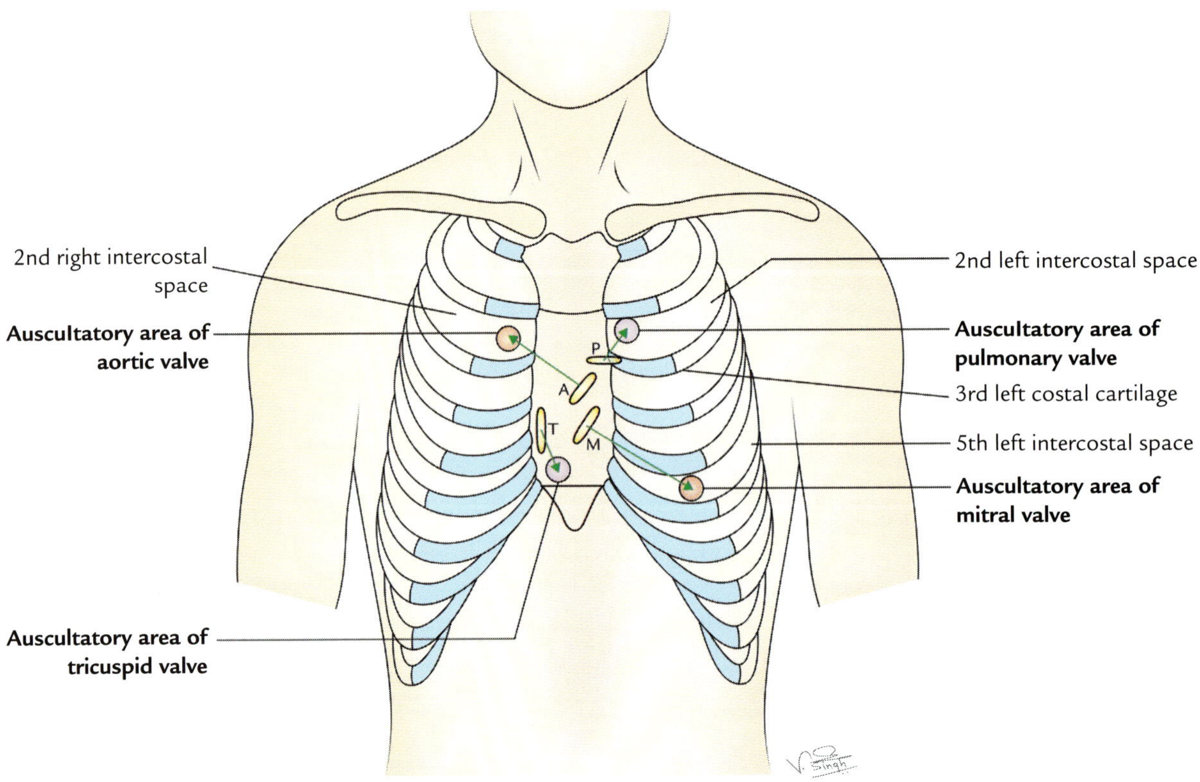

FIG. 21.18 ■ Surface projection of cardiac valves and sites of their auscultatory areas (P = pulmonary valve, A = aortic valve, T = tricuspid valve, M = mitral valve).

TABLE 21.6 Surface markings of the cardiac valves and the sites of their auscultatory areas

Valve	Surface marking	Site of auscultatory area
Pulmonary valve	A horizontal line (2.5 cm long) behind the medial end left third costal cartilage and adjoining part of the sternum	Second left intercostal space near the sternum
Aortic valve	A lightly oblique line (2.5 cm long) behind the left half of the sternum opposite to the third intercostal space	Second right intercostal space near the sternum
Mitral valve	An oblique line (3 cm long) behind the left half of the sternum opposite to the left fourth costal cartilage	Left fifth intercostal space 31/2 in (9 cm) from the midline, that is over the apex beat
Tricuspid valve	Nearly vertical oblique line (4 cm long) behind the right half of the sternum opposite the fourth and fifth intercostal spaces	Right half of the lower end of the body of the sternum

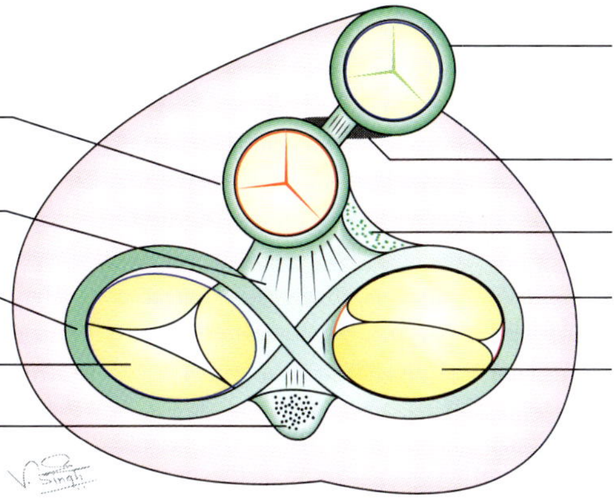

FIG. 21.19 Skeleton of the heart.

FIBROUS SKELETON/SKELETON OF THE HEART **AN 22.6**

The so called '***skeleton of the heart***' is composed of fibrous tissue which anchors the valves of the heart and gives attachment to myocardium of the heart (Fig. 21.19). It consists of 4 fibrous rings. These fibrous rings surround the AV, pulmonary, and aortic orifices. These rings provide a circular form and rigidity to the AV orifices and roots of the aorta and pulmonary trunk. They also provide attachment to the valves and prevent dilatation of these orifices. The cardiac valves are firmly attached to this skeleton. The cardiac skeleton along with the membranous part of the interventricular septum also provides attachments to the cardiac muscle fibres.

The two fibrous rings around the AV orifices separate the muscle fibres of the atria from those of the ventricles, but provide attachment to these fibres. Thus, there is no muscular continuity between the atria and ventricles, except for the atrio-ventricular bundle (bundle of His) of the conducting system.

Functional significance:

1. The skeleton of the heart allows the controlled contraction of heart, i.e. allows the cardiac muscle to contract against the rigid base.
2. The fibrous rings support the bases of the cusps of the valves and prevent the valves from stretching and becoming incompetent. The aortic ring is the strongest.

N.B.

- The AV fibrous rings (AV rings) form the figure of '8'.
- The large mass of the fibrous tissue between AV rings and aortic ring is called the *trigonum fibrosum dextrum*. In some mammals such as sheep and elephant, a bone—the *os cordis*—develops in it.
- The small mass of the fibrous tissue between the fibrous rings around semilunar valves is called the *trigonum fibrosum sinistrum*.
- The tendon of the infundibulum binds the posterior surface of the infundibulum to the aortic ring.

CONDUCTING SYSTEM OF THE HEART **AN 22.7**

COMPONENTS

The conducting system of the heart is made up of specialized cardiac muscle fibres (not the nervous tissue) and is responsible for the initiation and conduction of cardiac impulses (Fig. 21.20). They initiate normal cardiac cycle and coordinate the contraction of heart chambers.

The conducting system of the heart consists of the following five components:

1. SA node
2. AV node
3. AV bundle (of His)
4. Right and left branches of the bundle of His
5. Purkinje fibres

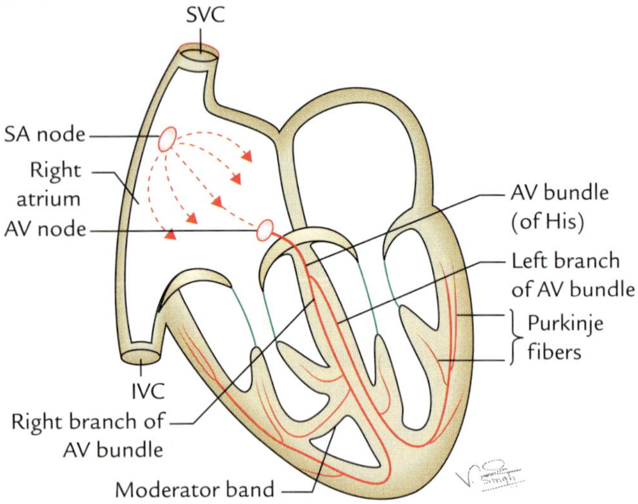

FIG. 21.20 ■ Conducting system of the heart (SA = sinuatrial, AV = atrioventricular).

LOCATION

SA node or the node of Keith Flack: It is a small horseshoe-shaped mass having specialized myocardial fibres, situated in the wall of the right atrium in the upper part of the sulcus terminalis just below the opening of SVC.

It is also known as the **'pacemaker of the heart'** because it generates impulses (about 70–100 beats/min) and initiates the contraction of the cardiac muscle producing the heartbeat.

N.B.

Autonomic nerve fibres controls the firing of SA node.

AV node (node of Tawara): It is smaller than the SA node and is located in the lower part of the atrial septum, just above the attachment of the septal cusp of the tricuspid valve/opening of the coronary sinus. It conducts the *cardiac impulse* to the ventricles by the *AV bundle*. The AV node is capable of generating impulses at the rate of about 40–60 beats/min. The speed of conduction of the cardiac impulse is slowed at AV node before they pass to ventricles (about 0.11 s). This provides sufficient time to the atria to empty their blood into the ventricles before they start contracting.

AV bundle (of His): It begins from the AV node, crosses the AV ring, and runs along the inferior part of the membranous part of the interventricular septum where it divides into the left and right branches.

N.B.

Since the skeleton (fibrous framework) of the heart separates the muscles of the atria from the muscles of the ventricles, the bundle of His is the only means of conducting impulses from the atria to the ventricles.

Right and left branches of the bundle (of His): The *right branch* passes down the right side of the interventricular septum and then becomes subendocardial on the right side of the septum. A large part of it continues in the septomarginal trabeculum (**moderator band**) to reach the anterior papillary muscle and anterior wall of the ventricle. Its Purkinje fibres then spread out beneath the endocardium.

The *left branch* descends on the left side of the ventricular septum, divides into Purkinje fibres that are distributed to the septum and left ventricle.

Purkinje fibres: They are the terminal branches of the right and left branches of the bundle of His and spread subendocardially over the septum and the rest of the ventricular wall.

ARTERIAL SUPPLY OF THE CONDUCTING SYSTEM AN 22.7

The whole of the conducting system of the heart is supplied by the right coronary artery except a part of the left branch of the AV bundle that is supplied by the left coronary artery.

Summary

The conducting system and mode of contraction of the cardiac muscle are summarized as follows:

The SA node (a spontaneous source of cardiac impulse) initiates an impulse that rapidly spreads to the muscle fibres of the atria, making them to contract. The AV node picks up the cardiac impulse from the atria and conducts it through the AV bundle and its branches to the papillary muscles and the walls of the ventricles. The papillary muscles contract first to tighten the chordae tendinae, and then the contraction of the ventricular muscle occurs to pump the blood.

CLINICAL CORRELATION

Conducting system defects: The defect/damage of the conducting system causes cardiac arrhythmias.

The SA node is the spontaneous source of generation of cardiac impulses. The AV node picks up these impulses from the atria and sends them to the ventricles through the AV bundle, the only means through which impulses can spread from the atria to ventricles.

If the AV bundle fails to conduct normal impulses, there occurs alteration in the rhythmic contraction of the ventricles (arrhythmias). If a complete bundle block occurs, there is complete dissociation in the rate of contraction of atria and ventricles. The most common cause of defective conduction through the AV bundle is atherosclerosis of the coronary arteries that leads to diminished blood supply to the conducting system.

N.B.

The rapid pulse is called **tachycardia**, the slow pulse is called **bradycardia**, whereas the irregular pulse is called **arrhythmia**.

ARTERIAL SUPPLY OF THE HEART AN 22.3

The heart is mostly supplied by the two coronary arteries called **right and left coronary arteries**. They arise from the ascending aorta immediately above the aortic valve (Fig. 21.21).

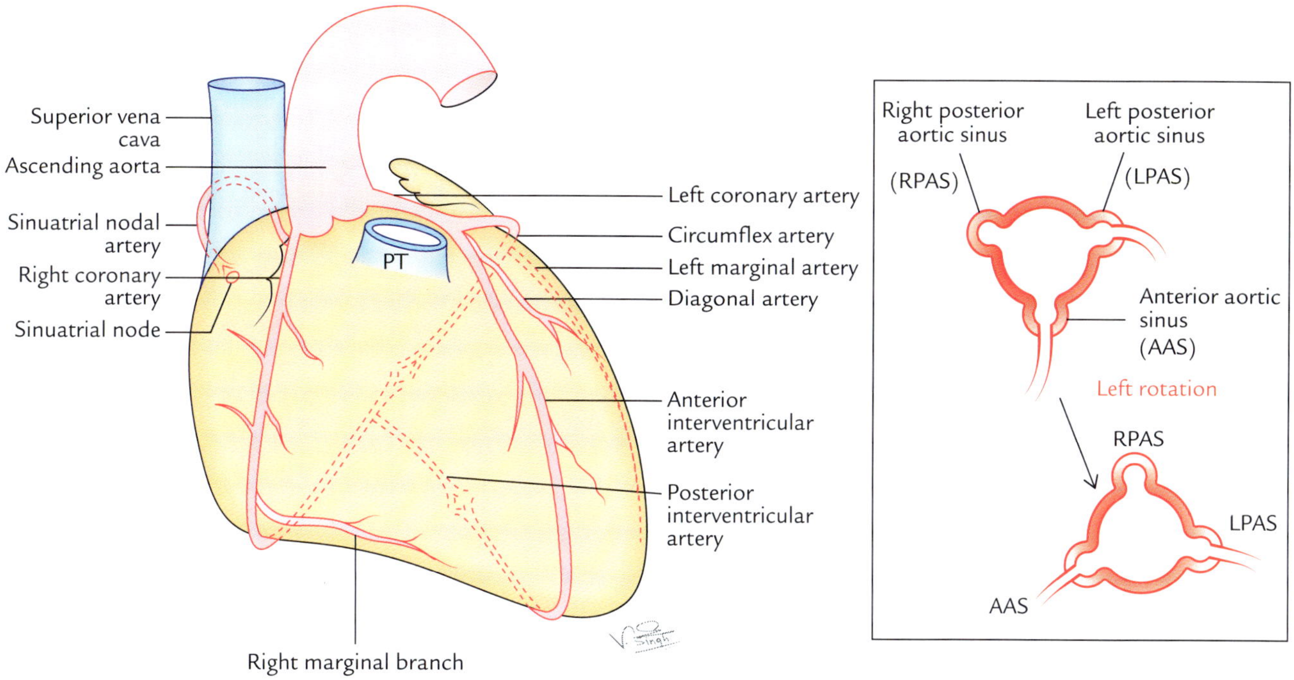

FIG. 21.21 Arterial supply of the heart (PT = pulmonary trunk). Figure in the inset on the right shows location of aortic sinuses (sinuses of Valsalva) before and after rotation; and origin of coronary arteries.

The coronary arteries and their branches run on the surface of the heart lying within the subpericardial fibrofatty tissue.

- Coronary arteries are the *vasa vasorum* of the heart.
- Anatomically, coronary arteries are not end arteries but functionally they behave like end arteries.

N.B.

Third coronary artery: It is an accessory coronary artery in about 10%–20% cases and arises directly from anterior aortic sinus.

RIGHT CORONARY ARTERY

AN 22.3

Origin

The right coronary artery arises from the *anterior aortic sinus* of the ascending aorta, immediately above the aortic valve.

Course

After arising from the ascending aorta, the right coronary artery first runs forward between the pulmonary trunk and the right auricle, and then it descends almost vertically in the right AV groove (right anterior coronary sulcus) up to the junction of the right and the inferior borders of the heart. At the inferior border of the heart, it turns posteriorly and runs in the posterior AV groove (right posterior coronary sulcus) up to the posterior interventricular groove where it terminates by anastomosing with the left coronary artery.

Branches and Distribution

1. **Right conus artery:** It supplies the anterior surface of the pulmonary conus (infundibulum of the right ventricle).
2. **Atrial branches:** They supply the atria. One of the atrial branches—the *artery of SA node* (also called *sinuatrial nodal artery*) supplies the SA node in 60% cases. In 40% of individuals, it arises from the left coronary artery.
3. **Anterior ventricular branches:** They are two or three and supply the anterior surface of the right ventricle. The *marginal branch* is the largest and runs along the lower margin of the sternocostal surface to reach the apex.
4. **Posterior ventricular branches:** They are usually two and supply the diaphragmatic surface of the right ventricle.
5. **Posterior interventricular artery:** It runs in the posterior interventricular groove up to the apex. It supplies the:
   a. Posterior part of the interventricular septum
   b. AV node in 60% of the cases, and
   c. Right and left ventricles.

N.B.

In 10% individuals, the posterior interventricular artery arises from the left coronary artery.

LEFT CORONARY ARTERY

AN 22.3

Origin

The left coronary artery arises from the *left posterior aortic sinus* of the ascending aorta, immediately above the aortic valve. It is larger than the right coronary artery.

Course

After arising from the ascending aorta, the left coronary artery runs forward and to the left between the pulmonary trunk and the left auricle. It then divides into an anterior interventricular and circumflex artery. The anterior interventricular artery (left anterior descending/LAD) runs downward in the anterior interventricular groove to the apex of the heart. It then passes posteriorly around the apex of the heart to enter the posterior interventricular groove to terminate by anastomosing with the posterior interventricular artery—a branch of the right coronary artery.

The circumflex artery winds around the left margin of the heart and continues in the left posterior coronary sulcus up to the posterior interventricular groove where it terminates by anastomosing with the right coronary artery.

Branches and Distribution

1. **Anterior interventricular artery/left anterior descending (LAD) artery:** It supplies (a) an anterior part of the interventricular septum, (b) a greater part of the left ventricle and part of the right ventricle, and (c) a part of the left bundle branch (of His).
2. **Circumflex artery:** It gives a *left marginal artery* that supplies the left margin of the left ventricle up to the apex of the heart.
3. **Diagonal artery:** It may arise directly from the trunk of the left coronary artery.
4. **Conus artery:** It supplies the pulmonary conus.
5. **Atrial branches:** They supply the left atrium.

The major branches of the right and left coronary arteries are summarized in Table 21.7.

N.B.

Clinically there are four main coronary arteries:

1. Right coronary artery
2. Left main coronary artery
3. Left circumflex artery
4. Left anterior descending artery

TABLE 21.7 Major branches of the right and left coronary arteries

Right coronary artery	Left coronary artery
Right marginal artery	Anterior interventricular artery
Posterior interventricular artery	Circumflex artery
Sinuatrial nodal artery	Diagonal artery

CORONARY DOMINANCE

The origin, course, and distribution of the posterior interventricular artery are variable.

If posterior interventricular artery arises from right coronary artery, it is called *right coronary dominance*. On the other hand, if posterior interventricular artery arises from circumflex branch of left coronary artery, then it is called *left coronary dominance*.

In right coronary dominance, the posterior interventricular artery is a branch of the right coronary artery. It is found in 90% of the individuals.

In left coronary dominance, the posterior interventricular artery arises from the circumflex branch of the left coronary artery. It is found in 10% of the individuals.

Anastomoses of the Coronary Arteries

Anastomoses exist between the terminal branches of the coronary arteries at the arteriolar level (collateral circulation). The time factor in occlusion of an artery is very important. If occlusion occurs slowly, there is time for the healthy arterioles to open up and collateral circulation is established, that is the anastomoses become functional. But if the sudden occlusion of one of the large branches (coronary artery) occurs, the arterioles do not get time to open up to provide collateral circulation.

CLINICAL CORRELATION

AN 22.4

- **Ischaemic heart disease**
  a) ***Angina pectoris:*** If the coronary arteries are narrowed, the blood supply to the cardiac muscles is reduced. As a result, on exertion, the patient feels moderately severe pain in the region of the left precordium that may last as long as 20 min. The pain is often referred to the left shoulder and the medial side of the left arm and the forearm.

  In angina pectoris, pain occurs on exertion and relieved by rest. This is because the coronary arteries are so narrowed that the ischaemia of the cardiac muscle occurs only on exertion.

  b) ***Myocardial infarction (MI):*** A sudden block (thrombosis) of coronary artery or one of its larger branches usually leads to the myocardial ischaemia followed by the myocardial necrosis (**myocardial infarction**). The part of the heart suffering from MI stops functioning and often causes death. This condition is termed *heart attack* or *coronary attack*. It is common cause of sudden death after 50 years of age.

  The clinical features of MI are as follows:

  1. A sensation of pressure/sinking and pain in the chest that lasts longer than 30 min.
  2. Nausea or vomiting, sweating, shortness of breath, and tachycardia.
  3. Pain radiates to the medial side of the arm, forearm, and hand. Sometimes, it may be referred to the jaw or the neck.

  c) **Common sites of coronary artery occlusion:** The three most common sites of the coronary artery occlusion are as follows:

  (a) **Anterior interventricular artery/LAD artery** = 40%–50%.
  (b) **Right coronary artery** = 30%–40%.
  (c) **Circumflex branch of the left coronary artery** = 15%–20%.

N.B.

- Anterior interventricular artery/LAD artery is most commonly blocked.
- The MI mostly occurs at rest, whereas angina occurs on exertion.

- **Widow maker's artery:** Left anterior descending artery (LAD) supplies most area of the heart (left ventricle). Its blockage often leads to death, hence it is also called as **widow maker's artery**.
- **Coronary angiography:** The coronary angiography is a radiological procedure to visualize the coronary arteries

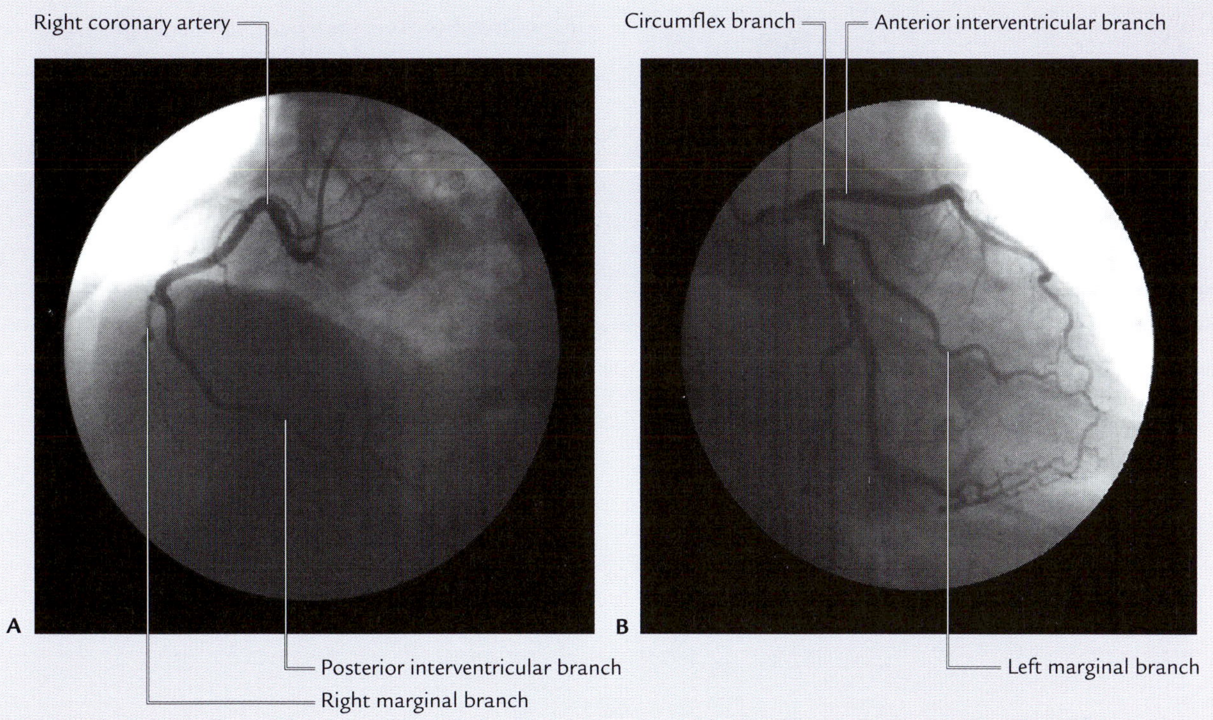

FIG. 21.22 ■ Normal coronary angiogram. (**A**) Of the right coronary artery (left anterior oblique view) and (**B**) of the left coronary artery (right anterior oblique view).

after injecting contrast medium in their lumen (Fig. 21.22). The coronary angiography is useful in localizing the site/sites of the blockage in the coronary arteries.

- **Coronary bypass surgery:** The coronary bypass surgery has become common in recent times in patients with unstable/severe angina due to the obstruction of the coronary artery. A segment of a vein or an artery is connected to the ascending aorta (or to the proximal part of the coronary artery) and then to the coronary artery distal to the obstruction (Fig. 21.23). A coronary bypass graft shunts blood from the aorta to the coronary artery distal to the blockage to increase the circulation.

N.B.

- The great saphenous vein is commonly used for grafting because (a) it is easily dissected, (b) it has diameter equal to or greater than that of the coronary artery, and (c) it provides lengthy portions with a minimum occurrence of valves or branching.
- The use of the left internal mammary artery graft (LIMA graft) and radial artery graft (RA graft) has also become increasingly common.

- **Coronary angioplasty:** In this process, the cardiologists pass a stent (a small catheter with a small inflatable balloon attached to its tip) into the obstructed coronary artery. As the catheter reaches the obstruction, the balloon in inflated. As a result, an atherosclerotic plaque is flattened against the vessel wall and the vessel is stretched to increase the lumen. Consequently, the blood flow is increased. Sometimes transluminal instruments with rotating blades and lasers are used to cut the clot. After the artery is dilated, an *intravascular stent* is introduced to maintain the dilatation.

  It is done to remove the small blockage. However, if there is blockage of large segment or at multiple sites, the **coronary bypass surgery** is done.

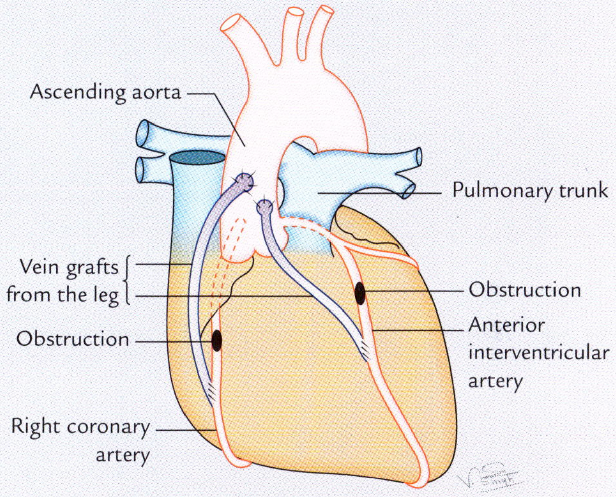

FIG. 21.23 ■ Double coronary artery bypass.

VENOUS DRAINAGE OF THE HEART **AN 22.5**

Venous blood from the heart is drained into the right atrium by the following (Fig. 21.24):

1. Coronary sinus
2. Anterior cardiac veins
3. Venae cordis minimae (Thebesian veins)

Coronary sinus: It is the principal vein of the heart. Most of the venous blood from the walls of the heart is drained into the right atrium through the coronary sinus. The coronary sinus is the largest vein of the heart and lies in the posterior part of the AV groove (left posterior coronary sulcus). *It develops from the left*

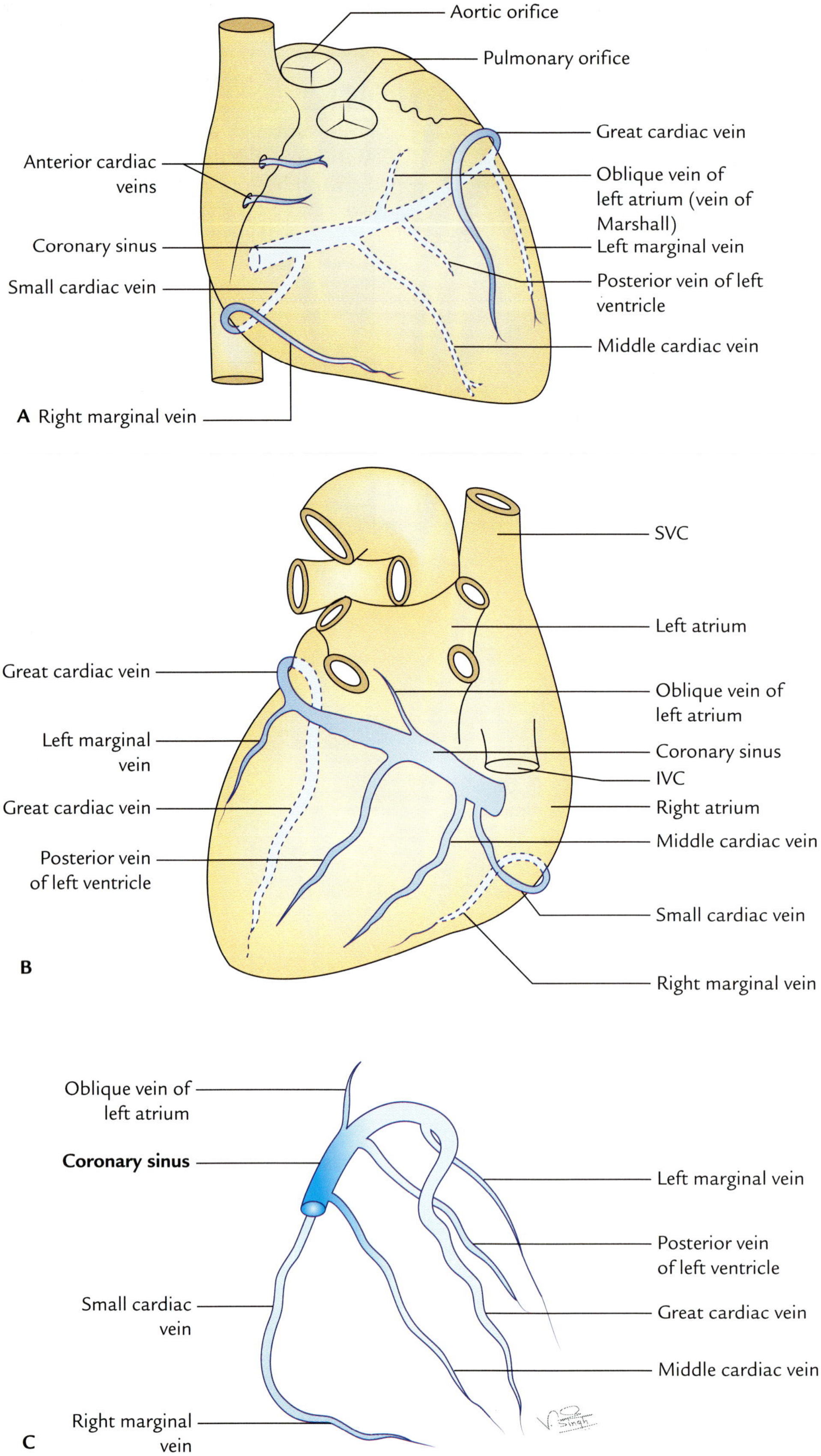

FIG. 21.24 ■ Veins of the heart. (**A**) An anterior view of the heart showing cardiac veins, (**B**) a posteroinferior view of the heart showing the cardiac veins, and (**C**) tributaries of the coronary sinus viewed from the front.

horn of the sinus venosus and a part of the left common cardinal vein.

Tributaries: The coronary sinus receives the following tributaries (Fig. 21.24A–C):

1. **Great cardiac vein:** It begins at apex of heart. Then accompanies the anterior interventricular and circumflex arteries to join the left end of the coronary sinus.
2. **Middle cardiac vein:** It accompanies the posterior interventricular artery and joins the coronary sinus near its termination.
3. **Small cardiac vein:** It accompanies the right ventricular artery in the right posterior coronary sulcus and the right end of the coronary sinus.
4. **Posterior vein of the left ventricle:** It runs on the diaphragmatic surface of the left ventricle and joins the sinus to the left of the middle cardiac vein.
5. **Oblique vein of the left atrium (vein of Marshall):** It is a small vein that runs downward on the posterior surface of the left atrium to enter the left end of the coronary sinus. It develops from the left common cardinal vein (duct of Cuvier).
6. **Right marginal vein:** It accompanies the marginal branch of the right coronary artery and joins the small cardiac vein or drains directly into the right atrium.
7. **Left marginal vein:** It accompanies the marginal branch of the left coronary artery and drains into the coronary sinus.

Anterior cardiac veins: These are series of small veins (three or four in number) which run parallel to each other across the surface of the right ventricle to open into the right atrium.

Venae cordis minimae (Thebesian veins): These are extremely small veins in the walls of all the four chambers of the heart. They open directly into the respective chambers. They are most numerous in the right atrium.

LYMPHATIC DRAINAGE OF THE HEART

The lymphatics of the heart accompany the coronary arteries, emerge from the fibrous pericardium along with the ascending aorta and pulmonary trunk in the form of two trunks. The **right trunk** drains into brachiocephalic nodes and the **left trunk** drains into tracheobronchial nodes (at the bifurcation of the aorta).

NERVE SUPPLY OF THE HEART

The heart is supplied by the sympathetic and parasympathetic fibres via the superficial and deep cardiac plexuses formed by the parasympathetic and sympathetic fibres.

The parasympathetic fibres are derived from the vagus nerves. They are *cardioinhibitory*; hence, their stimulation causes slowing of the heart rate and constriction of the coronary arteries.

The sympathetic fibres are derived from upper three to five thoracic spinal segments. They are *cardioacceleratory*; hence, their stimulation increases the heart rate and causes the dilatation of the coronary arteries. The sympathetic fibres also cause the dilatation of the coronary arteries.

A brief account of the formation and distribution of cardiac plexuses is given in the following section.

CARDIAC PLEXUSES

Superficial Cardiac Plexus

The superficial cardiac plexus (Fig. 21.25) lies below the arch of the aorta in front of the bifurcation of the pulmonary trunk, just to the right of the ligamentum arteriosum.

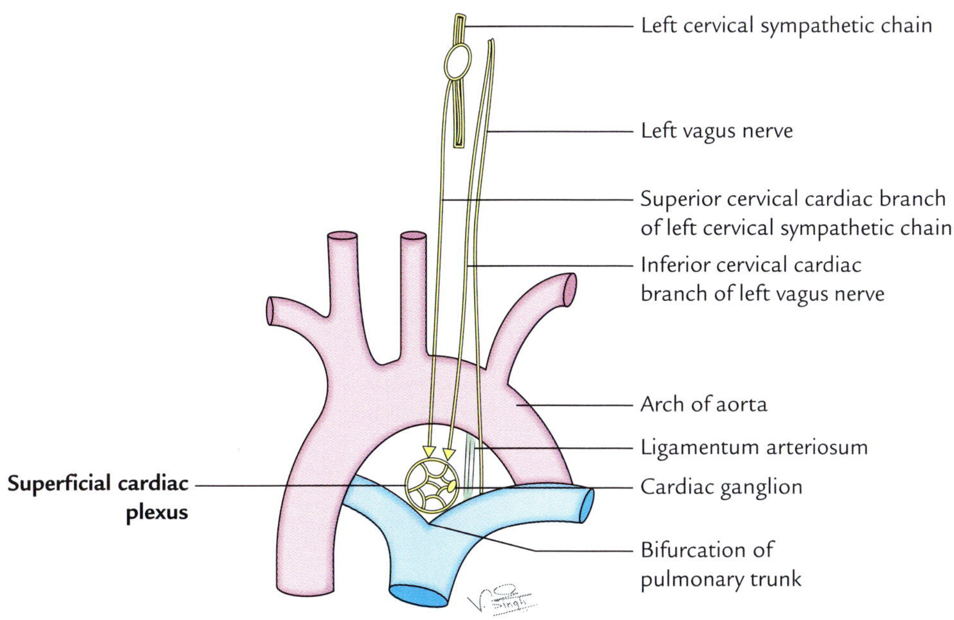

FIG. 21.25 ■ Superficial cardiac plexus.

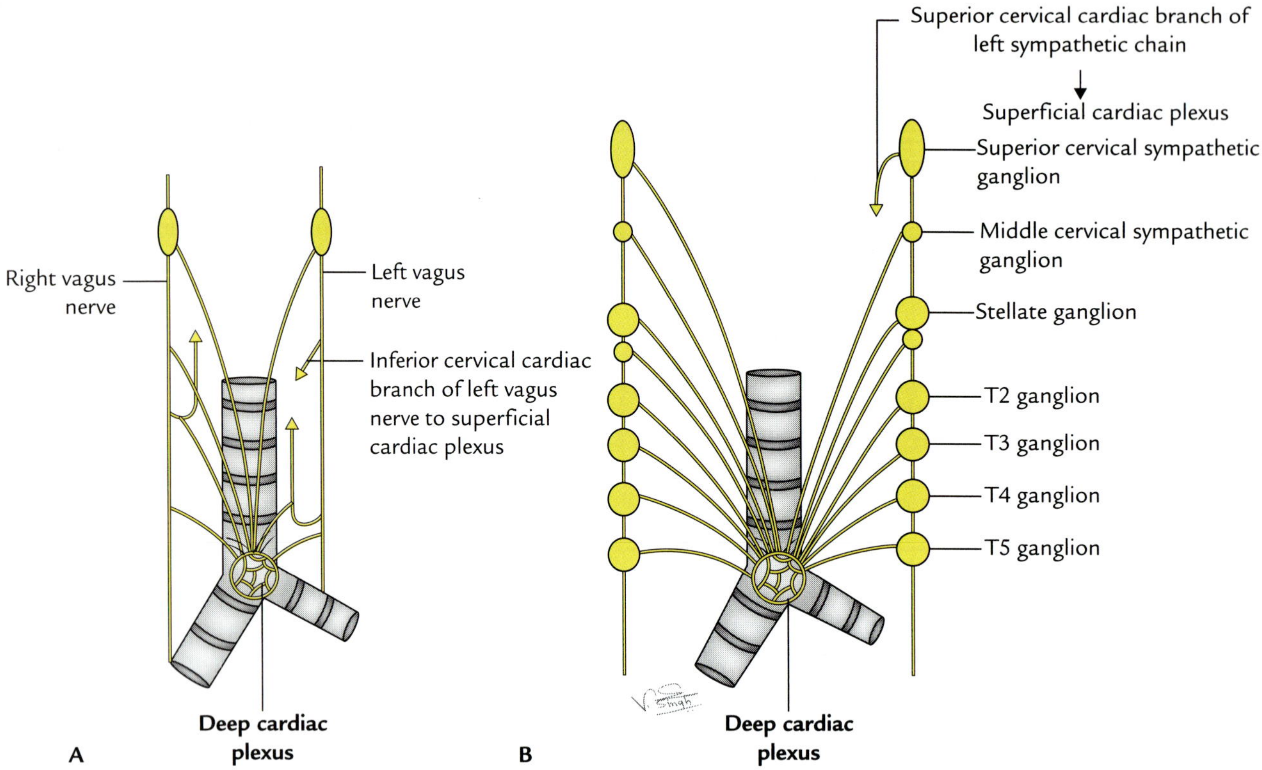

FIG. 21.26 ■ Deep cardiac plexus. (**A**) Parasympathetic contribution and (**B**) sympathetic contribution.

The cardiac ganglion (of Wrisberg) lies close to the ligamentum arteriosum.

It is formed by the:

(a) Superior cervical cardiac branch of the left cervical sympathetic trunk and
(b) Inferior cervical cardiac branch of the left vagus nerve.

Distribution

The superficial cardiac plexus gives branches to (a) the deep cardiac plexus, (b) right coronary artery, and (c) left anterior pulmonary plexus.

Deep Cardiac Plexus

The deep cardiac plexus lies in front of the bifurcation of the trachea, behind the arch of the aorta (Fig. 21.26).

It is formed by:

(a) All the cardiac branches derived from three cervical and upper four or five thoracic ganglia of the sympathetic chains except the *superior cervical cardiac branch* of the left cervical sympathetic chain and
(b) All the cardiac branches of the vagus and recurrent laryngeal nerves except the *inferior cervical cardiac branch* of the left vagus nerve.

Distribution

The right and left halves of the plexus distributes branches to (a) corresponding coronary arteries and pulmonary plexus, and (b) separate branches to the atria.

PAIN AND REFLEX PATHWAYS OF THE HEART

PAIN PATHWAYS

The sensations of pain arising due to the ischaemia of the heart pass through the sympathetic fibres to reach the upper five thoracic spinal segments (T1–T5) through the cervical and thoracic sympathetic ganglia and follow the usual somatosensory pathway to the central nervous system. The pain fibres pass from the thoracic ganglia to the spinal nerves via white rami communicantes. The cell bodies of the first-order sensory neurons are located in the dorsal root ganglia of the T1–T5 spinal nerves. Hence, cardiac pain is referred mainly in the area of the distribution of these nerves, that is the pectoral region and medial aspect of the arm and the forearm.

N.B.

Sometimes cardiac pain is referred to the neck and mandible. It is because of the connection of the sympathetic fibres with the cervical nerves.

PATHWAYS FOR CARDIOVASCULAR REFLEXES

The afferent fibres from heart subserving the cardiovascular reflexes pass by the parasympathetic fibres of the vagal nerves to reticular formation.

ACTION OF THE HEART

The heart is actually a double muscular pump. The right side pumps blood to the lungs and left side pumps blood to all the parts of the body. Each pump is made up of an atrium and a ventricle.

Cardiac cycle: The contraction of the heart followed by relaxation is one cardiac cycle. The contraction of the heart is termed systole and relaxation is known as diastole. During a cardiac cycle, series of changes take place as it fills with blood and empties the same. Normally, the heart beats 70–90 times per minute in adults and 130–150 times per minute in a newborn baby.

CLINICAL CORRELATION

- **Tachycardia and bradycardia:** The increased heart rate (rapid pulse) is called *tachycardia* and the decreased heart rate (slow pulse) is called *bradycardia*.
- **Arrhythmia:** The irregular heart rate (irregular pulse) is called arrhythmia.

Golden Facts to Remember

• Most fixed part of the heart	Base of the heart
• Most common stenosis of the heart valves	Mitral stenosis
• Strongest fibrous ring of the skeleton of the heart	Fibrous ring around the aortic orifice of the heart
• Pacemaker of the heart	SA node
• Most commonly blocked artery leading to MI	Anterior interventricular artery (LAD artery)
• Largest/widest/principal vein of the heart	Coronary sinus
• Unique feature of coronary arteries	They fill during ventricular diastole as a result of the aortic recoil
• Whole of the conducting system of the heart is supplied by the right coronary artery except	A part of the left branch of the AV bundle which is supplied by the left coronary artery
• Third coronary artery	Right conus artery arising directly from the aortic sinus
• Kugel's artery	An atrial branch of the circumflex artery which anastomoses with a similar atrial branch of the right coronary artery
• Annulus of Vieussens	Circular anastomotic channel around the infundibulum between the right and left conus arteries
• Triangle of Koch	Small triangular area located in the lower part of the septal area of right atrium. It is bounded in front by the septal cusp of the tricuspid valve, behind by the anteromedial margin of the coronary sinus and above by the tendon of Todaro (a subendocardial ridge)
• Heart attack	Acute MI
• Only way to conduct impulses from atria to ventricles	AV bundle of His
• Largest vein of the heart	Coronary vein

CLINICAL CASE STUDY

A 60-year-old man visited a cardiologist and complained that he was feeling pressure/tightness within his chest, accompanied by profuse sweating and pain in the left precordium that is radiating along the medial side of the arm and the forearm. On questioning, he told that earlier also he suffered from such symptoms which always occurred on exertion, for example when climbing stairs or digging in the garden. He also told that these symptoms disappear after resting. **He was diagnosed as a case of angina pectoris.**

Questions

1. What is angina pectoris?
2. Mention the anatomical basis of pain felt in the region of the left precordium and medial side of the arm and the forearm.
3. Name the arteries that supply the cardiac muscle and mention their origin.
4. What is the difference between the angina pectoris and myocardial infarction (MI)?

Answers

1. It is cardiac pain that occurs on exertion due to the narrowing of the coronary artery/arteries or their major branches. The pain is relieved by resting.
2. The afferent pain fibres from the heart reach the upper four or five thoracic spinal segments through the cardiac branches of the sympathetic trunks usually on the left side. Pain is referred in the left pericardium—T4 and T3 dermatomes and medial side of the arm (T2 dermatome) and medial side of the forearm (T1 dermatome).
3. Right and left coronary arteries. The right coronary artery arises from the anterior aortic sinus at the root of the ascending aorta, while the left coronary artery arises from the left posterior aortic sinus at the root of the ascending aorta.
4. The differences between the angina pectoris and MI are as follows:

Angina pectoris	MI (heart attack)
Occurs due to narrowing of the coronary artery/arteries causing myocardial ischaemia	Occurs due to a complete block of the coronary artery/arteries causing myocardial ischaemia that induces myocardial necrosis
Occurs on exertion and is relieved on rest	Occurs on rest and is not relieved on rest
Sensation of pressure or burning in the chest that may last as long as 20 min	Sensation of pressure or burning in the chest that lasts longer than 30 min

CHAPTER 22

Superior Vena Cava, Aorta, Pulmonary Trunk, and Thymus

SPECIFIC LEARNING OBJECTIVES

After studying this chapter, the student should be able to:

- Describe the arch of the aorta and descending thoracic aorta under the following headings: (a) course, (b) relations, (c) branches, and (d) applied anatomy. AN 23.4
- Describe the formation, course, relations, tributaries, and termination of superior vena cava. Discuss the effects of its blockage. AN 23.4
- Write short notes on: (a) ascending aorta, (b) pulmonary trunk, (c) thymus, (d) coarctation of the aorta, and (e) descending thoracic aorta.

The knowledge of the anatomy of the superior vena cava (SVC), aorta, and pulmonary trunk is clinically important because of their involvement in various disease processes such as the obstruction of SVC, aortic aneurysm, and pulmonary embolism.

SUPERIOR VENA CAVA AN 23.3

SVC is about 7 cm long and 1.25 cm in diameter (Fig. 22.1). It lies in the superior and middle mediastina. Its extrapericardial part lies in the superior mediastinum and its intrapericardial part lies in the middle mediastinum.

It is a large venous channel which drains venous blood from the upper half of the body (i.e. head and neck, upper limbs, thoracic wall, and upper abdominal wall) and drains it into the right atrium. Depending upon the site of obstruction, different collateral pathways develop. In mediastinal syndrome, the signs of obstruction of SVC appear first.

FORMATION, COURSE, AND TERMINATION

SVC is formed at the lower border of the first right costal cartilage by the union of the right and left brachiocephalic (innominate) veins. It passes vertically downward behind the right border of the sternum and pierces the pericardium at the level of the right second costal cartilage, and opens/terminates into the upper part of the right atrium at the lower border of the right third costal cartilage. It has no valves in its lumen because gravity facilitates the blood flow in it.

N.B.

There are no valves in (a) SVC and (b) brachiocephalic veins.

SUBDIVISIONS

SVC is subdivided into the following two parts:

1. Extrapericardial part (in superior mediastinum)
2. Intrapericardial part (in middle mediastinum)

RELATIONS (FIGS. 22.1B AND 22.2)

Anterior:

1. Right internal thoracic vessels
2. Margin of right lung and pleura
3. Chest wall

Posterior:

1. Trachea (posteromedial)
2. Right pulmonary artery and right bronchus

To the left:

1. Ascending aorta (anteromedial)
2. Pulmonary trunk

To the right:

1. Right phrenic nerve and pericardiophrenic vessels
2. Right lung and pleura

TRIBUTARIES

1. Right and left brachiocephalic veins.
2. Azygos vein, which arches over the root of the right lung and opens into SVC just before it pierces the fibrous pericardium.
3. Mediastinal and pericardial veins.

BRACHIOCEPHALIC VEINS

There are two brachiocephalic veins: (a) right and (b) left. Each of them is formed behind the sternoclavicular joint by the union of the corresponding internal jugular and subclavian veins. They unite to form SVC. Both are devoid of valves. Differences between the right and left brachiocephalic veins are enumerated in Table 22.1.

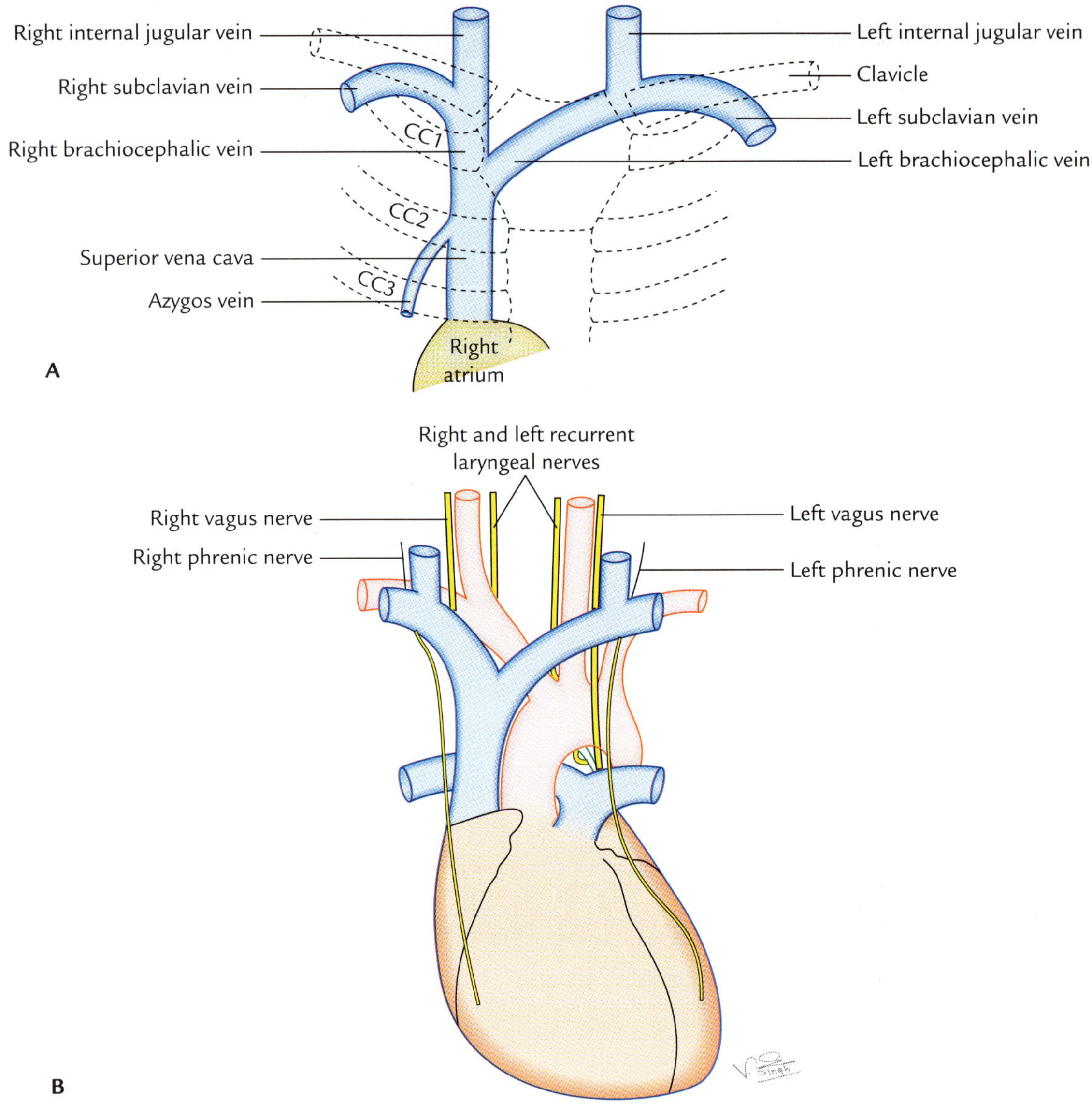

FIG. 22.1 ■ Superior vena cava. (**A**) Formation, course, and termination, and (**B**) relations (CC = costal cartilage).

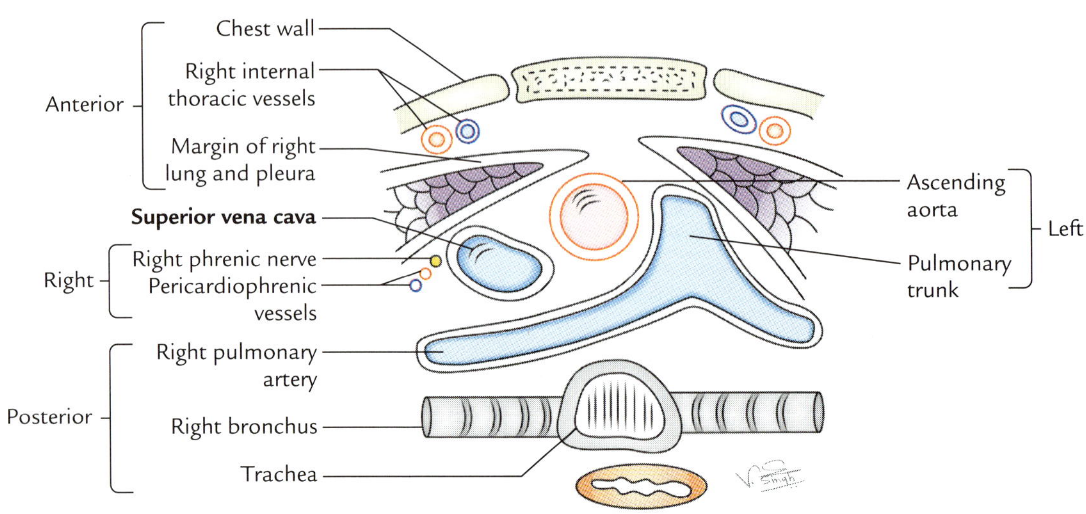

FIG. 22.2 ■ Relations of superior vena cava as seen in the cross section of the thorax.

TABLE 22.1 Differences between right and left brachiocephalic veins

	Right brachiocephalic vein	Left brachiocephalic vein
Length	Short (2.5 cm)	Long (6 cm)
Course	Vertical (runs vertically downward from the right sternoclavicular joint to the lower margin of the right first costal cartilage)	Oblique (runs obliquely across the superior mediastinum from the left sternoclavicular joint to the lower margin of the right first costal cartilage)
Tributaries	• Right vertebral vein • Right internal thoracic vein • Right inferior thyroid vein • First right posterior intercostal vein	• Left vertebral vein • Left internal thoracic vein • Left inferior thyroid vein • First left posterior intercostal vein • Left superior intercostal vein

CLINICAL CORRELATION

Obstruction of SVC and development of collateral pathways: SVC may be obstructed (compressed) at two sites: (a) above the opening of the azygos vein (i.e. in superior mediastinum) and (b) below the opening of the azygos vein (i.e. in the middle mediastinum).

- *If SVC is obstructed above the opening of the azygos vein*, the venous blood from the upper half of the body is shunted to the right atrium through development of collaterals including the *azygos vein* and its tributaries. The main collateral pathways are provided by the superior intercostal veins. The superficial veins of the chest wall do not receive sufficient blood to cause their prominence. If at all they become prominent, the prominence is limited up to the costal margin only (Fig. 22.3A).
- *If SVC is obstructed below the opening of the azygos vein*, the venous blood from the upper half of the body is returned to the right atrium through the inferior vena cava through the *collateral pathways, formed between the tributaries of the superior and inferior vena cavae (caval-caval shunt).* Clinically, under this condition, a subcutaneous anastomotic channel between the *superficial epigastric vein and lateral thoracic vein* (thoracoepigastric vein) is seen on the anterior aspect of the thoracoabdominal wall (Fig. 22.3B).

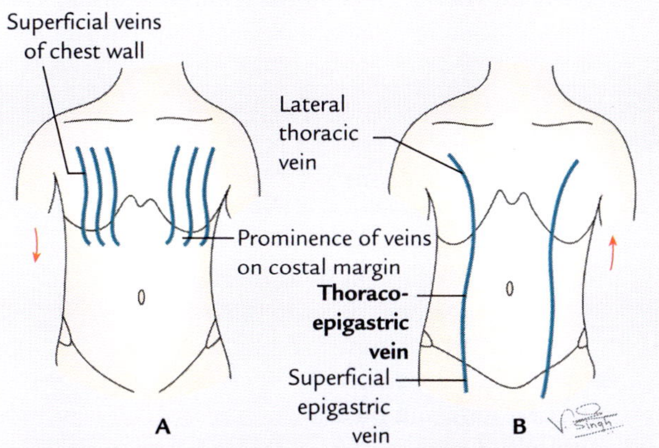

FIG. 22.3 ■ Prominence veins on the front of the trunk in the obstruction of the superior vena cava. (**A**) Obstruction above the opening of the azygos vein and (**B**) obstruction below the opening of the azygos vein.

AORTA

AN 23.4

The aorta is the largest artery (arterial trunk) of the body that carries the oxygenated blood from the left ventricle and distributes it to all the parts of the body.

PARTS OF AORTA

For the convenience of description, the aorta is divided into the following four parts (Fig. 22.4):

1. Ascending aorta
2. Arch of the aorta
3. Descending thoracic aorta
4. Abdominal aorta

N.B.

The first three parts are confined to the thoracic cavity and together form the thoracic aorta.

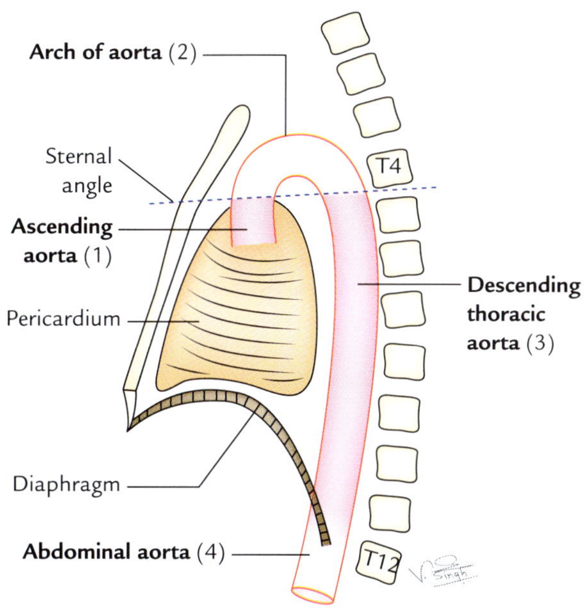

FIG. 22.4 ■ Parts of the aorta.

ASCENDING AORTA

AN 23.4

Origin and Course

1. Ascending aorta arises from the upper end of the left ventricle (i.e. aortic vestibule) and continues as an arch of the aorta at the level of sternal angle.
2. It is about 5 cm long and its diameter is about 3 cm. It is completely enclosed in the pericardium. It begins behind the left half of the sternum at the level of the lower border of left third costal cartilage, runs upward, forward, and to the right to continue as the arch of the aorta at the level of the sternal angle.

Aortic Sinuses (Sinuses of the Valsalva)

The root of the aorta presents three dilatations called the *aortic sinuses of Valsalva* (Fig. 22.5). These dilatations are just above the cusps of the aortic valve. Their positions are: anterior, left posterior, and right posterior.

- Anterior aortic sinus gives origin to the right coronary artery; hence, it is also called the **right coronary sinus**.
- The left posterior aortic sinus gives origin to the **left coronary artery**; hence, it is also called the left coronary sinus.
- The right posterior aortic sinus is termed the **non-coronary sinus**.

Aortic bulb (Fig. 22.5) is a bulge in the right wall of the ascending aorta at its union with the arch of the aorta.

Relations

Anterior: From below upward, these are as follows:

1. Infundibulum of right ventricle
2. Pulmonary trunk
3. Pericardium

Posterior: From before backwards and to right, these are as follows:

1. Transverse sinus of the pericardium.
2. Right pulmonary artery.
3. Right principal bronchus.
   (a) To the right:
      (i) Right atrium.
      (ii) SVC.
   (b) To the left:
      (i) Left atrium.
      (ii) Pulmonary trunk.

Branches

1. Right coronary artery from the anterior aortic sinus.
2. Left coronary artery from the left posterior aortic sinus.

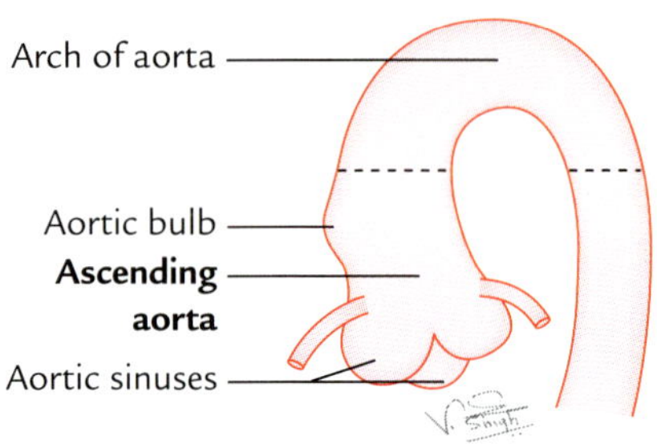

FIG. 22.5 Ascending aorta showing the aortic sinuses (sinuses of the Valsalva) and aortic bulb.

Development

The ascending aorta develops from the truncus arteriosus after its partition by the spiral septum.

CLINICAL CORRELATION

Aneurysm of the ascending aorta: It occurs at the bulb of the ascending aorta. The bulb of the aorta is a dilatation in the right wall of the ascending aorta that is subjected to a constant thrust of the forceful blood current ejected from the left ventricle. It may compress the right atrium, SVC, or right principal bronchus. Its rupture (a serious complication) leads to the accumulation of blood in the pericardial cavity (hemopericardium).

ARCH OF AORTA

AN 23.4

The arch of the aorta is the continuation of the ascending aorta at the level of the sternal angle and continues as the descending thoracic aorta at the level of the sternal angle. Thus, it (both) begins as well as terminates at the level of the sternal angle. It is situated in the superior mediastinum. At the beginning, the arch is anteriorly located while its termination is posteriorly located, very close to the left side of the T4 vertebra. The summit of the arch reaches the level of the middle of the manubrium sterni.

Extent and Course

The arch of the aorta begins at the level of the right second costal cartilage and runs upward, backward, and to the left, in front of the bifurcation of the trachea. Having reached the back of the middle of the manubrium, it turns backward and downward behind the left bronchus up to the level of the lower border of the T4 vertebra where it continues as the descending thoracic aorta.

N.B.

- The arch of the aorta arches over the root of the left lung.
- It begins and ends at the same level, that is at the sternal angle.
- It begins anteriorly and ends posteriorly.
- Ligamentum arteriosum (a fibrous remnant of ductus arteriosus) passes from the commencement of the left pulmonary artery to the concavity of arch of the aorta (Fig. 22.6C)

Relations (Figs. 22.6 and 22.7)

Posterior and to the right:

1. Trachea
2. Oesophagus
3. Left recurrent laryngeal nerve
4. Thoracic duct
5. Vertebral column

Anterior and to the left:

1. Left lung and pleura
2. Left phrenic nerve
3. Left vagus nerve
4. Left cardiac nerves (i.e. superior cervical cardiac branch of the left sympathetic chain and inferior cardiac branch of the left vagus nerve)
5. Left superior intercostal vein

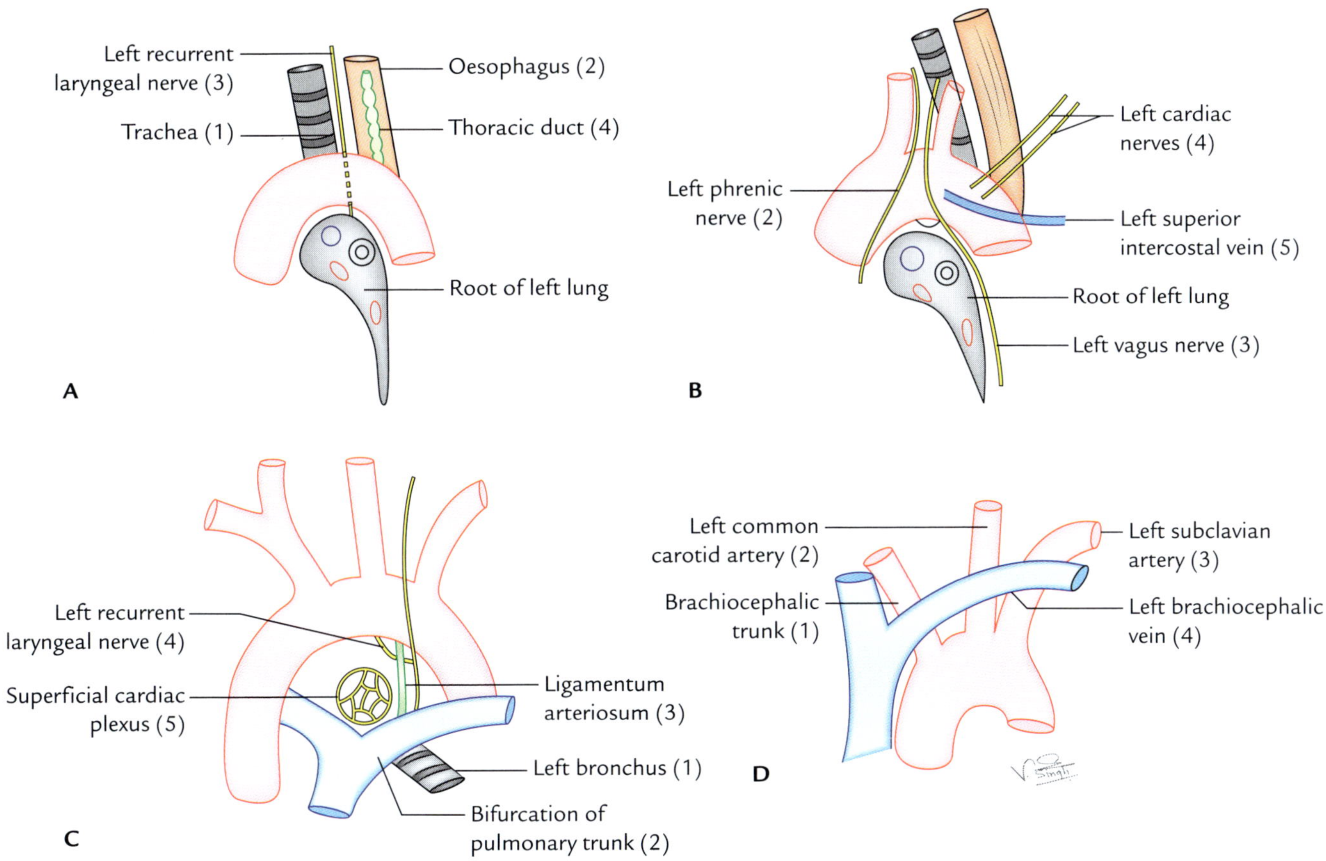

FIG. 22.6 ■ Relations of the arch of the aorta. (**A**) Posterior and to the right [vertebral column (5) is not shown], (**B**) anterior and to the left [left lung and pleura (1) are not shown], (**C**) inferior, and (**D**) superior [thymus (5) is not shown].

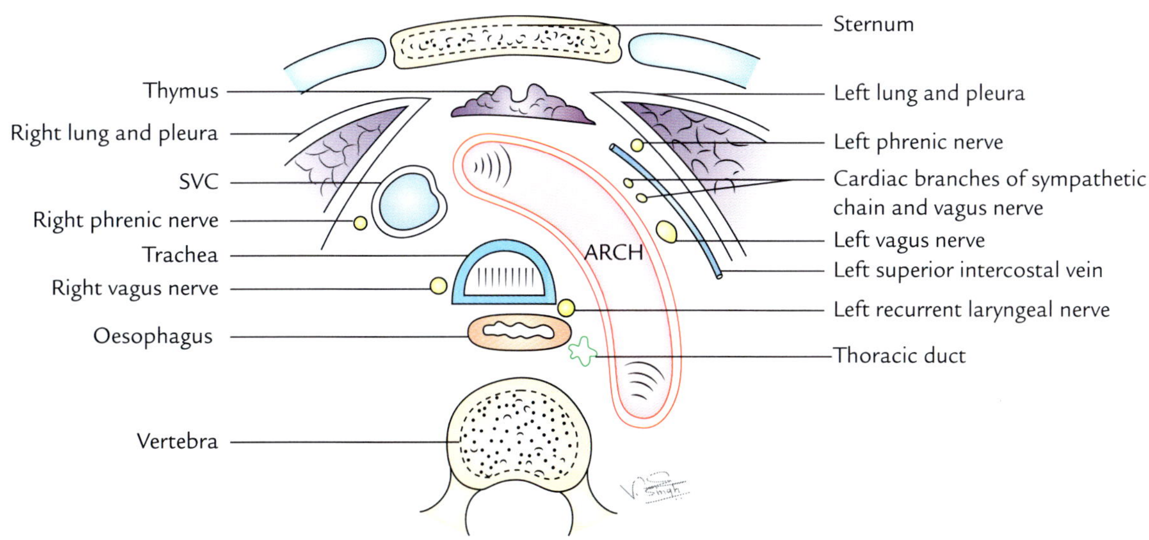

FIG. 22.7 ■ Cross section of the superior mediastinum showing relations of the arch of the aorta (SVC = superior vena cava).

Inferior:

1. Left bronchus
2. Bifurcation of the pulmonary trunk
3. Ligamentum arteriosum
4. Left recurrent laryngeal nerve
5. Superficial cardiac plexus

Superior:

1. Brachiocephalic trunk
2. Left common carotid artery
3. Left subclavian artery
4. Left brachiocephalic vein
5. Thymus

N.B.

The arch of the aorta is related to five structures on each aspect.

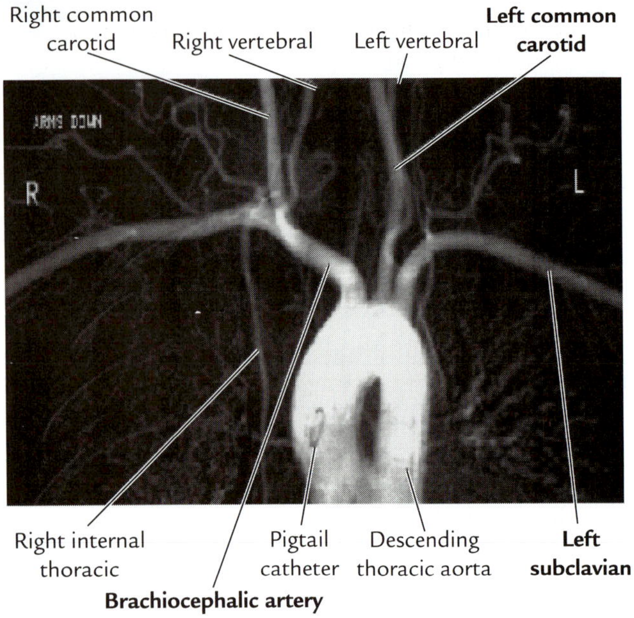

FIG. 22.8 ■ Branches of arch of the aorta as seen in the digital subtraction angiogram of the aortic arch. (*Source: Integrated Anatomy*, 1st ed.: David Heylings, Roy Spence, and Barry E. Kelly, Fig. 4.27, Page 107, Churchill Livingstone (Elsevier), 2007.)

Branches (Fig. 22.8)

1. Brachiocephalic (innominate) artery
2. Left common carotid artery
3. Left subclavian artery

The **brachiocephalic trunk** arises from the arch of the aorta a little to the left of the midline. It passes upward and to the right across the trachea to reach the back of the right sternoclavicular joint, where it divides into the right common carotid and right subclavian arteries.

The **left common carotid artery** arises from the upper convexity of the aortic arch just left to the brachiocephalic trunk. It passes straight upward alongside the trachea.

The **left subclavian artery arises** behind and left to the common carotid artery. It passes upward and then arches to the left over the pleura covering the apex of the left lung that it grooves markedly.

N.B.

None of three branches of the arch of the aorta (vide supra) gives any branch in the mediastinum except rare **thyroidea ima artery** that may arise from the brachiocephalic trunk or directly from the arch of the aorta.

Development

The arch of the aorta develops from the following sources:

1. Aortic sac
2. Left horn of the aortic sac
3. Left fourth aortic arch artery
4. Left dorsal aorta [between the attachment of the fourth aortic arch (artery) and seventh cervical intersegmental artery]

CLINICAL CORRELATION

- **Aortic knuckle:** In an X-ray of the chest (PA view), the shadow of the arch of the aorta appears as small bulb-like projection at the upper end of the left margin of the cardiac shadow called the *aortic knuckle*. The aortic knuckle may become prominent in old age due to *undue folding* of the arch caused by atherosclerosis.
- **Coarctation of aorta (Fig. 22.9):** It is congenital narrowing of the arch of the aorta just proximal or just distal to the entrance of the *ductus arteriosus*. The collateral circulation develops between the branches of the subclavian arteries and those of the descending aorta, namely, anastomosis between anterior and posterior intercostal arteries.

  Clinical features:

  1. There is a **difference in the blood pressure of the upper and lower limbs** (i.e. high blood pressure in upper limbs and low unrecordable blood pressure in the lower limbs).
  2. **Notching of the lower borders of the ribs** due to the dilatation of engorged posterior intercostal arteries (Fig. 22.10).
  3. Pulsating scapula due to development of collateral through intercostal arteries in the scapular anastomosis.
- **Patent ductus arteriosus (Fig. 22.11):** In foetal life, the pulmonary trunk is connected to the arch of the aorta (just distal to the origin of the left subclavian artery) by a short wide channel called the *ductus arteriosus*. Normally, after birth, it closes functionally within a week and anatomically within 4–12 weeks. The obliterated ductus arteriosus is called the *ligamentum arteriosum*. Nonobliterated ductus arteriosus is called patent ductus arteriosus.
- **Aneurysm of the arch of the aorta:** It is the localized dilatation of the arch and causes the compression of neighbouring structures in the superior mediastinum producing *mediastinal syndrome*. The characteristic clinical sign under this condition is '*tracheal-tug*', which is a feeling of tugging sensation in the suprasternal notch.

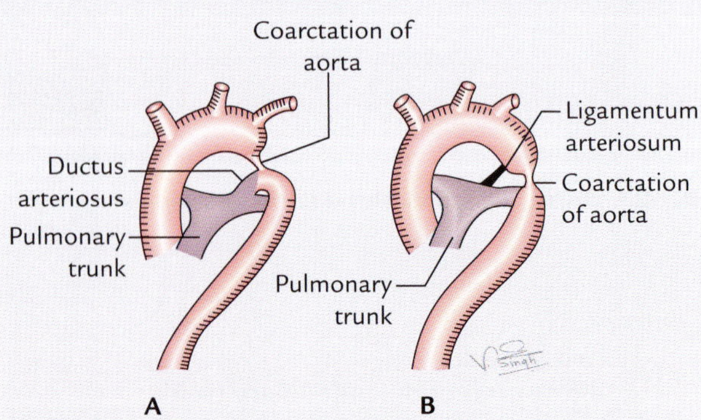

FIG. 22.9 ■ Coarctation of the aorta. (**A**) Preductal type and (**B**) postductal type. (*Source: Clinical and Surgical Anatomy*, 2 ed.: Vishram Singh, Fig. 9.24, p. 474, Elsevier, 2007.)

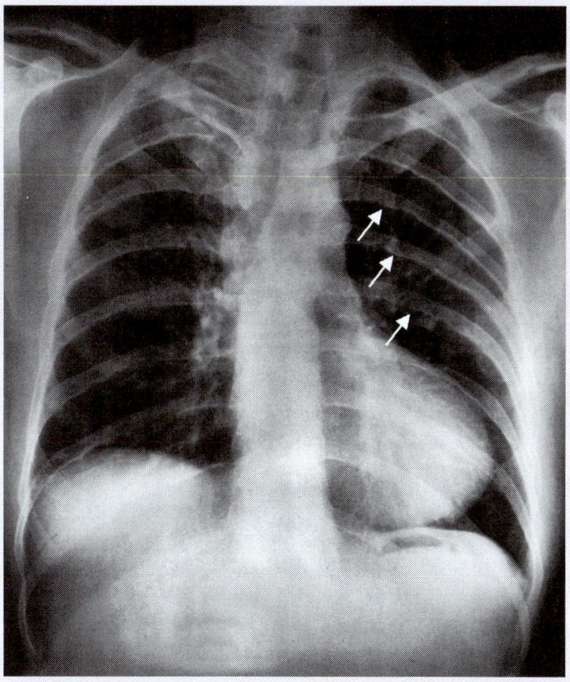

FIG. 22.10 ■ X-ray chest showing notches seen as small translucent shadows (white arrows) along the inferior borders of ribs (fifth to seventh). (*Source: Gray's Anatomy for Students*, 3 ed.: Richard L Drake, Wayne Vogl, Adam WM Mitchell, Fig. 3.111, Page 247, Elsevier Inc. 2015.)

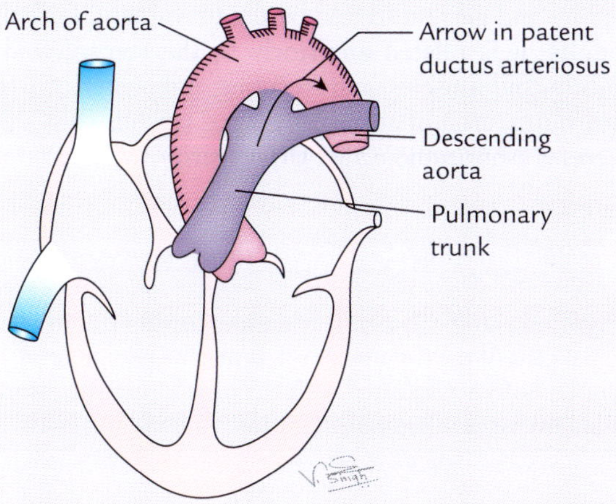

FIG. 22.11 ■ Patent ductus arteriosus. (*Source: Clinical and Surgical Anatomy*, 2ed.: Vishram Singh, Fig. 9.23, p. 474, Elsevier, 2007.)

DESCENDING THORACIC AORTA AN 23.4

The descending thoracic aorta is the continuation of the arch of the aorta in the posterior mediastinum.

Extent and Course

It begins on the left side of the lower border of the fourth thoracic (T4) vertebra and descends in the posterior mediastinum with an inclination towards the right. As a result, it terminates in front of the lower border of the body of the 12th thoracic (T12) vertebra.

At its lower end, it passes through the aortic opening of the diaphragm to continue as the abdominal aorta.

Relations

Anterior: From above downwards it is related to:

1. Left lung root
2. Pericardium (enclosing heart)
3. Oesophagus (in the lower part)
4. Diaphragm

Posterior:

1. Vertebral column
2. Hemiazygos and accessory hemiazygos veins

To the right side:

1. Oesophagus (in the upper part)
2. Thoracic duct
3. Azygos vein
4. Right lung and pleura

To the left side: Left lung and pleura

(*Note:* Descending thoracic aorta produces a deep vertical groove on the mediastinal surface of the left lung posterior to the hilum of the lung.)

Branches (Fig. 22.12)

Parietal Branches

1. Nine (3rd–11th) posterior intercostal arteries on each side.
2. Subcostal artery on each side.
3. Superior phrenic artery on each side.

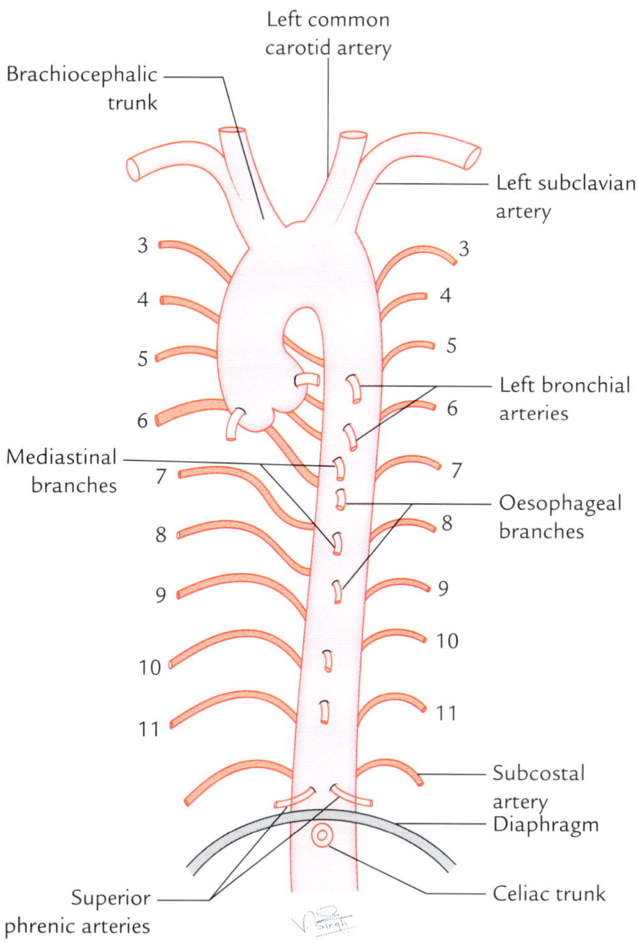

FIG. 22.12 ■ Branches of the thoracic aorta.

Visceral Branches

1. Pericardial branches, to the posterior surface of the pericardium.
2. Mediastinal branches, to the lymph nodes and areolar tissue of the posterior mediastinum.
3. Two left bronchial arteries (upper and lower).
4. Oesophageal branches, supplying the middle one-third of the oesophagus.

CLINICAL CORRELATION

Dissecting aneurysm: Under this condition, the blood from the aortic lumen enters into its wall through a tear in the tunica intima creating a channel of blood in the tunica media that leads to the dilatation of the aorta. Clinically, it presents as pain in the back due to the compression of intercostal nerves. Occasionally, the aorta may rupture into the left pleural cavity.

PULMONARY TRUNK

ORIGIN

The pulmonary trunk is about 5 cm long and arises from the upper part (infundibulum) of the right ventricle at the level of the sternal end of the left third costal cartilage.

COURSE

After arising from infundibulum in the middle mediastinum, it passes backward and to the left and terminates below the arch of the aorta and in front of the left principal bronchus by dividing into the right and left pulmonary arteries.

RELATIONS

Anterior:

1. Sternal end of the left second intercostal space
2. Left lung and pleura

Posterior:

1. Ascending aorta
2. Commence of the left coronary artery
3. Transverse sinus of the pericardium

To the right:

1. Ascending aorta
2. Origin of the right coronary artery
3. Right auricle

To the left:

1. Left coronary artery
2. Left auricle

BRANCHES

Right and left pulmonary arteries.

N.B.

The right pulmonary artery is longer than the left and lies slightly at a lower level.

CLINICAL CORRELATION

- **Pulmonary artery catheterization:** Various aspects of cardiopulmonary functions are monitored by the cardiologists by pulmonary artery catheterization.
  The catheter is passed successively as follows:
  Internal jugular vein/subclavian vein → Right atrium → Right ventricle → Pulmonary trunk → Pulmonary artery.
- **Sudden occlusion of pulmonary trunk** by an embolus may be a sequel to the thrombosis of deep veins of the calf (viz. popliteal/femoral vein) or large pelvic vein following operation or immobilization in the sick bed. When the blockage is complete, death ensues rapidly.

THYMUS

The thymus is a **central lymphoid organ** responsible for production of mature T-lymphocytes.

It is unequal bilobed gland situated in the superior mediastinum and often extends above in the root of the neck and below in the upper part of the anterior mediastinum (Fig. 22.13).

It plays a prominent role in the development of the **immune system** by producing T-lymphocytes hence, it is usually prominent in children and gradually increases in size till puberty, when it weighs about 40 g. Thereafter it atrophies and gets infiltrated by the fibrous and fatty tissue. In adults, it is related anteriorly to the sternohyoid and sternothyroid muscles, and sternum; and posteriorly to the pericardium, arch of aorta, SVC, and trachea (Fig. 22.14). It secretes a hormone called **thymosin.**

CLINICAL CORRELATION

Thymoma (Fig. 22.14): It is tumour arising from the epithelial cells of the thymus gland. It may be benign or malignant and often associated with the neuromuscular disorder called **myasthenia gravis** that causes muscle weakness.

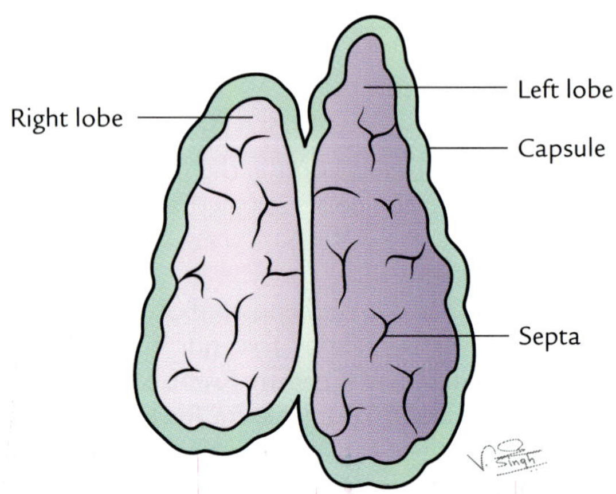

FIG. 22.13 ■ Thymus—an unequal bilobed gland.

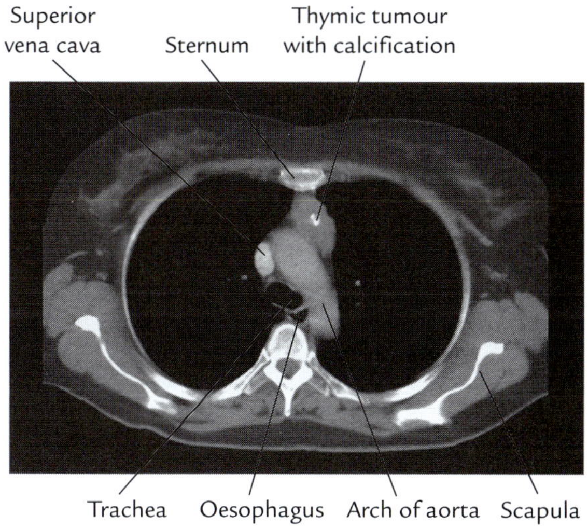

FIG. 22.14 ■ CT scan chest showing thymoma (benign thymic tumour). (*Source*: *Integrated Anatomy*, 3 ed.: David Heylings, Roy Spence, and Barry E. Kelly, Fig. 4.43, Page 118, Churchill Livingstone (Elsevier), 2007.)

Golden Facts to Remember

• Largest artery of the body	Aorta
• Bulb of aorta	Dilatation in the right wall of the ascending aorta at its union with the arch of the aorta
• Largest branch of the arch of the aorta	Brachiocephalic trunk
• Commonest variation in the origin of great arteries from the arch of the aorta	Origin of left common carotid artery from the brachiocephalic trunk
• Aortic knuckle	Projection at the upper end of the left margin of the cardiac shadow in the PA view of X-ray chest
• Part of the aorta mostly affected by dissecting aneurysm	Descending thoracic aorta
• Smallest part of the aorta	Ascending aorta
• Sinuses of Valsalva	Three dilatations in the ascending aorta above the semilunar valves

CLINICAL CASE STUDY

A mother took her 12-year-old son to the hospital and complained that he feels weakness even after slight exertion (reduced exercise tolerance), leg cramps on walking, and shortness of the breath. On examination, the doctors noticed radiofemoral delay. Blood pressure was 126/20 mmHg in upper limbs and 80/60 mmHg in the lower limbs. The X-ray of the chest showed notching of the lower borders of the ribs. **Clinically, he was diagnosed as a case of coarctation of the aorta**, which was confirmed later by echocardiography.

Questions

1. What is coarctation of the aorta?
2. Why there is delay in radial and femoral pulses?
3. What is the cause of high blood pressure in the upper limbs and low blood pressure in the lower limbs?
4. Mention the reason for notching of the ribs.

Answers

1. It is congenital stenosis of the arch of the aorta, usually distal to the origin of the left subclavian artery.
2. Because subclavian arteries supplying upper limbs arise proximal to the site of stenosis, whereas femoral arteries supplying lower limbs arise from aorta far distal to the site of obstruction.
3. Answer is the same as that of Question No. 2.
4. Due to the dilatation and tortuosity of the posterior intercostal arteries that erode the costal groove of the ribs.

CHAPTER

23 Trachea and Oesophagus

SPECIFIC LEARNING OBJECTIVES

After studying this chapter, the student should be able to:

- Describe the trachea under the following headings: (a) introduction, (b) extent, (c) length, (d) relations, (e) blood supply, (f) lymphatic drainage, (g) nerve supply, and (h) applied anatomy. AN 24.6
- Describe the microscopic structure of trachea. AN 25.1
- Describe the oesophagus under the following headings: (a) introduction, (b) curvatures, (c) constrictions, (d) blood supply, (e) nerve supply, (f) lymphatic drainage, and (g) applied anatomy. AN 23.1
- Give the anatomical/embryological basis of (a) achalasia cardia, (b) tracheoesophageal fistula, and (c) oesophageal varices.
- Enumerate oesophageal constrictions and discuss their clinical significance.

TRACHEA AN 24.6

The trachea (syn. windpipe; Fig. 23.1) is a flexible fibrocartilaginous tube forming the beginning of the lower respiratory tract. Its lumen is kept patent by 16–20 C-shaped rings of the hyaline cartilage. The gap between the posterior free ends of C-shaped cartilages is bridged by a band of smooth muscle (trachealis) and a fibroelastic ligament, which permit the expansion of the oesophagus during the passage of bolus of food.

The arrangement of cartilages and elastic tissue in the tracheal wall prevents its kinking and obstruction during the movements of the head and the neck.

LOCATION

The trachea extends from the lower border of the cricoid cartilage (corresponding to the lower border of the C6 vertebra) in the neck to the lower border of the T4 vertebra in the thorax. Thus, the upper half of the trachea is located in the neck (cervical part) and the lower half in the superior mediastinum (thoracic part).

N.B.

The extent of the trachea varies as follows:
- C6–T4 in the cadaver placed in supine position
- C6–T6 in living individuals in standing position
- C6–T3 in newborn

DIMENSIONS

Length: 10–12 cm
External diameter: 2 cm in males and 1.5 cm in females
Internal diameter: 12 mm in adult, 3 mm in newborn
Lumen of trachea:

1. The lumen of the trachea is smaller in living human beings than in the cadavers.
2. It is 3 mm at 1 year of age; during childhood, it corresponds to the age in years (i.e. a 5-year-old child will have a tracheal diameter of 5 mm) with a maximum of 12 mm in adults. For this reason, endotracheal tubes are graduated in mm.

COURSE

The trachea is the continuation of the larynx and begins at the lower border of the cricoid cartilage at the level of the C6 vertebra, about 5 cm above the jugular notch.

It enters the thoracic inlet in the midline and passes downward and backward behind the manubrium to terminate by bifurcating into two principal bronchi, a little to the right side at the lower border of the T4 vertebra corresponding to the sternal angle in the cadaver (Fig. 23.2). However, in living person in erect posture, it bifurcates into two principal bronchi at the lower border of T6 vertebra and descends still further during inspiration.

RELATIONS

Relations of the Cervical Part

The relations of the cervical part of the trachea are described in detail in *Textbook of Anatomy: Head, Neck and Brain, Vol. III* by Vishram Singh.

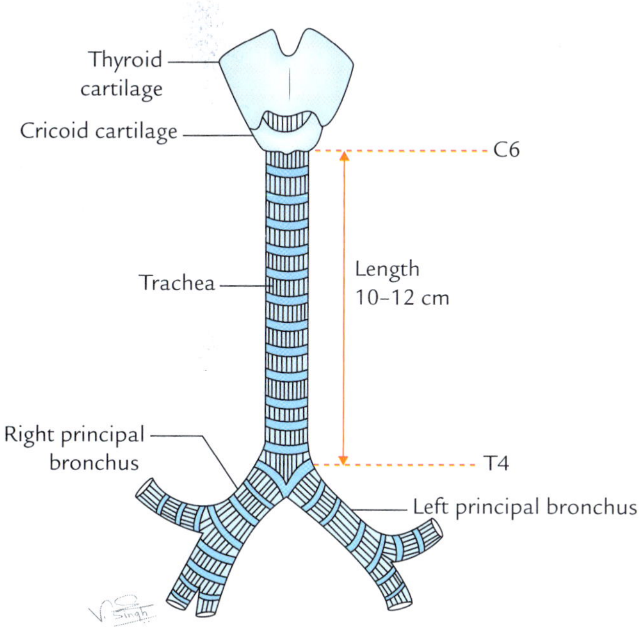

FIG. 23.1 ■ Trachea.

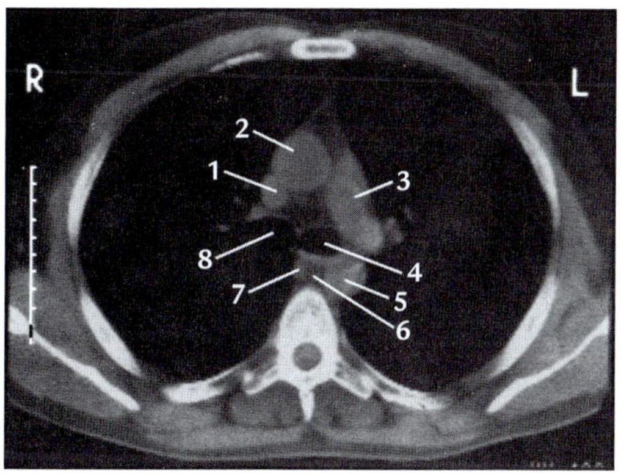

FIG. 23.2 ■ CT scan at T5 vertebral level. Just below the tracheal bifurcation, viewed from below: 1 = superior vena cava; 2 = ascending aorta; 3 = left pulmonary artery; 4 = left main bronchus; 5 = thoracic aorta; 6 = oesophagus; 7 = azygos vein; 8 = right main bronchus. (*Source: Last's Anatomy: Regional and Applied*, 12 ed.: Chummy S. Sinnatamby, Fig. 4.14, Page 194, Churchill Livingstone (Elsevier), 2011.)

Relations of the Thoracic Part (Figs. 23.3 and 23.4)

Anterior:

1. Arch of aorta
2. Brachiocephalic trunk and left common carotid artery
3. Left brachiocephalic vein
4. Superior vena cava (anterolateral)
5. Deep cardiac plexus

Posterior:

1. Oesophagus
2. Vertebral column
3. Left recurrent laryngeal nerve (it ascends up between the trachea and the oesophagus)

To the right:

1. Right lung and pleura
2. Azygous vein
3. Right vagus nerve

To the left:

1. Arch of aorta
2. Left common carotid artery
3. Left subclavian artery
4. Left vagus nerve
5. Left phrenic nerve

MICROSCOPIC STRUCTURE (FIG. 23.5) AN 25.1

Histologically, the tracheal tube from within outward is made up of the following layers:

1. **Mucosa:** It consists of the lining epithelium and lamina propria.
   (a) *Lining epithelium* is pseudostratified ciliated columnar with few goblets cells.
   (b) *Lamina propria* consists of longitudinal elastic fibres.
2. **Submucosa:** It consists of loose areolar tissue containing a large number of serous and mucous glands.
3. **Cartilage and smooth muscle layer:** It is made up of horseshoe-shaped (C-shaped) hyaline cartilaginous rings that are deficient posteriorly. The posterior gap is filled chiefly by the smooth muscle (trachealis) and fibroelastic fibres.
4. **Perichondrium:** It encloses the cartilage.
5. **Fibrous membrane:** It is a layer of dense connective tissue, containing a neurovascular structure.

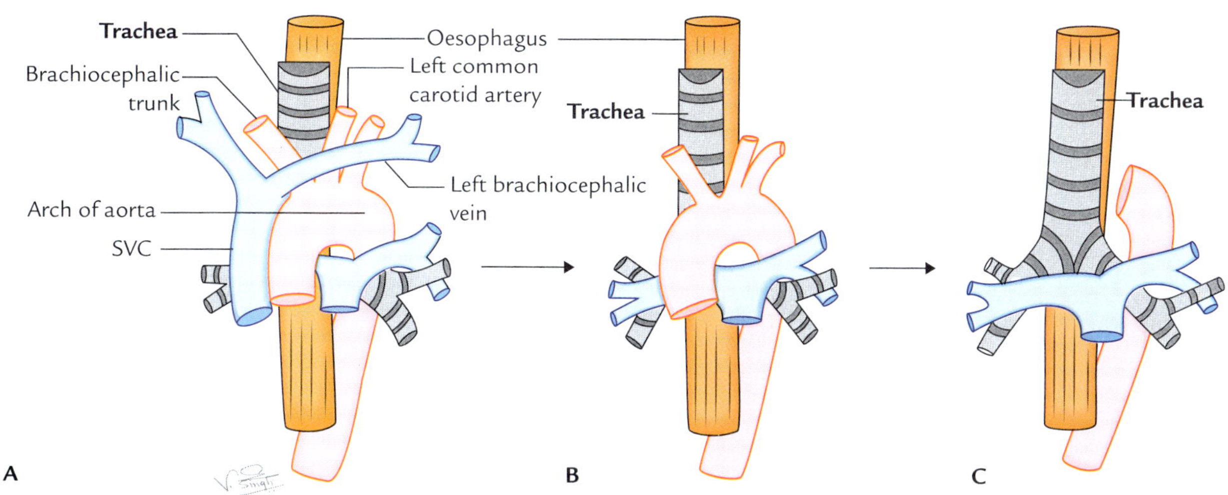

FIG. 23.3 ■ Anterior relations (A–C) of the trachea from superficial to deep (SVC = superior vena cava).

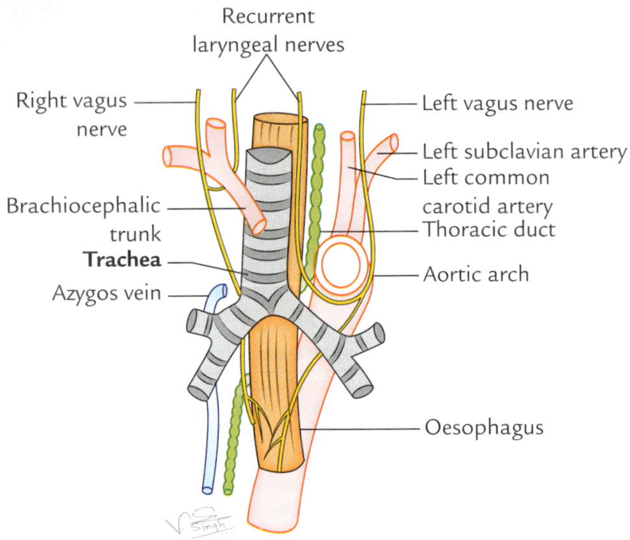

FIG. 23.4 ■ Posterior and lateral relations of the trachea.

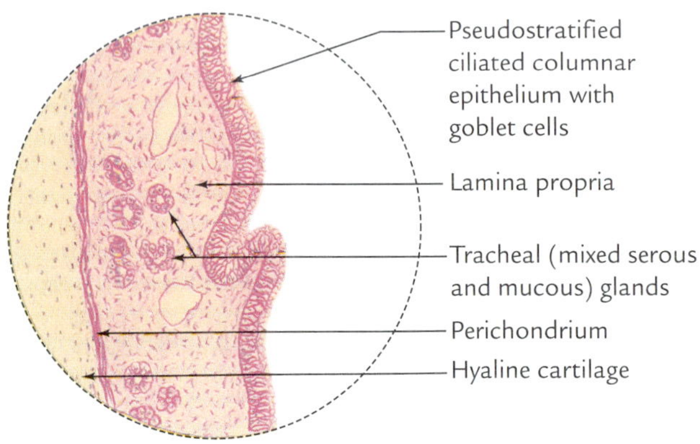

FIG. 23.5 ■ Microscopic structure of trachea. (*Source: Textbook of Histology and a Practical Guide,* 2 ed.: J.P. Gunasegaran, Box 16.2, p. 349, Elsevier, 2010.)

N.B.

There is no clear demarcation between lamina propria and submucosa.

VASCULAR SUPPLY AND LYMPHATIC DRAINAGE

- Blood supply to the trachea is by inferior thyroid and bronchial arteries.
- Venous drainage of the trachea occurs into the left brachiocephalic (innominate) vein.
- Lymphatic drainage of the trachea is into pretracheal and paratracheal lymph nodes.

NERVE SUPPLY

Nerve supply occurs by the autonomic nerve fibres:

- Parasympathetic fibres are sensory and secretomotor to the mucous membrane, and motor to the trachealis muscle.
- Sympathetic fibres are vasomotor.

CLINICAL CORRELATION

- **Tracheal shadow in a radiograph:** It is seen as a *vertical translucent shadow* in front of cervicothoracic spine. The translucency is due to the presence of air in the tracheal lumen.
- **Palpation of trachea:** Clinically, the trachea is palpated in the suprasternal notch. Normally, it is median in position but an appreciable shift of the trachea to the right or left side indicates the *mediastinal shift*.
- **Importance of carina:** It is a keel-like median ridge in the lumen at the bifurcation of the trachea. The lowest tracheal ring at the bifurcation of the trachea is thick in its central part. From the lower margin of this thick central part, a keel-shaped (hook-shaped) process projects downward and backward between the right and left principal bronchi. It has both functional and pathological importance.
  - *Functional importance:* The mucosa of the trachea over the carina is *most sensitive*. The cough reflex is usually initiated here, which helps to clear the sputum.
  - *Pathological significance:* It is visible as a sharp sagittal ridge at the tracheal bifurcation during *bronchoscopy*, hence serves as a useful landmark. It is located about 25 cm from the incisor teeth and 30 cm from the nostrils. If the tracheobronchial lymph nodes in the angle between the main (principal) bronchi are enlarged due to spread of *bronchiogenic carcinoma*, the carina becomes distorted and flattened.
- **Importance of mucous secretion in the tracheal lumen:** It helps to trap the inhaled foreign particles and solid mucous is then expelled during coughing. The *cilia of lining epithelium of the mucous membrane* also beat upward pushing the mucous upward. The *fibroelastic ligament* prevents overdistension of the tracheal lumen, while the *trachealis muscle* reduces the diameter on contraction during coughing that involves the increased velocity of expired air required for cleaning the air passages.

OESOPHAGUS AN 23.1

The oesophagus (Fig. 23.6) is a narrow muscular tube extending from the pharynx to the stomach. It is about 25 cm long and provides a passage for chewed food (bolus) and liquids during the third stage of deglutition. The anatomy of the oesophagus is clinically important because of its involvement in various diseases such as oesophagitis, oesophageal varices, and cancer. It begins in the lower part of the neck and terminates in the upper part of the abdomen by joining the upper end of the stomach.

DIMENSIONS AND LUMEN

Length: 25 cm (10 in)
Width: 2 cm
Lumen: It is flattened anteroposteriorly. Normally, it is kept closed (collapsed) and opens (dilates) only during the passage of the food.

COURSE

The oesophagus begins in the neck at the lower border of the cricoid cartilage (at the lower border of the C6 vertebra), descends in front of the vertebral

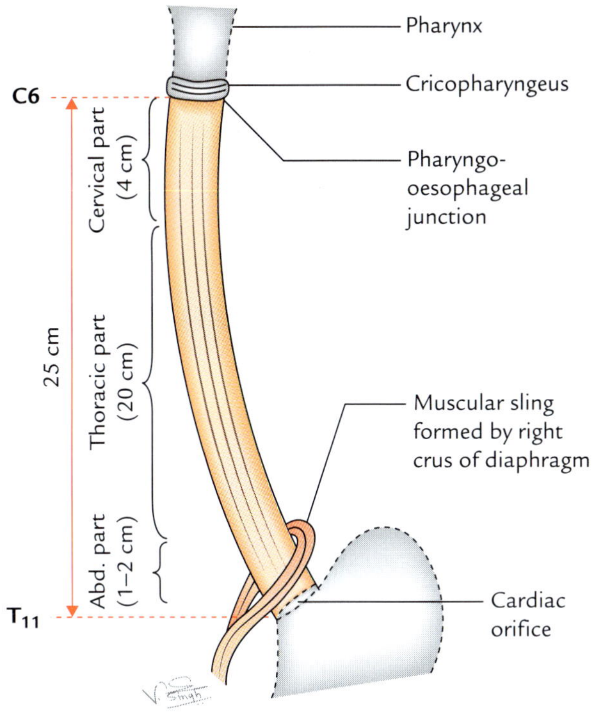

FIG. 23.6 Oesophagus (Abd. = abdominal).

column passes through superior and posterior mediastina, pierces the diaphragm at the level of T10 vertebra, and ends in the abdomen at the cardiac orifice of the stomach at the level of the T11 vertebra (Fig. 23.6).

CURVATURES

The cervical portion of oesophagus commences in the midline, then inclines slightly to the left of the midline at the root of the neck, enters the thoracic inlet, and passes through the superior mediastinum. At the level of the T5 vertebra, it returns to the midline, but at T7, it again deviates to the left and inclines forward to pass in front of the descending thoracic aorta and pierces the diaphragm 2.5 cm to the left of the midline (a thumb's breadth from the side of the sternum), at the level of the seventh left costal cartilage. Here fibres of the right crus of the diaphragm sweep around the oesophageal opening, forming a sling around the oesophagus. It enters the abdomen to join the stomach at the level of the T11 vertebra. Thus, oesophagus presents the following curvatures:

1. Two side-to-side curvatures, both toward the left:
   (a) First at the root of the neck, before entering the thoracic inlet.
   (b) Second at the level of the T7 vertebra, before passing in front of the descending thoracic aorta.
2. Two anteroposterior curvatures.
   (a) First corresponding to the curvature of the cervical spine.
   (b) Second corresponding to the curvature of the thoracic spine.

CONSTRICTIONS

Normally, there are four sites of anatomical constrictions/narrowings in the oesophagus. The distance of each constriction is measured from the upper incisor teeth. The constrictions are as follows (Fig. 23.7):

1. **First constriction**, at the pharyngo-oesophageal junction, 15 cm (6 in) from the incisor teeth.
2. **Second constriction**, where it is crossed by the arch of aorta, 22.5 cm (9 in) from the incisor teeth.
3. **Third constriction**, where it is crossed by the left principal bronchus, 27.5 cm (11 in) from the incisor teeth.
4. **Fourth constriction**, where it pierces the diaphragm, 40 cm (16 in) from the incisor teeth.

The sites of constriction, their respective distances from the upper incisor teeth and their vertebral level are given in Table 23.1.

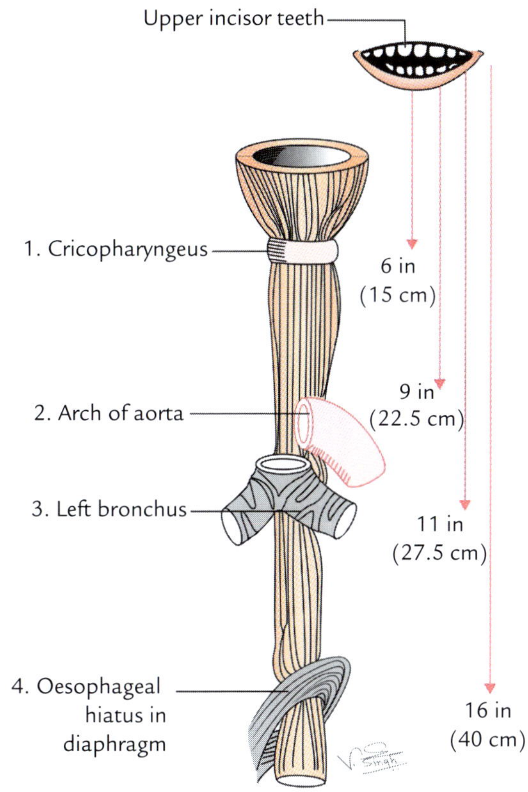

FIG. 23.7 Anatomical sites of constrictions in the oesophagus. On the right side, distances of these sites from the upper incisor teeth are given.

TABLE 23.1 Sites of constriction in the oesophagus

Site of constriction	Vertebral level	Distance from upper incisor teeth
At the pharyngo-oesophageal junction (cervical constriction)	C6	6 in (15 cm)
At crossing of the arch of aorta (aortic constriction)	T4	9 in (22.5 cm)
At crossing of the left principal bronchus (bronchial constriction)	T6	11 in (27.5 cm)
At the opening in the diaphragm (diaphragmatic constriction)	T10	16 in (40 cm)

N.B.

The *narrowest part of the oesophagus* is its commencement at the cricopharyngeal sphincter.

CLINICAL CORRELATION

Clinical significance of oesophageal constrictions: The anatomical constrictions of the oesophagus are of considerable clinical importance due to the following reasons:

1. These are the sites where swallowed foreign bodies are most likely to be lodged/stuck in the oesophagus.
2. These are the sites where strictures develop after the ingestion of corrosive substances.
3. These sites have predilection for the carcinoma of the oesophagus.
4. These are sites through which it may be difficult to pass oesophagoscope/gastric tube (Fig. 23.8).

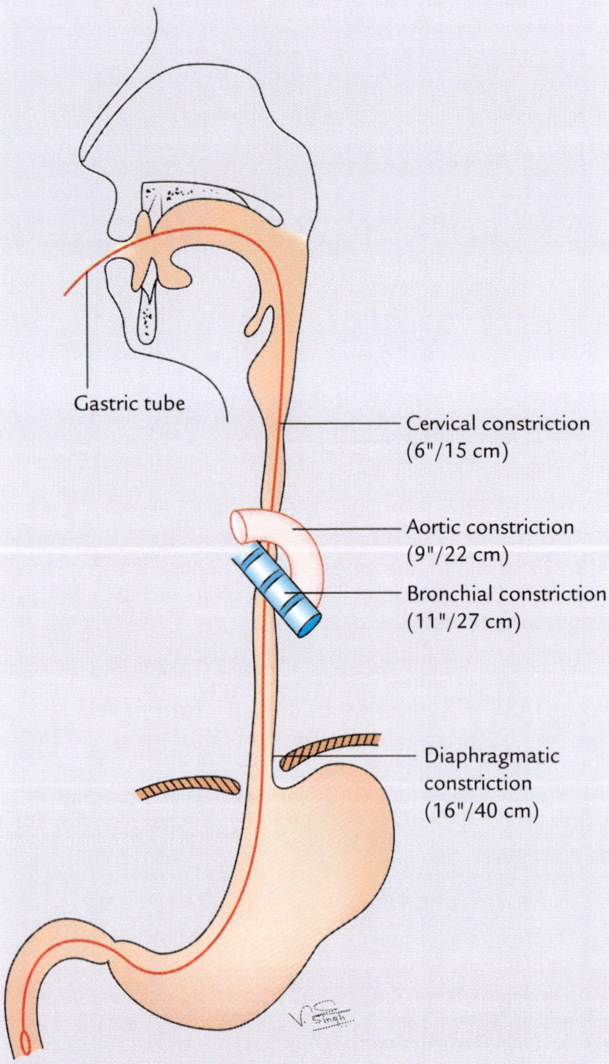

FIG. 23.8 ■ Anatomical sites of the oesophageal constrictions and passage of the gastric tube.

PARTS OF THE OESOPHAGUS

The oesophagus is divided into the following three parts:

1. Cervical part (4 cm in length)
2. Thoracic part (20 cm in length)
3. Abdominal part (1–2 cm in length)

The cervical part extends from the lower border of the cricoid cartilage to the superior border of the manubrium sterni (described in detail in the *Textbook of Anatomy: Head, Neck and Brain, Vol. III* by Vishram Singh).

The thoracic part extends from the superior border of the manubrium sterni to the oesophageal opening in the diaphragm.

The abdominal part extends from the oesophageal opening in the diaphragm to the cardiac end of the stomach.

RELATIONS (FIGS. 23.9 AND 23.10)

Relation of the Cervical Part of the Oesophagus

For description, refer to the *Textbook of Anatomy: Head, Neck and Brain, Vol III* by Vishram Singh, Chapter.

Relations of the Thoracic Part of the Oesophagus

Anterior: From above downward, these are as follows:

1. Trachea
2. Arch of aorta
3. Right pulmonary artery
4. Left principal bronchus
5. Left atrium enclosed in the pericardium
6. Diaphragm

Posterior:

1. Vertebral column
2. Right posterior intercostal arteries
3. Thoracic duct
4. Azygos vein
5. Hemiazygos veins (terminal parts)
6. Descending thoracic aorta

To the right:

1. Right lung and pleura
2. Azygos vein
3. Right vagus nerve

To the left:

1. Arch of aorta
2. Left subclavian artery
3. Thoracic duct
4. Left lung and pleura
5. Left recurrent laryngeal nerve
6. Descending thoracic aorta

N.B.

In the oesophageal aperture of the diaphragm, the left vagus nerve (now called the anterior gastric nerve) is related anteriorly and the right vagus nerve (now called the posterior gastric nerve) is related posteriorly.

Relations of Abdominal Part of the Oesophagus

Anterior:

1. Posterior surface of the left lobe of the liver
2. Anterior gastric nerve

Posterior:

1. Left crus of diaphragm
2. Posterior gastric nerve

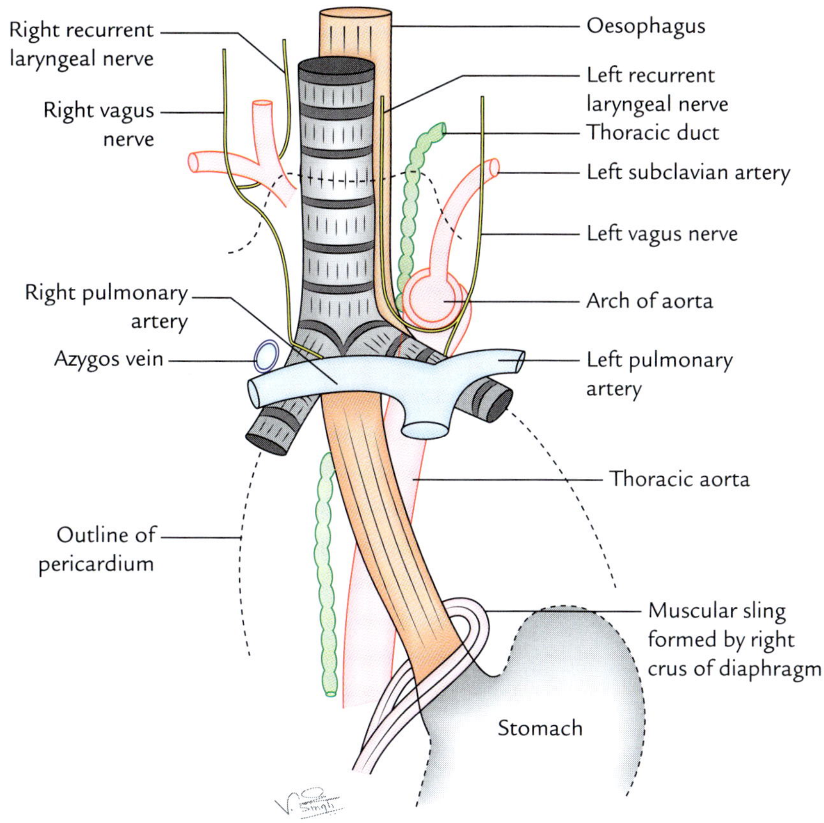

FIG. 23.9 Anterior and lateral relations of the oesophagus.

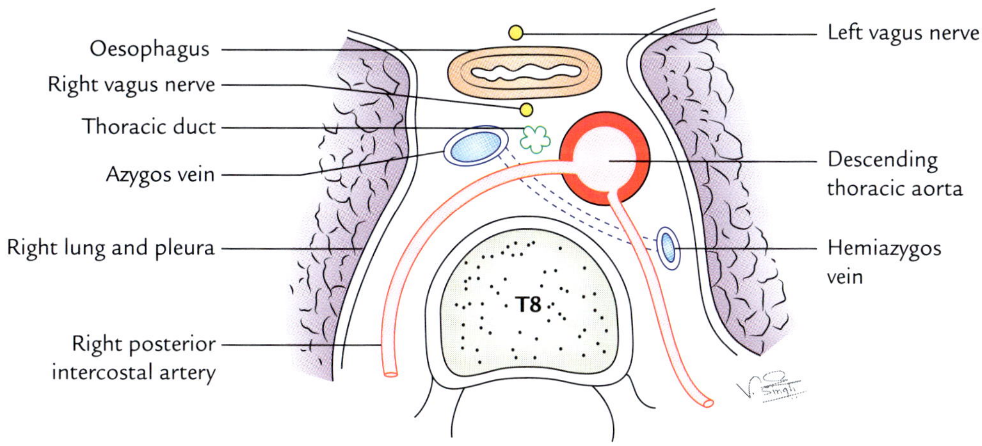

FIG. 23.10 Cross section of the posterior mediastinum at the level of the T8 vertebra showing posterior relations of the oesophagus.

N.B.

The abdominal part of the oesophagus is shortest (1–2 cm long) and is the only part covered with the serous membrane—the peritoneum.

ARTERIAL SUPPLY

- Blood supply to the **cervical part** is by inferior thyroid arteries.
- Blood supply to the **thoracic part** is by oesophageal branches of
  (a) descending thoracic aorta and
  (b) bronchial arteries
- Blood supply to the **abdominal part** is by oesophageal branches of
  (a) left gastric artery and
  (b) left inferior phrenic artery

VENOUS DRAINAGE

- Cervical part is drained by inferior thyroid veins.
- Thoracic part is drained by azygos and hemiazygos veins.

- Abdominal part is drained by two venous channels, *namely*,
  (a) hemiazygos vein, a tributary of superior vena cava and
  (b) left gastric vein, a tributary of the portal vein.

Thus, the abdominal part of the oesophagus is the site of portocaval anastomosis.

CLINICAL CORRELATION

Oesophageal varices: The lower end of the oesophagus is one of the important sites of *portocaval anastomosis*. In portal hypertension, for example, due to the cirrhosis of liver there is back pressure in portal circulation. As a result, collateral channels of portocaval anastomosis not only open up but become dilated and tortuous to form *oesophageal varices*. The ruptured oesophageal varices cause *haematemesis* (vomiting of blood).

LYMPHATIC DRAINAGE

From the cervical part, the lymph is drained into deep cervical lymph nodes.

From the thoracic part, the lymph is drained into posterior mediastinal lymph nodes.

From the abdominal part, the lymph is drained into left gastric and coeliac lymph nodes.

NERVE SUPPLY

The oesophagus is supplied by both the parasympathetic and sympathetic fibres.

The parasympathetic fibres are derived from recurrent laryngeal nerves and oesophageal plexuses formed by vagus nerves. They provide sensory, motor, and secretomotor supply to the oesophagus.

The sympathetic fibres are derived from T5 to T9 spinal segments are sensory and vasomotor.

CLINICAL CORRELATION

Referred pain of oesophagus: The pain sensations mostly arise from the lower part of the oesophagus as it is vulnerable to acid-peptic oesophagitis. Pain sensations are carried by sympathetic fibre to the T5 to T9 spinal segments.

Therefore, oesophageal pain is referred to the lower thoracic region and epigastric region of the abdomen, and at times it becomes difficult to differentiate oesophageal pain from the anginal pain.

MICROSCOPIC STRUCTURE

Histologically, oesophageal tube from within outward is made up of the following four basic layers (Fig. 23.11):

1. **Mucosa:** It is composed of the following components:
   (a) *Epithelium*—highly stratified squamous and nonkeratinized.
   (b) *Lamina propria*—contains connective tissue with plenty of lymphocytes. It may contain ***cardiac oesophageal glands*** (oesophageal mucous glands) in the lower part only.

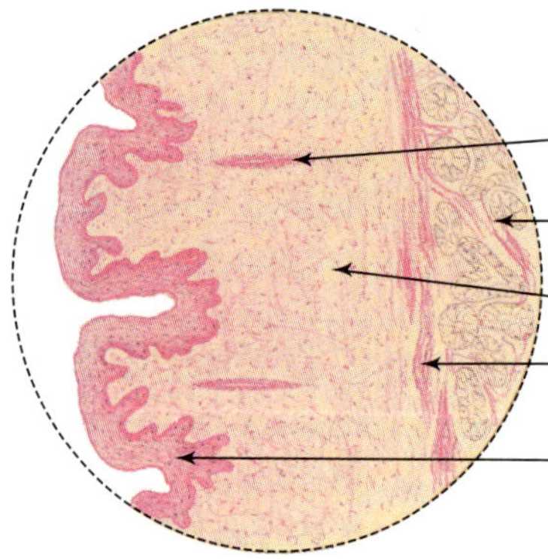

FIG. 23.11 ■ Microscopic structure of the oesophagus. (*Source: Textboook of Histology and a Practical Guide,* 2 ed.: J.P. Gunasegaran, Box 12.6, p. 223, Elsevier, 2010.)

   (c) *Muscularis mucosa*—extremely thick and made up of only longitudinal layer of smooth muscle fibres.
2. **Submucosa:** It contains mucous oesophageal glands. They secrete neutral mucous which protects oesophagus from reflex entry of acidic gastric juice.
3. **Muscular layer:**
   (a) ***In upper one-third***, it is made up of **skeletal muscle**.
   (b) ***In middle one-third***, it is made up of **both skeletal and smooth muscles**.
   (c) ***In lower one-third***, it is made up of **smooth muscle**.
4. **Fibrous membrane (adventitia):** It consists of dense connective tissue with many elastic fibres.

N.B.

A clinical condition in which the stratified squamous epithelium of the oesophagus is replaced by the gastric epithelium is called the *Barrett oesophagus*. It may lead to *oesophageal carcinoma*.

Development of the Oesophagus and Trachea

Oesophagus develops from the foregut. The respiratory tract develops from foregut diverticulum called the laryngotracheal diverticulum/tube. The following two important events occur in the development of the oesophagus:

(a) Separation of the laryngotracheal tube by the formation of the laryngotracheal septum.
(b) Recanalization of the obliterated lumen.

N.B.

The failure of the canalization of the oesophagus leads to the *oesophageal atresia*, and the maldevelopment of the laryngotracheal septum between the oesophagus and trachea leads to the *tracheoesophageal fistula*.

CLINICAL CORRELATION AN 25.8

- **Radiological examination of the oesophagus by barium swallow:** *It* is performed to detect (a) the enlargement of the left atrium due to mitral stenosis, (b) oesophageal strictures, and (c) carcinoma and achalasia cardia.

N.B.

In a normal case, the barium swallow examination presents three indentations in its outline caused by the aortic arch, left principal bronchus, and left atrium.

- **Oesophagoscopy:** *It* is performed to visualize the interior of the oesophagus; while passing oesophagoscope, the sites of normal constrictions should be kept in mind.
- **Achalasia cardia** (Fig. 23.12): It is a clinical condition in which the sphincter at the lower end of the oesophagus fails to relax when the food is swallowed. As a result, food accumulates in the oesophagus and its regurgitation occurs. This condition occurs probably due to the congenital absence of ganglion cells in the myenteric plexus of nerves in the oesophageal wall. A radiographic barium swallow examination of the oesophagus reveals a characteristic *bird's beak/rat tail appearance*.

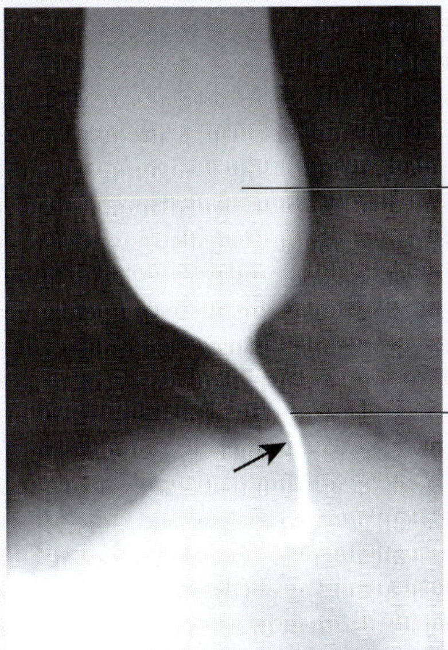

FIG. 23.12 Barium meal swallow in achalasia cardia showing characteristic bird's beak/rat tail appearance of oesophagus, as shown by black arrow. (*Source: Radiology in Medical Practice*, 5 ed.: ABM Abdullah, Plate 3.1B, P. 155, Elsevier Inc. 2016.)

- **Dysphagia (difficulty in swallowing):** It occurs due to:
  (a) compression of the oesophagus from outside by the aortic arch aneurysm, enlargement of lymph nodes, abnormal right subclavian artery (passing posterior to the oesophagus), etc., and
  (b) narrowing of the lumen due to stricture or carcinoma.
- **Tracheoesophageal fistula** (Fig. 23.13): It is the most common congenital anomaly of the oesophagus that occurs due to the failure of the separation of the *lumen* of the *tracheal tube* from that of the *oesophagus* by a laryngotracheal septum. In the most common type of the tracheoesophageal fistula, the upper oesophagus ends blindly and the lower oesophagus communicates with the trachea at the level of the T4 vertebra. Clinically, it presents as: (a) hydramnios because the fetus is unable to swallow amniotic fluid, (b) stomach is distended with air, and (c) the infant vomit every feed given or may cough up bile. The fistula must be closed surgically to avoid the passage of swallowed liquids into the lungs.

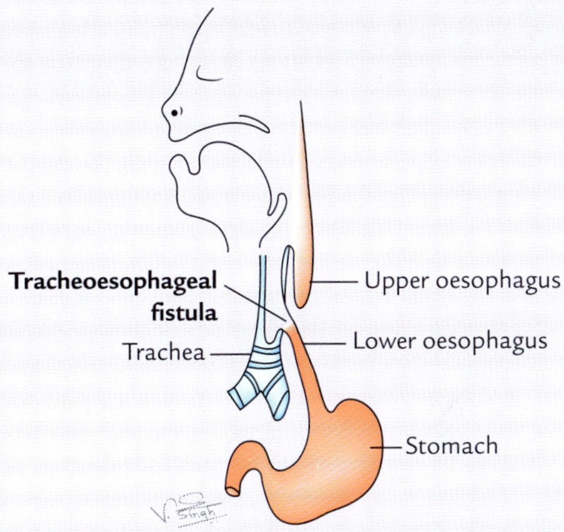

FIG. 23.13 Tracheoesophageal fistula.

- **Carcinoma of the lower third of the oesophagus:** It most commonly occurs in its lower one-third.
  The lymph vessels from the lower one-third of the oesophagus descend through the oesophageal opening of the diaphragm and drain into the coeliac lymph nodes around the coeliac trunk. A malignant tumour from the lower one-third of the oesophagus, therefore, spreads below the diaphragm into these lymph nodes. Consequently, **surgical resection of the lesion** includes not only the primary site (i.e. oesophagus) but also coeliac lymph nodes and all the regions that drain into these lymph nodes such as stomach, upper half of the duodenum, spleen, and omenta. The continuity of the gut is restored by performing an oesophagojejunostomy.

Golden Facts to Remember

• Most sensitive part of the trachea	Carina
• Commonest site of malignancy (cancer) in the oesophagus	Lower one-third
• Longest part of the oesophagus	Thoracic part
• Part of GIT having thickest muscularis mucosa in its wall	Oesophagus
• Most common motility disorder of the oesophagus	Achalasia cardia
• Most common congenital anomaly of the oesophagus	Tracheoesophageal fistula

CLINICAL CASE STUDY

A 65-year-old woman visited the hospital and complained of difficulty in swallowing (dysphagia) and marked loss of weight. The barium swallow revealed narrowing of the lower end of the oesophagus. The biopsy was taken from the end of the oesophagus and **it confirmed as the case of oesophageal malignancy**.

Questions

1. What are extent, length, and functions of oesophagus?
2. Name the three factors that can cause dysphagia.
3. Mention the lymphatic drainage of the oesophagus.
4. What is the most common site of the malignant tumour in oesophagus?

Answers

1. (a) It extends from the lower border of the cricoid cartilage in the neck (at the level of the C6 vertebra) to the cardiac orifice of stomach in abdomen at the level of the T11 vertebra.
   (b) It is 25 cm (10 in) in length.
   (c) It conducts the chewed food (bolus) from the pharynx to the stomach.
2. (a) Aneurysm of the arch of aorta, (b) enlarged lymph nodes, and (c) carcinoma of the oesophagus.
3. From the cervical part into deep cervical lymph nodes, from the thoracic part into posterior mediastinal lymph nodes, and from the abdominal part into the left gastric and coeliac lymph nodes.
4. Lower one-third of the oesophagus.

CHAPTER 24

Thoracic Duct, Azygos and Hemiazygos Veins, and Thoracic Sympathetic Trunks

SPECIFIC LEARNING OBJECTIVES

After studying this chapter, the student should be able to:

- Describe the thoracic duct under the following headings: (a) formation, (b) course, (c) termination, (d) relations, (e) tributaries, and (f) applied anatomy. AN 23.2
- Describe the origin, course, relations, tributaries, and termination of azygos and hemiazygos veins. AN 23.3
- Write short notes on: (a) thoracic duct, (b) azygos vein, and (c) hemiazygos vein.
- Draw a labelled diagram to show the relations of the thoracic duct in the root of the neck.
- Describe the location and extent of thoracic sympathetic chain. AN 23.5
- Describe the splanchnic nerves. AN 23.6

THORACIC DUCT AN 23.2

The thoracic duct is the largest lymphatic vessel (trunk or great lymph channel) that drains the lymph from most of the body into the blood stream. The lymph in the thoracic duct is milky-white in appearance because it contains a product of fat digestion (chyle) from the intestine. The duct appears beaded due to the presence of numerous valves within its lumen.

Area of drainage: The thoracic duct drains the lymph from all the parts of the body *except* the (a) right side of the head and neck, (b) right side of the chest wall, (c) right lung, (d) right side of the heart, (e) right surface of the liver, and (f) right upper limb.

N.B.

The lymph from right upper quadrant of the body, which is drained by the **right lymphatic duct** which opens in the angle between right subclavian and right internal jugular vein (Fig. 24.1). AN 23.7

Extent: The thoracic duct extends from the upper end of cisterna chyli on the posterior abdominal wall at the lower border of the T12 vertebra to the junction of the left internal jugular and left subclavian veins at the root of the neck.

N.B.

The *cisterna chyli* is a large lymphatic sac lying in front of L1 and L2 bodies, right to abdominal aorta, and behind right crus of diaphragm.

Measurements: The *measurements* of the thoracic duct are as follows:

Length: 45 cm (18 in).

Width of lumen: 5 mm (at the ends but narrow in the middle).

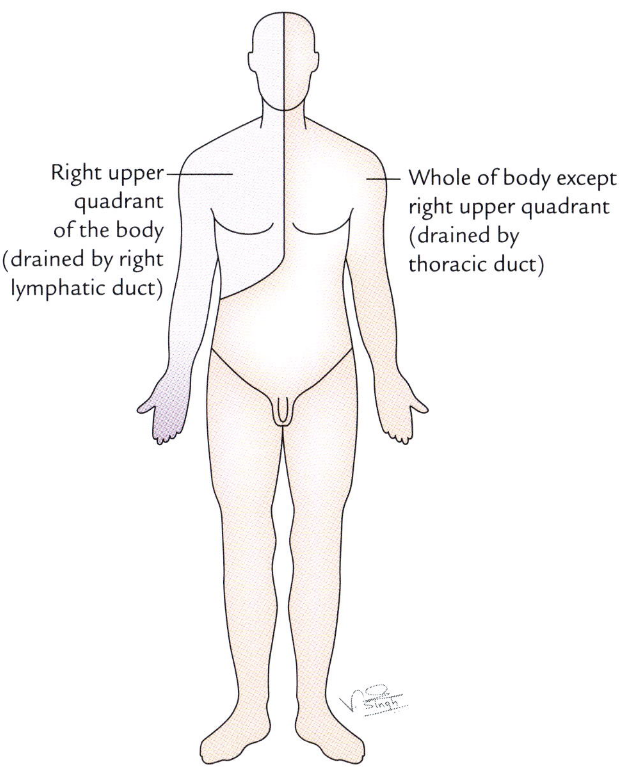

FIG. 24.1 Lymphatic drainage of the body. Note that the lymph from the right upper quadrant of the body is drained by the right lymphatic duct. The lymph from the remaining area of the body is drained by the thoracic duct.

FORMATION, COURSE, AND TERMINATION

The duct begins in the abdomen at the lower border of the T12 vertebra, as a continuation of cisterna chyli (the largest lymphatic sac, lying in front of the bodies of the L1 and L2 vertebrae) and enters the thorax through the aortic opening of the diaphragm. It then ascends in the posterior mediastinum to the right of the midline on the front of vertebral bodies.

On reaching the T5 vertebra, it crosses the midline from the right to left side and enters the superior mediastinum to run along the left border of the oesophagus and reaches the root of the neck.

At the root of the neck, it arches laterally at the level of the C7 vertebra—in front of the vertebral system (e.g. vertebral artery and vertebral vein) and the left cervical sympathetic trunk and behind the carotid system (e.g. left common carotid artery, left internal jugular vein, and left vagus nerve). The summit of the arch lies 3–4 cm above the clavicle. Finally, the duct descends in front of the first part of the left subclavian artery and finally terminates by opening into the junction of left subclavian and left internal jugular veins.

N.B.

The thoracic duct begins in abdomen, courses through the thorax, and terminates in the neck (Fig. 24.2).

RELATIONS

The relations of the thoracic duct are as follows:

A. **At the aortic orifice of the diaphragm:**
   Anterior: Median arcuate ligament of the diaphragm
   Posterior: T12 vertebra
   To the right: Azygos vein
   To the left: Aorta

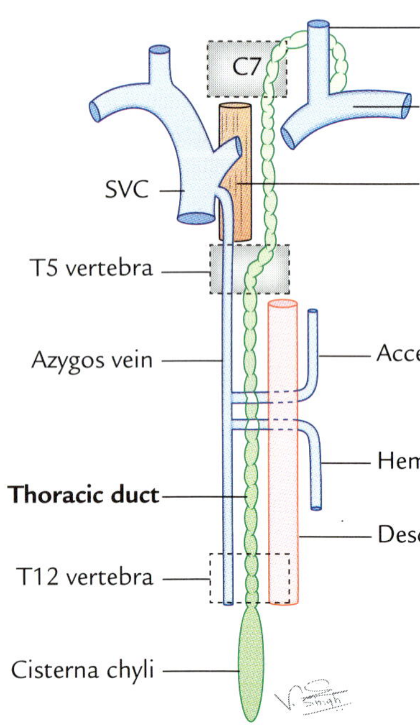

FIG. 24.2 ■ Formation, course, and termination of the thoracic duct.

B. **In the posterior mediastinum:**
   Anterior:
   1. Diaphragm
   2. Descending aorta (lower part)
   3. Oesophagus (upper part)

   Posterior:
   1. Vertebral column
   2. Anterior longitudinal ligament
   3. Terminal parts of hemiazygos and accessory hemiazygos veins
   4. Right posterior intercostal arteries

   To the right: Azygos vein
   To the left: Descending thoracic aorta

C. **In the superior mediastinum:**
   Anterior:
   1. Arch of the aorta
   2. Commencement of the left subclavian artery

   Posterior: Vertebral column
   To the right: Edge of the oesophagus
   To the left: Left lung and pleura

D. **In the root of the neck (Fig. 24.3):**
   Anterior: Carotid sheath containing the left common carotid artery, left internal jugular vein, and left vagus nerve.
   Posterior:
   1. Vertebral artery and vein
   2. Scalenus anterior muscle (medial border)
   3. Phrenic nerve
   4. Thyrocervical trunk and its branches (e.g. suprascapular, transverse cervical, and inferior thyroid arteries).

TRIBUTARIES

The tributaries of the thoracic duct are as follows (Fig. 24.4):

A. **In the thorax:**
   - A *pair of descending lymph trunks* from posterior intercostal lymph nodes of lower six spaces.
   - Lymph vessels from posterior mediastinal lymph nodes.
   - *Ascending lumbar lymph trunks* draining upper lateral aortic lymph nodes. These are bilateral and pierce the corresponding crus of diaphragm and eventually join the thoracic duct in the posterior mediastinum.

B. **In the neck:**
   1. Left jugular lymph trunk, draining lymph from the left half of head and neck.
   2. Left subclavian lymph trunk, draining lymph from the left upper limb.
   3. Left bronchomediastinal trunk.

CLINICAL CORRELATION

- **Injury of the thoracic duct:** The thoracic duct is thin walled and appears colourless during surgery therefore, it is sometimes injured inadvertently during surgical procedures in the posterior mediastinum. Laceration of the thoracic duct during lung surgery leads to leakage of

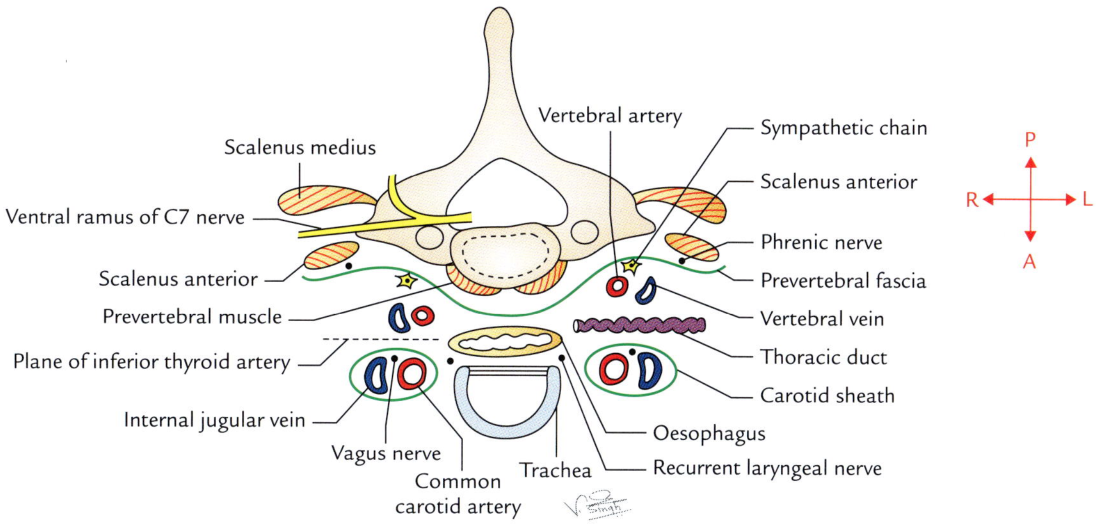

FIG. 24.3 ■ Relations of the thoracic duct in the root of the neck.

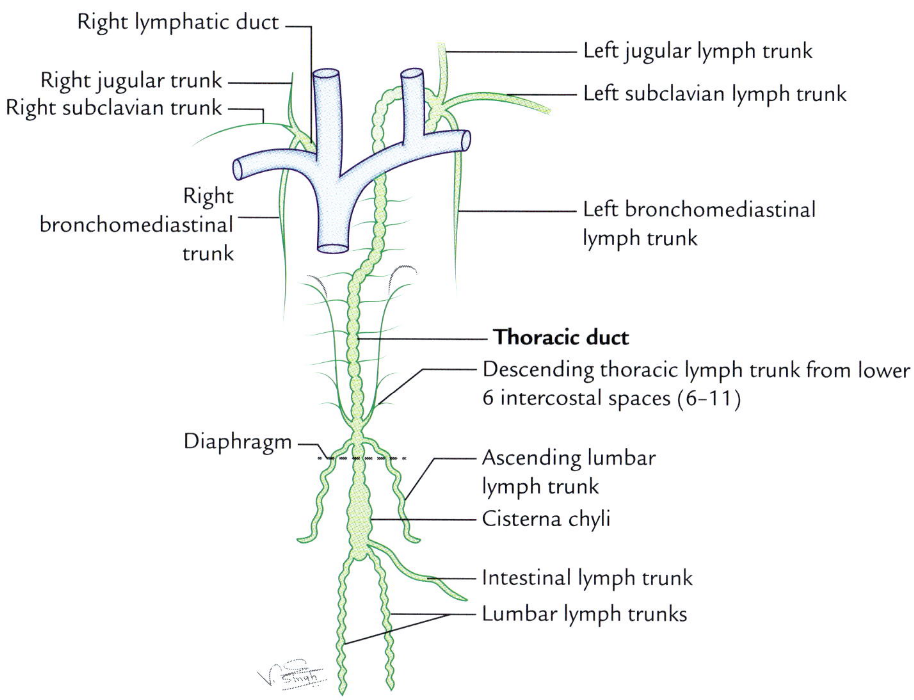

FIG. 24.4 ■ Tributaries of the thoracic duct.

chyle into the pleural cavity producing a clinical condition called *chylothorax*.

The cervical part of the thoracic duct may be damaged during the block dissection of the neck. It should be ligated immediately. If ligated, the lymph returns by anastomotic channels. But if the injury is not detected at the time of operation, and hence not ligated, it may cause an unpleasant *chylus fistula* and leakage of lymph. Immediate ligation of the duct is required to stop the leakage.

- **Obstruction of the thoracic duct:** Sometimes in filarial infection, the thoracic duct is obstructed by microfilarial parasites (*Wuchereria bancrofti*) leading to widespread effects, such as *chylothorax*, *chyloperitoneum*, *chyluria*, and even the accumulation of chyle in the tunica vaginalis of testis (chylocele).

DEVELOPMENT

There are three stages in the development of the thoracic duct (Fig. 24.5).

Stage I: In this stage, the network of the lymph channels is seen in front of the thoracic part of the vertebral column.

Stage II: In this stage, two longitudinal lymph channels appear, in the network of lymph channels, one on the left and another on the right with a number of cross communications.

Stage III: In this stage, the cross communication appears opposite to the T5 vertebra, right longitudinal channel below this cross communication, and left longitudinal channel above this cross communication persists and form the thoracic duct. All the other parts disappear.

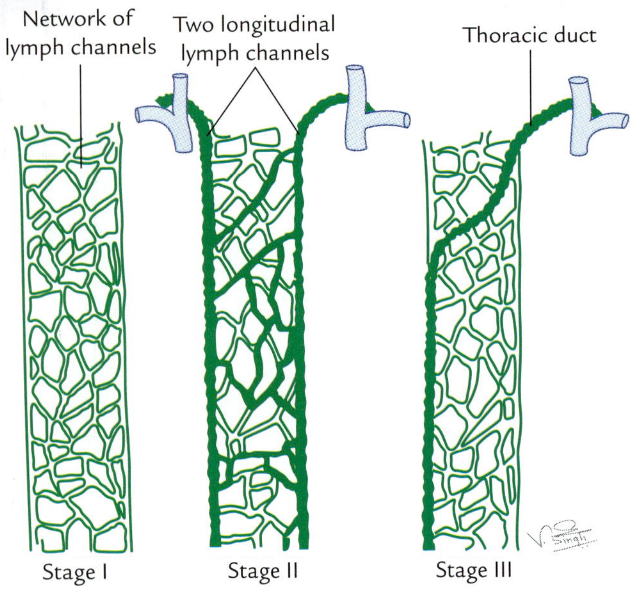

FIG. 24.5 ■ Development of the thoracic duct.

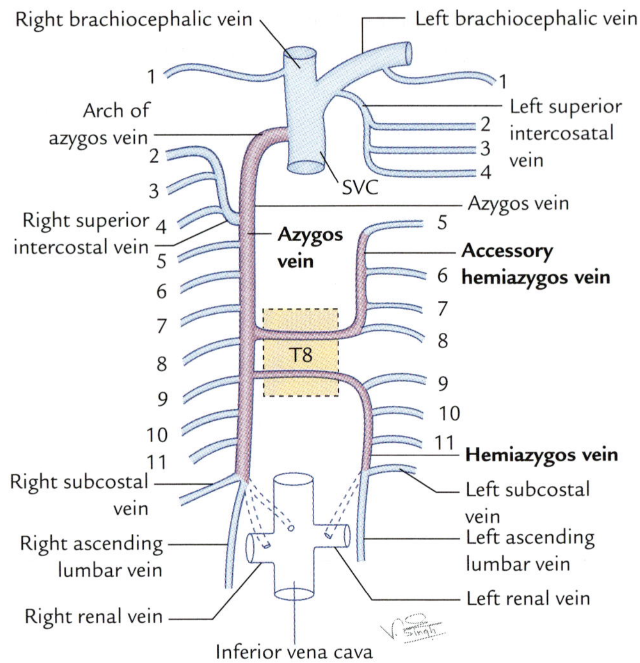

FIG. 24.6 ■ Azygos, hemiazygos, and accessory hemiazygos veins. Numbers 1 to 11 represent posterior intercostal veins.

AZYGOS AND HEMIAZYGOS VEINS AN 23.3

The term azygos means single, that is without a companion. The azygos system of veins consists of azygos, hemiazygos, and accessory hemiazygos veins. These veins lie in front of the thoracic part of the vertebral column and play an important role in the venous drainage of the thorax.

AZYGOS VEIN AN 23.3

The azygos vein is present on the right side of the thoracic vertebral column in the posterior mediastinum (Fig. 24.6). It connects the inferior vena cava (IVC) with the superior vena cava (SVC). It is provided with valve/valves halfway along azygos arch (between vertical azygos vein and point where the azygos vein enters the SVC). This part may appear tortuous.

The functions of the azygos vein are as follows:

1. It drains venous blood from the upper part of posterior abdominal wall and thoracic wall.
2. It connects SVC with IVC. Thus, it forms an important collateral channel connecting the SVC and IVC.

Formation

The formation of the azygos vein is variable. It is formed in one of the following ways:

1. Formed by the union of the *right subcostal* and the *right ascending lumbar vein* at the level of the T12 vertebra (common).
2. Arises from the *posterior aspect of the IVC* near the renal veins.
3. As a continuation of the right subcostal vein.
4. Occasionally, it may arise from the right renal or right first lumbar vein.

Course and Termination

The azygos vein after formation ascends up and leaves the abdomen by passing through the aortic opening of the diaphragm and enters the posterior mediastinum. There it ascends vertically lying in front of the vertebral column up to the level of the T4 vertebra, where it arches forward above the hilum of the right lung to terminate in the SVC at the level of the second costal cartilage.

Relations

Anterior: Oesophagus (right edge)

Posterior:
1. Lower eighth thoracic vertebrae
2. Right posterior intercostal arteries

To the right:
1. Right lung and pleura
2. Greater splanchnic nerve

To the left:
1. Thoracic duct
2. Descending thoracic aorta
3. Oesophagus (right border)

The arch of the azygos vein is related *below* to the root of the right lung, on the *right side* to the right lung and the pleura, and the *left side* to the right border of the oesophagus, trachea, and right vagus nerve.

Tributaries

The tributaries of the azygos vein are as follows:

1. *Right superior intercostal vein* (formed by the union of the second, third, and fourth right posterior intercostal veins).
2. *Fifth to eleventh right posterior intercostal veins.*
3. *Hemiazygos vein* (at the level of the lower border of T8 vertebra).
4. *Accessory hemiazygos vein* (at the level of the upper border of T8 vertebra).
5. *Right subcostal vein.*

6. Right ascending lumbar vein.
7. Right bronchial vein (near the terminal end of azygos vein).
8. Oesophageal veins with the exception of those at its lower end.
9. Mediastinal veins.
10. Pericardial veins.

CLINICAL CORRELATION

In the case of obstruction of SVC, the azygos vein serves as the main collateral channel to shunt the blood from the upper half of the body to IVC (for details, see clinical correlation on page 289, Chapter 22).

HEMIAZYGOS VEIN AN 23.3

The hemiazygos vein (syn. inferior hemiazygos vein) lies on the left side thoracic vertebral column and corresponds to the lower part of the azygos vein (i.e. mirror image of the lower part of the azygos vein) (Fig. 24.6).

Formation

The hemiazygos vein formed on the left, similar to the azygos vein, by the union of the left ascending lumbar vein and the left subcostal vein. It may arise from the posterior surface of the left renal vein.

Course and Termination

It pierces the left crus of the diaphragm and ascends vertically in front of the left side of the vertebral column up to the level of the T8 vertebra. At the T8 vertebra, it turns to the right and crosses in front of the vertebral column posterior to the aorta, oesophagus, and thoracic duct to terminate in the azygos vein.

Tributaries

The tributaries of the hemiazygos vein are as follows:

1. Lower three (9th–11th) left posterior intercostal veins.
2. Left subcostal vein.
3. Left ascending lumbar vein.
4. Small oesophageal and mediastinal veins.

ACCESSORY HEMIAZYGOS VEIN

The accessory hemiazygos vein (syn. superior hemiazygos vein; Fig. 24.6) lies on the left side thoracic vertebral column and corresponds to the upper part of the azygos vein (i.e. mirror image of the upper part of the azygos vein).

Course and Termination

The accessory hemiazygos vein begins at the medial end of the left fourth or fifth intercostal space and descends to the left side of the vertebral column. At the level of the T8 vertebra, it turns to the right passes in front of the vertebral column posterior to the aorta, oesophagus, and thoracic duct to terminate in the azygos vein.

N.B.

Sometimes the terminal parts of hemiazygos and accessory hemiazygos veins join together to form a common trunk that crosses across the vertebral column to open into the azygos vein.

Tributaries

The following are the tributaries of the accessory hemiazygos vein:

1. Fifth to eighth left posterior intercostal veins
2. Left bronchial veins (sometimes)

THORACIC SYMPATHETIC TRUNKS AN 23.5, AN 23.6

The thoracic sympathetic trunk is a ganglionated chain situated on either side of the vertebral column (Fig. 24.7). Superiorly it is continuous with the cervical sympathetic chain at the thoracic inlet and inferiorly with the lumbar sympathetic chain after passing behind the medial arcuate ligament of the diaphragm.

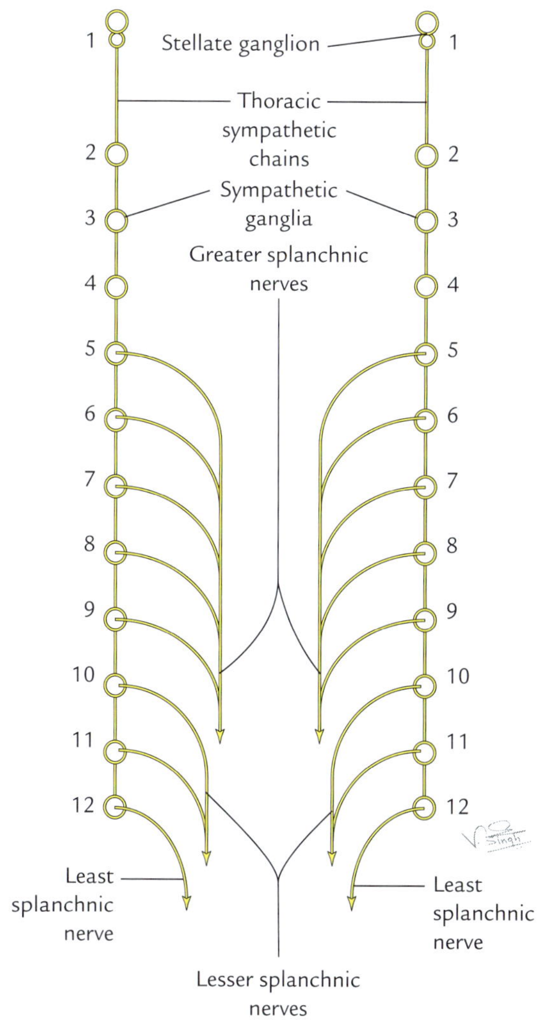

FIG. 24.7 ■ Thoracic sympathetic trunks and splanchnic nerves.

COURSE AND RELATIONS

The thoracic sympathetic chain begins at stellate ganglion (cervicothoracic ganglion), and descends in the thorax in front of the neck of the first rib, head of the 2nd–10th ribs and along the bodies of the T11 and T12 vertebrae, in front of the posterior intercostal nerves and vessels. On the side of body of 12th thoracic vertebra it passes behind the *medial arcuate ligament* to become continuous with the *lumbar sympathetic trunk*.

GANGLIA

Initially, each thoracic sympathetic trunk has 12 ganglia, corresponding to the 12 thoracic spinal nerves. Later, the first thoracic ganglion commonly fuses with the inferior cervical sympathetic ganglion to form the *cervicothoracic/stellate ganglion*. The second ganglion also may occasionally fuse with the first ganglion. Thus, there are usually 11 ganglia in the thoracic sympathetic trunk; sometimes there may be only 10 ganglia (vide supra). Each ganglion lies at the level of the corresponding intervertebral disc and is connected to the corresponding spinal nerve by the white and grey ramus communicans.

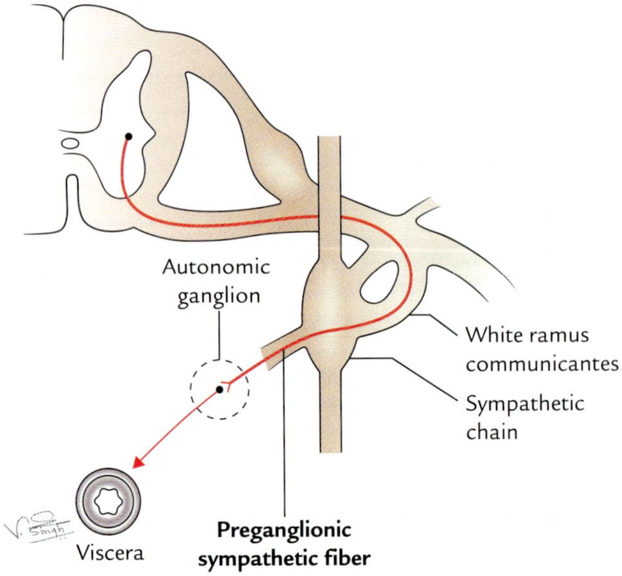

FIG. 24.8 ■ Origin of preganglionic fibres of thoracic splanchnic nerve.

BRANCHES

The branches of thoracic sympathetic trunks are divided into two groups: medial and lateral.

A. **Medial branches:**

The medial branches supply the viscera. They are as follows:

1. The medial branches from the first to fifth ganglia consist of postganglionic fibres and are distributed to the heart, great vessels, lungs, and oesophagus through the following plexuses:
   (a) *Pulmonary plexus*
   (b) *Cardiac plexus*
   (c) *Aortic plexus*
   (d) *Oesophageal plexus*
2. Medial branches from the 5th to 12th thoracic ganglia consist of preganglionic fibres and form **three splanchnic nerves**.
   (a) ***Greater splanchnic nerve***: It is formed by the preganglionic fibres arising from the *fifth to ninth thoracic sympathetic ganglia*. It descends obliquely on the vertebral bodies, pierces the corresponding crus of the diaphragm, and terminates mainly in the celiac ganglion. Partly it also terminates in the *aorticorenal ganglion* and the *suprarenal gland*. It provides sympathetic supply to foregut and adrenal medulla.
   (b) ***Lesser splanchnic nerve:*** It is formed by the preganglionic fibres from the *10th and 11th ganglia*. Its course is obliquely similar to the greater splanchnic nerve, pierces the corresponding crus of the diaphragm, and terminates in the *superior mesenteric ganglion*.
   It provides sympathetic supply to midgut.
   (c) ***Least (lowest) splanchnic nerve:*** It is also called the *renal nerve*. This tiny nerve arises from the 12th thoracic ganglion and may even be absent. It descends obliquely as greater and lesser splanchnic nerves, pierces either the crus or passes behind the medial arcuate ligament of the diaphragm, and terminates in the renal plexus/ganglions.
   It provides sympathetic supply to kidneys.

Further details about thoracic splanchnic nerves. These are as follows:

- These nerves provide sympathetic supply to the organs of abdomen.
- Their fibres originate from thoracic spinal segments from T5 to T12. Then travel through white rami communicants and pass through sympathetic ganglia without synapsing, and join together to form a splanchnic nerve (Fig. 24.8).
- Thus they are made up of preganglionic fibres which synapse with coeliac, superior mesenteric and aorticorenal ganglia. From them postganglionic fibres arise and supply abdominopelvic organs.
- There are three sets of paired thoracic splanchnic nerves:
  - Greater splanchnic nerves
  - Lesser splanchnic nerves
  - Least splanchnic nerves

  They are already described in detail earlier.

B. **Lateral branches:**

The lateral branches supply limbs and body wall. Their supply is *pilomotor*, *sudomotor*, and *vasomotor* to the skin of these regions.

The preganglionic fibres arise from the lateral horns of the spinal segments and enter the sympathetic ganglion via white *rami communicantes* of the spinal nerve. The postganglionic fibres from the ganglion reenter the spinal nerve via grey rami communicantes and supply the corresponding dermatome of the upper limb and the body wall.

N.B.

Lumbar splanchnic nerves: They arise from lumbar part of the sympathetic trunk. The nerve fibres arising from trunk synapse in inferior mesenteric ganglion. The postsynaptic fibres arising from this ganglion supplied smooth muscle and glands of the pelvic viscera.

CLINICAL CORRELATION

- **Thoracoabdominal sympathectomy:** The bilateral thoracoabdominal sympathectomy is done to relieve **severe hypertension.** The surgical procedure involves the removal of the sympathetic trunk from T5 to L2 ganglia and excision of the splanchnic nerves. As a result, there occurs splanchnic vasodilatation and consequent fall in the blood pressure.
- The ***upper limb sympathectomy*** is used to treat the *Raynaud's disease*. In this, part of thoracic sympathetic chain is excised below the level of stellate ganglion.

N.B.

Injury to stellate ganglion may cause ipsilateral Horner's syndrome.

- **Hypotension during spinal anaesthesia:** Sometimes ***hypotension*** occurs during high spinal anaesthesia due to the paralysis of sympathetic outflow to the splanchnic nerves.
- **Referred pain of the diaphragm:** The irritation of the diaphragm secondary to peritonitis causes pain due to the stimulation of the phrenic nerve (root value C3–C5). The pain is referred to the corresponding tip of the shoulder, being supplied by the supraclavicular nerve (root value C3–C5).

Golden Facts to Remember

• Largest lymphatic channel in the body	Thoracic duct
• Chylothorax	Accumulation of chyle in the pleural cavity
• Chylocele	Accumulation of chyle in the tunica vaginalis
• Chyluria	Presence of chyle in urine
• Renal nerve	Least splanchnic nerve
• Commonest cause of damage of thoracic duct at the root of the neck	Block dissection of the neck
• Largest collateral channel connecting superior and inferior vena cavae	Azygos vein
• Largest splanchnic nerve	Greater splanchnic nerve
• Most posterior intercostal veins drain into	Azygos venous system

CLINICAL CASE STUDY

A 50-year-old male visited the hospital and complained of swelling of the scrotum associated with periodic fever and passage of milky urine. On examination, the doctor found that scrotum as a whole was enlarged. The scrotal skin was thickened mainly at the bottom. On aspiration of scrotum, a milky fluid came out. **He was diagnosed as a case of chylocele and chyluria due to obstruction of thoracic duct.**

Questions

1. What is chylocele?
2. What is the cause of chylocele?
3. What is the cause of thickening of scrotal skin?

Answers

1. Accumulation of chyle in the tunica vaginalis around the testis.
2. When the thoracic duct is obstructed by the microfilaria (*Wuchereria bancrofti*). It leads to widespread effects such as chylothorax, chyloperitoneum, and chyluria.
3. Lymphostasis.

CHAPTER 25

Surface Anatomy of the Thorax

SPECIFIC LEARNING OBJECTIVES

After studying this chapter, the student should be able to:

- Palpate the important surface landmarks on the front of thorax.
- To do the surface marking of lung and pleura. AN 25.9
- To do surface marking of the heart and its associated vessels. AN 25.9
- To do the surface markings of trachea and oesophagus.

The surface marking deals with projections of deeper structures on the surface of the body. For convenience of understanding the **surface landmarks have been described with the concerned chapters**. The present chapter deals only with the surface marking of only important structures.

SURFACE MARKINGS OF PLEURA AND LUNGS AN 25.9

Parietal pleura: It has been described in detail in Chapter 18 (Fig. 18.6).

Visceral pleura: The surface marking of the visceral pleura coincides with that of the lungs. The surface markings of the lung is described in Chapter 19 (Fig. 19.9).

For easy recall, Fig. 25.1 reveals the surface projections of the lungs and the pleura.

SURFACE MARKING OF THE HEART/STERNOCOSTAL SURFACE OF THE HEART ON THE ANTERIOR CHEST WALL (FIG. 25.2) AN 25.9

1. **Right border**
   - Mark a point 'a' on the upper border of the right third costal cartilage, about 1 cm from the margin of the sternum.
   - Mark a point 'b' in the right fourth intercostal space, 4 cm from the median plane.
   - Mark a point 'c' on the lower border of the right sixth cartilage, 2 cm from the sternal margin.

   The right border is marked by a line joining these points with slight convexity to the right.
2. **Lower border**
   - Mark a point 'd' on the xiphisternal joint in the median plane.
   - Mark a point 'e' in the left fifth intercostal space, 9 cm from the midsternal line.

   The line joining the points 'c', 'd', and 'e' marks the lower border of the heart.
3. **Left border**

   Mark a point 'f' on the lower border of the left second costal cartilage, about 1.25 cm from the sternal margin.

   The line joining the points 'd' and 'e' marks the left border.
4. **Upper border**

   The line joining the points 'a' and 'f' marks the upper border.

SURFACE MARKING OF THE CARDIAC VALVES AND AUSCULTATORY AREAS AN 25.9

It is described in detail in Chapter 21 (Fig. 21.18).

SURFACE MARKING OF THE AORTA (FIG. 25.3)

A. **Ascending aorta:** It is marked by drawing two parallel lines 2.5 cm apart. These lines start from the medial end of the left third intercostal space, go upward, and to the right up to the right half of the sternal angle.

B. **Arch of the aorta:** It lies behind the lower half of the manubrium sterni. It is marked on the surface as under:
   - Mark a point 'a' at the right end of the sternal angle.
   - Mark a point 'b' at the centre of the manubrium sterni.
   - Mark a point 'c' on the sternal end of the left second costal cartilage.

   The aortic arch marked on the surface by two parallel lines 2.5 cm apart, joining these points with upward/outer convexity.

C. **Descending thoracic aorta (DTA)**
   - Mark a point 'c' at the sternal end of the left second costal cartilage.
   - Mark a point 'd' 2 cm above the transpyloric plane in the median plane.

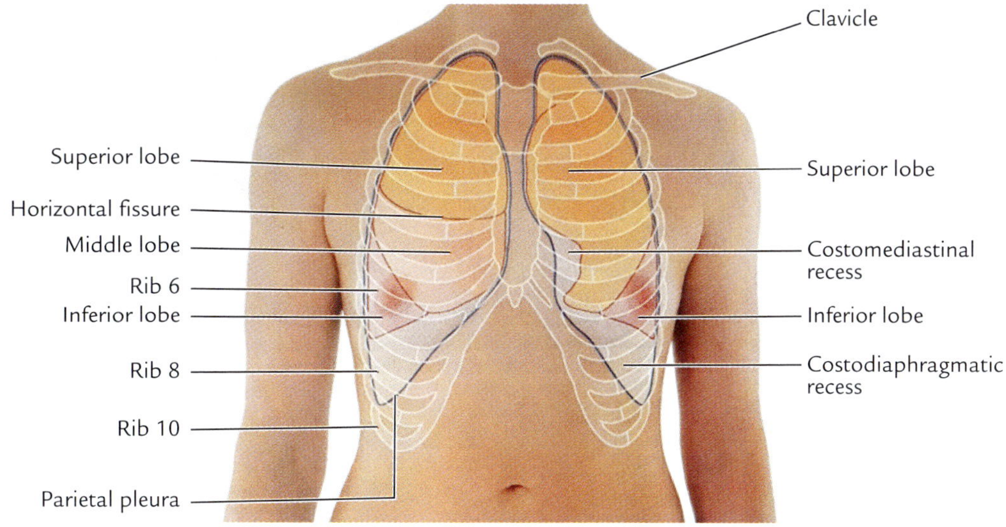

FIG. 25.1 ■ Surface markings of the lungs and pleura on the anterior aspect of female chest. (*Source: Gray's Anatomy for Students*, 3 ed.: Richard L Drake, Wayne Vogl, Adam WM Mitchell, Fig. 3.103A, p. 237, Elsevier Inc., 2005.)

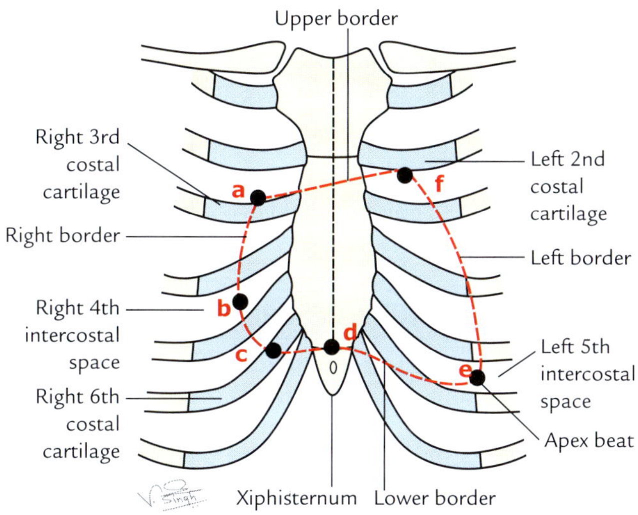

FIG. 25.2 ■ Surface markings of the heart on the anterior chest wall/sternocostal surface of the heart.

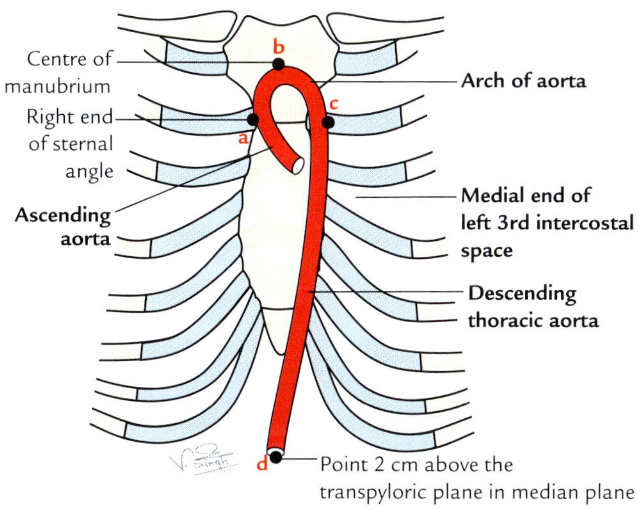

FIG. 25.3 ■ Surface markings of the aorta.

The DTA is drawn on the surface by two parallel lines 2.5 cm apart, which extends downward and slightly medially from the first to the second point.

SURFACE MARKING OF THE INTERNAL MAMMARY (INTERNAL THORACIC) ARTERY (FIG. 25.4)

- Mark a point 'a' 1 cm above the sternal end of the clavicle, 3.5 cm from the median plane.
- Mark a point 'b' on the sixth costal cartilage, 1.25 cm lateral to the sternal margin.
- Mark a point 'c' in the sixth intercostals space, 1.25 cm lateral to the sternal margin. The internal mammary artery is marked by joining above points.

SURFACE MARKINGS OF THE TRACHEA AND BRONCHI (FIG. 25.5)

Trachea (cervical and thoracic parts; Fig. 25.5)

The cervical and thoracic parts of trachea are marked on the surface as follows:

- Mark a point 'a' on the lower border of the cricoid cartilage (arch) in the median plane.
- Mark a point 'b' on the sternal angle, 1 cm to the right of its centre.

Now, draw two parallel lines 2 cm apart joining points 'a' and 'b' to mark the trachea. They should commence at the first point and should incline slightly to the right at the sternal angle.

Right principal bronchus (Fig. 25.5)

- Mark a point 'b' on sternal angle 1 cm to the right of its centre.
- Mark a point 'c' at the sternal end of the right third costal cartilage.

Now, join these points by a 2.5-cm-long line to mark the right bronchus on the surface.

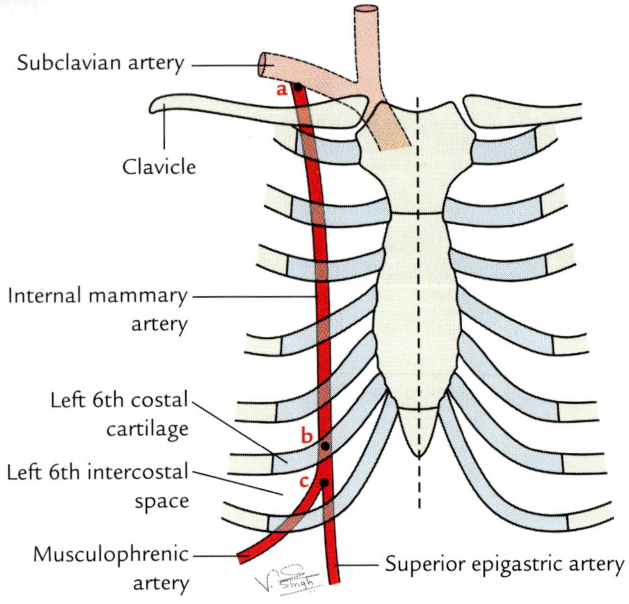

FIG. 25.4 ■ Surface markings of the internal mammary (internal thoracic) artery.

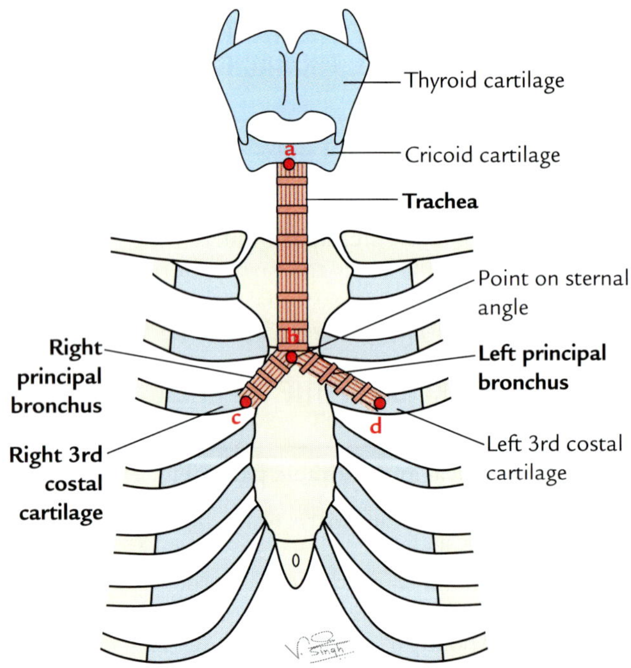

FIG. 25.5 ■ Surface markings of the trachea and bronchi.

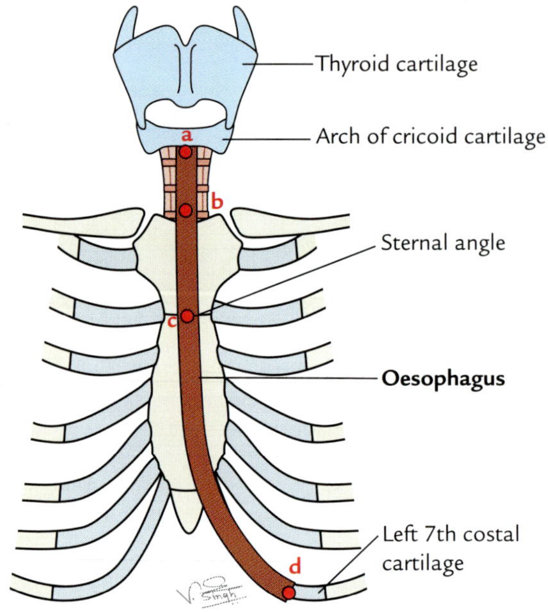

FIG. 25.6 ■ Surface marking of the oesophagus.

Left principal bronchus (Fig. 25.5)

- Mark a point 'b' on sternal angle 1 cm to the right of its centre.
- Mark a point 'd' on the left third costal cartilage, 3.5 cm from the median plane.

Now, join these points by a 5-cm-long line to mark the left principal bronchus on the surface.

SURFACE MARKING OF OESOPHAGUS (FIG. 25.6)

It is marked on the surface as follows (Fig. 25.6):

- Mark a point 'a' at the lower border of the cricoid cartilage anteriorly in the median plane.
- Mark a point 'b' at the root of the neck, a little to the left of the median plane.
- Mark a point 'c' at the sternal angle.
- Mark a point 'd' on the left seventh costal cartilage, 2.5 cm away from the midline.

Now join these points by two parallel lines 2.5 cm apart.

N.B.

While connecting the first two points (a and b), the line should incline slightly to the **l**eft and then slightly to the **r**ight and finally while joining the last three points, the line should incline slightly to the **l**eft again.

Mnemonic: **L**eft-**R**ight-**L**eft.

Multiple Choice Questions: Upper Limb and Thorax

UPPER LIMB

CHAPTER 1

1. The most important function of the hand in humans is
   (a) Power grip
   (b) Hook grip
   (c) Precision grip
   (d) None of the above
2. Evolutionary changes occurred in human upper limb include all ***except***
   (a) Appearance of joints permitting rotatory movements of the forearm
   (b) Addition of clavicle to act as a strut
   (c) Rotation of thumb to 180° for opposition
   (d) Rotation of thumb to 90° for opposition
3. Shoulder region includes all of the following regions ***except***
   (a) Pectoral region
   (b) Axilla
   (c) Arm
   (d) Scapular region

Answers
1. ***c***, 2. ***c***, 3. ***c***

CHAPTER 2

1. Select the incorrect statement about the clavicle:
   (a) It is only a long bone which lies horizontally
   (b) It has no medullary cavity
   (c) It ossifies mainly in cartilage
   (d) It ossifies by two primary centres
2. All the statements about clavicle are correct ***except***
   (a) It is the first bone to start ossifying
   (b) It acts like a strut to keep upper limb away from the trunk
   (c) It commonly fractures at the junction of its lateral two-third and medial one-third
   (d) It can be palpated throughout its extent
3. All the statements about scapula are correct ***except***
   (a) It has three processes
   (b) It has head and neck
   (c) It extends vertically from first to eighth rib
   (d) Its lateral border is thickest
4. All the structures are attached to coracoid process ***except***
   (a) Coracohumeral ligament
   (b) Coracoacromial ligament
   (c) Rhomboid ligament
   (d) Long head of biceps brachii
5. Select the ***incorrect statement*** about the surgical neck of humerus:
   (a) It is commonest site of fracture of humerus
   (b) It is related to axillary nerve
   (c) It is a short constriction at the upper end of the shaft below the greater and lesser tubercles
   (d) It is related to posterior and anterior circumflex humeral arteries
6. Select the ***incorrect statement*** about the lower end of radius:
   (a) It is the widest part of the bone
   (b) Its posterior surface presents Lister's tubercle
   (c) Groove lateral to Lister's tubercle lodges the tendon of extensor pollicis longus
   (d) Its medial surface presents the ulnar notch
7. All of the following statements about ulna are correct ***except***
   (a) It stabilizes the forearm during supination and pronation
   (b) Its head is directed upwards
   (c) Its posterior border provides attachment to three muscles by a common aponeurosis
   (d) Its upper end presents two notches
8. Select the ***incorrect statement*** about carpal bones:
   (a) Scaphoid is the most commonly fractured carpal bone
   (b) Capitate is the largest carpal bone
   (c) Pisiform is the first bone to ossify
   (d) Lunate is the most commonly dislocated carpal bone
9. All are the peculiar features of first metacarpal bone ***except***
   (a) Its dorsal surface faces laterally
   (b) Its base possesses saddle-shaped articular surface
   (c) Its head is related to two sesamoid bones
   (d) Its epiphysis is at its distal end

10. Select the ***incorrect statement*** about the phalanges:
    (a) They are 14 in number
    (b) They are short long bones
    (c) All the digits have three phalanges
    (d) Heads of proximal and middle phalanges are pulley shaped

Answers

1. ***c***, 2. ***c***, 3. ***c***, 4. ***d***, 5. ***a***, 6. ***c***, 7. ***b***, 8. ***c***, 9. ***d***, 10. ***c***

CHAPTER 3

1. Muscles of pectoral region include all ***except***
    (a) Pectoralis major
    (b) Serratus anterior
    (c) Pectoralis minor
    (d) Subclavius
2. Select the ***incorrect statement*** about the pectoralis major muscle:
    (a) It arises from lateral half of the anterior surface of the clavicle
    (b) It is supplied by all the five spinal segments of the brachial plexus
    (c) Its clavicular head flexes the arm
    (d) Its sternocostal head adducts and medially rotates the arm
3. Select the ***incorrect statement*** about the serratus anterior muscle:
    (a) It arises by eight digitations from upper eight ribs
    (b) It is inserted into the costal surface of scapula along its lateral border
    (c) It is supplied by long thoracic nerve
    (d) It is the chief protractor of the scapula
4. Regarding clavipectoral fascia, all of the following statements are correct ***except***
    (a) It lies deep to sternocostal head of the pectoralis major
    (b) It encloses subclavius and pectoralis minor muscles
    (c) Vertically it extends from clavicle and axillary fascia
    (d) Its thick upper part is called costoclavicular ligament
5. Clavipectoral fascia is pierced by all of the following structures ***except***
    (a) Cephalic vein
    (b) Thoracoacromial artery
    (c) Medial pectoral nerve
    (d) Lymph vessels from the breast
6. All of the following statements regarding breast are correct ***except***
    (a) It lies in the superficial fascia of the pectoral region
    (b) It is a modified sebaceous gland
    (c) Vertically, it extends from second to sixth rib
    (d) Horizontally, it extends from sternum to midaxillary line
7. The deep aspect of breast is related to all of the following muscles ***except***
    (a) Pectoralis major
    (b) Pectoralis minor
    (c) Serratus anterior
    (d) Aponeurosis of external oblique muscle of abdomen
8. Regarding breast cancer, which of following statements is ***incorrect***:
    (a) It mostly occurs in its superolateral quadrant
    (b) It is immobile and fixed
    (c) It produces retraction of nipple
    (d) Its spread to vertebral column occurs through lymphatics

Answers

1. ***b***, 2. ***a***, 3. ***b***, 4. ***a***, 5. ***c***, 6. ***b***, 7. ***b***, 8. ***d***

CHAPTER 4

1. The axillary sheath is derived from:
    (a) Investing layer of deep cervical fascia
    (b) Pretracheal fascia
    (c) Prevertebral fascia
    (d) Deep fascia of the axilla
2. The apex of axilla is bounded by all of the following structures ***except***
    (a) Clavicle
    (b) Upper border of scapula
    (c) Neck of humerus
    (d) Outer border of the first rib
3. Which of the following structures is ***not*** a content of the axilla?
    (a) Axillary vessels
    (b) Roots of brachial plexus
    (c) Axillary tail of the mammary gland
    (d) Intercostobrachial nerve
4. Select the ***incorrect statement*** about the axillary artery:
    (a) It extends from outer border of first rib to the lower border of teres major muscle
    (b) It is divided into three parts of the pectoralis minor muscle
    (c) It usually gives rise to five branches
    (d) It is the 'key structure' of the axilla
5. Select the ***incorrect statement*** about the axillary vein:
    (a) It is continuation of subclavian vein
    (b) It lies medial to the axillary artery
    (c) It lies outside the axillary sheath
    (d) It receives venae comitantes of the brachial artery
6. Select the ***incorrect statement*** about the Erb's point:
    (a) It is the point on the upper trunk of brachial plexus where six nerves meet
    (b) Traction injury of Erb's point involves C5 and C6 fibres
    (c) Suprascapular and nerve to subclavius arise at this point
    (d) Dorsal scapular and long thoracic nerves arise at this point

7. Which of the following parts of the brachial plexus is involved in Klumpke's paralysis?
   (a) Upper trunk
   (b) Middle trunk
   (c) Lower trunk
   (d) None of the above
8. Klumpke's paralysis presents all of the following clinical features ***except***
   (a) Claw hand
   (b) Sensory loss along the medial border of forearm and hand
   (c) Horner's syndrome
   (d) Wrist drop

Answers

1. ***c***, 2. ***c***, 3. ***b***, 4. ***c***, 5. ***a***, 6. ***d***, 7. ***c***, 8. ***d***

CHAPTER 5

1. Which of the following two muscles contract together while climbing a tree?
   (a) Latissimus dorsi and trapezius
   (b) Teres major and minor
   (c) Teres major and pectoralis major
   (d) Latissimus dorsi and pectoralis major
2. All of the following muscles are supplied by dorsal scapular nerve ***except***
   (a) Supraspinatus
   (b) Rhomboideus minor
   (c) Rhomboideus major
   (d) Levator scapulae
3. All of the following structures form the boundary of triangle of auscultation ***except***
   (a) Trapezius
   (b) Rhomboideus major
   (c) Latissimus dorsi
   (d) Medial border of the scapula
4. All of the following arteries take part in the formation of anastomosis around scapula ***except***
   (a) Deep branch of the transverse cervical artery
   (b) Suprascapular artery
   (c) Lateral thoracic artery
   (d) Circumflex scapular artery
5. Select the ***incorrect statement*** about the deltoid muscle:
   (a) It is shaped like an inverted Greek letter delta
   (b) It is supplied by axillary nerve
   (c) It abducts the arm from 0° to 90°
   (d) Its middle fibres are multipennate
6. All of the following structures pass through quadrangular intermuscular space ***except***
   (a) Axillary nerve
   (b) Circumflex scapular artery
   (c) Posterior circumflex humeral artery
   (d) Posterior circumflex humeral vein
7. Which of the following structures pass through the upper triangular intermuscular space?
   (a) Anterior circumflex humeral artery
   (b) Posterior circumflex humeral artery
   (c) Profunda brachii artery
   (d) Circumflex scapular artery
8. Which of the following nerves traverse through lower triangular intermuscular space:
   (a) Axillary nerve
   (b) Thoracodorsal nerve
   (c) Radial nerve
   (d) Median nerve

Answers

1. ***d***, 2. ***a***, 3. ***b***, 4. ***c***, 5. ***c***, 6. ***b***, 7. ***d***, 8. ***c***

CHAPTER 6

1. All of the following statements about sternoclavicular joint are true ***except***
   (a) It is a saddle type of synovial joint
   (b) Its articular surfaces are covered with fibrocartilage
   (c) It is frequently involved in dislocation
   (d) Its joint cavity is divided into two parts by an articular disc
2. Musculotendinous cuff is formed by all the muscles ***except***
   (a) Supraspinatus
   (b) Teres major
   (c) Infraspinatus
   (d) Teres minor
3. Anatomically the shoulder joint is most commonly dislocated:
   (a) Superiorly
   (b) Inferiorly
   (c) Anteriorly
   (d) Posteriorly
4. The synovial bursa, which commonly communicates with the cavity of the shoulder joint is
   (a) Subscapular bursa
   (b) Infraspinatus bursa
   (c) Subacromial bursa
   (d) None of the above
5. Which of the following nerves is commonly injured in inferior dislocation of shoulder joint?
   (a) Radial nerve
   (b) Ulnar nerve
   (c) Thoracodorsal nerve
   (d) Axillary nerve
6. Shoulder movements occur at
   (a) Glenohumeral joint only
   (b) Sternoclavicular joint only
   (c) Acromioclavicular joint only
   (d) Scapulothoracic joint only
   (e) All of the above joints
7. Which of the following structures prevent superior dislocation of head of humerus?
   (a) Coracoclavicular ligament
   (b) Coracohumeral ligament
   (c) Coracoacromial arch
   (d) Transverse humeral ligament

8. Chief articulation of shoulder is
   (a) Sternoclavicular joint
   (b) Acromioclavicular joint
   (c) Glenohumeral joint
   (d) Scapulothoracic joint
9. The term ***shoulder separation*** is used for
   (a) Dislocation of shoulder joint
   (b) Dislocation of acromioclavicular joint
   (c) Dislocation of sternoclavicular joint
   (d) None of the above

Answers

1. ***c***, 2. ***b***, 3. ***b***, 4. ***a***, 5. ***d***, 6. ***e***, 7. ***c***, 8. ***c***, 9. ***b***

CHAPTER 7

1. The group of spinal segments supplying cutaneous innervation to upper limb is
   (a) C5 to T1
   (b) C4 to C8
   (c) C3 to T3
   (d) C4 to T2
2. The spinal segment providing dermatomal supply to the little finger is
   (a) C4
   (b) T4
   (c) C8
   (d) C6
3. All of the following structures are present in the deltopectoral groove ***except***
   (a) Cephalic vein
   (b) Deltopectoral lymph node
   (c) Basilic vein
   (d) Deltoid branch of thoracoacromial artery
4. The lymph vessels from thumb drain into which group of lymph nodes:
   (a) Supraclavicular lymph nodes
   (b) Posterior axillary
   (c) Lateral axillary
   (d) Infraclavicular lymph nodes
5. Most commonly used vein for intravenous injection is
   (a) Cephalic vein
   (b) Basilic vein
   (c) Median cubital vein
   (d) Median vein of the forearm
6. Which of the following statements about cephalic vein is ***incorrect?***
   (a) Cephalic vein corresponds to the great saphenous vein of the lower limb
   (b) It is the postaxial vein of the upper limb
   (c) It pierces clavipectoral fascia to drain into axillary vein
   (d) Greater part of its blood is drained into basilic vein through median cubital vein
7. Select the *incorrect statement* about the basilic vein:
   (a) It is the postaxial vein of the upper limb
   (b) It begins from the medial end of the dorsal venous plexus
   (c) It continues upwards as axillary vein at the upper border of teres major
   (d) It is accompanied by medial cutaneous nerve of the forearm
8. All of the following cutaneous nerves are derived from radial nerve ***except***
   (a) Lower lateral cutaneous nerve of arm
   (b) Upper lateral cutaneous nerve of arm
   (c) Superficial terminal branch of radial nerve
   (d) Posterior cutaneous nerve of arm

Answers

1. ***a***, 2. ***c***, 3. ***c***, 4. ***d***, 5. ***c***, 6. ***b***, 7. ***c***, 8. ***b***

CHAPTER 8

1. All of the following muscles are present in the anterior compartment of the arm ***except***
   (a) Brachialis
   (b) Brachioradialis
   (c) Coracobrachialis
   (d) Biceps brachii
2. The only muscle of anterior compartment of arm that is inserted into the humerus is
   (a) Biceps brachii
   (b) Coracobrachialis
   (c) Brachialis
   (d) None of the above
3. All transitions which occur at the level of insertion of coracobrachialis are correct ***except***
   (a) Median nerve crosses brachial artery from lateral to medial side
   (b) Ulnar pierces medial intermuscular septum to enter the posterior compartment of the arm
   (c) Cephalic vein pierces the deep fascia
   (d) Radial nerve pierces the lateral intermuscular septum to enter the anterior compartment of the arm
4. The nerve that lies in the groove behind the medial epicondyle of humerus is
   (a) Median
   (b) Ulnar
   (c) Radial
   (d) Musculocutaneous
5. Which of the following muscles is innervated by both musculocutaneous and radial nerve?
   (a) Biceps brachii
   (b) Coracobrachialis
   (c) Brachialis
   (d) Brachioradialis
6. Select the ***incorrect statement*** about the coracobrachialis:
   (a) It arises from tip of coracoid process of scapula
   (b) It has more morphological than functional significance
   (c) The ligament of Struthers' represents its third head
   (d) It is pierced by ulnar nerve

7. All of the following are branches of brachial artery ***except***
   (a) Profunda brachii artery
   (b) Main humeral nutrient artery
   (c) Radial collateral artery
   (d) Superior ulnar collateral artery
8. Select the ***incorrect statement*** about the biceps brachii muscle:
   (a) It normally has two heads
   (b) Its long head arises from infraglenoid tubercle of scapula
   (c) It is capable of affecting movements at glenohumeral, elbow and superior radioulnar joints
   (d) It is supplied by musculocutaneous nerve

Answers
1. ***b***, 2. ***b***, 3. ***c***, 4. ***b***, 5. ***c***, 6. ***d***, 7. ***c***, 8. ***b***

CHAPTER 9

1. All of the following are superficial muscles on the front of forearm ***except***
   (a) Flexor carpi radialis
   (b) Pronator teres
   (c) Palmaris longus
   (d) Flexor pollicis longus
2. Select the ***incorrect statement*** about the pronator teres:
   (a) It is the smallest superficial flexor of the forearm
   (b) Its medial border forms the medial boundary of cubital fossa
   (c) Median nerve passes between its two heads
   (d) Ulnar nerve is separated from median nerve by its deep head
3. The radial artery on the front of wrist lies lateral to the tendon of:
   (a) Brachioradialis
   (b) Abductor pollicis longus
   (c) Flexor carpi radialis
   (d) Flexor carpi ulnaris
4. The anterior interosseous nerve is a branch of:
   (a) Superficial branch of radial nerve
   (b) Deep branch of radial nerve
   (c) Median nerve
   (d) Ulnar nerve
5. All of the following deep muscles on the back of the forearm outcrop in the distal third of the forearm ***except***
   (a) Abductor pollicis longus
   (b) Extensor carpi radialis longus
   (c) Extensor pollicis longus
   (d) Extensor pollicis brevis
6. All of the following structures pass through the fourth compartment of extensor retinaculum on the dorsal aspect of wrist ***except***
   (a) Extensor digitorum
   (b) Extensor pollicis longus
   (c) Anterior interosseous artery
   (d) Posterior interosseous nerve
7. The supinator muscle is supplied by
   (a) Ulnar nerve
   (b) Anterior interosseous nerve
   (c) Median nerve
   (d) Posterior interosseous nerve
8. Which of the following statements is ***not correct?***
   (a) Ulnar nerve passes between the two heads of flexor carpi ulnaris
   (b) Median nerve passes between the two heads of pronator teres
   (c) Median nerve passes between the two head of flexor digitorum superficialis
   (d) Radial nerve passes between the two heads of flexor digitorum superficialis

Answers
1. ***d***, 2. ***b***, 3. ***c***, 4. ***c***, 5. ***b***, 6. ***b***, 7. ***d***, 8. ***d***

CHAPTER 10

1. Select the ***incorrect statement*** about the elbow joint:
   (a) It is a hinge type of synovial joint
   (b) It consists of two articulations, humeroradial and humeroulnar
   (c) It usually dislocates anteriorly
   (d) Effusion within joint cavity distends elbow posteriorly
2. Medial collateral ligament of elbow joint is closely related to:
   (a) Radial nerve
   (b) Ulnar artery
   (c) Ulnar nerve
   (d) Median nerve
3. Clinically most important synovial bursa around elbow joint is
   (a) Subtendinous olecranon bursa
   (b) Subcutaneous olecranon bursa
   (c) Bicipitoradial bursa
   (d) Bursa between biceps tendon and oblique cord
4. Select the ***incorrect statement*** about superior radioulnar joint:
   (a) It is a pivot type of synovial joint
   (b) Its cavity does not communicate with the cavity of elbow joint
   (c) It permits movements of supination and pronation
   (d) Its prime stabilizing factor is its annular ligament
5. Most common nerve entrapments around the elbow is
   (a) Median nerve entrapment
   (b) Ulnar nerve entrapment
   (c) Radial nerve entrapment
   (d) Posterior interosseous nerve entrapment
6. Select the ***incorrect statement*** about the inferior radioulnar joint:
   (a) It is a pivot type of synovial joint
   (b) Its cavity communicates with the cavity of wrist joint
   (c) Its prime stability is provided by its articular disc
   (d) It permits supination and pronation of forearm

7. Select the ***incorrect statement*** about the interosseous membrane of the forearm:
   (a) It is a fibrous membrane, which stretches between interosseous border of radius and ulna
   (b) Its fibres run downwards and laterally from ulna to the radius
   (c) Its posterior surface is related to anterior interosseous artery and posterior interosseous nerve
   (d) Its anterior surface is related to anterior interosseous artery and anterior interosseous nerve
8. All are correct statements about oblique cord of forearm ***except***
   (a) It is fibrous band extending between radial and ulnar tuberosities
   (b) Its fibres are directed opposite to those of interosseous membrane
   (c) Posterior interosseous nerve enters the back of forearm through gap between oblique cord and interosseous membrane
   (d) Morphologically, it represents the degenerated part of the flexor pollicis longus

Answers
1. ***c***, 2. ***c***, 3. ***b***, 4. ***b***, 5. ***b***, 6. ***b***, 7. ***b***, 8. ***c***

CHAPTER 11

1. Select the ***incorrect statement*** about the palmaris brevis muscle:
   (a) It is subcutaneous muscle
   (b) It arises from flexor retinaculum and palmar aponeurosis
   (c) It is innervated by median nerve
   (d) Its contraction causes wrinkling of medial palmar skin
2. All of the following structures pass superficial to the flexor retinaculum ***except***
   (a) Ulnar nerve
   (b) Superficial radial nerve
   (c) Tendon of palmaris longus
   (d) Ulnar artery
3. All the structures pass through carpal tunnel ***except***
   (a) Tendons of flexor digitorum superficialis
   (b) Tendon of flexor digitorum profundus
   (c) Tendon of flexor carpi radialis
   (d) Tendon of flexor pollicis longus
4. Select the ***true statement*** about the adductor pollicis:
   (a) It is a muscle of thenar eminence
   (b) It is a content of thenar space
   (c) It transmits ulnar artery between its two heads
   (d) It is innervated by ulnar nerve
5. Select the ***incorrect statement*** about an anatomical snuff-box:
   (a) It is bounded posteromedially by the tendon of extensor pollicis longus
   (b) Its roof is crossed by cephalic vein
   (c) Pulsations of radial artery can be felt in its floor
   (d) Tenderness in the anatomical snuff-box indicates fracture of capitate bone
6. First lumbrical canal is a diverticulum of
   (a) Thenar space
   (b) Midpalmar space
   (c) Space of Parona
   (d) None of the above
7. Radial bursa is the synovial sheath enclosing the tendon of
   (a) Flexor carpi radialis
   (b) Flexor pollicis longus
   (c) Extensor carpi radialis longus
   (d) Extensor carpi radialis brevis
8. All the statements about the palmar interossei are correct ***except***
   (a) They are unipennate
   (b) They take origin from all the five metacarpals
   (c) They are innervated by ulnar nerve
   (d) They adduct the digits
9. All the statements about ulnar bursa are correct ***except***
   (a) It encloses tendons of flexor digitorum superficialis and flexor digitorum profundus
   (b) It communicates with the digital synovial sheath of little finger
   (c) Distally it extends in the palm up to the heads of metacarpals
   (d) Proximally, it extends into the forearm about a finger breadth above the flexor retinaculum
10. Select the ***incorrect statement*** about the superficial palmar arterial arch:
   (a) It is a direct continuation of ulnar artery
   (b) It lies proximal to the deep palmar arch
   (c) It lies deep to the palmar aponeurosis
   (d) It lies superficial to long flexor tendons

Answers
1. ***c***, 2. ***b***, 3. ***c***, 4. ***d***, 5. ***d***, 6. ***a***, 7. ***b***, 8. ***b***, 9. ***c***, 10. ***b***

CHAPTER 12

1. Select the ***incorrect statement*** about the wrist joint:
   (a) It is a synovial joint of saddle variety
   (b) It is a synovial joint of ellipsoid variety
   (c) Ulna does not take part in this articulation
   (d) Its cavity does not communicate with the cavity of inferior radioulnar joint
2. Select the ***incorrect statement*** about the wrist joint:
   (a) Its upper articular surface is formed by radius and ulna
   (b) Its lower articular surface is formed by scaphoid, lunate, and triquetral bones
   (c) It is an ellipsoidal joint
   (d) It permits free rotatory movements
3. All of the following bones form the proximal row of carpal bones ***except***
   (a) Lunate
   (b) Pisiform
   (c) Trapezium
   (d) Scaphoid

4. All the carpometacarpal joints are plane type of synovial joint ***except***
   (a) First carpometacarpal
   (b) Second carpometacarpal
   (c) Third carpometacarpal
   (d) Fourth carpometacarpal
5. All are the features of 'position of rest of hand' ***except***
   (a) Forearm is in semiprone position
   (b) Wrist joint is slightly extended
   (c) Fingers are partially flexed
   (d) Plane of thumb-nail lies parallel to the plane of finger-nails
6. Flexion of thumb is produced by all muscles ***except***
   (a) Flexor pollicis longus
   (b) Opponens pollicis
   (c) Flexor carpi radialis
   (d) Flexor pollicis brevis
7. The following muscles cause abduction of wrist ***except***
   (a) Extensor carpi radialis longus
   (b) Extensor carpi radialis brevis
   (c) Abductor pollicis longus
   (d) Abductor pollicis brevis
8. Which finger is ***not abducted*** by dorsal interossei:
   (a) Second
   (b) Third
   (c) Fourth
   (d) Fifth

Answers

1. ***a***, 2. ***a***, 3. ***c***, 4. ***a***, 5. ***d***, 6. ***c***, 7. ***d***, 8. ***d***

CHAPTER 13

1. Select the ***incorrect statement*** about the radial nerve:
   (a) It arises from posterior cord of the brachial plexus
   (b) It gives lateral and posterior cutaneous nerves of arm in spiral groove
   (c) It supplies flexor carpi radialis
   (d) Its lesion in radial groove causes wrist drop
2. Skin over the thenar eminence is supplied by
   (a) Palmar cutaneous branch of median nerve
   (b) Palmar cutaneous branch of ulnar nerve
   (c) Recurrent branch of ulnar nerve
   (d) None of the above
3. All the statements about superficial radial nerve are true *except*
   (a) It arises from radial nerve in the spiral groove
   (b) It is entirely sensory
   (c) It arises from radial nerve in cubital fossa
   (d) It provides sensory innervation to skin on the root of thumb
4. Which of the following statements is *incorrect*?
   (a) Median nerve is called 'labourer's nerve'
   (b) Ulnar nerve is called 'musician's nerve'
   (c) Ulnar nerve in the hand is called 'eye of the hand'
   (d) Median nerve in the hand is called 'eye of the hand'
5. Sensory innervation to the skin on the dorsum of hand is provided by
   (a) Radial nerve
   (b) Median nerve
   (c) Ulnar nerve
   (d) All of the above
6. The 'ape-thumb deformity' occurs due to lesion of
   (a) Radial nerve
   (b) Median nerve
   (c) Ulnar nerve
   (d) Musculocutaneous nerve
7. All are signs of ulnar nerve lesion *except*
   (a) Wasting of hypothenar eminence
   (b) Loss of abduction and adduction of fingers
   (c) Absence of flexion of ring and little fingers
   (d) Absence of flexion of index finger
8. A median nerve palsy causes all signs *except*
   (a) Wasting of thenar eminence
   (b) Loss of opposition of thumb
   (c) Pointing index finger
   (d) Loss of sensation on the palmar aspect of medial 1½ fingers
9. Forearm has all of the following cutaneous nerves *except*
   (a) Lateral cutaneous nerve of forearm
   (b) Medial cutaneous nerve of forearm
   (c) Anterior cutaneous nerve of forearm
   (d) Posterior cutaneous nerve of the forearm

Answers

1. ***c***, 2. ***a***, 3. ***a***, 4. ***c***, 5. ***d***, 6. ***b***, 7. ***d***, 8. ***d***, 9. ***c***

THORAX

CHAPTER 15

1. Select the ***incorrect statement*** about the thoracic inlet:
   (a) It communicates with the root of the neck
   (b) It is roofed on either side by suprapleural membrane
   (c) It is circular in shape
   (d) Its plane slops downwards and forwards
2. All the statements about Sibson's fascia are correct *except*
   (a) Forms the diaphragm of thoracic inlet
   (b) Its apex is attached to the tip of the transverse process of T1 vertebra
   (c) Its base is attached to the inner border of the first rib
   (d) It protects the underlying cervical pleura
3. All the nerves pass through thoracic inlet *except*
   (a) Right and left phrenic nerves
   (b) Right and left first thoracic nerves
   (c) Right recurrent laryngeal nerve
   (d) Right and left vagus nerves
4. Which of the following structures does not pass through the aortic orifice of the diaphragm?
   (a) Aorta
   (b) Thoracic duct
   (c) Hemiazygos vein
   (d) Azygos vein

5. Caval opening of diaphragm lies at the level of
   (a) Body of T6 vertebra
   (b) Body of T8 vertebra
   (c) Body of T10 vertebra
   (d) Body of T12 vertebra
6. Congenital posterolateral defect of diaphragm occurs due to failure of development of
   (a) Mesoderm of body wall
   (b) Dorsal mesentery of oesophagus
   (c) Septum transversum
   (d) Pleuroperitoneal membrane
7. All of the following structures pass through the crura of diaphragm *except*
   (a) Greater splanchnic nerve
   (b) Lesser splanchnic nerve
   (c) Hemiazygos vein
   (d) Sympathetic chain
8. Sympathetic chain enters the abdomen by passing deep to
   (a) Median arcuate ligament
   (b) Medial arcuate ligament
   (c) Aortic opening
   (d) Lateral arcuate ligament

Answers

1. ***c***, 2. ***b***, 3. ***c***, 4. ***c***, 5. ***b***, 6. ***d***, 7. ***d***, 8. ***b***

CHAPTER 16

1. Select the ***incorrect statement*** about the manubrium sterni:
   (a) It is the thickest and strongest part of the sternum
   (b) It is the commonest site for bone marrow aspiration
   (c) It articulates below with body of sternum to form primary cartilaginous joint
   (d) Upper half of its posterior surface is related to the arch of aorta
2. All the statements about the sternal angle are correct ***except***
   (a) It is formed by the articulation of the manubrium with the body of the sternum
   (b) It lies at the level of second costal cartilage
   (c) It lies opposite the intervertebral disc between the T3 and T4 vertebrae
   (d) Ascending aorta ends at this level
3. All are the atypical ribs ***except***
   (a) 1st rib
   (b) 2nd rib
   (c) 9th rib
   (d) 10th rib
4. Anterior aspect of the neck of first rib is related to all structures ***except***
   (a) Sympathetic chain
   (b) Superior intercostal vein
   (c) Superior intercostal artery
   (d) Ventral ramus of first thoracic nerve
5. Select the ***incorrect statement*** about the 12th thoracic vertebrae:
   (a) It appears like first lumbar vertebra
   (b) Its transverse process presents three tubercles
   (c) Its transverse process has small articular facet
   (d) Its pedicle presents circular articular facet on each side
6. First costosternal/chondrosternal joint is a
   (a) Synovial joint
   (b) Primary cartilaginous joint
   (c) Secondary cartilaginous joint
   (d) Fibrous joint
7. The rib commonly fractures:
   (a) At its posterior angle
   (b) At the middle of its shaft
   (c) At its neck
   (d) At its anterior angle
8. All are the atypical features of first rib ***except***
   (a) Its shaft has upper and lower surfaces
   (b) Its angle and tubercle coincide
   (c) Its head bears two articular facets
   (d) It is the most curved rib

Answers

1. ***c***, 2. ***c***, 3. ***c***, 4. ***b***, 5. ***c***, 6. ***b***, 7. ***a***, 8. ***c***

CHAPTER 17

1. Which of the following muscles is attached on the inner aspects of the ribs?
   (a) External intercostal
   (b) Internal intercostal
   (c) Intercostalis intimus
   (d) None of the above
2. Anterior intercostal membrane is the continuation of
   (a) External intercostal muscle
   (b) Internal intercostal muscle
   (c) Intercostalis intimi muscle
   (d) Subcostalis muscle
3. All of the following are parts of transverse thoracis muscle ***except***
   (a) Intercostalis intimus
   (b) Subcostalis
   (c) Levatores costarum
   (d) Sternocostalis
4. Typical intercostal nerves are
   (a) 3rd–6th intercostal nerves
   (b) 7th–11th intercostal nerves
   (c) 7th–10th intercostal nerves
   (d) 1st and 2nd intercostal nerves
5. The branches of all of the following arteries supply blood to intercostal spaces ***except***
   (a) Descending thoracic aorta
   (b) Internal thoracic artery
   (c) Superior epigastric artery
   (d) Musculophrenic artery
6. Increase in vertical diameter of thoracic cavity is brought about by
   (a) Pump-handle movement of the sternum
   (b) Bucket-handle movement of the ribs
   (c) Contraction of diaphragm
   (d) (a) and (b)
7. During quiet respiration, the elevation of ribs is done mostly by the contraction of
   (a) Internal intercostal muscles
   (b) External intercostal muscles

(c) Intercostalis intimi muscles
(d) Subcostalis muscles

8. Select the ***incorrect statement*** about the increase in various diameters of thoracic cavity:
   (a) Pump-handle movement of sternum increases its anteroposterior diameter
   (b) Contraction of diaphragm increases its vertical diameter
   (c) Bucket-handle movement of ribs increases its transverse diameter
   (d) Pump-handle movement of sternum increases its vertical diameter

Answers
1. ***c***, 2. ***a***, 3. ***c***, 4. ***a***, 5. ***c***, 6. ***c***, 7. ***b***, 8. ***d***

CHAPTER 18

1. Select the ***incorrect statement*** about the parietal pleura:
   (a) It develops from somatopleuric mesoderm
   (b) It is supplied by somatic nerves
   (c) It develops from splanchnopleuric mesoderm
   (d) It is sensitive to pain and touch
2. All the statements about visceral pleura are correct ***except***
   (a) It develops from splanchnopleuric mesoderm
   (b) It is innervated by autonomic nerves
   (c) It lines the thoracic wall
   (d) It is insensitive to touch and temperature
3. Pleura extends beyond the thoracic cage on all of the following sites ***except***
   (a) Root of the neck
   (b) Costovertebral angles
   (c) Right xiphisternal angle
   (d) Left xiphisternal angle
4. Select the ***incorrect statement*** about the summit of cervical pleura:
   (a) It lies 2.5 cm above the medial end of the clavicle
   (b) It lies 2.5 cm above the first costal cartilage
   (c) It lies 5 cm above the first costal cartilage
   (d) It is covered by Sibson's fascia
5. In the midaxillary line, the inferior margin of parietal pleura crosses:
   (a) 6th rib
   (b) 8th rib
   (c) 10th rib
   (d) 12th rib
6. All arteries supply the pleura ***except***
   (a) Internal thoracic
   (b) Intercostal
   (c) Bronchial
   (d) Pulmonary
7. Select the ***incorrect statement*** about the pulmonary ligament:
   (a) It is a fold of the visceral pleura
   (b) It provides a dead space for expansion of pulmonary veins
   (c) It extends from root of lung as far down as diaphragm
   (d) It extends between mediastinum and the lung
8. Select the ***incorrect statement*** about the costodiaphragmatic recess:
   (a) It is the lower part of pleural cavity between the diaphragmatic and costal pleura
   (b) It is the least dependent part of the pleural cavity
   (c) Vertically it extends from 8th to 10th ribs along the midaxillary line
   (d) It measures about 5 cm

Answers
1. ***c***, 2. ***c***, 3. ***d***, 4. ***b***, 5. ***c***, 6. ***d***, 7. ***a***, 8. ***b***

CHAPTER 19

1. Mediastinal surface of right lung is related to all ***except***
   (a) Right atrium
   (b) Arch of aorta
   (c) Arch of azygos vein
   (d) Inferior vena cava
2. Mediastinal surface of the left lung is related to all ***except***
   (a) Left ventricle
   (b) Ascending aorta
   (c) Superior vena cava
   (d) Arch of aorta
3. Uppermost structure in the hilum of right lung is
   (a) Pulmonary artery
   (b) Superior pulmonary vein
   (c) Eparterial bronchus
   (d) Hyparterial bronchus
4. During quiet respiration, the posterior end of lower border of lung passes across
   (a) 6th rib
   (b) 8th rib
   (c) 10th rib
   (d) T12 spine
5. Nutrition to the nonrespiratory portions of lung is supplied by
   (a) Pulmonary artery
   (b) Pulmonary vein
   (c) Bronchial arteries
   (d) (a) and (c)
6. All are characteristic features of a bronchopulmonary segment ***except***
   (a) It is pyramidal in shape
   (b) It is aerated by a tertiary bronchus
   (c) It has its own segmental vein
   (d) It is surrounded by the connective tissue
7. Number of bronchopulmonary segments in lower lobe of each lung is
   (a) Two
   (b) Three
   (c) Four
   (d) Five
8. The lingula is a tongue-shaped projection from
   (a) Upper lobe of right lung
   (b) Upper lobe of left lung
   (c) Lower lobe of right lung
   (d) Lower lobe of left lung

Answers
1. ***b***, 2. ***c***, 3. ***c***, 4. ***c***, 5. ***c***, 6. ***c***, 7. ***d***, 8. ***b***

CHAPTER 20

1. All are correct statements about mediastinum ***except***
   (a) It is a broad septum within thoracic cavity, which separates two pleural cavities
   (b) It contains all the thoracic viscera and structures except lungs
   (c) Structures forming mediastinum are bound together by loose connective tissue
   (d) It is rigid and nonmovable septum in living people
2. All form the boundaries of superior mediastinum ***except***
   (a) Manubrium sterni
   (b) Upper four thoracic vertebrae
   (c) Diaphragm
   (d) Plane of superior thoracic aperture
3. All are the contents of superior mediastinum ***except***
   (a) Arch of aorta
   (b) Pulmonary trunk
   (c) Superior vena cava
   (d) Brachiocephalic trunk
4. All structures traverse the whole length of mediastinum ***except***
   (a) Oesophagus
   (b) Trachea
   (c) Thoracic duct
   (d) Sympathetic trunks
5. All are contents of middle mediastinum ***except***
   (a) Heart
   (b) Pulmonary arteries
   (c) Brachiocephalic veins
   (d) Pulmonary veins
6. All the statements regarding posterior mediastinum are wrong ***except***
   (a) Pus in the posterior mediastinum can enter the thighs
   (b) Neck infection behind prevertebral layer of deep cervical fascia cannot extend into the posterior mediastinum
   (c) Neck infection in the retropharyngeal space can extend into the posterior mediastinum
   (d) Its superior boundary is formed by superior thoracic aperture
7. Posterior mediastinum provides passage to all structures ***except***
   (a) Oesophagus
   (b) Trachea
   (c) Descending thoracic aorta
   (d) Azygos veins
8. The thymus is located in
   (a) Superior mediastinum
   (b) Middle mediastinum
   (c) Posterior mediastinum
   (d) Anterior mediastinum

Answers

1. ***d***, 2. ***c***, 3. ***b***, 4. ***b***, 5. ***c***, 6. ***d***, 7. ***b***, 8. ***a***

CHAPTER 21

1. Pericardial cavity lies between
   (a) Fibrous pericardium and serous pericardium
   (b) Fibrous pericardium and epicardium
   (c) Parietal pericardium and visceral pericardium
   (d) Epicardium and myocardium
2. Select the ***correct statement*** about the transverse pericardial sinus:
   (a) It lies in front of superior vena cava
   (b) It lies in front of pulmonary veins
   (c) It lies behind the ascending aorta and pulmonary trunk
   (d) It lies in front of ascending aorta and pulmonary trunk
3. Sternocostal surface of the heart is mainly formed by
   (a) Right atrium
   (b) Right ventricle
   (c) Left ventricle
   (d) (a) and (b)
4. Apex beat in adults is normally felt in the
   (a) Left fourth intercostal space in the midclavicular line
   (b) Left fifth intercostal space just medial to the midclavicular line
   (c) Left sixth intercostal space just medial to the midclavicular line
   (d) Left third intercostal space just lateral to the midclavicular line
5. Select the ***incorrect statement*** about the oblique pericardial sinus:
   (a) It is the recess of pericardial cavity
   (b) It lies behind the left atrium
   (c) It lies behind the right atrium
   (d) It is closed on all sides except below
6. All the statements are correct about the conducting system of the heart ***except***
   (a) It is made up of specialized cardiac muscle fibres
   (b) It is responsible for initiation and conduction of impulses
   (c) Nearly whole of the conducting system is supplied by left coronary artery
   (d) Its SA node is known as the pacemaker of the heart
7. Select the ***incorrect statement*** about the area of superficial cardiac dullness:
   (a) It lies in front of right ventricle
   (b) It is related to the left fourth and fifth intercostal spaces
   (c) It is covered by lung and pleura
   (d) It can be used as a site of aspiration of fluid in pericardial effusion
8. The base of the heart is formed by
   (a) Right and left ventricles
   (b) Right and left atria
   (c) Right atrium and right ventricle
   (d) Left atrium and left ventricle

9. All structures meet at the crux of the heart ***except***
   (a) Posterior interventricular groove
   (b) Posterior atrioventricular groove
   (c) Interatrial groove
   (d) Sulcus terminalis
10. Most anteriorly located valve of the heart is
   (a) Pulmonary
   (b) Aortic
   (c) Tricuspid
   (d) Bicuspid
11. Conducting system of the heart is a modification of:
   (a) Epicardium
   (b) Myocardium
   (c) Endocardium
   (d) None of the above

Answers

1. ***c***, 2. ***c***, 3. ***d***, 4. ***b***, 5. ***c***, 6. ***c***, 7. ***c***, 8. ***b***, 9. ***d***, 10. ***a***, 11. ***b***

CHAPTER 22

1. All the statements about SVC are correct ***except***
   (a) It lies both in superior and middle mediastina
   (b) It is devoid of valves
   (c) It is formed at the lower border of the right first costal cartilage
   (d) It pierces pericardium at the level of the right fourth costal cartilage
2. All are the tributaries of SVC ***except***
   (a) Right brachiocephalic vein
   (b) Left brachiocephalic vein
   (c) Hemiazygos vein
   (d) Azygos vein
3. All the statements regarding SVC are correct ***except***
   (a) It is 7 cm long and 2 cm wide
   (b) It has no valves
   (c) Its lower half is covered by pericardium
   (d) It is completely enclosed in the pericardium
4. The ascending aorta gives origin to
   (a) Brachiocephalic trunk
   (b) Left common carotid artery
   (c) Left subclavian artery
   (d) Right and left coronary arteries
5. All are the branches of arch of aorta ***except***
   (a) Brachiocephalic trunk
   (b) Right common carotid artery
   (c) Left common carotid artery
   (d) Left subclavian artery
6. All are the branches of descending thoracic aorta ***except***
   (a) Superior intercostal arteries
   (b) Posterior intercostal arteries
   (c) Subcostal arteries
   (d) Left bronchial arteries
7. All are correct statements about pulmonary trunk ***except***
   (a) It is about 5 cm long
   (b) It arises from the infundibulum of the right ventricle
   (c) Its termination lies in front of the arch of aorta
   (d) It is completely enclosed within the fibrous pericardium
8. Select the ***incorrect statement*** about the pulmonary trunk:
   (a) It is completely enclosed within the fibrous pericardium
   (b) It along with ascending aorta is enclosed by a common sheath of visceral pericardium
   (c) It is intimately related to the two coronary arteries
   (d) It lies entirely to the right of ascending aorta
9. Aortic knuckle, a projection in the upper part of left margin of the cardiac shadow in X-ray chest PA view, is cast by
   (a) Ascending aorta
   (b) Arch of aorta
   (c) Aortic sinuses
   (d) Descending aorta

Answers

1. ***d***, 2. ***c***, 3. ***d***, 4. ***d***, 5. ***b***, 6. ***a***, 7. ***c***, 8. ***d***, 9. ***b***

CHAPTER 23

1. Select the ***incorrect statement*** about the oesophagus:
   (a) It is narrowest at its commencement
   (b) It is about 15 cm long
   (c) It ends at the level of T11 vertebra
   (d) It pierces diaphragm at the level of T10 vertebra
2. Constrictions of oesophagus are present at all sites ***except***
   (a) At cricopharyngeal junction
   (b) Where it is crossed by the arch of aorta
   (c) Where it is surrounded by right crus of diaphragm
   (d) Where it is crossed by the left principal bronchus
3. Select the ***incorrect statement*** about the distances of constrictions in oesophagus from upper incisor teeth:
   (a) First constriction is about 6 inches
   (b) Second constriction is about 9 inches
   (c) Third constriction is 11 inches
   (d) Fourth constriction is about 27 inches
4. Lymphatics from the lower end of oesophagus drains into
   (a) Deep cervical lymph nodes
   (b) Pretracheal lymph nodes
   (c) Posterior mediastinal lymph nodes
   (d) Celiac lymph nodes
5. Oesophagus is supplied by the oesophageal branches of all the arteries ***except***
   (a) Inferior thyroid
   (b) Descending thoracic aorta
   (c) Left gastric
   (d) Right gastric
6. All statements regarding trachea are true ***except***
   (a) It begins in the neck at the lower border of cricoid cartilage
   (b) It is about 20 cm long

(c) It is made up of 16–20 C-shaped hyaline cartilages
(d) It terminates in the thorax at the level of sternal angle

7. Select the *incorrect statement* about the trachea:
(a) It is flexible fibroelastic tube
(b) It extends from lower border C6 vertebra to the lower border of T4 vertebra
(c) Its external diameter in an adult male is about 2 cm
(d) Its internal diameter in an adult male is 15 mm

8. Anteriorly the trachea is related to all structures ***except:***
(a) Arch of aorta
(b) Left brachiocephalic vein
(c) Oesophagus
(d) Deep cardiac plexus

Answers
1. ***b***, 2. ***a***, 3. ***d***, 4. ***d***, 5. ***d***, 6. ***b***, 7. ***d***, 8. ***c***

CHAPTER 24

1. Select the ***incorrect statement*** about the thoracic duct:
(a) It begins as an upward continuation of cisterna chyli
(b) It enters the thoracic cavity through an aortic opening of the diaphragm
(c) It crosses the vertebral column from right to left side in front of T5 vertebra
(d) It terminates in the external jugular vein

2. All structures form posterior relations of the thoracic duct in the posterior mediastinum ***except***
(a) Right posterior intercostal arteries
(b) Terminal parts of hemiazygos and accessory hemiazygos veins
(c) Oesophagus
(d) Vertebral column

3. All structures lie behind the thoracic duct at the root of the neck ***except***
(a) Vertebral artery and vein
(b) Carotid sheath
(c) Phrenic nerve
(d) Thyrocervical trunk and its branches

4. All the statements about azygos veins are correct ***except***
(a) They are paravertebral in position
(b) They are not accompanied by corresponding arteries
(c) They have no valves in their lumen
(d) They may appear tortuous

5. All are the tributaries of azygos vein ***except***
(a) Hemiazygos vein
(b) Accessory hemiazygos vein
(c) Right first posterior intercostal vein
(d) Right bronchial vein

6. The left superior intercostal vein drains into
(a) Accessory hemiazygos vein
(b) Hemiazygos vein
(c) Azygos vein
(d) Left brachiocephalic vein

7. All the statements regarding accessory hemiazygos vein are correct ***except***
(a) It lies on left side only
(b) It receives left superior intercostal vein
(c) It receives left bronchial veins
(d) It drains into azygos vein

8. Select the ***incorrect statement*** about the thoracic sympathetic trunk:
(a) Its upper end lies in front of the neck of the first rib
(b) Its lower end passes behind the medial arcuate ligament of diaphragm
(c) It commonly possesses 12 ganglia
(d) It lies in front of posterior intercostal nerve and vessels

9. Regarding thoracic splanchnic nerves, which is the ***incorrect statement***:
(a) They consist of preganglionic sympathetic fibres
(b) They are three in number
(c) The lower splanchnic nerve is also called renal nerve
(d) Greater splanchnic nerve arises from first to fifth thoracic ganglia

Answers
1. ***d***, 2. ***c***, 3. ***b***, 4. ***c***, 5. ***c***, 6. ***d***, 7. ***b***, 8. ***c***, 9. ***d***

Index

N

O

P

R

S